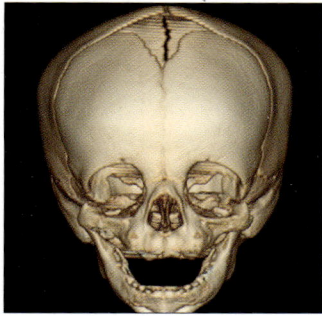

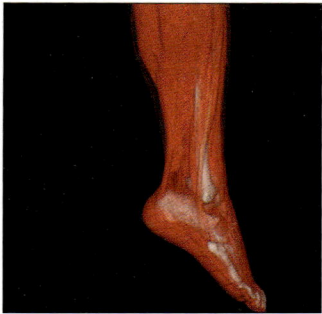

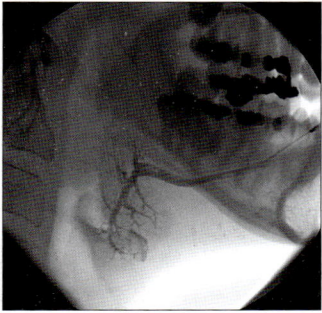

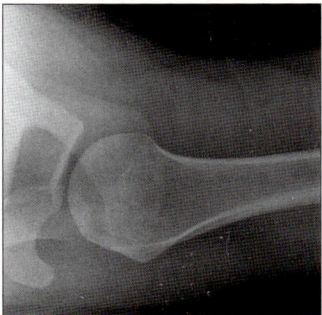

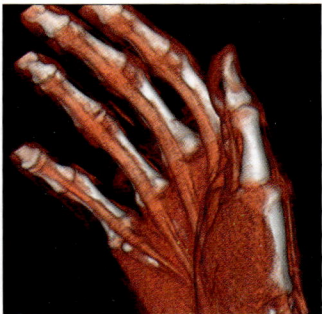

IMAGING

HUMAN
ANATOMY

FOUR
EDITI

Commissioning Editor: Madelene Hyde
Development Editor: Sharon Nash
Project Manager: Frances Affleck
Design: Kirsteen Wright
Marketing Managers: Jason Oberacker (US) and Ian Jordan (UK)

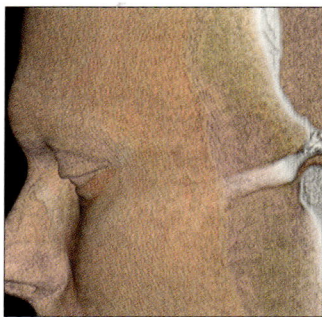

IMAGING ATLAS OF
HUMAN
ANATOMY

FOURTH EDITION

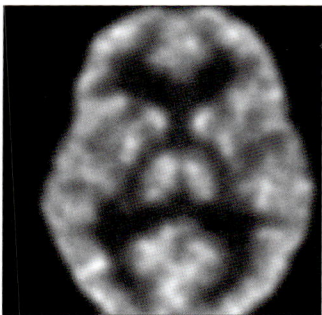

Jamie Weir MBBS, DMRD, FRCP(Ed), FRANZCR(Hon), FRCR

Emeritus Professor of Radiology
University of Aberdeen
Aberdeen, UK

Peter H Abrahams MBBS, FRCS(Ed), FRCR, DO(Hon)

Professor of Clinical Anatomy, Warwick Medical School, UK
Professor of Clinical Anatomy, St George's University, Grenada, West Indies
Extraordinary Professor, Department of Anatomy, University of Pretoria, South Africa
Fellow, Girton College, Cambridge, UK
Examiner, MRCS, Royal College of Surgeons, UK
Family Practitioner, Brent, London, UK

Jonathan D Spratt MBBChir, MA(Cantab), FRCS(Eng), FRCS(Glasg), FRCR

Chief Radiologist, County Durham and Darlington NHS Foundation Trust
Examiner in Anatomy, Royal College of Radiologists, UK
Examiner, MRCS, Royal College of Surgeons, UK
Fellow in Anatomical Radiology, Northumbria University, UK
Visiting Professor of Anatomy, St George's School of Medicine, Grenada and St Vincent

Lonie R Salkowski MD

Associate Professor of Radiology and Anatomy
University of Wisconsin School of Medicine and Public Health
Madison, Wisconsin, USA
Clinical Professor, College of Health Sciences
University of Wisconsin-Milwaukee
Milwaukee, Wisconsin, USA

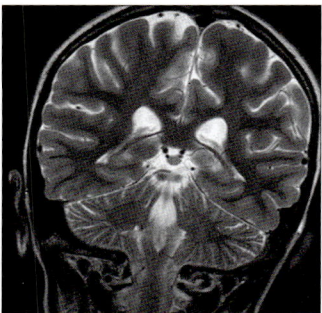

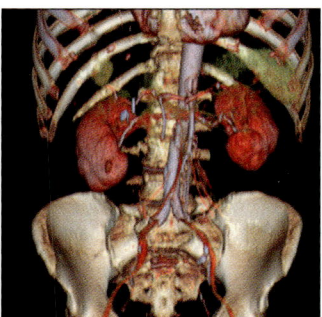

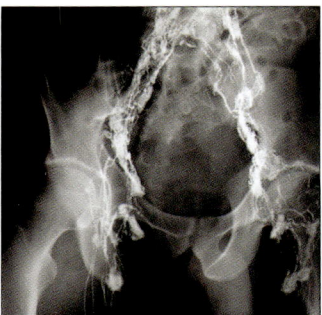

MOSBY

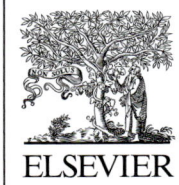

ELSEVIER

Contents

Preface to the Fourth edition   vii

Preface to the First edition   vii

Acknowledgements and Dedication   viii

Introduction   ix

1. Head, neck and brain   1

2. Vertebral column and spinal cord   55

3. Upper limb   67

4. Thorax   89

5. Abdomen and pelvis – Cross-sectional   123

6. Abdomen and pelvis – Non cross-sectional   171

7. Lower limb   207

8. Nuclear medicine   235

Index   241

Preface to the fourth edition

There is increasing importance placed on the interpretation of radiological anatomy in a world that has seen considerable changes in medical student training programmes over the last decade, combined with the reduction in cadaver dissection.

We have updated and revised this atlas, by the addition of new images and techniques, to reflect these trends. The 'Author' team has also changed. We wish to record our sincere thanks to Drs Hourihan, Belli, Moore and Owen for their previous contributions and introduce you to our two new co-authors, Dr Jonathan Spratt from Durham, UK and Dr Lonie Salkowski from Madison, WI, USA. Both are radiological anatomists of high repute and most of the new material emanates from their work.

The format for this fourth edition remains the same but the layout of the chapters on the abdomen and pelvis has been revised to reflect current radiological and anatomical practice; the new chapters being cross-sectional imaging of the abdomen and pelvis and non cross-sectional imaging of the abdomen and pelvis.

A new section on nuclear medicine, by Dr Salkowski, has also been added.

We are adding for the first time, a website of pathology to complement this radiological atlas. It consists of a series of 34 PowerPoint tutorials related to the eight anatomical chapters and based on nine 'concepts'. These 'concepts' have been designed to help you understand the relationship between normal anatomy and altered, abnormal anatomy that is the discipline of pathology. This material has been produced with the help of Dr Jennifer Allison who started this project as a medical student. A selection of these tutorials is available free with the atlas (please see inside front cover for access details) and the remainder will be available for a small charge from the same site.

The nine concepts are as follows:

1. 'things pushed'
2. 'things pulled'
3. 'things added'
4. 'things missing'
5. 'things larger than normal'
6. 'things smaller than normal'
7. 'things that have an abnormal structure, either locally or diffusely'
8. 'things that have an abnormal shape, either locally or generally'
9. 'things you cannot see despite knowing they are present pathologically, i.e. you are either using the wrong imaging technique or you will never see any abnormality because the disease is only microscopic and has not induced any visible anatomical (or physiological) change'.

Further explanations together with numerous examples to demonstrate these 'concepts' are on the website. We believe the ongoing reliance placed by clinicians on the imaging of pathological processes will be facilitated by this novel and exciting approach and the addition of pathology combined with this extensively revised radiological anatomy text will enhance the understanding of imaging to the benefit of both you, the reader, and your patient. As this book and accompanying website are for you, the student, we encourage and welcome corrections or suggestions and ideas for future editions.

Jamie Weir, Peter H Abrahams, Jonathan Spratt and Lonie Salkowski
January 2010

Preface to the first edition

Imaging methods used to display normal human anatomy have improved dramatically over the last few decades. The ability to demonstrate the soft tissues by using the modern technologies of magnetic resonance imaging, X-ray computed tomography, and ultrasound has greatly facilitated our understanding of the link between anatomy as shown in the dissecting room and that necessary for clinical practice. This atlas has been produced because of the new technology and the fundamental changes that are occurring in the teaching of anatomy. It enables the preclinical medical student to relate to basic anatomy while, at the same time, providing a comprehensive study guide for the clinical interpretation of imaging, applicable for all undergraduate and postgraduate levels.

Several distinguished authors, experts in their fields of imaging, have contributed to this book, which has benefited from editorial integration to ensure balance and cohesion. The atlas is designed to complement and supplement the *McMinn's Clinical Atlas of Human Anatomy* 6th edition.

Duplication of images occurs only where it is necessary to demonstrate anatomical points of interest or difficulty. Similarly, examples of different imaging modalities of the same anatomical region are only included if they contribute to a better understanding of the region shown. Radiographs that show important landmarks in limb ossification centre development, together with examples of some common congenital anomalies, are also documented. In certain sections, notably MR and CT, the legends may cover more than one page, so that a specific structure can be followed in continuity through various levels and planes.

Human anatomy does not alter, but our methods of demonstrating it have changed significantly. Modern imaging allows certain structures and their relationships to be seen for the first time, and this has aided us in their interpretation. Knowledge and understanding of radiological anatomy are fundamental to all those involved in patient care, from the nurse and the paramedic to medical students and clinicians.

Jamie Weir and Peter H Abrahams
February 1992

Acknowledgements

Thank you to all of our previous contributors of images to the previous editions of this atlas and to Dr Alison Murray who has kindly granted permission for use of images used in the online pathology tutorials. New material and labelling have been added by Dr Richard Wellings, University Hospital, Coventry and Warwickshire and Dr Andrew Hine, N.W. London Hospitals and we are very grateful for their help. The two images in the introduction, the body MRA and the MR tractography, were kindly supplied by Toshiba Medical Systems.

Dedication

To our students – past, present and future

Introduction

Guide to ossification tables

Ossification tables, such as the one shown on the right, appear throughout this book.

The key to these tables is as follows:

(c) = cartilage
(m) = membrane
miu = months of intrauterine life
wiu = weeks of intrauterine life
mths = months
yrs = years

And the rule to remember is: girls before boys.

Magnetic resonance imaging

Magnetic resonance imaging (MRI) produces images by magnetising the patient in the bore of a powerful magnet and broadcasting short pulses of radiofrequency (RF) energy at 46 MHz to resonate mobile protons (hydrogen nuclei) in fat, protein and water. The protons produce RF echoes when their resonant energy is released and their density and location can be exactly correlated by complex mathematical algorithms into an image matrix.

The spinning proton of the hydrogen nucleus acts like a tiny bar magnet, aligning either with or against the magnetic field producing a small net magnetic vector. RF energy is used to generate a second magnetic field, perpendicular to the static magnetic field, which rotate or 'flip' the protons away from the static magnetic field. Once the RF pulse is switched off, the protons flip back to their original position of equilibrium ('relaxation'), emitting the RF energy they had acquired into the antenna around the patient, which is then digitised, amplified and, finally, spatially encoded by the array processor.

MRI systems are graded according to the strength of the magnetic field they produce. Routine high-field systems are those capable of producing a magnetic field strength of 1.5–3 T (Tesla) using a superconducting electromagnet immersed in liquid helium. Open magnets for claustrophobic patients and limb scanners use permanent magnets between 0.2 and 0.75 T. For comparison, earth's magnetic field varies from 30 to 60 uT. MRI does not present any recognised biological hazard. Patients who have any form of pacemaker or implanted electro-inductive device must not be examined. Other prohibited items include ferromagnetic intracranial aneurysm slips, certain types of cardiac valve replacement and intra-ocular metallic foreign bodies. Many extra cranial vascular clips and orthopaedic prostheses are now 'MRI friendly', but these may cause local artefacts. Loose metal items must be excluded from the examination room – pillows containing metallic coiled springs have been known to near suffocate patients!

Although beyond the remit of the current edition of this book, new methods of analysing normal and pathologic brain anatomy are now

CLAVICLE (m)	Appears	Fused
Lateral end	5 wiu	20+ yrs
Medial end	15 yrs	20+ yrs
SCAPULA (c)		
Body	8 wiu	15 yrs
Coracoid	<1 yr	20 yrs
Coracoid base	Puberty	15–20 yrs
Acromion	Puberty	15–20 yrs

at the forefront of research, namely MRS, fMRI and mMRI, the latter taking on a new direction since the description of the human genome.

Magnetic resonance spectroscopic imaging (MRS) assesses function within the living brain. MRS takes advantage of the fact that protons

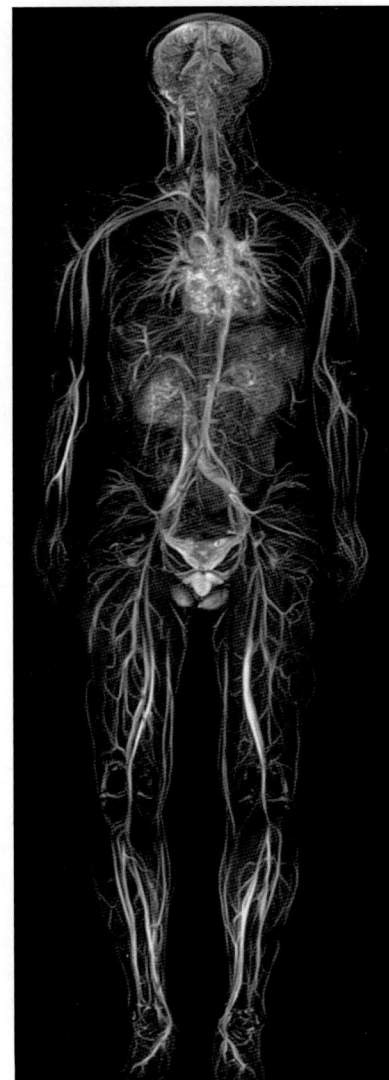

Body MRA.

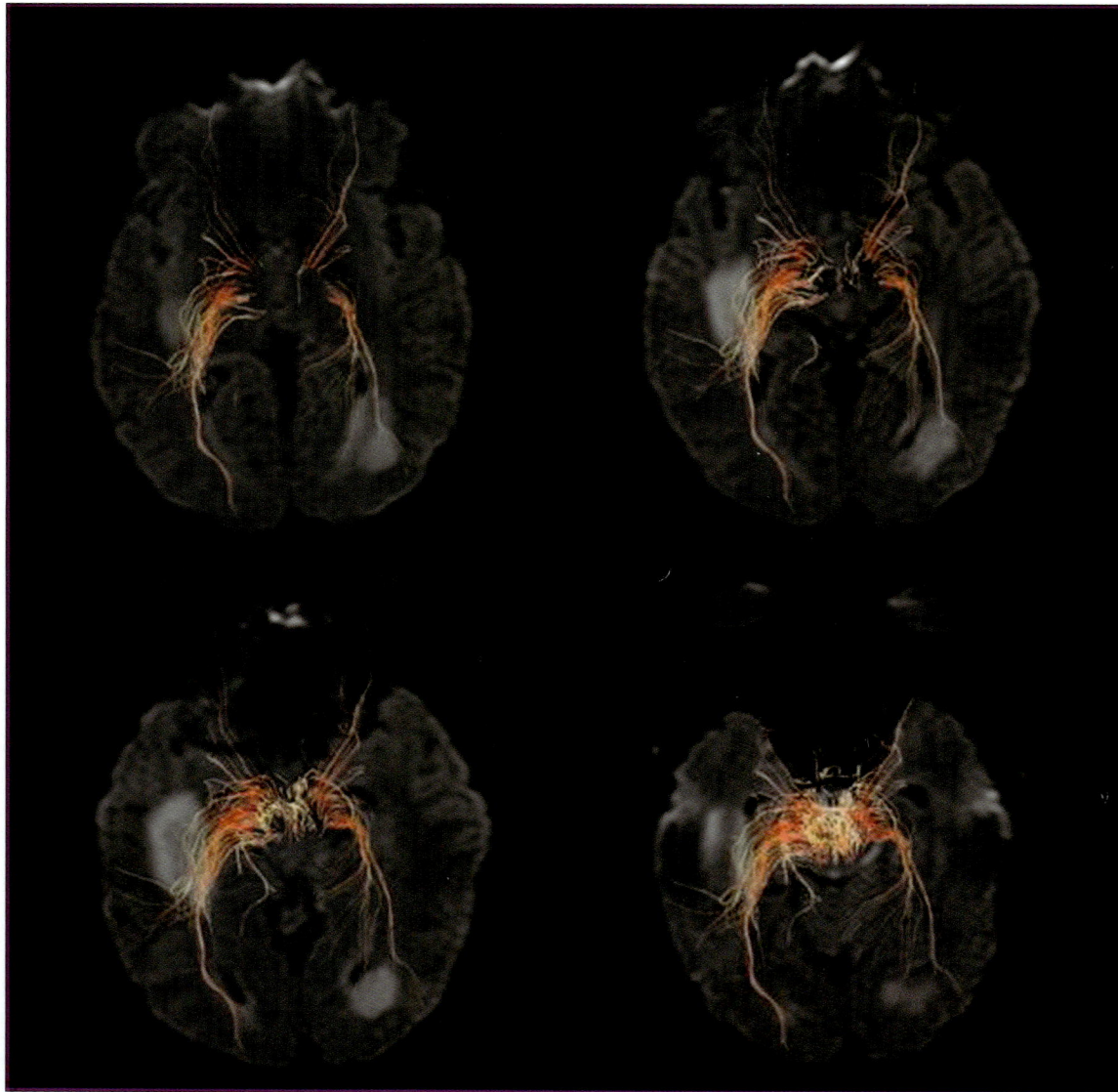

MR tractography.

residing in differing chemical environments possess slightly different resonant properties (chemical shift). For a given volume of brain the distribution of these proton resonances can be displayed as a spectrum. Discernible peaks can be seen for certain neurotransmitters: N-acetylaspartate varies in multiple sclerosis, stroke and schizophrenia while choline and lactate levels have been used to evaluate certain brain tumours.

Functional MRI (fMRI) depends on the fact that haemoglobin is diamagnetic when oxygenated but paramagnetic when deoxygenated. These different signals can be weighted to the smaller vessels, and hence closer to the active neurons, by using larger magnetic fields. In molecular imaging (mMRI) biomarkers interact chemically with their surroundings and alter the image according to molecular changes occurring within the area of interest, potentially enabling early detection and treatment of disease and basic pharmaceutical development, also allowing for quantitative testing.

High-field-strength magnets of course give significant improvement in spatial resolution and contrast. MR images have been acquired at 8 T of the microvasculature of the live human brain allowing close comparison to histology, having significant implications in the treatment of reperfusion injury and in the physiology of solid tumours and angiogenesis. There is every reason to believe that continued efforts to push the envelope of high-field-strength applications will open new vistas in what appears to be a never-ending array of potential clinical applications.

Ultrasound

In contrast with the other images in this book, ultrasound images do not depend on the use of electromagnetic wave forms. It is the properties of high-frequency sound waves (longitudinal waves) and their interaction with biological tissues that go to form these 'echograms'.

A sound wave of appropriate frequency (diagnostic range 3.5–20 MHz) is produced by piezo-electric principles, namely that certain crystals can change their shape and produce a voltage potential, and vice versa. As the beam passes through tissues, two important effects determine image production: attenuation and reflection. Attenuation is caused by the loss of energy due to absorption, reflection, refraction out of the capture of the receiver with resulting reduction in signal intensity. Reflection of sound waves within the range of the receiver produces the image, the texture of which is dependent upon tiny differences in acoustic impedance between different tissues. Blood flow and velocity can be measured (using the Doppler principle) in duplex mode.

Techniques such as harmonic imaging and the use of ultrasound contrast agents (stabilised microbubbles) have enabled non-invasive determination of myocardial perfusion to be recently discovered. These contrast agents clearly improve the detection of metastases in the liver and spleen. Ultrasound is the most common medical imaging technique for producing elastograms in which stiffness or strain images of soft tissue are used to detect or classify tumours. Cancer is 5–28 times stiffer than the background of normal soft tissue. When a mechanical compression or vibration is applied, the tumour deforms less than the surrounding tissue. Elastography can be used for example to measure the stiffness of the liver in vivo or in the detection of breast or thyroid tumours. A correlation between liver elasticity and the cirrhosis score has been shown.

Only a handful of key ultrasound images have been included in the book to illustrate a particular point or area, as the real-time nature of ultrasound precludes further coverage. Interpretation of the anatomy from static ultrasound images is more difficult than that from other imaging modalities because the technique is highly operator-dependent and provides information on tissue structure and form different from that of other imaging techniques.

Nuclear medicine

Historically the field of nuclear medicine began in 1946 when radioactive iodine was administered as an 'atomic cocktail' to treat thyroid cancer. Since that time, nuclear medicine has advanced and was recognized by the American Medical Association as a medical specialty in 1971.

Diagnostic radiology creates an image by passing radiation through the body from an external source. Nuclear medicine, unlike diagnostic radiology, creates an image by measuring the radiation emitted from tracers taken internally. Thus the image is created from the radiation emitted from the patient. Overall the radiation dosages are comparable and vary depending on the examination.

Nuclear medicine also differs from most other imaging modalities in that the tests demonstrate the physiological function of a specific area of the body. In some instances this physiological information can be fused with more anatomical imaging of CT or MRI thus combining the strengths of anatomy and function for diagnosis.

Rather than a contrast media for imaging, nuclear medicine uses radiopharmaceuticals, which are pharmaceuticals that have been labelled with a radionuclide. These radiopharmaceuticals are administered to patients by intravenous injection, ingestion, or inhalation. The method of administration depends on the type of examination and the organ or organ process to be imaged. By definition, all these radiopharmaceuticals emit radiation. This emitted radiation is detected and imaged with specialised equipment such as gamma cameras, positron emission tomography (PET), and single photon emission computed tomography (SPECT). Radiation in certain tests can be measured from parts of the body by the use of probes, or samples can be taken from patients and measured in counters.

The premise of nuclear medicine imaging involves functional biology, thereby not only can studies be done to image a disease process but they can also be used to treat diseases. Radiopharmaceuticals that are used for imaging emit a gamma ray (γ) and those used for treatment emit a beta (β) particle. Gamma rays are of higher energy to pass through the body and be detected by a detection camera, whereas beta particles travel only short distances and emit their radiation dose to the target organ. For example, technetium-99m or iodine-123 may be used to detect thyroid disease, but certain thyroid diseases or thyroid cancer may be treated solely or in part by treatment with iodine-131. The difference in the agent used depends on the type and energy levels of the radiation particle that the radioisotope emits.

Radionuclides, or the radioactive particle, used in nuclear medicine are often chemically bound to a complex called a tracer so that when administered it acts in a characteristic way in the body. The way the body handles this tracer can differ in disease or pathologic processes and thus demonstrate images different from normal in disease states. For example, the tracer used in bone imaging is methylene-diphosphonate (MDP). MDP is bound to technetium-99m for bone imaging. MDP attaches to hydroxyapatite in the bone. If there is a physiological change in the bone from a fracture, metastatic bone disease or arthritic change, there will be an increase in bone activity and thus more accumulation of the tracer in this region compared with the normal bone. This will result in a focal 'hot spot' of the radiopharmaceutical on a bone scan.

Technetium-99m is the major workhorse radioisotope of nuclear medicine. It can be eluted from a molybdenum/technetium generator stored within a nuclear medicine department allowing for easy access. It has a short half-life (6-hours), which allows for ease of medical imaging and disposal. Its pharmacological properties allow it to be easily bound to various tracers and it emits gamma rays that are of suitable energy for medical imaging.

In addition to technetium-99m the most common intravenous radionuclides used in nuclear medicine are iodine-123 and 131, thallium-201, gallium-67, 18-fluorodeoxyglucose (FDG) and indium-111 labeled leukocytes. The most common gaseous/aerosol radionuclides used are xenon-133, krypton-81m, technetium-99m (Technegas) and technetium-99m DTPA.

The images obtained from nuclear medicine imaging can be in the form of one or many images. Image sets can be represented as time sequence imaging (e.g. cine) such as dynamic imaging or cardiac gated sequences, or by spatial sequence imaging where the gamma camera is moved relative to the patient such as in SPECT imaging. Spatial sequence imaging allows the images to be presented as a slice-stack of images much like CT or MRI images are displayed. Spatial sequence imaging can also be fused with concomitant CT or MR imaging to provide combined physiologic and anatomical imaging. Time and spatial sequence imaging offer a unique perspective and information of physiological processes in the body.

A PET (positron emission tomography) scan is a specialised type of nuclear medicine imaging that measures important body functions, such as blood flow, oxygen use, and sugar (glucose) metabolism to evaluate how well organs and tissues are functioning. PET imaging involves short-lived radioactive tracer isotopes that are chemically incorporated into biologically active molecules. The most common molecule used is fluorodeoxyglucose (FDG), which is a sugar. After injection into the body, these active molecules become concentrated into the tissues of interest. After this waiting time, which is about an hour for FDG, imaging can proceed. Imaging of FDG occurs as the isotope decays. The isotope undergoes positron emission decay. As the positron is emitted, it travels only a few millimeters and annihilates with an electron and in so doing produce a pair of gamma photons moving in opposite directions. The PET scan detectors process only those photon pairs that are detected simultaneously (coincident detection). This data is then processed to create an image of tissue activity with respect to that particular isotope. These images can then be fused with CT or MR images.

A limitation of PET imaging is the short half-life of the isotopes. Thus close access to a cyclotron for generation of the isotopes plays an important role in the feasible location of PET imaging. Typical isotopes used in medical imaging and their half-lives are: carbon-11 (~20 min), nitrogen-13 (~10 min), oxygen-13 (~2 min) and fluorine-18 (~110 min).

Angiography/Interventional radiology

Angiographic imaging began in 1927 by Egas Moniz, a physician and neurologist, with the introduction of contrast X-ray cerebral angiography. In 1949 he was awarded the Nobel Prize for his work. The field of angiography however was revolutionised with the advent of the Seldinger technique in 1953, in which no sharp needles remained inside the vascular lumen during imaging.

Although the field of angiography began with X-ray and fluoroscopic imaging of blood vessels and organs of the body by injecting radio-opaque contrast agents in to the blood, it has evolved to so much more. Many of the procedures performed by angiography can be diagnostic, as newer techniques arose, it has allowed for the advent of minimally invasive procedures performed with image guidance and thus the name change of the discipline to Interventional radiology (or vascular and interventional radiology).

Angiograms are typically performed by gaining access to the blood vessels, whether this is through the femoral artery, femoral vein or jugular vein depends on the area of interest to be imaged. Angiograms can be obtained of the brain as cerebral angiograms, of the heart as coronary angiograms, of the lungs as pulmonary angiograms, and so on. Imaging of the arterial and venous circulation of the arms and legs can demonstrate peripheral vascular disease. Once vascular access is made, then catheters are directed to the specific location to be imaged in the body by the use of guide wires. Contrast agents are injected through these catheters to visualise the vessels or the organ with X-ray imaging.

In addition to diagnostic imaging, treatment and/or interventions can often be performed through similar catheter based examinations. Such procedures might involve angioplasties where a balloon mechanism is placed across an area of narrowing, or stenosis, in a vessel or lumen.

With controlled inflation of the balloon, the area of narrowing can be widened. Often to keep these areas from narrowing again, stents can be placed within the lumen of the vessel or even in the trachea or oesophagus.

Imaging in diagnostic or interventional procedures can be still images or motion (cine) images. The technique often used is called digital subtraction angiography (DSA). In this type of imaging, images are taken at 2–30 frames per second to allow imaging of the flow of blood through vessels. A preliminary image of the area is taken before the contrast is injected. This 'mask' image is then electronically subtracted from all the images leaving behind only the vessels filled with contrast. This technique requires the patient to remain motionless for optimal subtraction.

Angiograms can be performed of the heart to visualise the size and contractility of the chambers and anatomy of the coronary vessels. The thorax can also be studied to evaluate the pulmonary arteries and veins for vascular malformations, blood clots and possible origins of hemoptysis. The neck is often imaged to visualise the vessels that supply the brain as they arise from the aortic arch to the cerebral vessels, in the investigation of atherosclerotic disease, vascular malformations and tumoral blood supplies. Renal artery imaging can elucidate the cause of hypertension in selected patients, as can imaging of the mesenteric vessels discover the origin of gastrointestinal bleeding or mesenteric angina.

In addition to angiograms and venograms, the field of interventional radiology also performs such procedures as coil-embolisation of aneurysms and vascular malformations, balloon angioplasty and stent placement, chemoembolisation directly into tumours, drainage catheter insertions, embolisations (e.g. uterine artery embolisation for treatment of uterine fibroids), thrombolysis to dissolve blood clots, tissue biopsy (percutaneous or transvascular), radiofrequency ablation and cryoablation of tumours, line insertions for specialised vascular access, inferior vena cava filter placements, vertebroplasty, nephrostomy placement, gastrostomy tube placement for feeding, dialysis access, TIPS (transjugular intrahepatic porto-systemic shunt) placement, biliary interventions, and, most recently, endovenous laser ablation of varicose veins.

Computed tomography

The limitation of all plain radiographic techniques is the two dimensional representation of three dimensional structures: the linear attenuation co-efficient of all the tissues in the path of the X-ray beam form the image.

Computed tomography (CT) obtains a series of different angular X-ray projections that are processed by a computer to give a section of specified thickness. The CT image comprises a regular matrix of picture elements (pixels). All of the tissues contained within the pixel attenuate the X-ray projections and result in a mean attenuation value for the pixel. This value is compared with the attenuation value of water and is displayed on a scale (the Hounsfield Scale). Water is said to have an attenuation of 0 Hounsfield units (HU); air typically has an HU number of –1000; fat is approximately –100 HU; soft tissues are in the range +20 to +70 HU; and bone is usually greater than +400 HU.

Modern multislice helical CT scanners can obtain images in sub-second times and imaging of the whole body from the top of the head to the thighs can take as little as a single breath hold of only a few seconds. The fast scan times allow dynamic imaging of arteries and veins at different times after the injection of intravenous contrast agents. The continuous acquisition of data from a helical CT scanner allows reconstruction of an image in any plane, commonly sagittal and coronal, as displayed in many of the forthcoming chapters. This orthogonal imaging greatly improves the understanding of the three dimensional aspects of radiological anatomy and now forms part of the standard practice of assessing disease.

Digital images are stored in an archive and form part of an electronic storage record that is becoming commonplace throughout the world, namely a PACS (Picture Archiving and Communication System). PACS allows interrogation of images via an electronic network so that those images (and reports) may be visualised at a distance, for example, on the wards or at another hospital. The Electronic Patient Record (EPR), where all patient information is stored, is developing rapidly and gaining acceptance allowing a marked improvement in data handling.

No specific preparation is required for CT examinations of the brain, spine or musculoskeletal system. Studies of the chest, abdomen and pelvis usually require intravenous contrast medium that contains iodine, so enhancing the arteries and veins and defining their relationships to a greater extent. Opacification of the bowel in CT studies of the abdomen and pelvis can be accomplished by oral ingestion of a water-soluble contrast medium from 24 hours prior to the examination to show the colon, combined with further oral intake 0–60 minutes prior to the scan, for outlining the stomach and small bowel. Occasionally, direct insertion of rectal contrast to show the distal large bowel may be required.

Generally all studies are performed with the patient supine and images are obtained in the transverse or axial plain. Modern CT scanners allow up to 25 degrees of gantry angulation, which is particularly valuable in spinal imaging. Occasionally, direct coronal images are obtained in the investigation of cranial and maxillofacial abnormalities; in these cases the patient lies prone with the neck extended and the gantry appropriately angled, but this technique has largely been superseded by the orthogonal imaging described above.

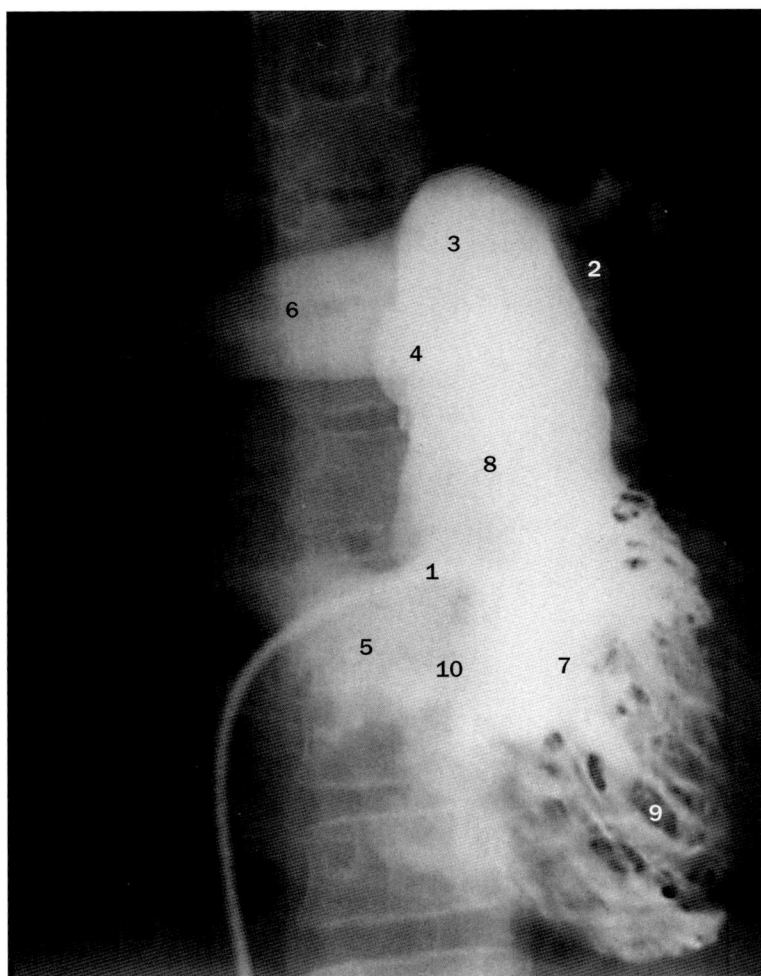

Right ventricular angiogram (p. 112).

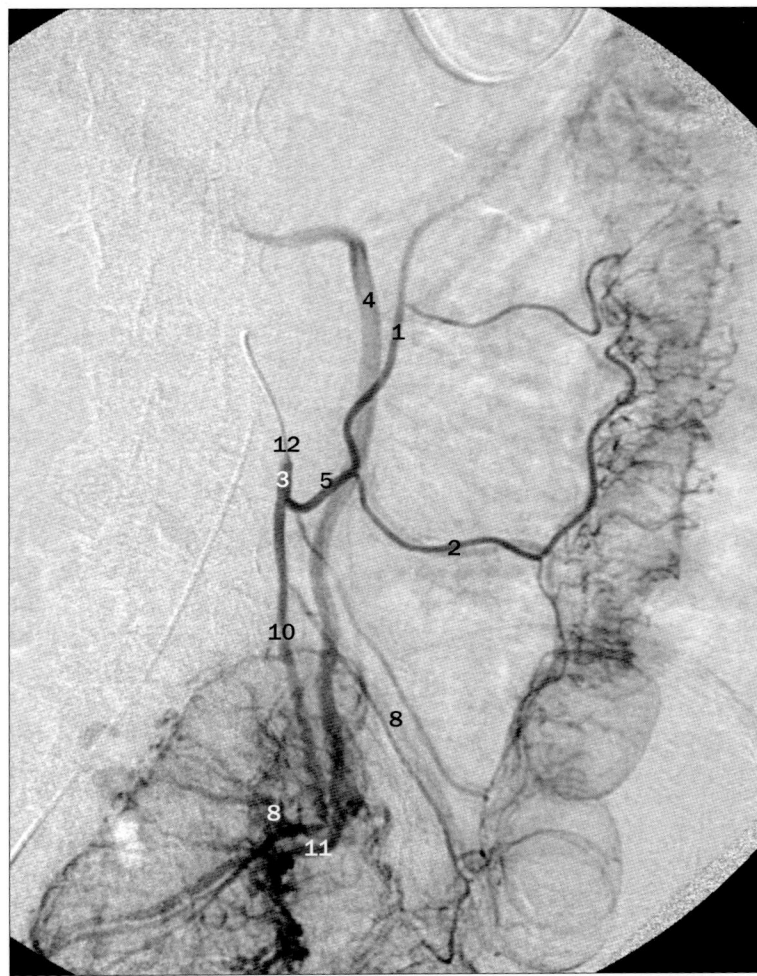

Inferior mesenteric arteriogram (p. 186).

1 Head, neck and brain

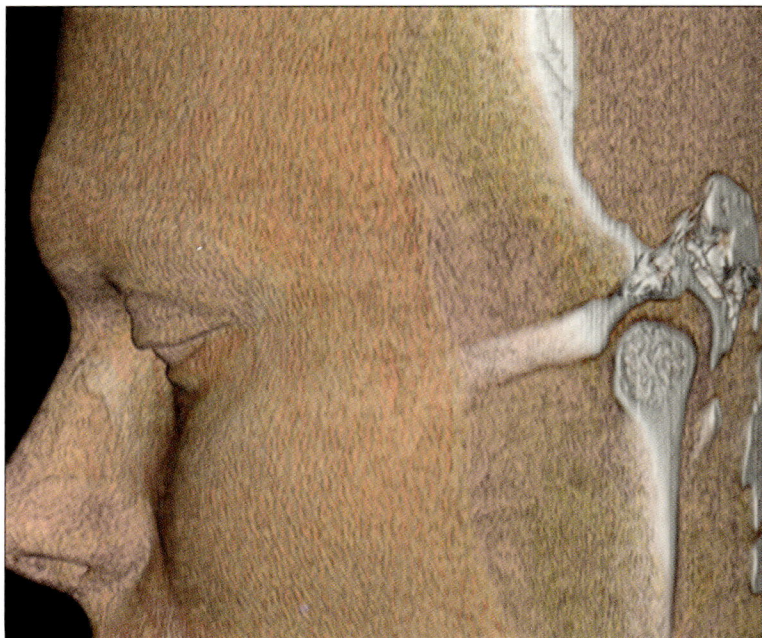

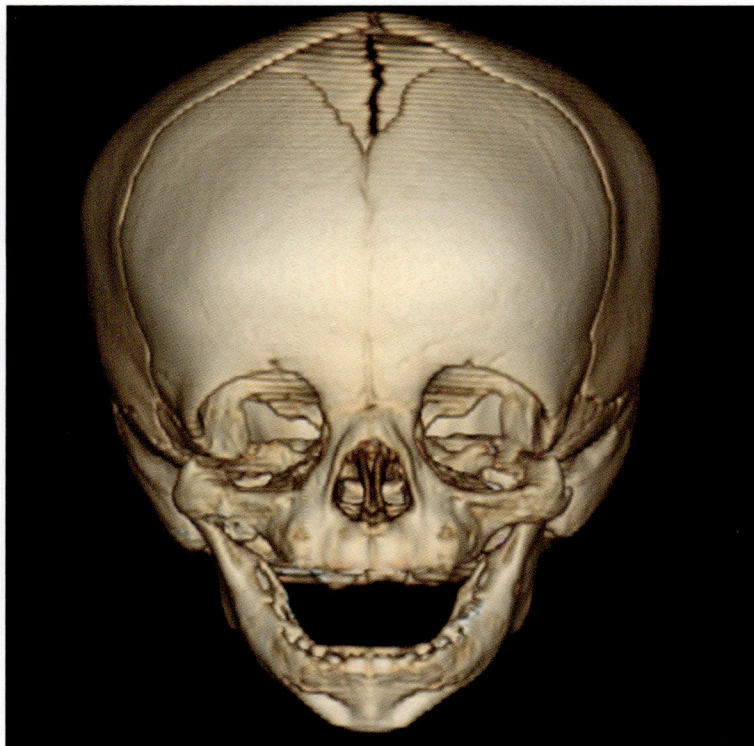

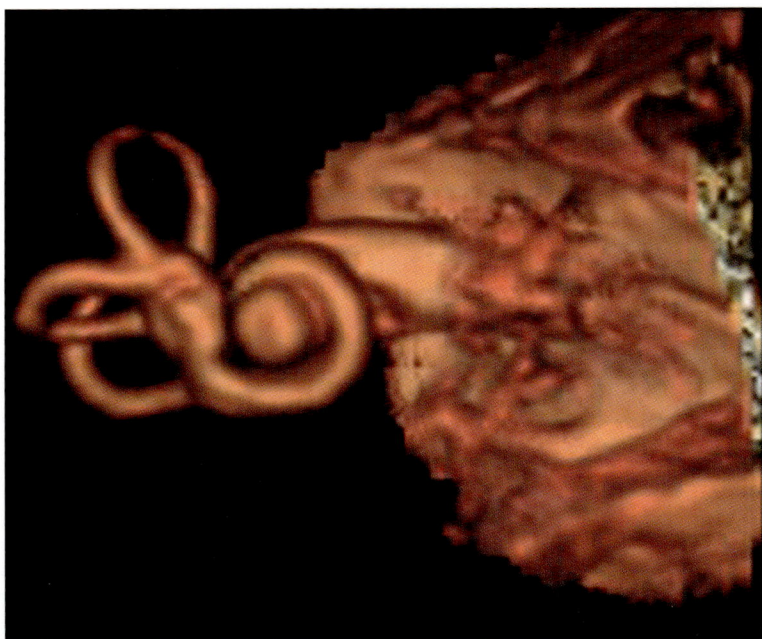

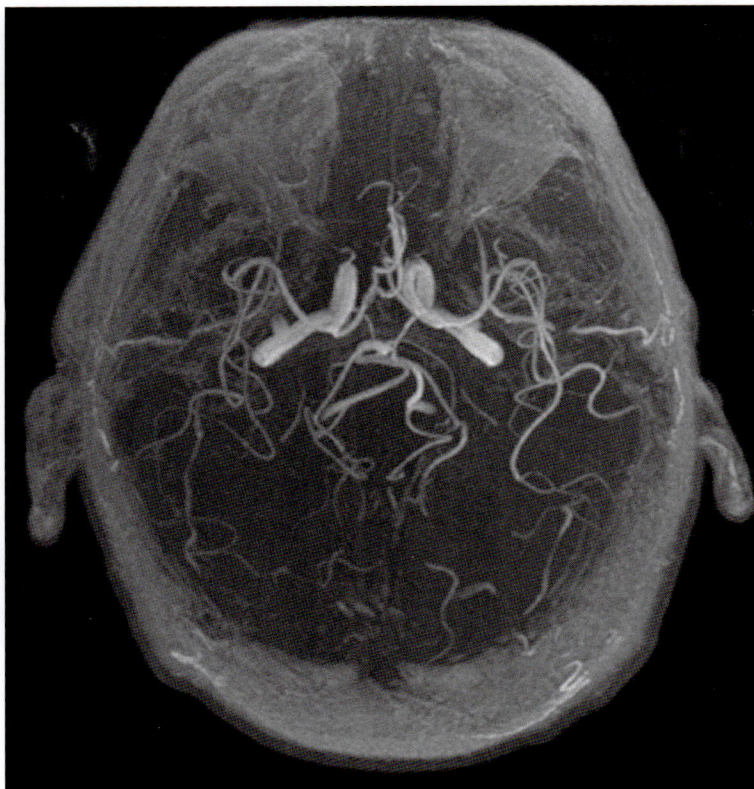

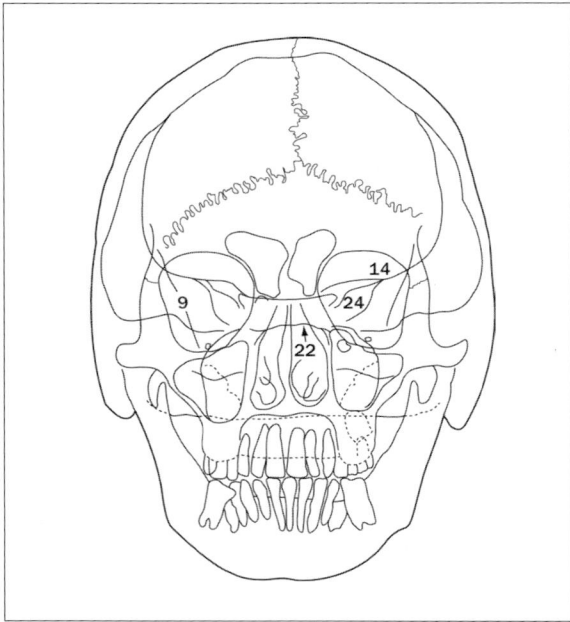

(a) Skull, occipitofrontal projection.
(b) Skull, demonstrating the foramina rotunda, occipitofrontal projection.

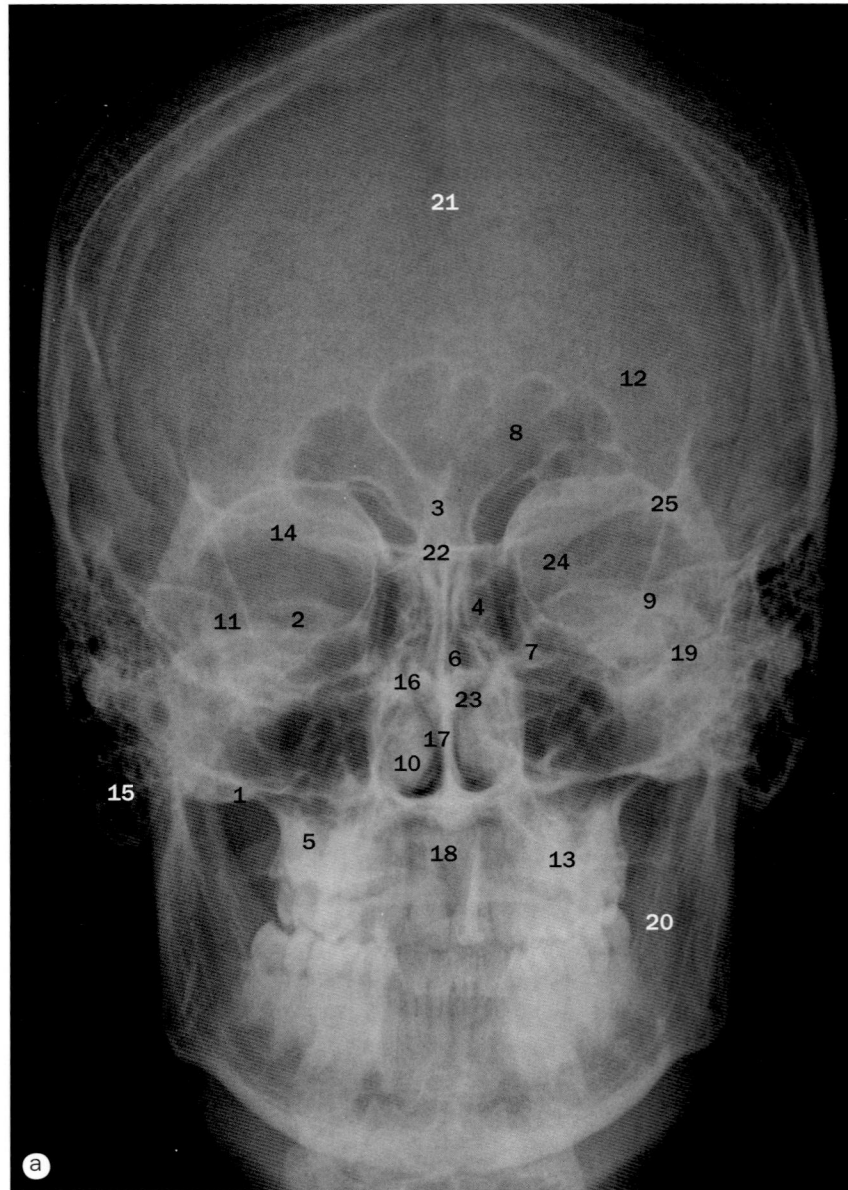

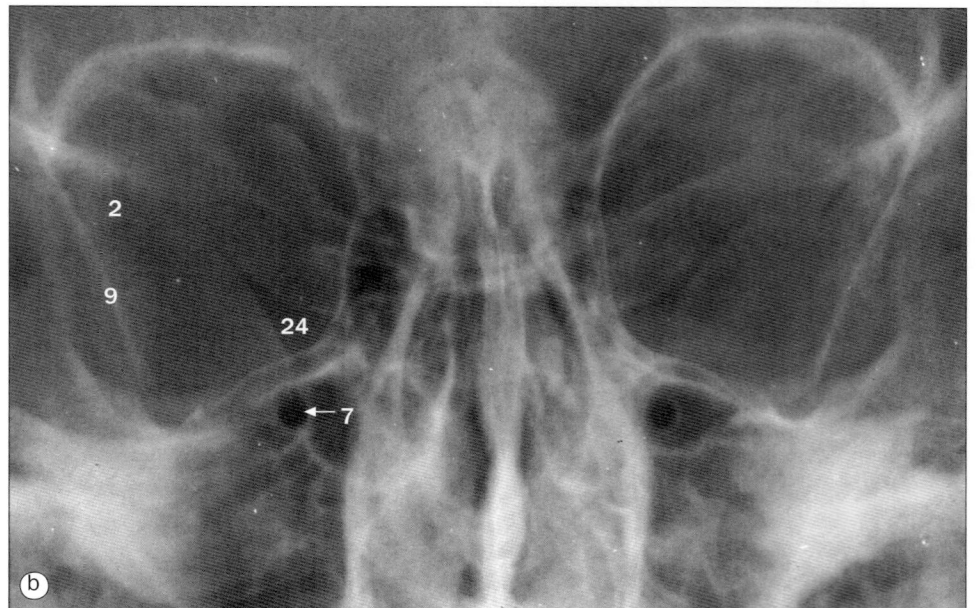

 1 Basi-occiput
 2 Body of sphenoid
 3 Crista galli
 4 Ethmoidal air cells
 5 Floor of maxillary sinus (antrum)
 6 Floor of pituitary fossa
 7 Foramen rotundum
 8 Frontal sinus
 9 Greater wing of sphenoid
10 Inferior turbinate
11 Internal acoustic meatus
12 Lambdoid suture
13 Lateral mass of atlas (first cervical vertebra)
14 Lesser wing of sphenoid
15 Mastoid process
16 Middle turbinate
17 Nasal septum
18 Odontoid process (dens) of axis
    (second cervical vertebra)
19 Petrous part of temporal bone
20 Ramus of mandible
21 Sagittal suture
22 Planum sphenoidale
23 Sphenoid air sinus
24 Superior orbital fissure
25 Temporal surface of greater wing of sphenoid

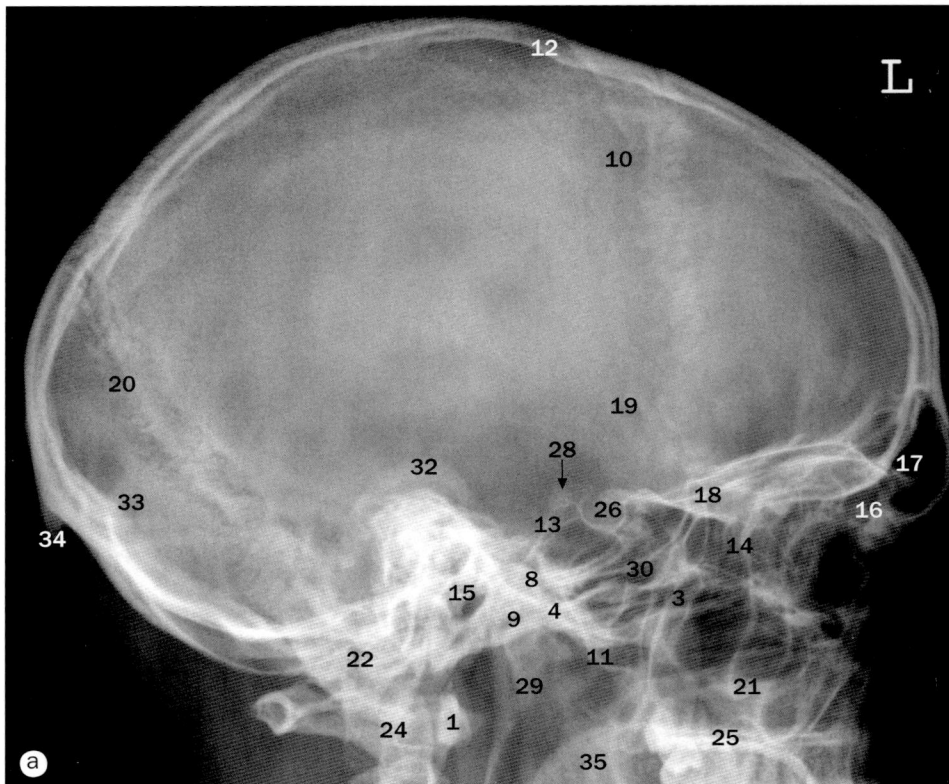

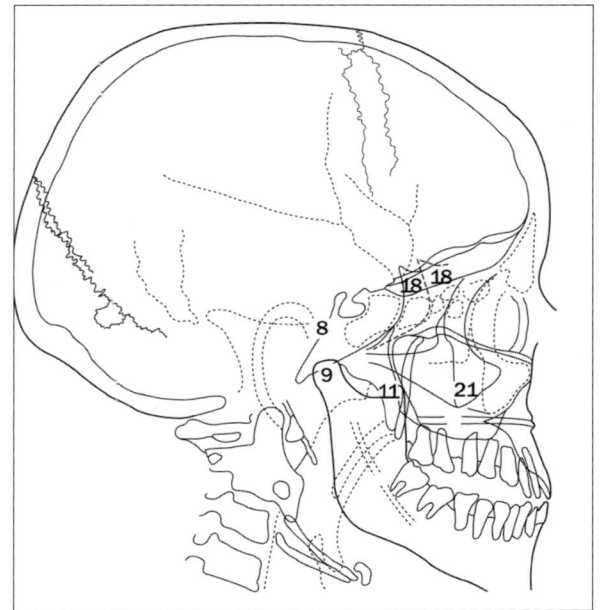

(a) Skull, lateral projection.

Pituitary fossa (sella turcica), (b) of a 7-year-old child, (c) of a 23-year-old woman, lateral projections.

1 Anterior arch of atlas (first cervical vertebra)
2 Anterior clinoid process
3 Arch of zygoma
4 Articular tubercle for temporomandibular joint
5 Basilar part of occipital bone
6 Basisphenoid/basi-occiput synchondrosis
7 Carotid sulcus
8 Clivus
9 Condyle of mandible
10 Coronal suture
11 Coronoid process of mandible

12 Diploë
13 Dorsum sellae
14 Ethmoidal air cells
15 External acoustic meatus
16 Frontal process of zygoma
17 Frontal sinus
18 Greater wing of sphenoid
19 Grooves for middle meningeal vessels
20 Lambdoid suture
21 Malar process of maxilla
22 Mastoid air cells
23 Middle clinoid process

24 Odontoid process (dens) of axis (second cervical vertebra)
25 Palatine process of maxilla
26 Pituitary fossa (sella turcica)
27 Planum sphenoidale
28 Posterior clinoid process
29 Ramus of mandible
30 Sphenoidal sinus
31 Tuberculum sellae
32 Pinna of ear
33 Inion
34 External occipital protruberance
35 Soft palate

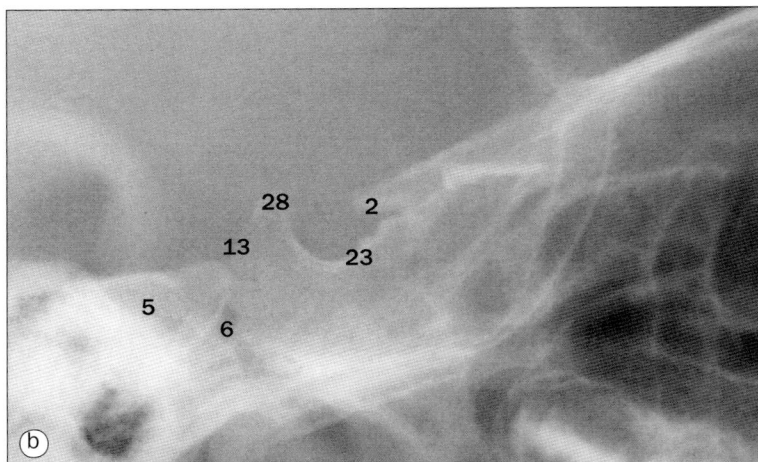

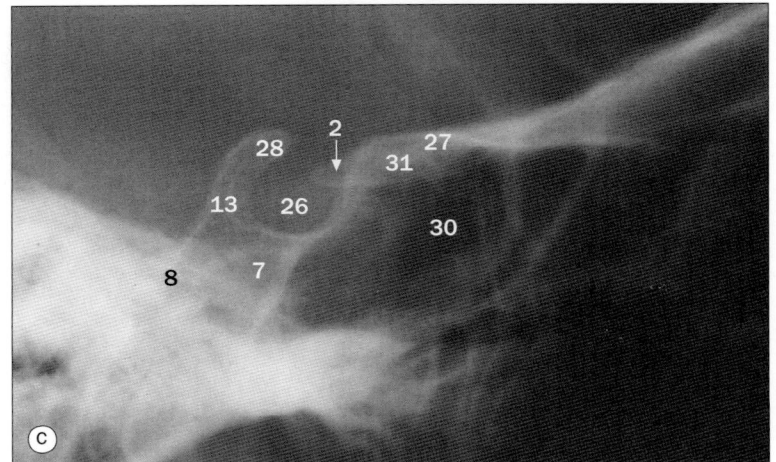

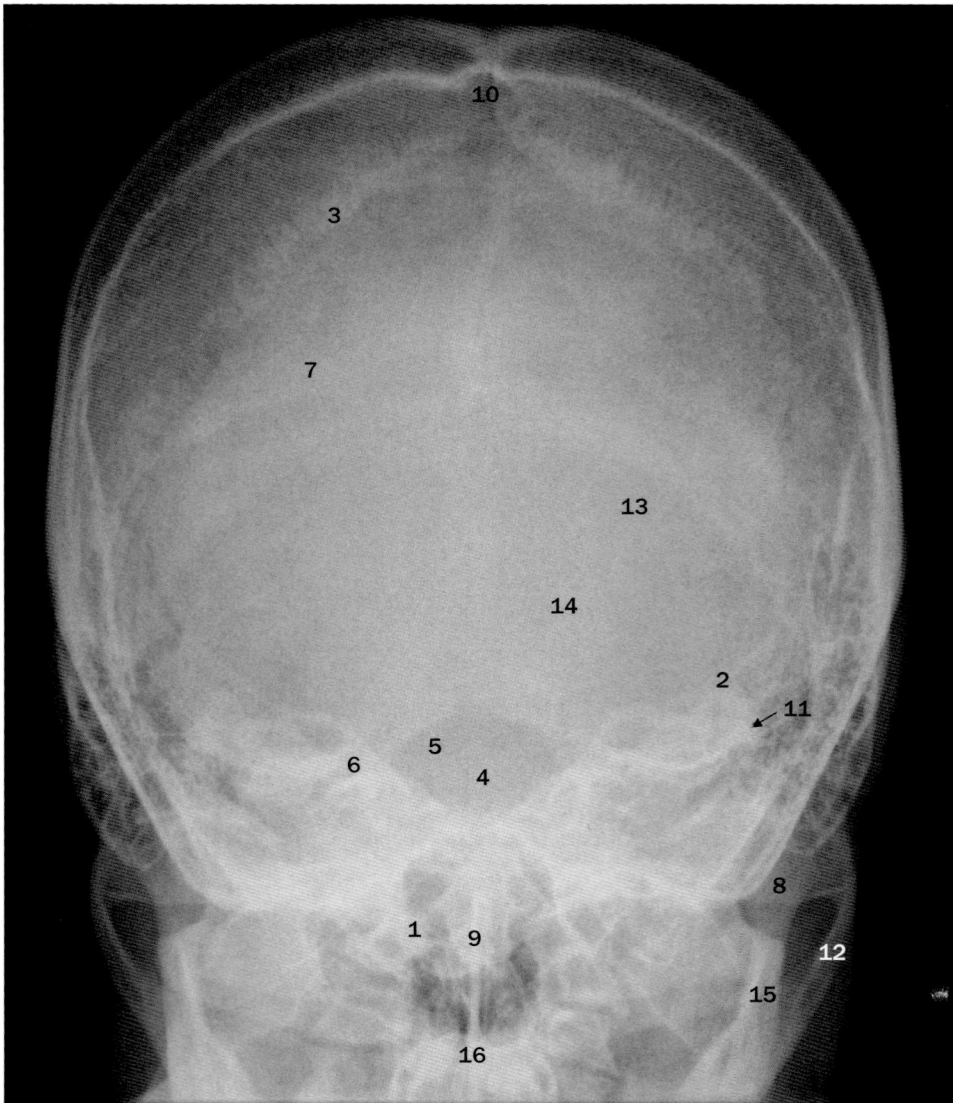

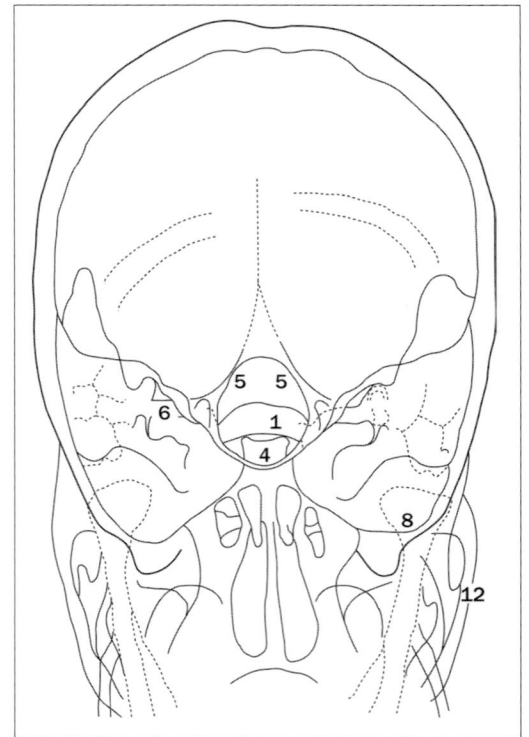

Skull, 30° fronto-occipital (Townes') projection.

 1 Arch of atlas (first cervical vertebra)
 2 Arcuate eminence of temporal bone
 3 Coronal suture
 4 Dorsum sellae
 5 Foramen magnum
 6 Internal acoustic meatus
 7 Lambdoid suture
 8 Mandibular condyle
 9 Odontoid process (dens) of axis (second cervical vertebra)
10 Sagittal suture
11 Superior semicircular canal
12 Zygomatic arch
13 Groove for transverse sinus
14 Squamous occipital bone
15 Mandible
16 Nasal septum

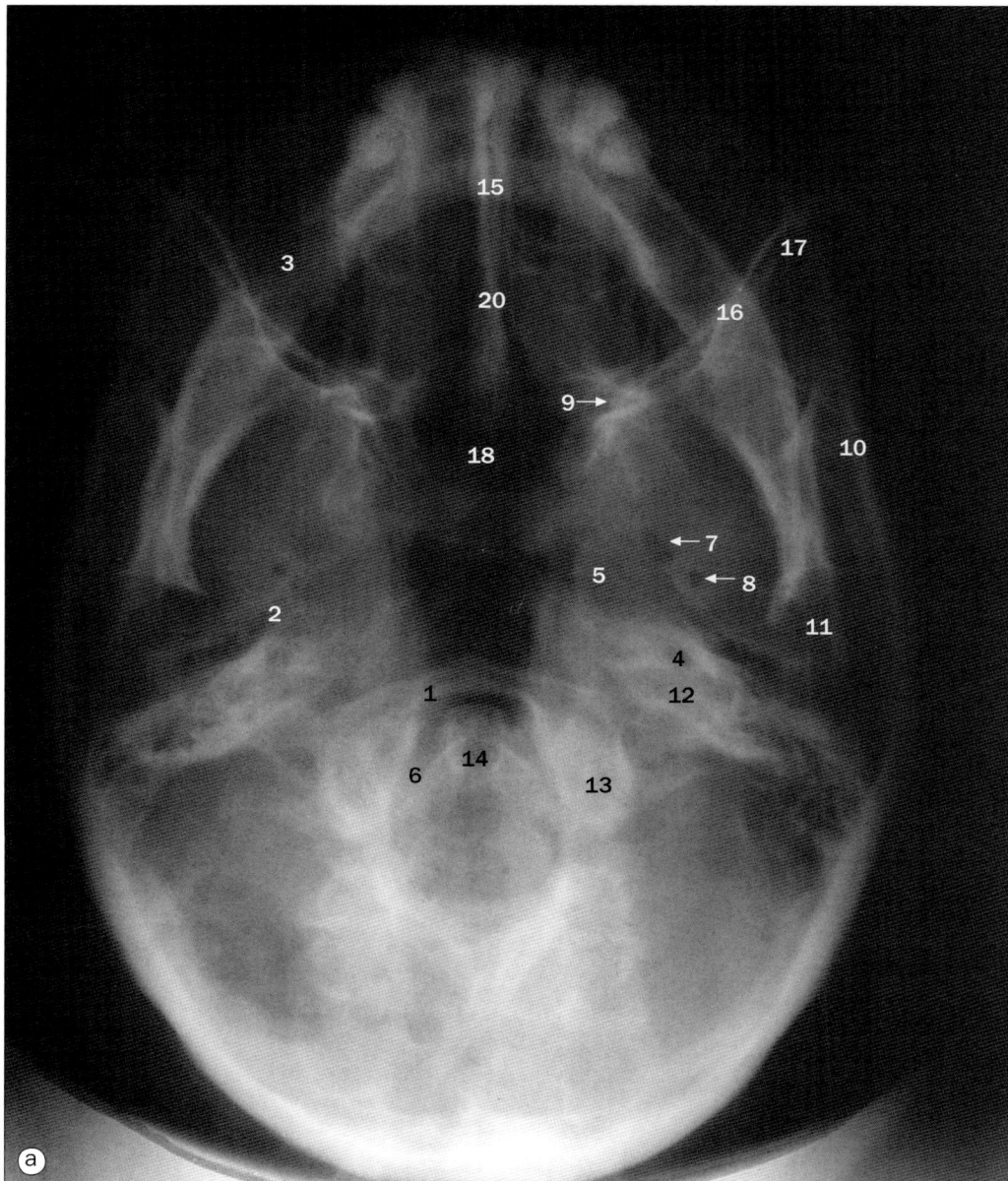

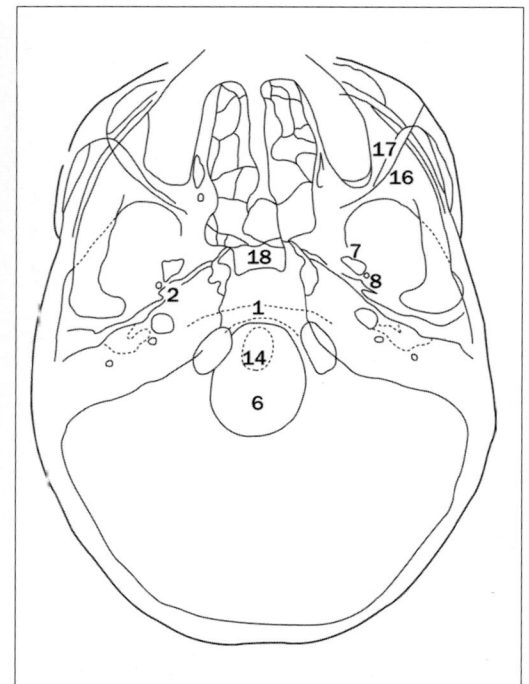

(a) Skull, submentovertical projection.
(b) Skull, with additional angulation for zygomatic arches, submentovertical projection.

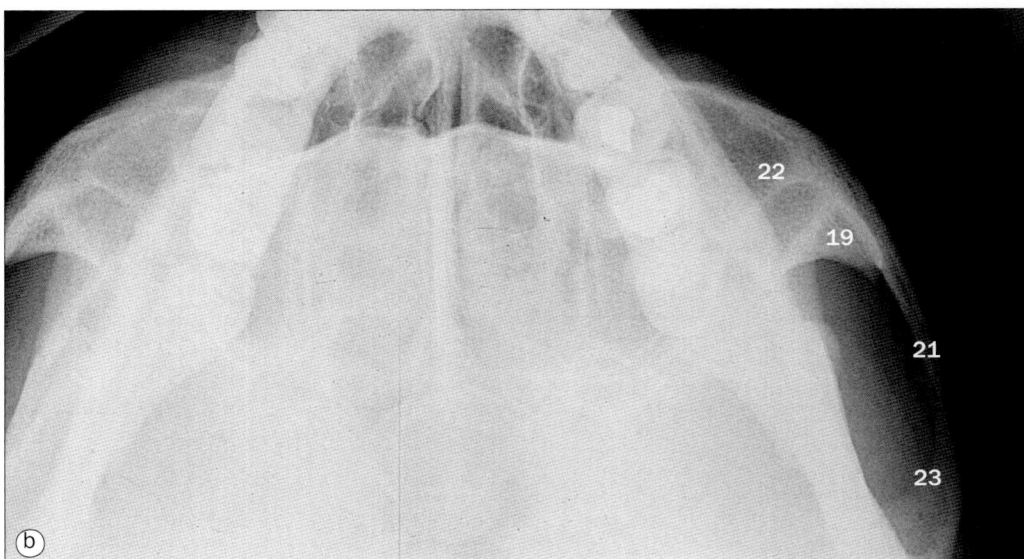

1 Anterior arch of atlas (first cervical vertebra)
2 Auditory (Eustachian) tube
3 Body of mandible
4 Carotid canal
5 Foramen lacerum
6 Foramen magnum
7 Foramen ovale
8 Foramen spinosum
9 Greater palatine foramen
10 Greater wing of sphenoid
11 Head of mandible
12 Jugular foramen
13 Occipital condyle
14 Odontoid process (dens) of axis (second cervical vertebra)
15 Perpendicular plate of ethmoid
16 Posterior margin of orbit
17 Posterior wall of maxillary sinus (antrum)
18 Sphenoidal sinus
19 Temporal process of zygomatic bone
20 Vomer
21 Zygomatic arch
22 Zygomatic bone
23 Zygomatic process of temporal bone

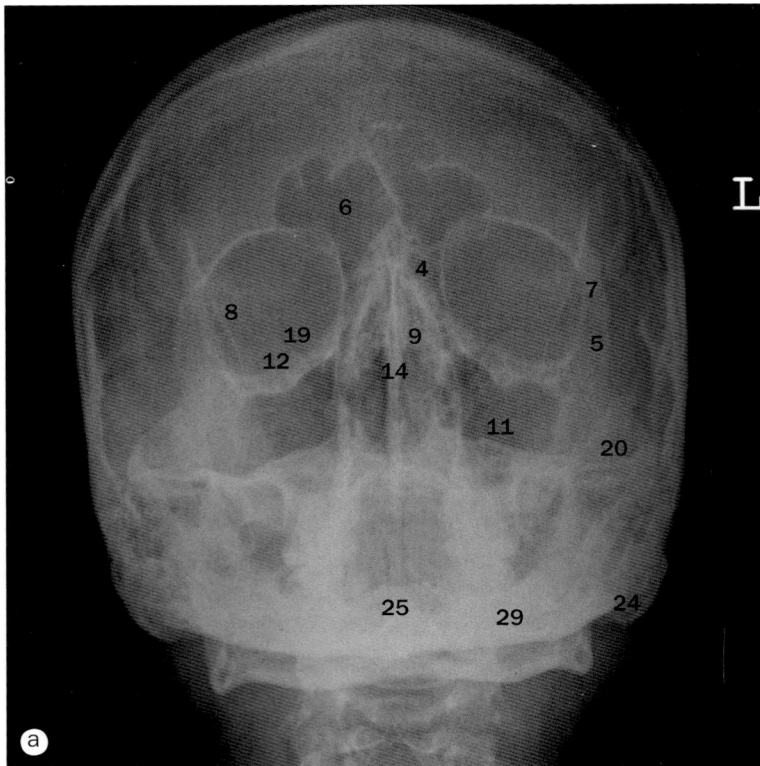

(a) Modified occipito frontal projection.

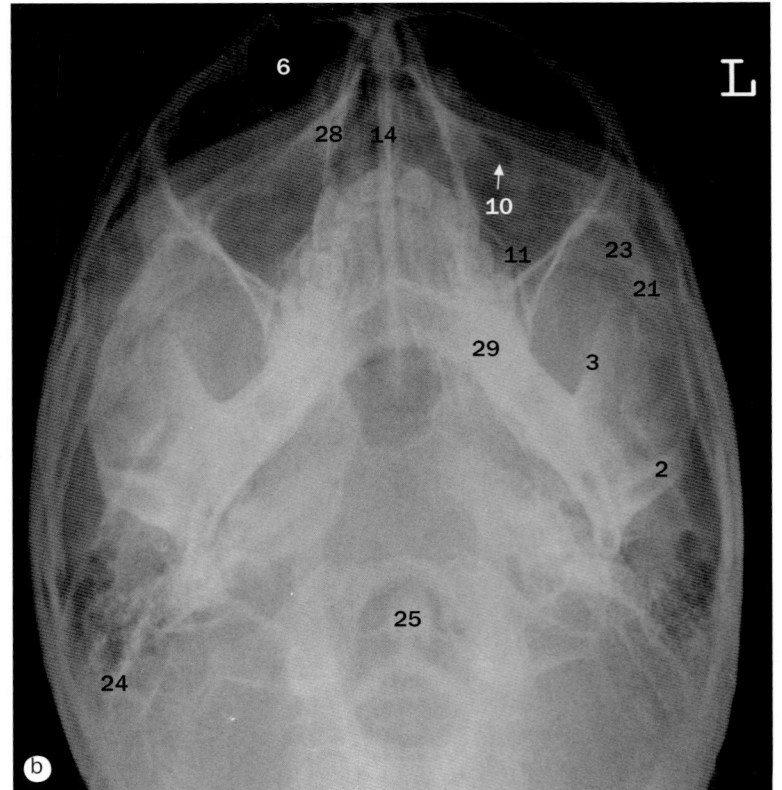

(b) Occipito mental projection.

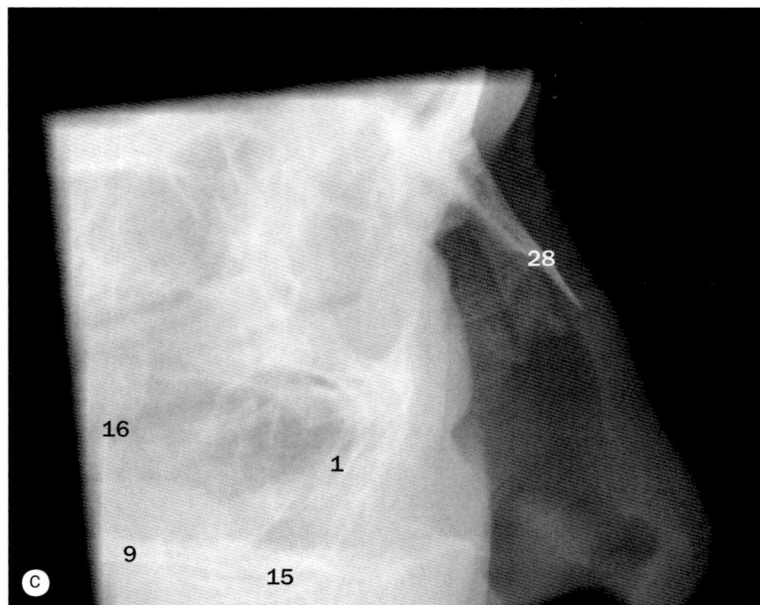

(c) Lateral nasal bones projection.

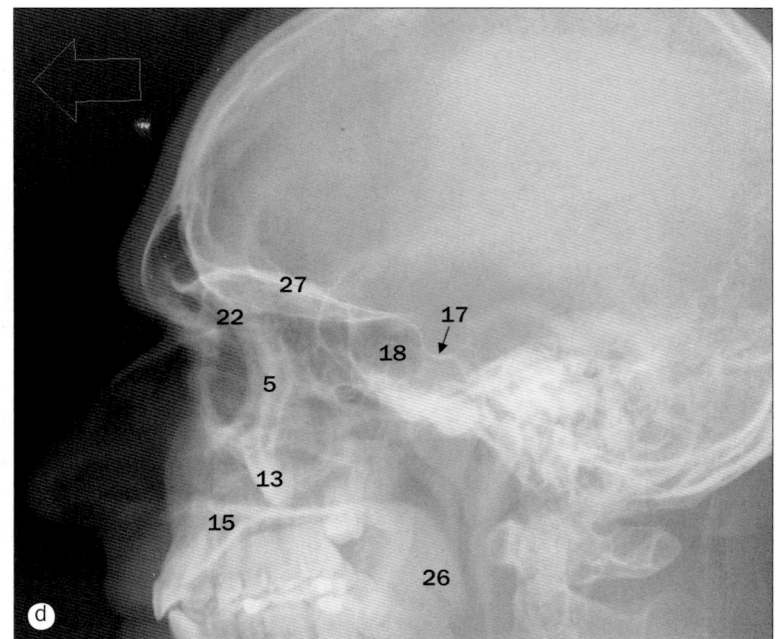

(d) Lateral sinus projection.

1 Anterior wall of maxillary sinus (antrum)	11 Left maxillary sinus (antrum)	21 Zygomatic arch
2 Condyle of mandible	12 Lesser wing of sphenoid	22 Zygomatic process of frontal bone
3 Coronoid process of mandible	13 Malar process of maxilla	23 Zygomatic process of temporal bone
4 Ethmoidal sinuses	14 Nasal septum	24 Mastoid process
5 Frontal process of zygomatic bone	15 Palatine process of maxilla	25 Odontoid peg
6 Frontal sinuses	16 Posterior wall of maxillary sinus (antrum)	26 Soft palate
7 Frontozygomatic suture	17 Sella turcica	27 Floor of anterior cranial fossa
8 Greater wing of sphenoid	18 Sphenoidal sinus	28 Nasal bones
9 Horizontal plate of palatine bone	19 Superior orbital fissure	29 Mandible
10 Infra-orbital foramen	20 Temporal process of zygomatic bone	

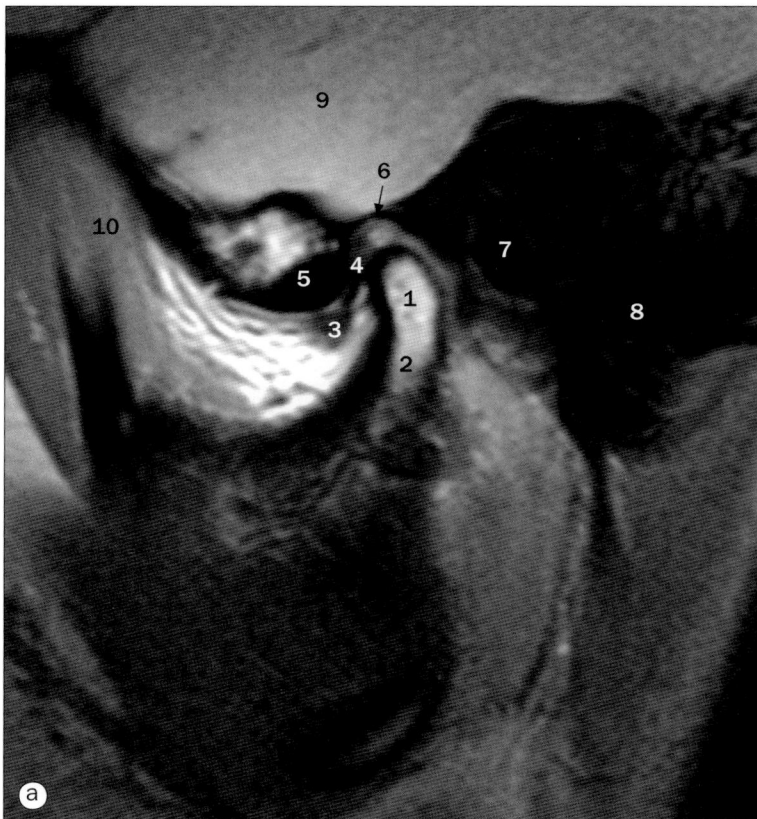

(a) Temporomandibular joint MR: closed.

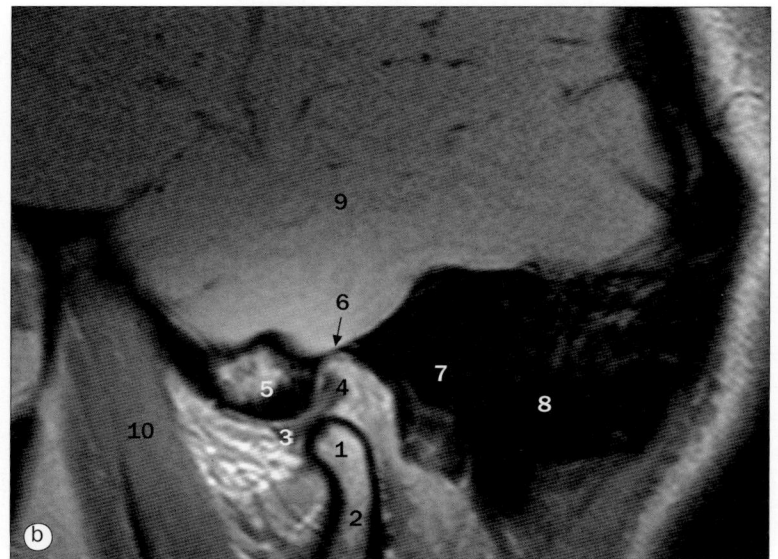

(b) Temporomandibular joint MR: open.

MR of the temporomandibular joint with the subject looking to the left.

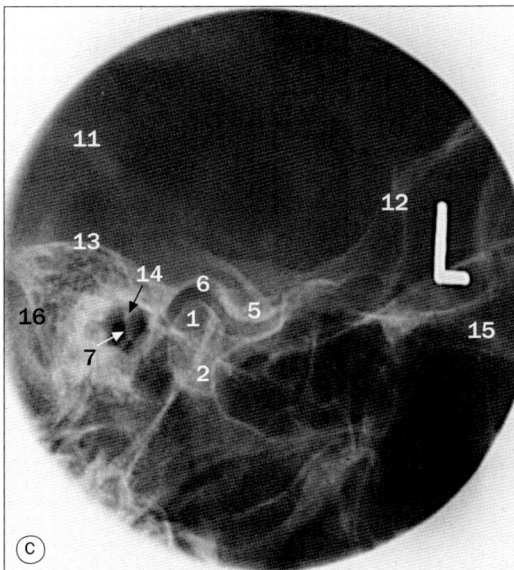

(c) Radiograph of temporomandibular joint: closed.

1 Condylar head
2 Condylar neck
3 Anterior band of disc
4 Posterior band of disc
5 Articular eminence
6 Mandibular fossa
7 External auditory canal
8 Mastoid process of temporal bone
9 Temporal lobe of brain
10 Temporalis muscle
11 Pinna of ear
12 Greater wing of sphenoid
13 Tegmen tympani
14 Malleus
15 Zygomatic process of temporal bone
16 Sinus plate

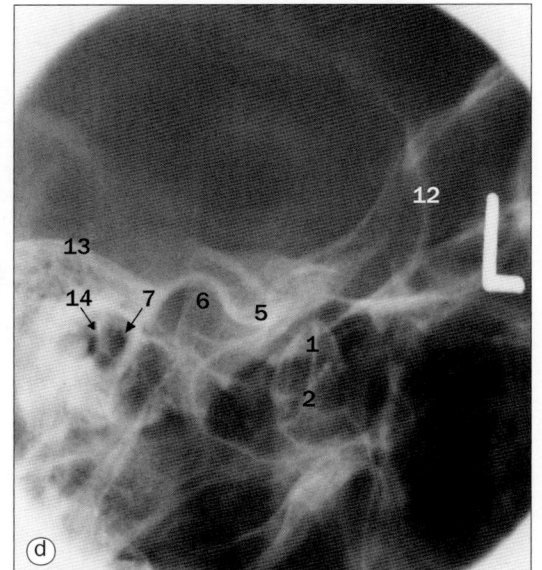

(d) Radiograph of temporomandibular joint: open.

Radiographs of the temporomandibular joint with the subject looking to the right.

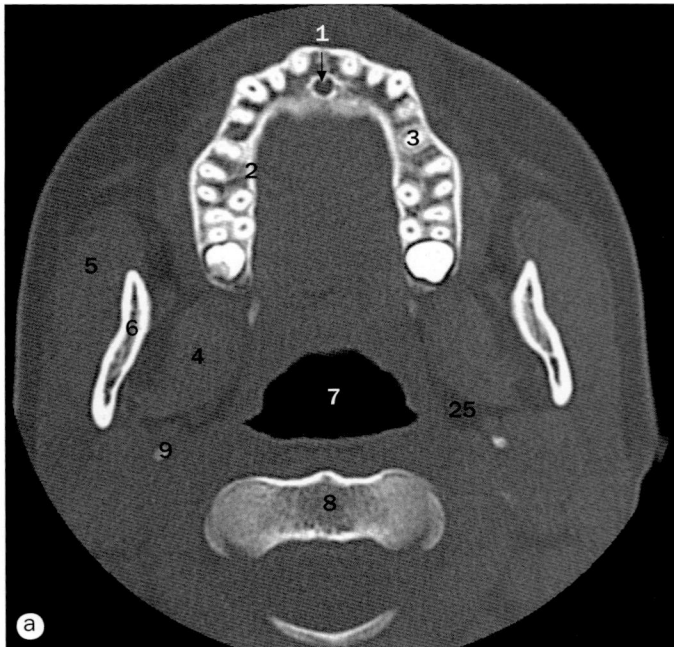

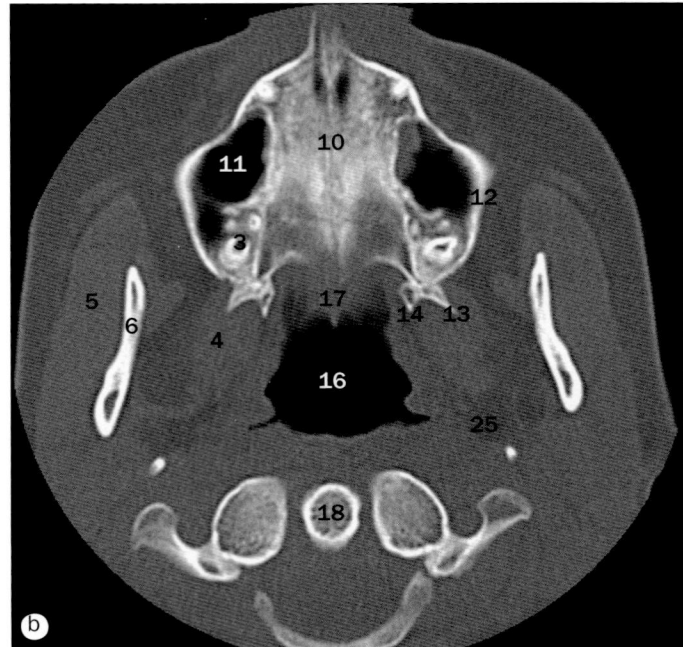

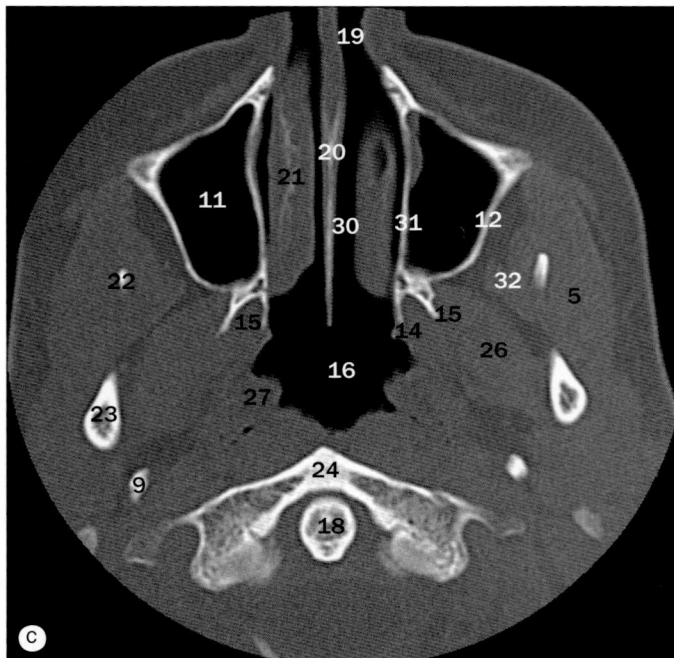

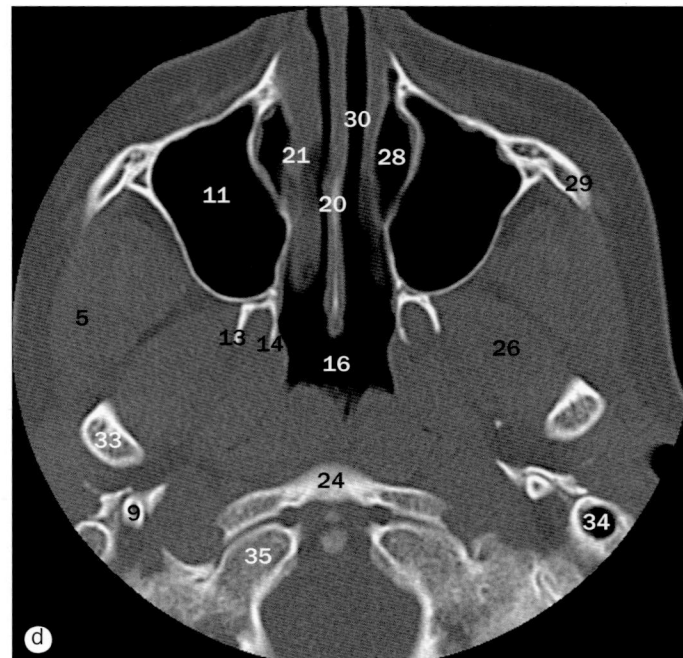

Facial bones and paranasal sinuses, axial CT images demonstrated at the following levels: **(a)** alveolar process of the maxilla, **(b)** hard palate, **(c)** nares, **(d)** maxillary sinus, **(e)** middle turbinate, **(f)** zygomatic arch, **(g)** sphenoid sinus, **(h)** ethmoid sinus.

1 Incisive canal	**14** Medial pterygoid plate	**26** Lateral pyterygoid muscle
2 Alveolar rim	**15** Pterygoid fossa	**27** Torus tubarius
3 Alveolar recess	**16** Nasopharynx	**28** Inferior meatus (at location of
4 Medial pterygoid muscle	**17** Vomer	nasolacrimal opening)
5 Masseter muscle	**18** Odontoid process (dens)	**29** Zygoma
6 Ramus of mandible	**19** Nares	**30** Nasal cavity
7 Oropharynx	**20** Nasal septum	**31** Medial wall of maxillary sinus (antrum)
8 Body of C2	**21** Inferior turbinate	**32** Temporalis muscle
9 Styloid process	**22** Coronoid process of mandible	**33** Condylar head of mandible
10 Hard palate	**23** Condylar neck of mandible	**34** Mastoid air cells
11 Maxillary sinus (antrum)	**24** Anterior arch of atlas (first cervical	**35** Occipital condyle
12 Lateral wall of maxillary sinus (antrum)	vertebra)	**36** Middle turbinate
13 Lateral pterygoid plate	**25** Parapharyngeal space	**37** Middle meatus

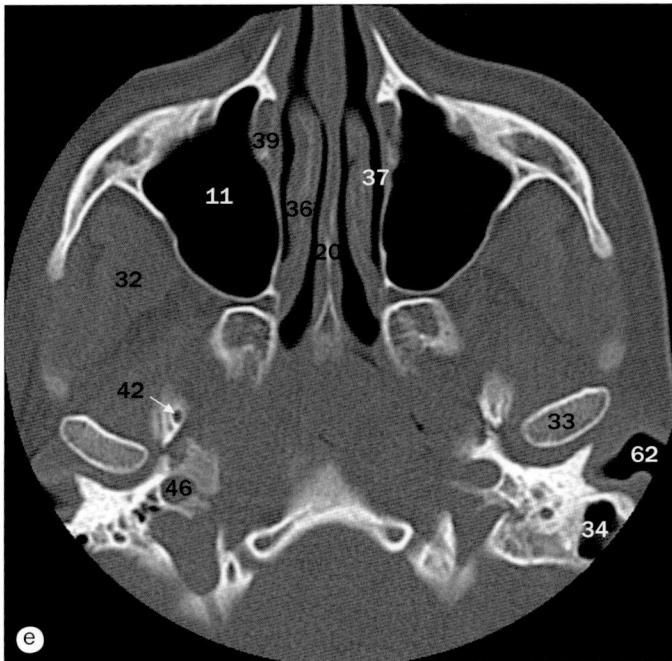

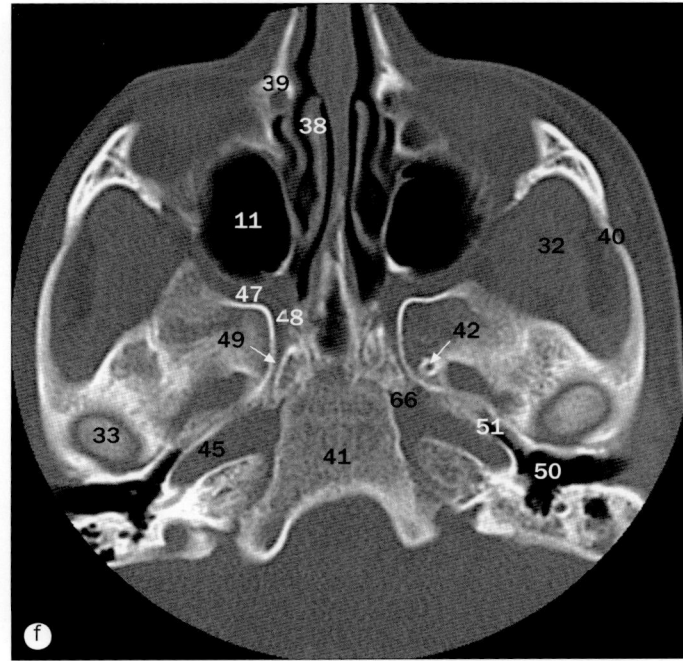

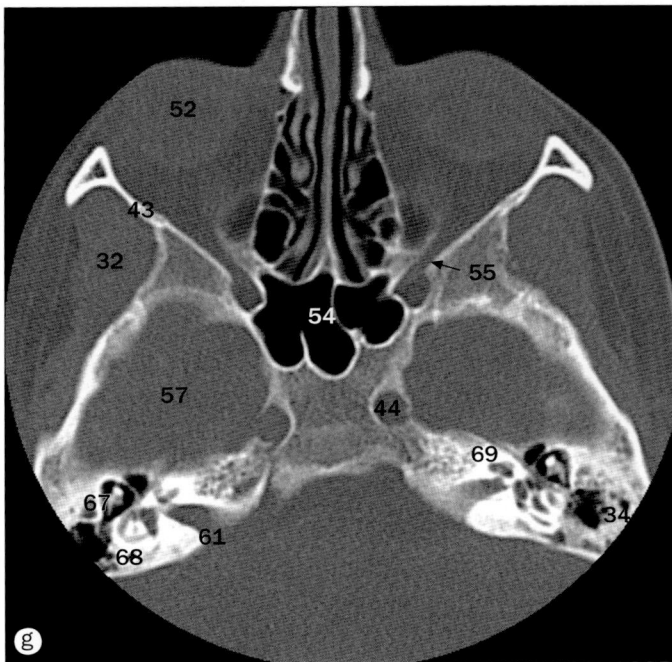

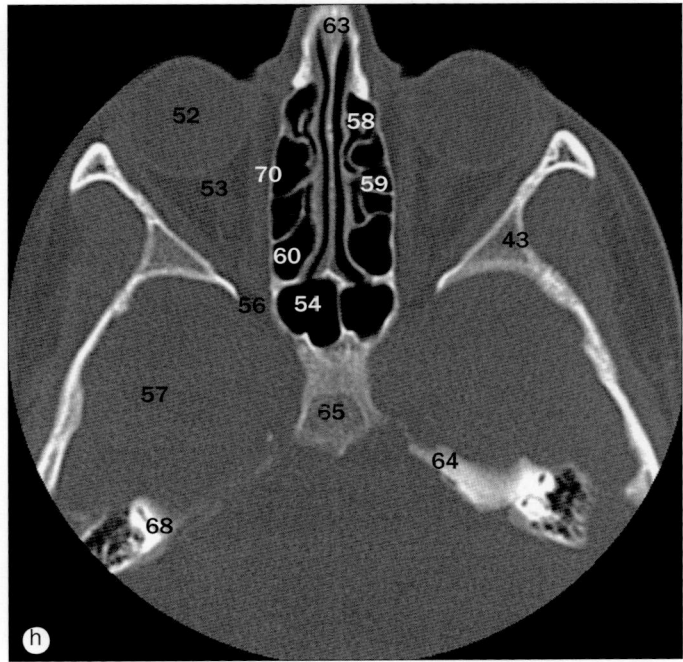

38 Superior turbinate
39 Nasolacrimal duct
40 Zygomatic arch
41 Clivus
42 Foramen spinosum
43 Greater wing of sphenoid
44 Cavernous internal carotid artery
45 Horizontal petrous internal carotid artery canal
46 Vertical petrous internal carotid artery canal
47 Pterygopalatine fossa

48 Foramen rotundum
49 Vidian canal
50 Middle ear cavity
51 Eustachian tube
52 Globe of eye
53 Optic nerve
54 Sphenoid sinus (antrum)
55 Inferior orbital fissure
56 Superior orbital fissure
57 Temporal lobe
58 Anterior ethmoidal air cells
59 Middle ethmoidal air cells

60 Posterior ethmoidal air cells
61 Internal auditory canal
62 External auditory canal
63 Nasal bone
64 Petrous apex
65 Floor of sella
66 Foramen lacerum
67 Ossicles of middle ear (incus and malleus)
68 Semicircular canals of inner ear
69 Cochlea of inner ear
70 Lamina papyracea

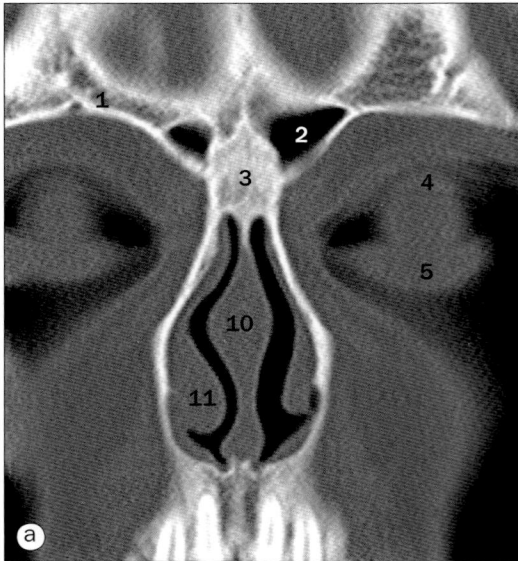

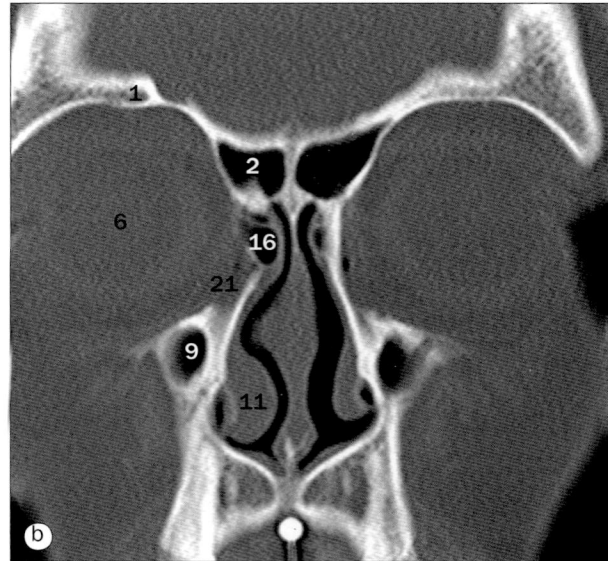

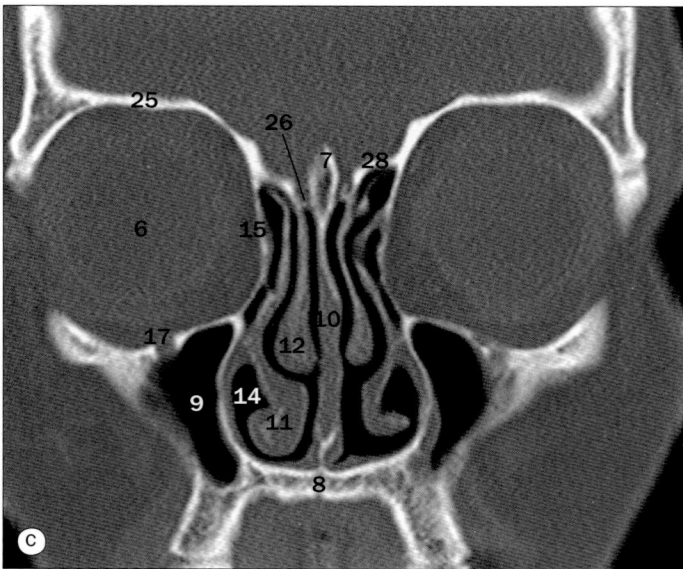

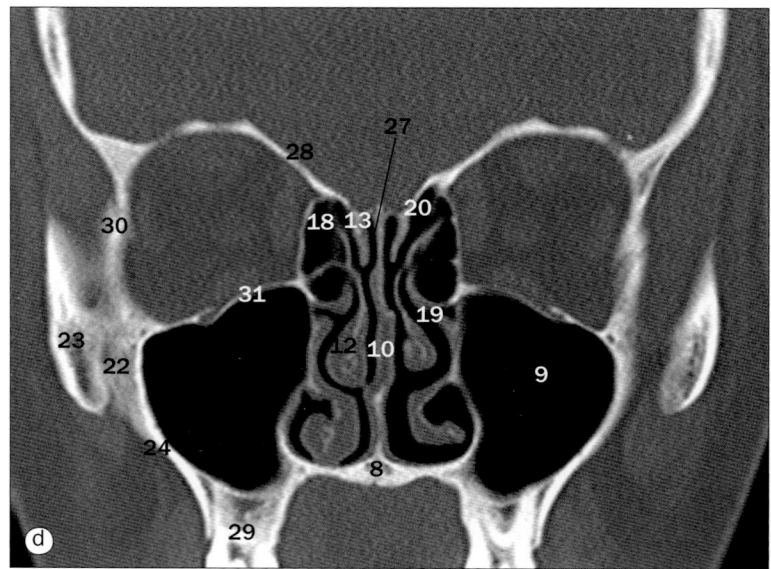

Paranasal sinuses, coronal CT images demonstrated at the following levels: (a) frontal sinuses, (b) nasolacrimal duct, (c) cribriform plate, (d) anterior ethmoids, (e) middle ethmoids, (f) pterygopalatine fossa, (g) sphenoid sinus, (h) nasopharynx.

1 Frontal bone	**11** Inferior turbinate (concha)
2 Frontal sinus (antrum)	**12** Middle turbinate (concha)
3 Nasal bone	**13** Superior turbinate (concha)
4 Upper eyelid	**14** Inferior meatus
5 Lower eyelid	**15** Lamina papyracea
6 Globe of eye	**16** Air in nasolacrimal sac
7 Crista galli	**17** Inferior orbital canal
8 Hard palate	**18** Anterior ethmoid air cells
9 Maxillary sinus (antrum)	**19** Middle meatus
10 Nasal septum	**20** Superior meatus

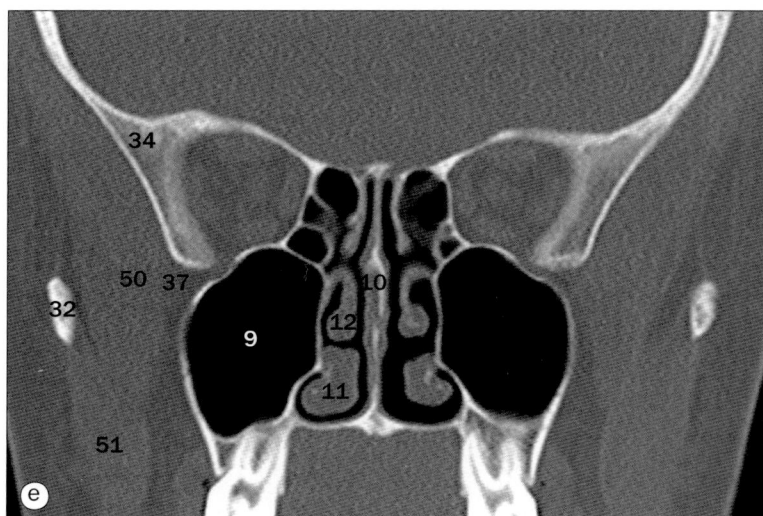

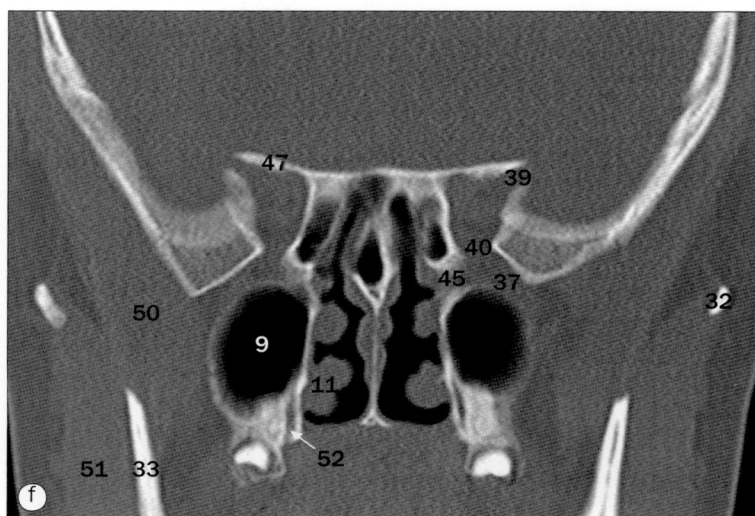

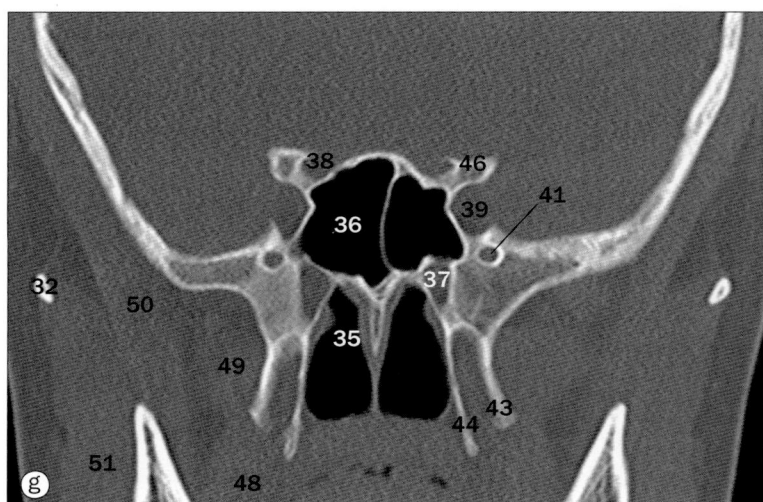

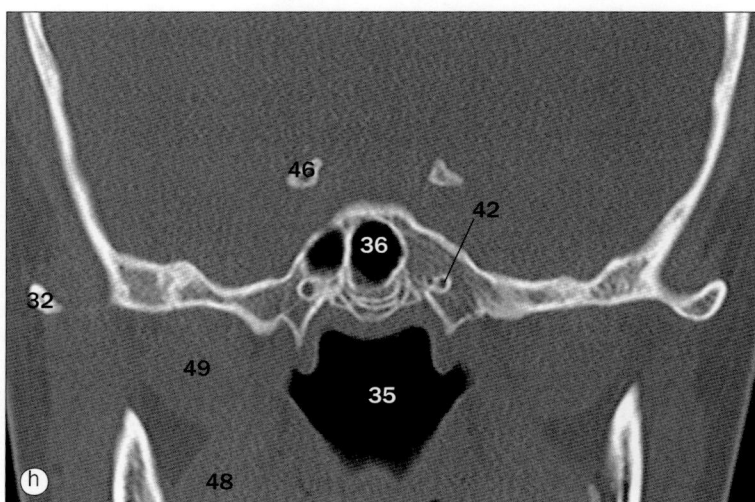

Paranasal sinuses, coronal CT images demonstrated at the following levels: (a) frontal sinuses, (b) nasolacrimal duct, (c) cribriform plate, (d) anterior ethmoids, (e) middle ethmoids, (f) pterygopalatine fossa, (g) sphenoid sinus, (h) nasopharynx.

21 Nasolacrimal duct	32 Zygomatic arch	43 Lateral pterygoid plate
22 Maxilla	33 Ramus of mandible	44 Medial pterygoid plate
23 Zygoma	34 Greater wing of sphenoid	45 Sphenopalatine foramen
24 Lateral wall of maxillary sinus	35 Nasopharynx	46 Anterior clinoid process
25 Orbital roof, frontal bone	36 Sphenoid sinus (antrum)	47 Lesser wing of sphenoid
26 Cribriform plate, ethmoid bone	37 Pterygopalatine fossa	48 Medial pterygoid muscle
27 Perpendicular plate, ethmoid bone	38 Optic canal	49 Lateral pterygoid muscle
28 Fovea ethmoidalis, frontal bone	39 Superior orbital fissure	50 Temporalis muscle
29 Upper alveolar ridge of maxilla	40 Inferior orbital fissure	51 Masseter muscle
30 Lateral orbital wall, zygomatic bone	41 Foramen rotundum	52 Greater palatine foramen
31 Orbital floor, maxillary bone	42 Vidian canal	

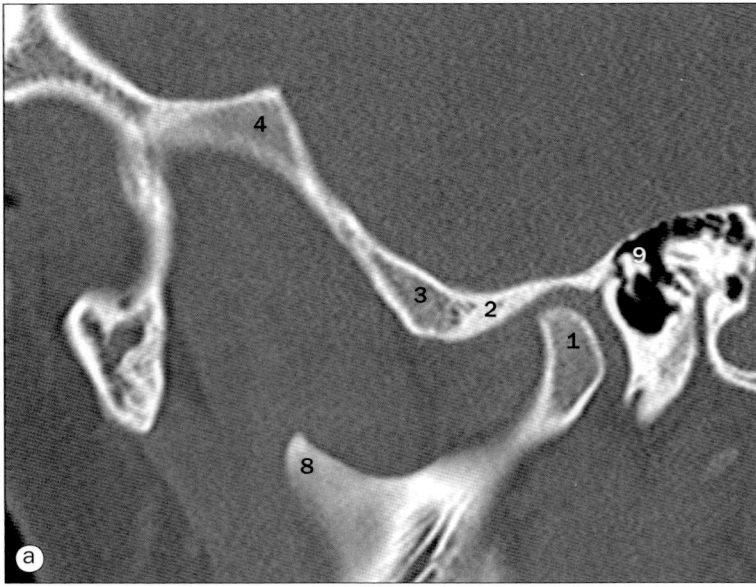

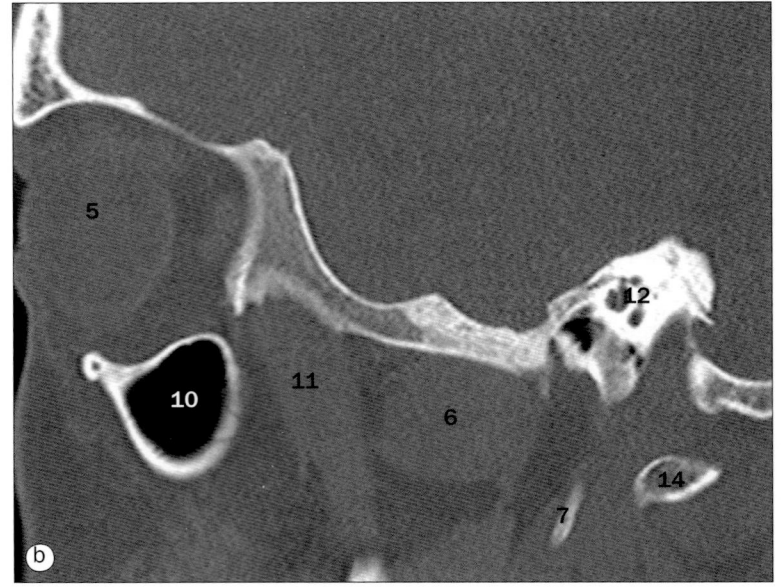

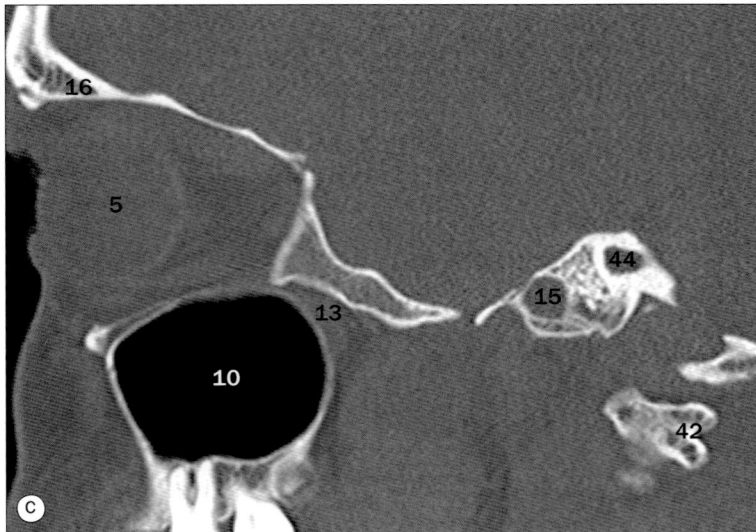

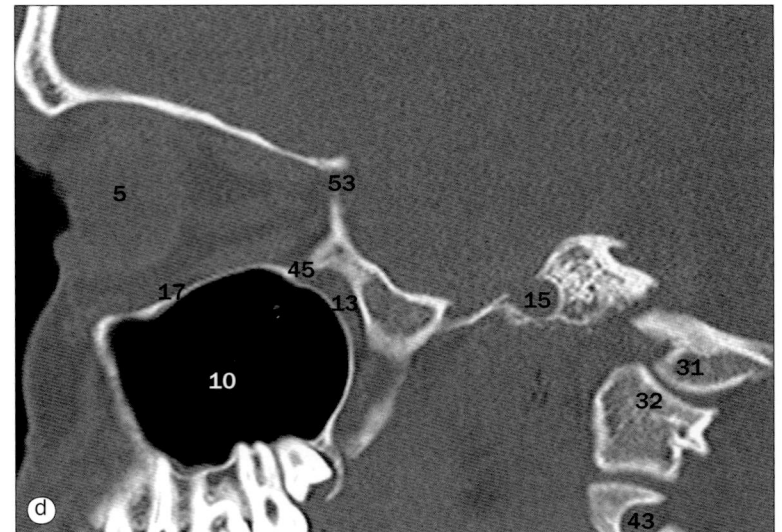

(a)–(h) Paranasal sinuses, sagittal CT images, from lateral to midline.

1	Condyle of mandible	**15**	Horizontal petrous internal carotid artery canal
2	Articular eminence	**16**	Frontal bone, orbital roof
3	Zygomatic arch	**17**	Maxillary bone, orbital floor
4	Zygoma	**18**	Hard palate
5	Globe of eye	**19**	Soft palate
6	Lateral pterygoid muscle	**20**	Tongue
7	Styloid process	**21**	Oropharynx
8	Coronoid process of mandible	**22**	Nasopharynx
9	Middle ear	**23**	Sphenoid sinus (antrum)
10	Maxillary sinus (antrum)	**24**	Frontal sinus (antrum)
11	Masseter muscle	**25**	Posterior ethmoid air cells
12	Inner ear	**26**	Anterior ethmoid air cells
13	Pterygopalatine fossa	**27**	Greater palatine foramen
14	Transverse process of C1	**28**	Inferior turbinate (concha)

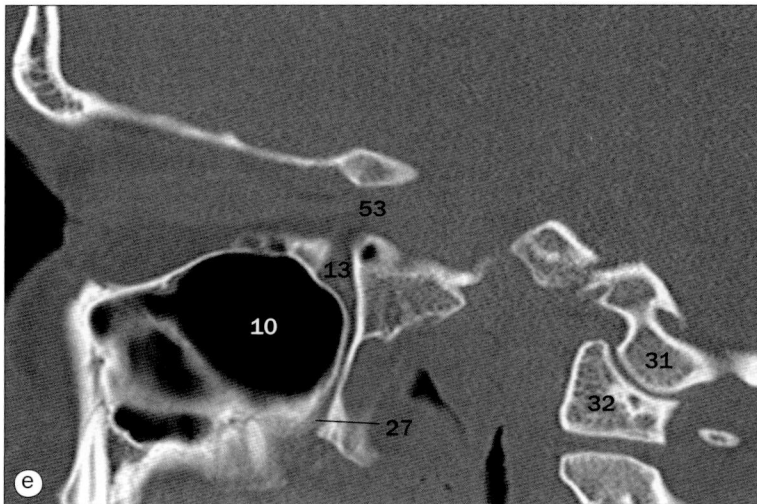

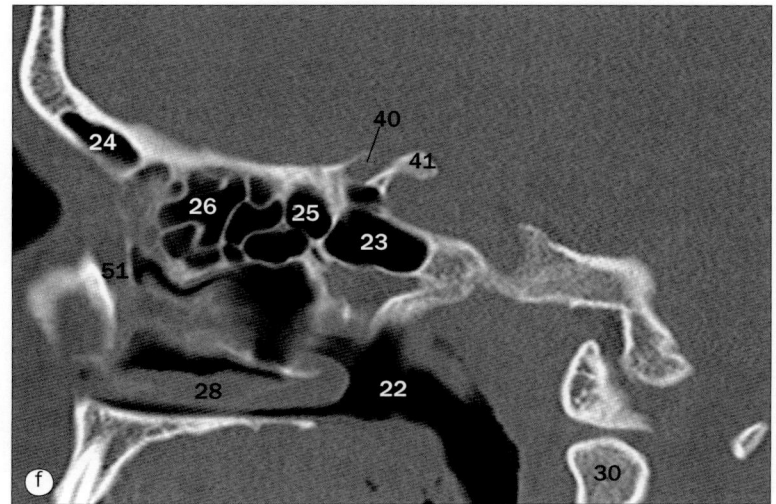

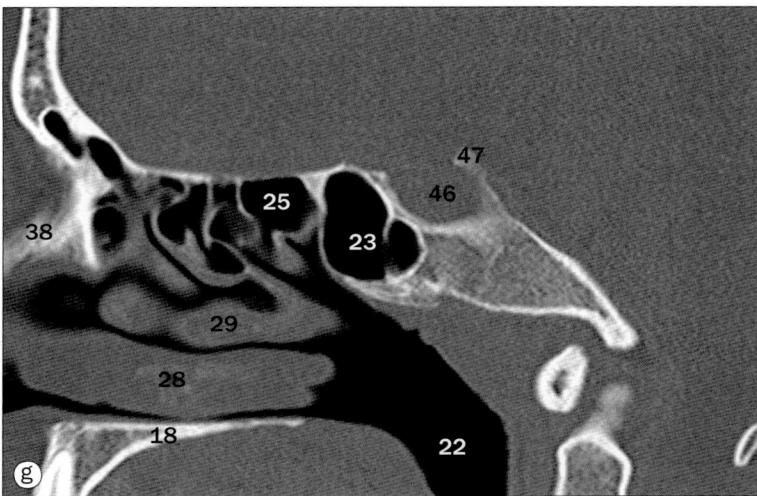

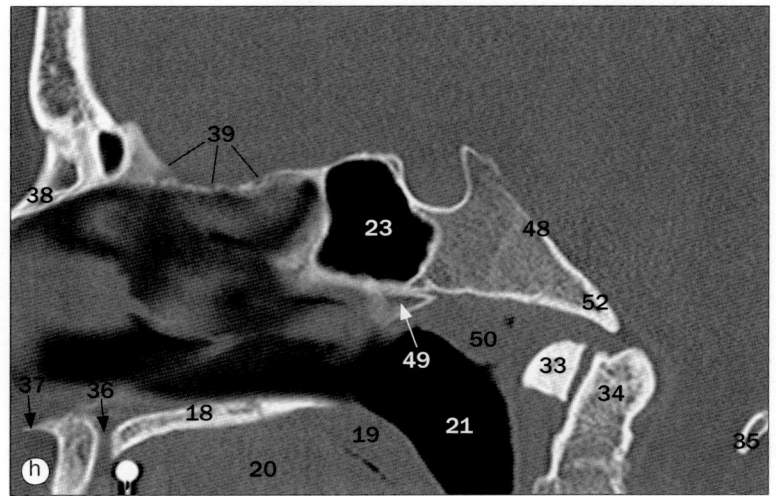

(a)–(h) Paranasal sinuses, sagittal CT images, from lateral to midline.

29 Middle turbinate (concha)
30 Base of C2
31 Occipital condyle
32 Lateral mass of C1
33 Anterior arch of C1
34 Dens (odontoid process)
35 Posterior arch of C1
36 Incisive foramen (contains nasopalatine nerve – V2 sensory branch)
37 Anterior nasal spine of maxillae
38 Nasal bone
39 Cribriform plate
40 Optic canal

41 Anterior clinoid
42 Tubercles of transverse process of C1
43 Transverse foramen of C2
44 Internal auditory canal
45 Inferior orbital fissure
46 Hypophyseal fossa
47 Dorsum sellae
48 Clivus
49 Vomer
50 Pharyngeal tonsil
51 Nasolacrimal duct
52 Basion
53 Superior orbital fissure

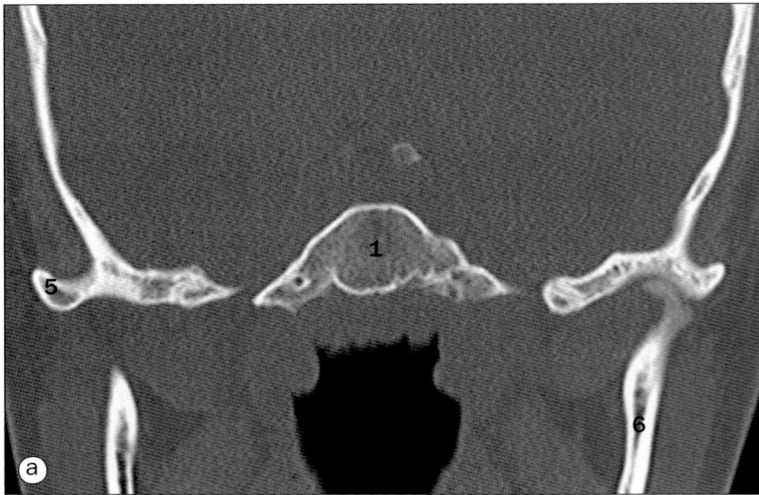

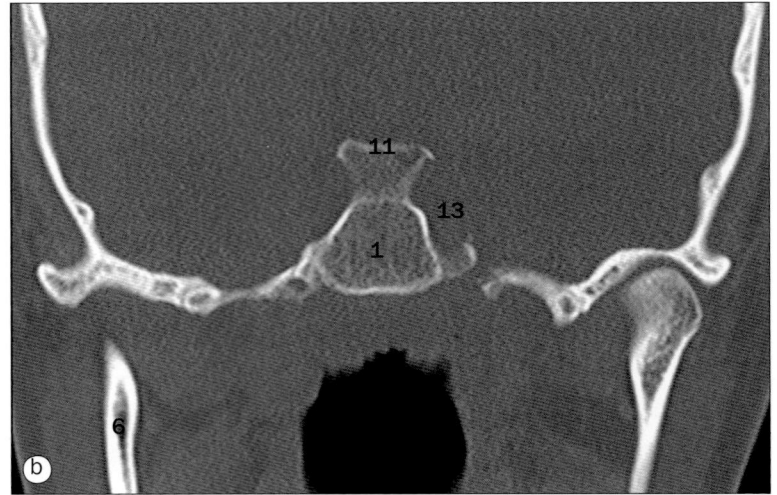

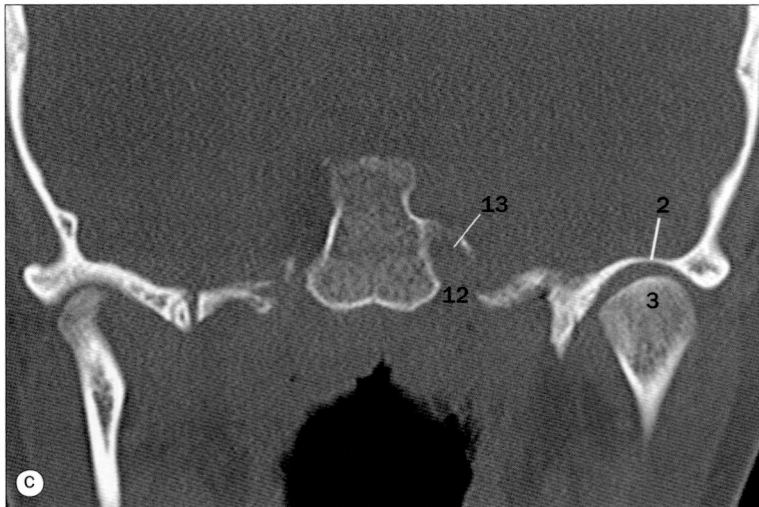

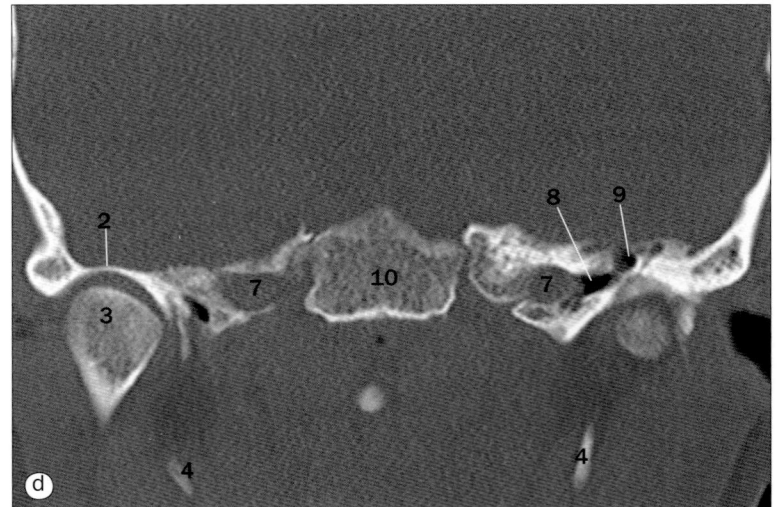

(a)–(h) Coronal CT images, from anterior to posterior.

1 Sphenoid body	9 Epitympanum
2 Condylar fossa of temporomandibular joint	10 Basi-occiput (lower clivus)
3 Mandibular condyle head	11 Dorsum sellae
4 Styloid process	12 Foramen lacerum
5 Zygomatic arch	13 Location of vertical portion of internal carotid artery
6 Mandibular ramus	14 Anterior arch of C1
7 Horizontal petrous internal carotid artery	15 Dens (odontoid process)
8 Hypotympanum	16 Body of C2

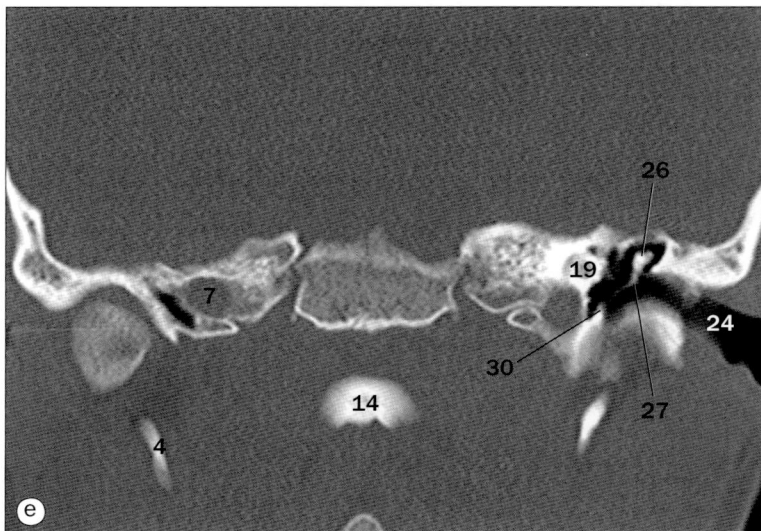

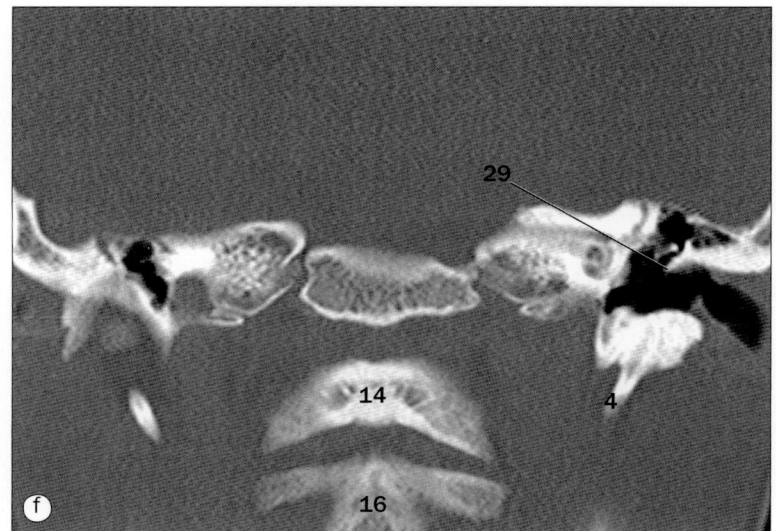

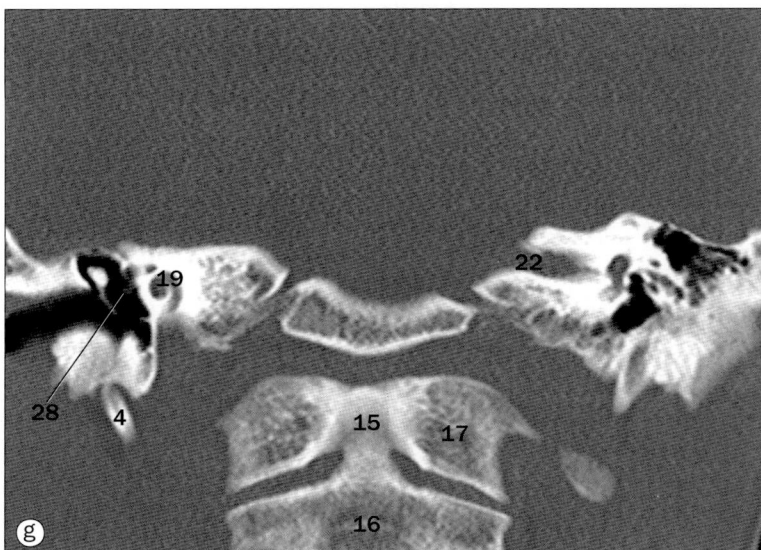

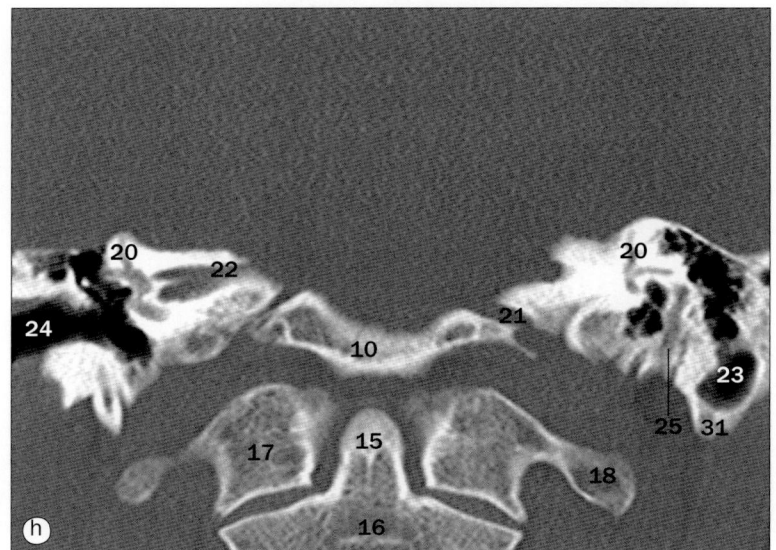

(a)–(h) Coronal CT images, from anterior to posterior.

17 Transverse process of C1
18 Lateral mass of C1
19 Cochlea
20 Semicircular canal
21 Jugular foramen
22 Internal acoustic canal
23 Mastoid air cells
24 External auditory canal

25 Stylomastoid foramen (location of mastoid segment of CN7)
26 Incus
27 Malleus
28 Tendon of tensor tympani muscle
29 Scutum
30 Tympanic annulus
31 Mastoid tip

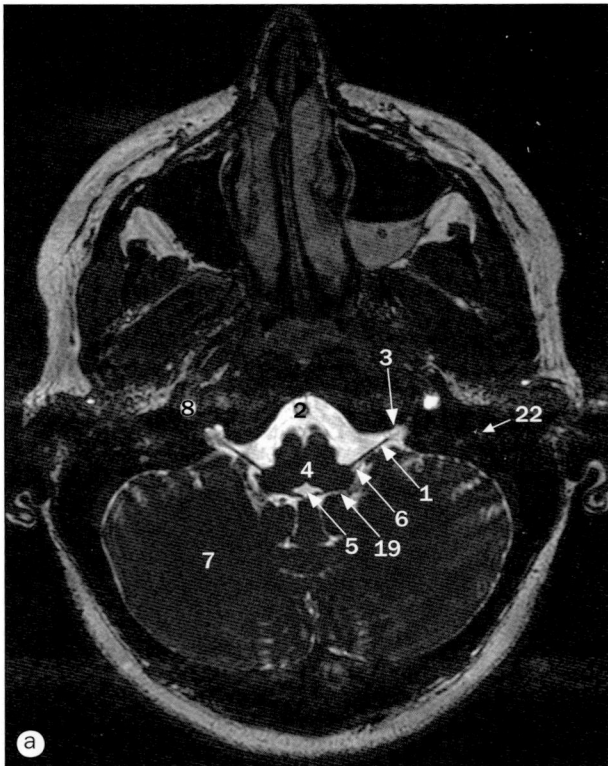

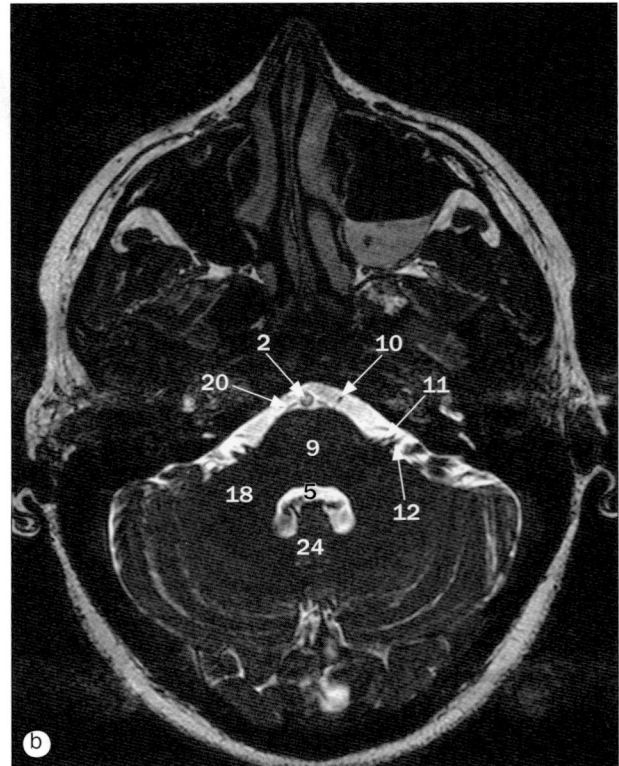

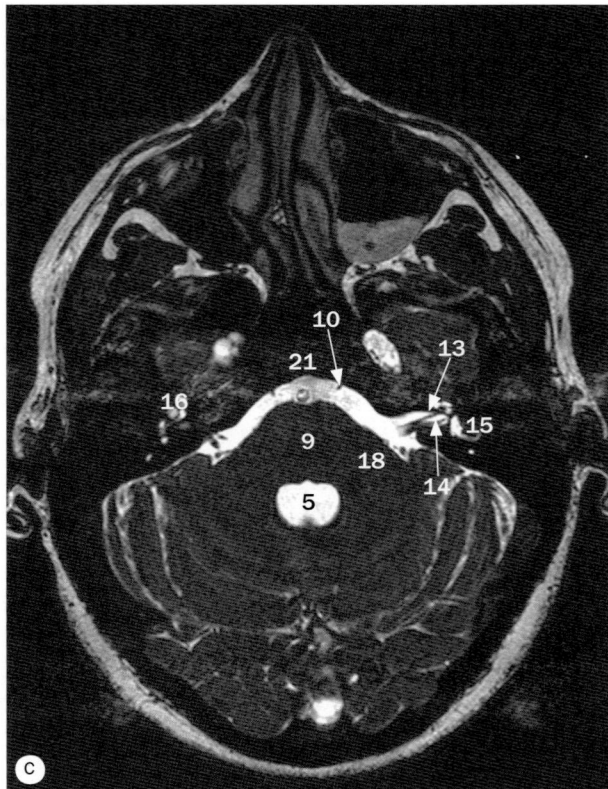

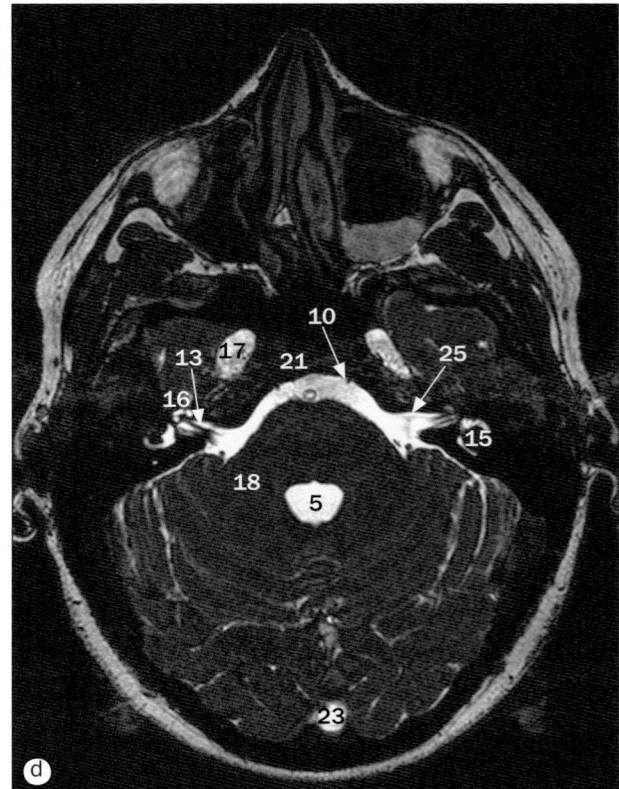

(a)–(h) Axial MR images, from inferior to superior.

1 Glossopharyngeal nerve (CN9)	5 Fourth ventricle	9 Pons
2 Basilar artery	6 Vagus nerve (CN10)	10 Abducens nerve (CN6)
3 Jugular foramen	7 Cerebellar hemisphere	11 Facial nerve (CN7)
4 Medulla	8 Internal carotid artery	12 Vestibulocochlear nerve (CN8)

The legends for pages 16–19 are common for all 4 pages.

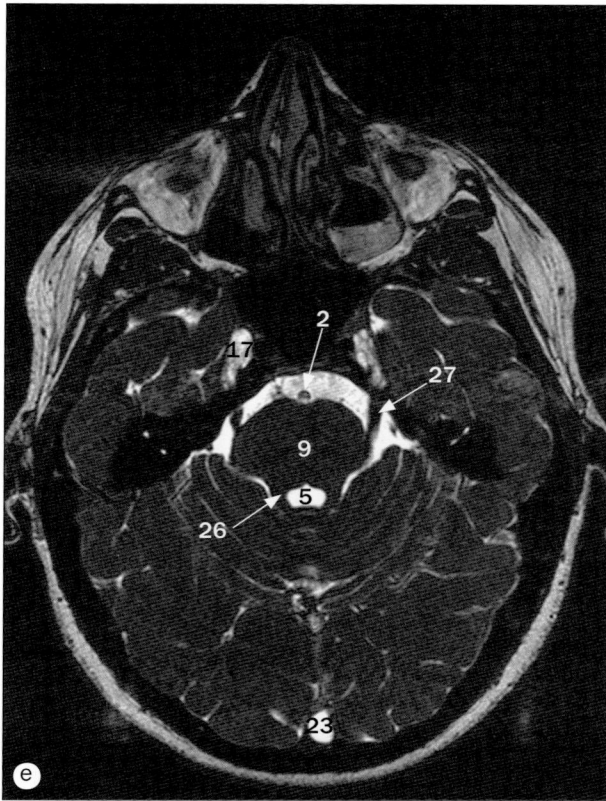

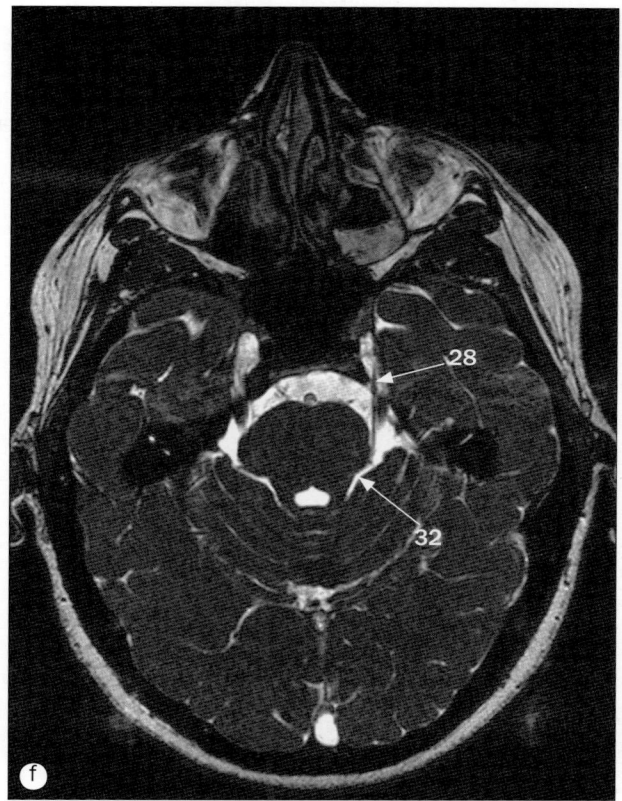

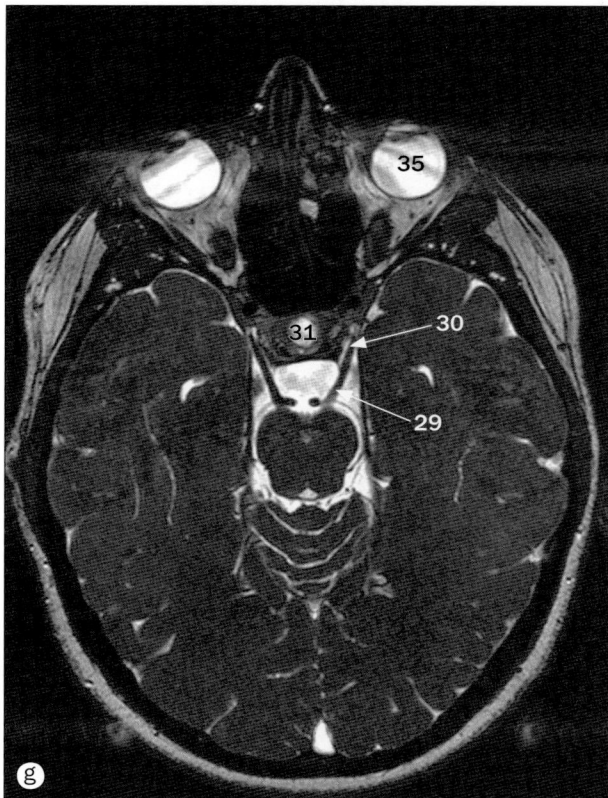

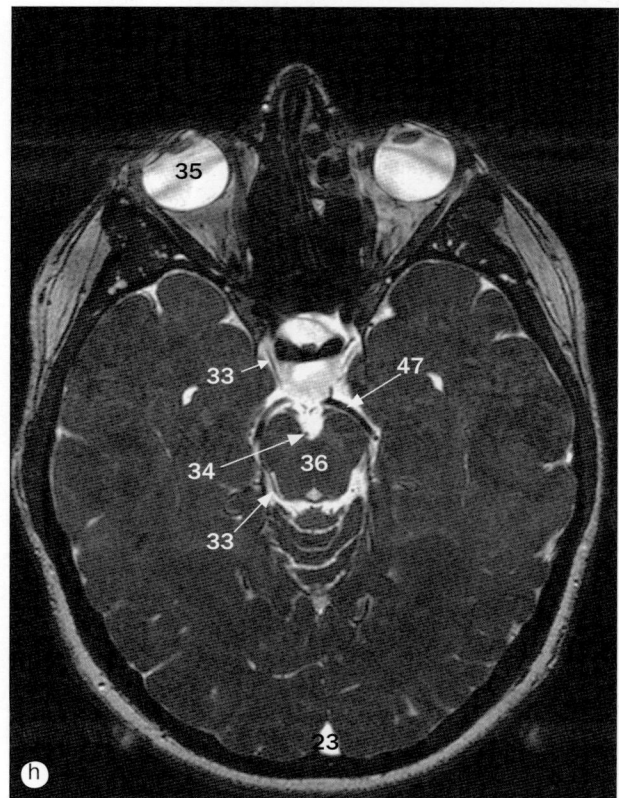

(a)–(h) Axial MR images, from inferior to superior.

13 Cochlear nerve	**17** Meckel's cave	**21** Clivus
14 Vestibular nerve	**18** Middle cerebellar peduncle	**22** Facial nerve in stylomastoid foramen
15 Semicircular canals	**19** Foramen of Luschka	**23** Superior sagittal sinus
16 Cochlea	**20** Anterior inferior cerebellar artery	**24** Vermis

The legends for pages 16–19 are common for all 4 pages.

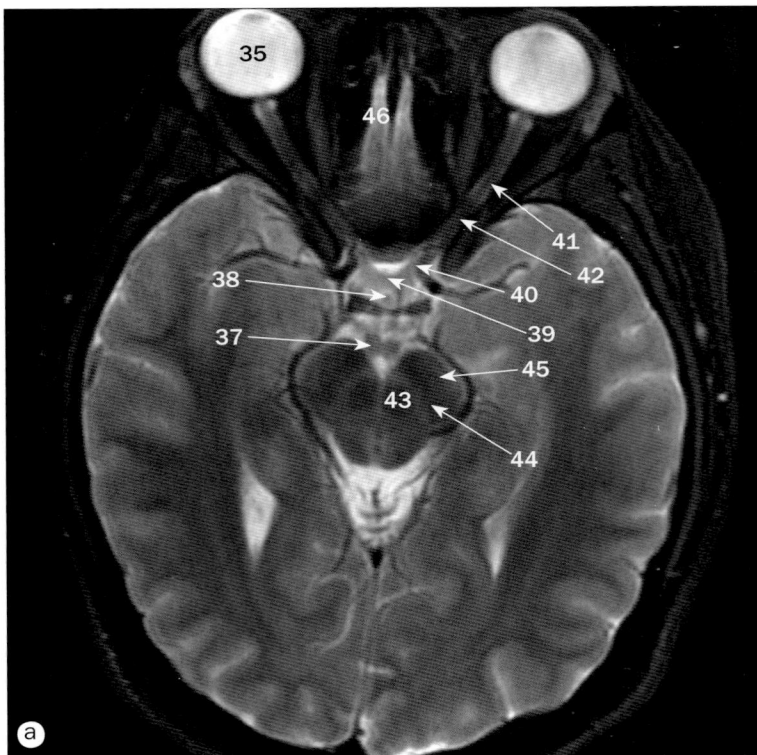

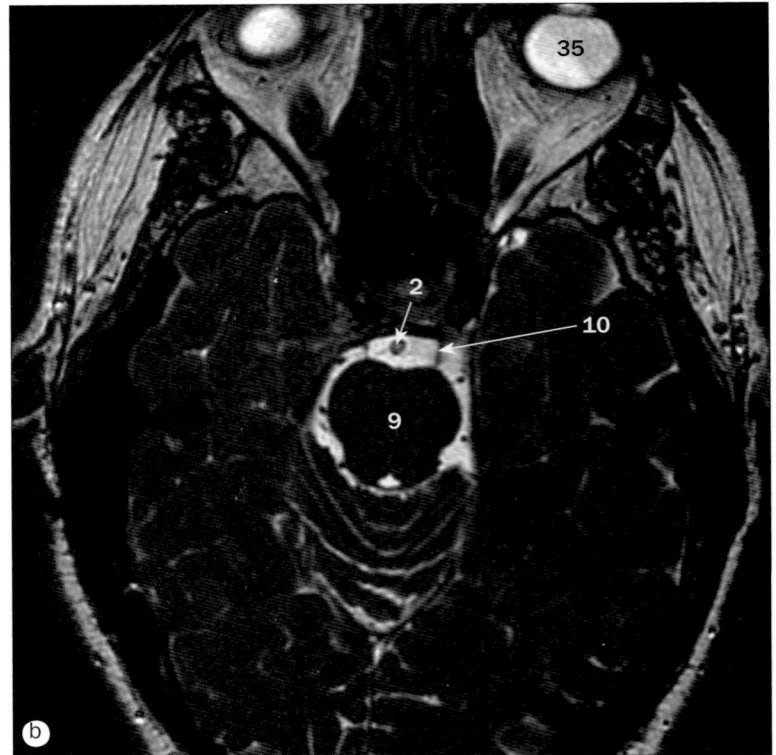

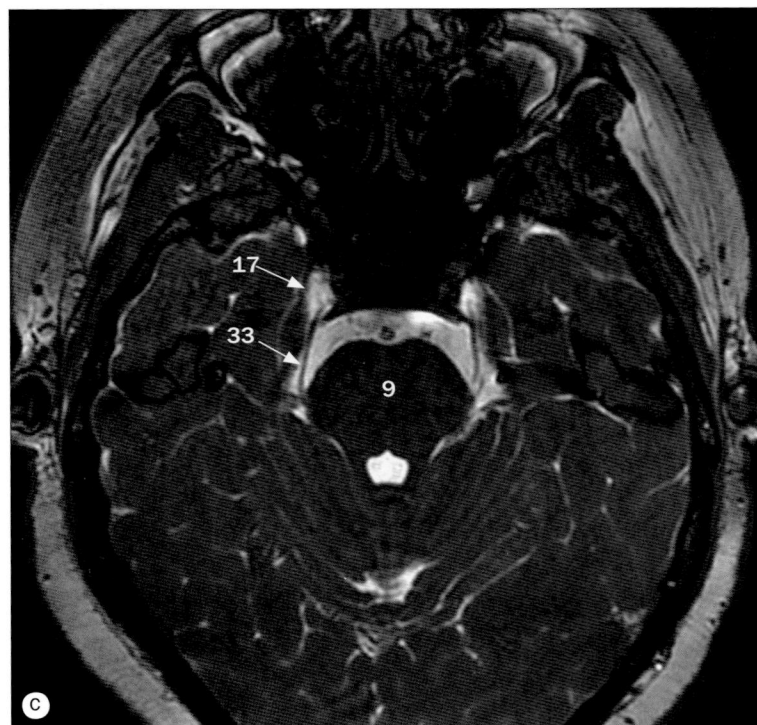

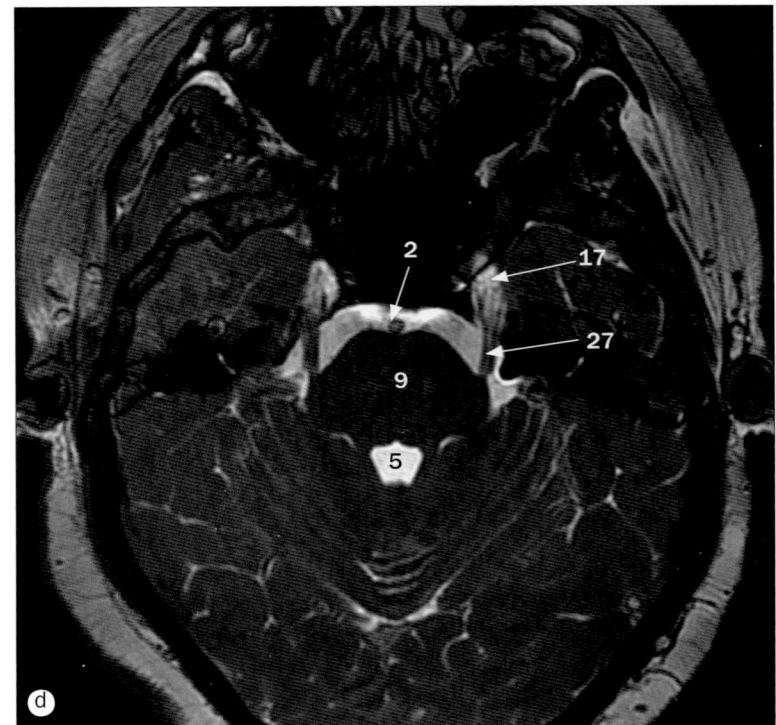

Cranial nerves, MR images of (a) olfactory and optic nerves, (b) oculomotor nerve, (c) trochlear nerve, (d) trigeminal nerve, (e) and (f) abducens, facial and auditory nerves, (g) glossopharyngeal nerve, (h) hypoglossal nerve.

25 Internal auditory canal	31 Pituitary
26 Superior cerebellar peduncle	32 Ambient cistern
27 Preganglionic segment of CN5 (trigeminal)	33 Trochlear nerve (CN4)
28 CN5 enters Meckel's cave	34 Interpenduncular cistern
29 Oculomotor nerve (CN3)	35 Globe of eye
30 CN3 in oculomotor cistern	36 Midbrain

The legends for pages 16–19 are common for all 4 pages.

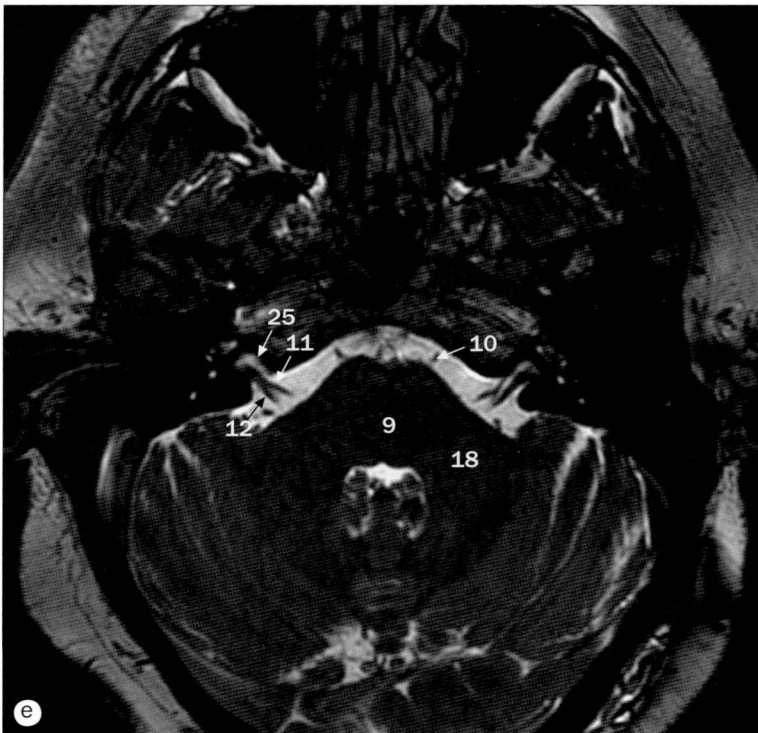

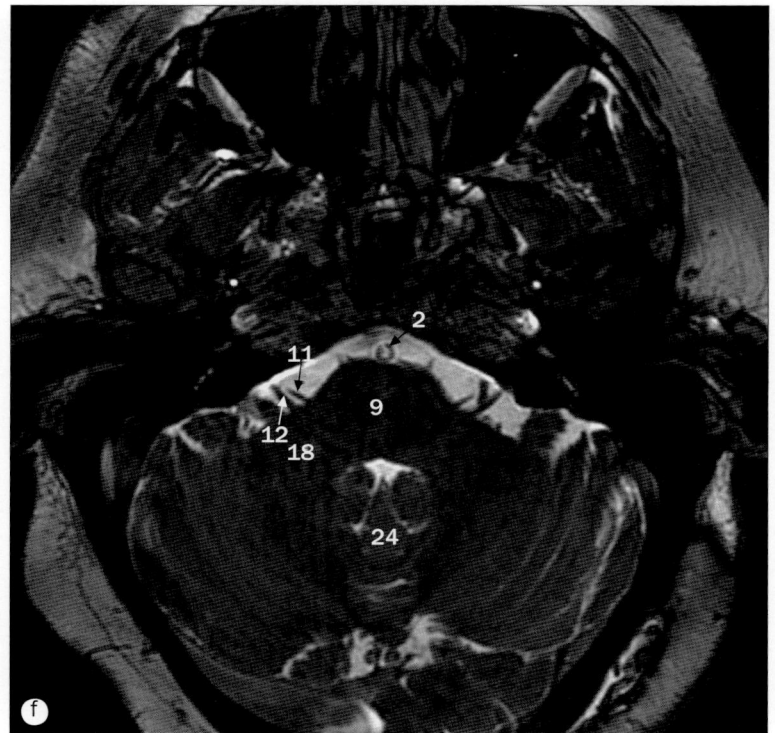

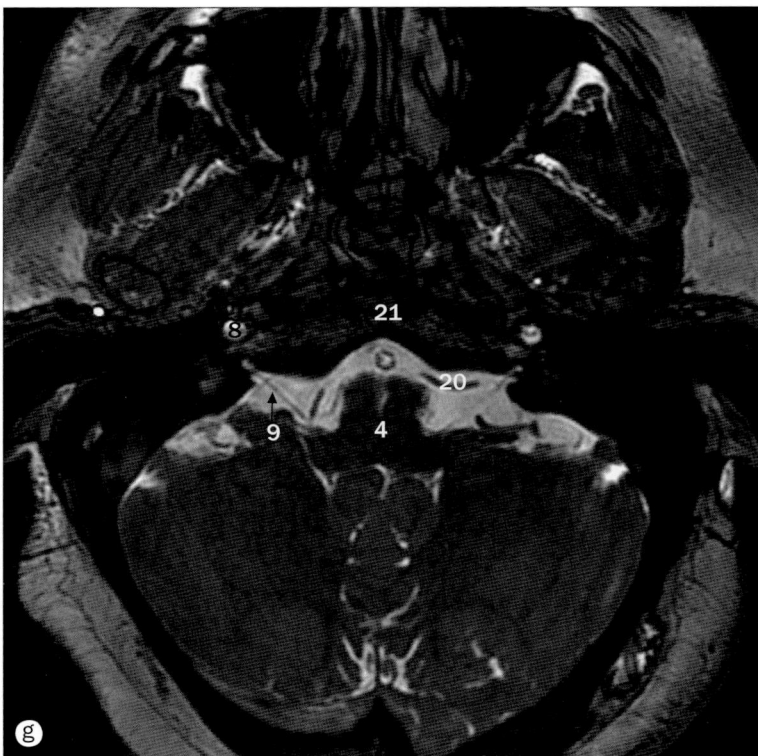

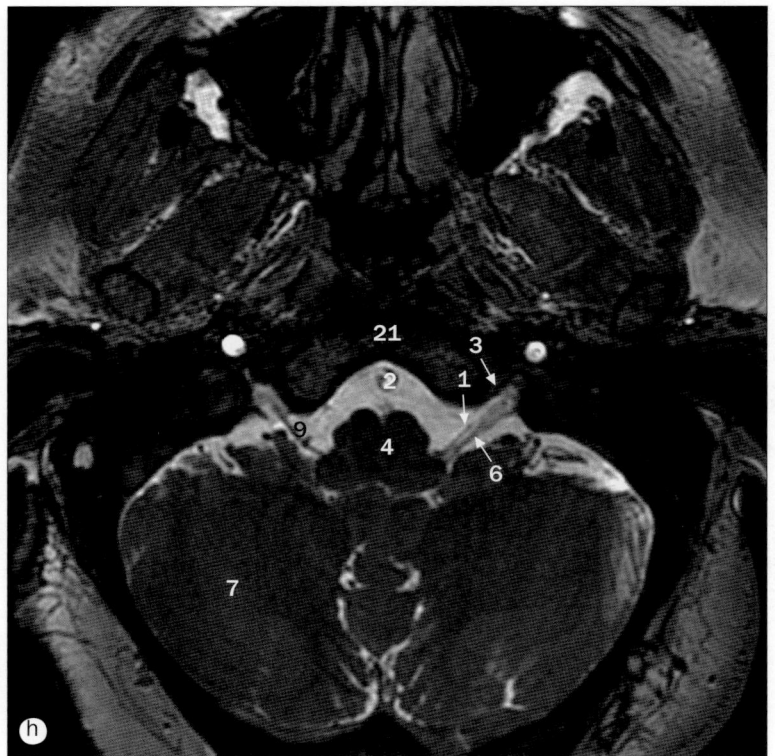

Cranial nerves, MR images of (a) olfactory and optic nerves, (b) oculomotor nerve, (c) trochlear nerve, (d) trigeminal nerve, (e) and (f) abducens, facial and auditory nerves, (g) glossopharyngeal nerve, (h) hypoglossal nerve.

37 Mammillary body
38 Infundibulum
39 Optic chiasm
40 Optic nerve, intracranial portion
41 Optic nerve, intra-ocular segment
42 Optic nerve, intracanalicular segment

43 Red nucleus of midbrain
44 Substantia nigra
45 Cerebral peduncle
46 Olfactory tract and bulb (CN1)
47 Posterior cerebral artery

The legends for pages 16–19 are common for all 4 pages.

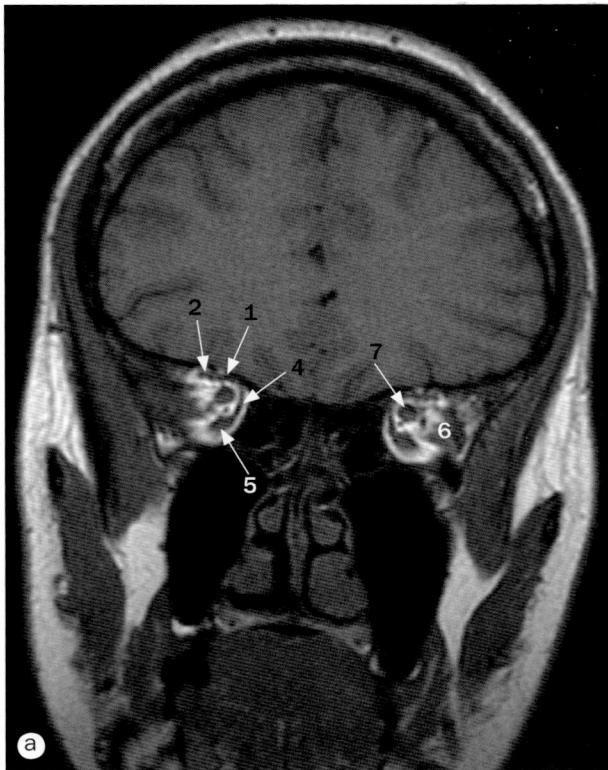

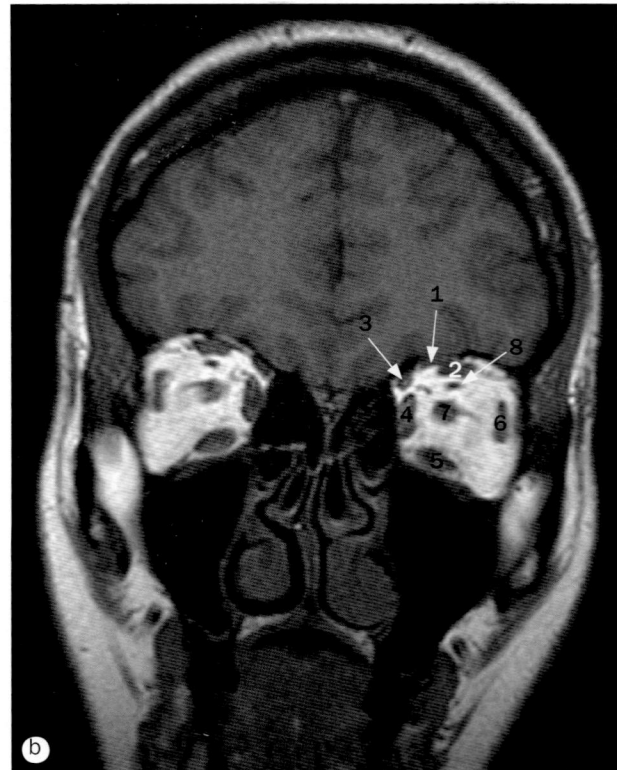

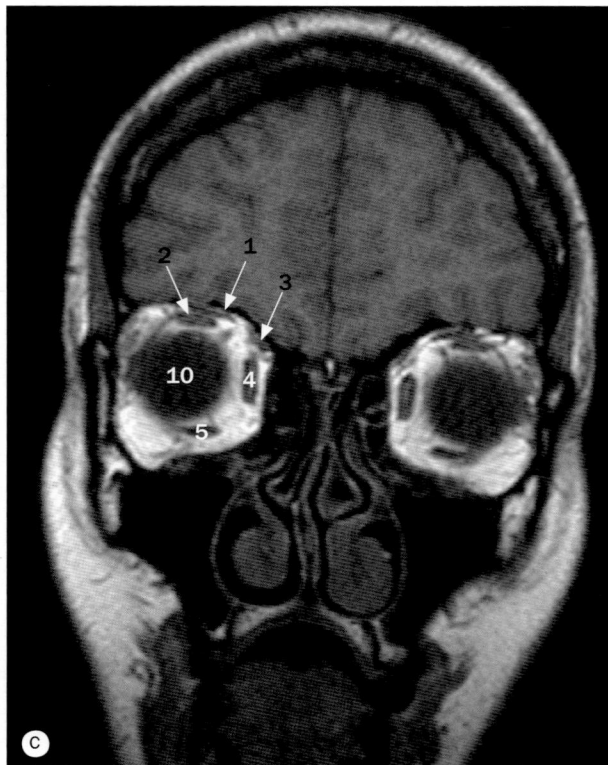

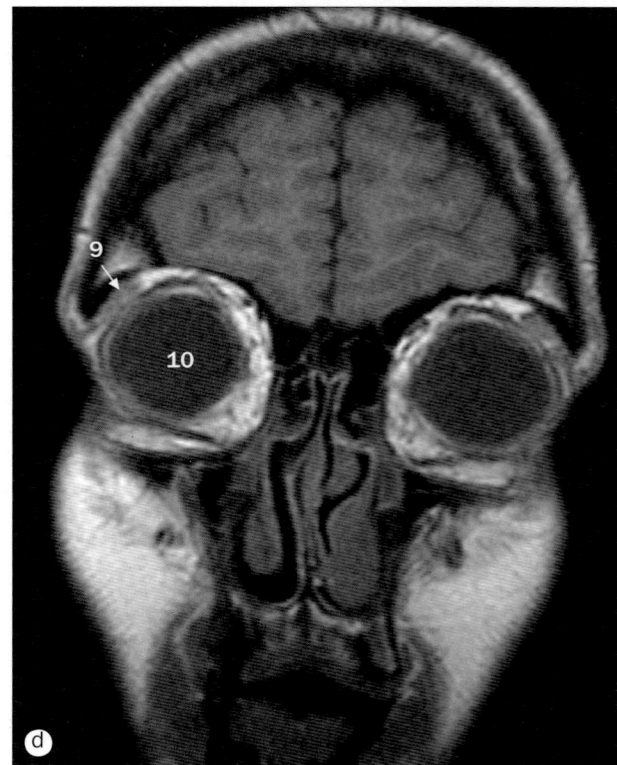

(a)–(d) Coronal MR images, from posterior to anterior.

1 Levator palpebrae superioris muscle	6 Lateral rectus muscle
2 Superior rectus muscle	7 Optic nerve/sheath complex
3 Superior oblique muscle	8 Superior ophthalmic vein
4 Medial rectus muscle	9 Lacrimal gland
5 Inferior rectus muscle	10 Globe of eye

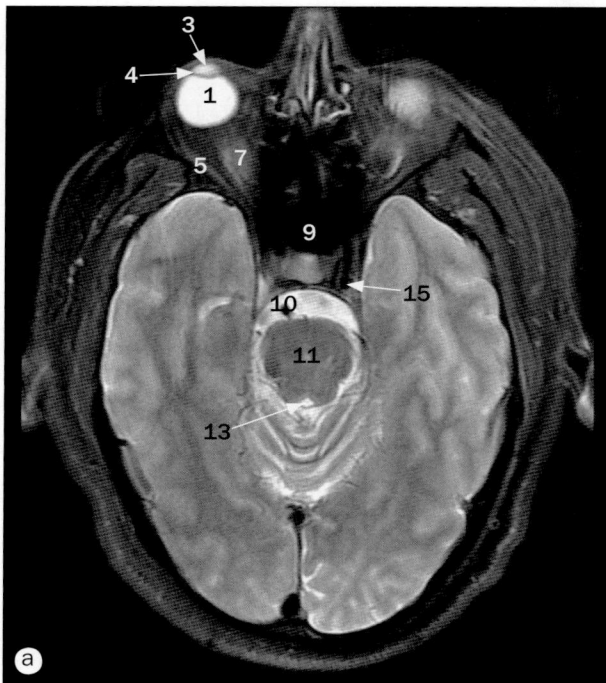

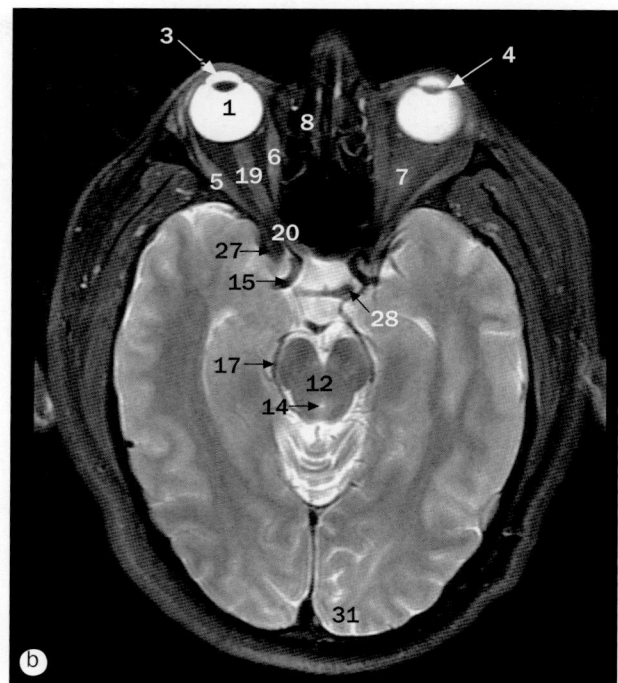

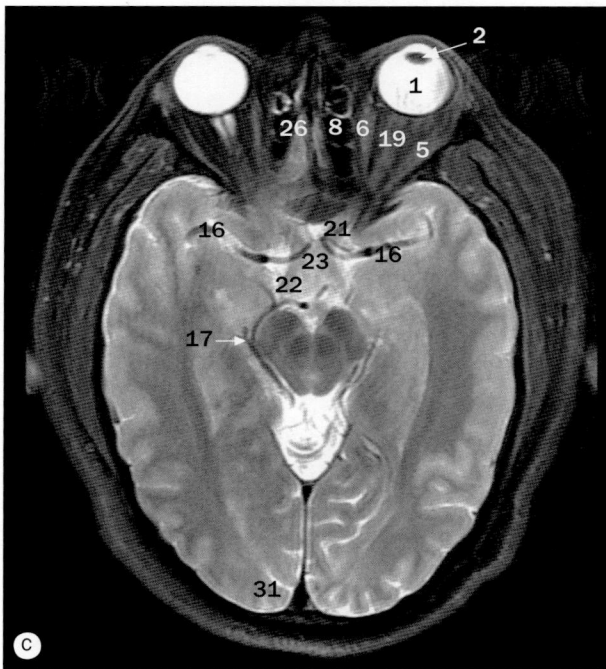

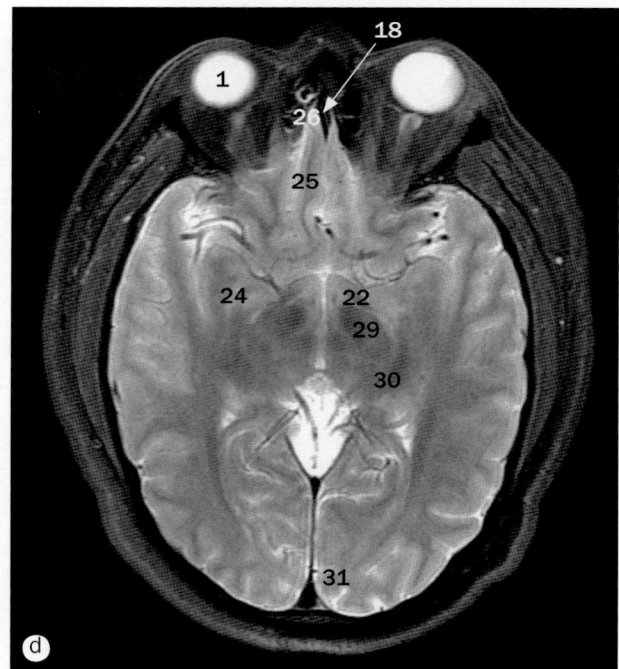

(a)–(d) Orbit, axial MR images, from inferior to superior.

1 Vitreous chamber of globe	12 Midbrain	23 Optic chiasm
2 Lens	13 Superior recess fourth ventricle	24 Anterior commissure
3 Anterior chamber of globe	14 Cerebral aqueduct	25 Gyrus rectus
4 Ciliary body	15 Internal carotid artery	26 Olfactory nerve (CN1)
5 Lateral rectus muscle	16 Middle cerebral artery	27 Anterior clinoid process
6 Medial rectus muscle	17 Posterior cerebral artery	28 Dorsum sellae
7 Superior rectus muscle	18 Crista galli	29 Cerebral peduncle
8 Ethmoid air cells	19 Optic nerve (intra-orbital segment)	30 Medial and lateral geniculate bodies
9 Sphenoid sinus (antrum)	20 Optic nerve (intracanalicular segment)	31 Visual (calcarine) cortex
10 Basilar artery	21 Optic nerve (intracranial segment)	
11 Pons	22 Optic tract	

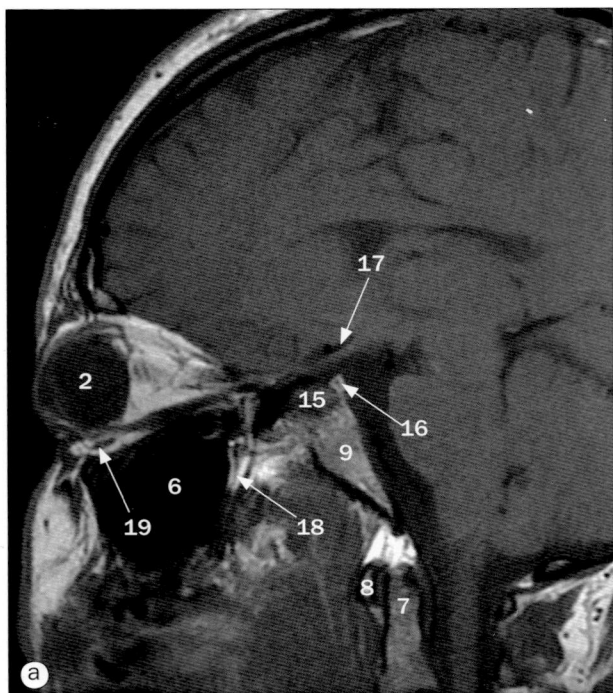

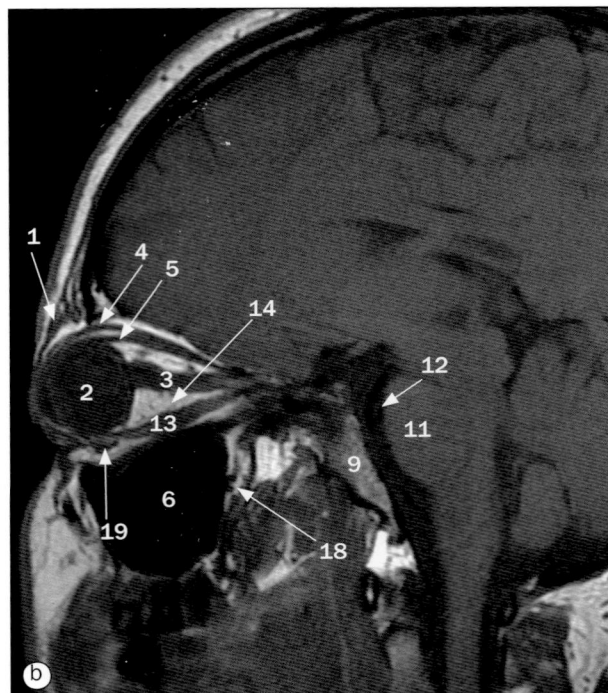

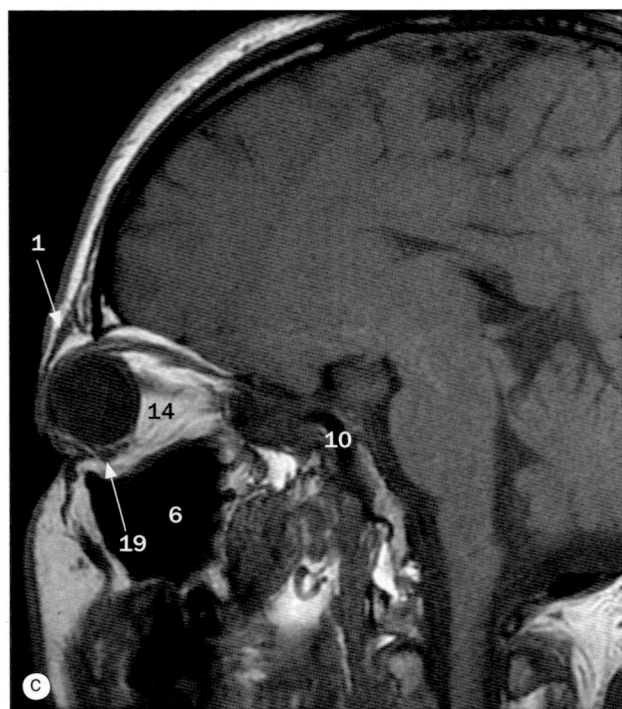

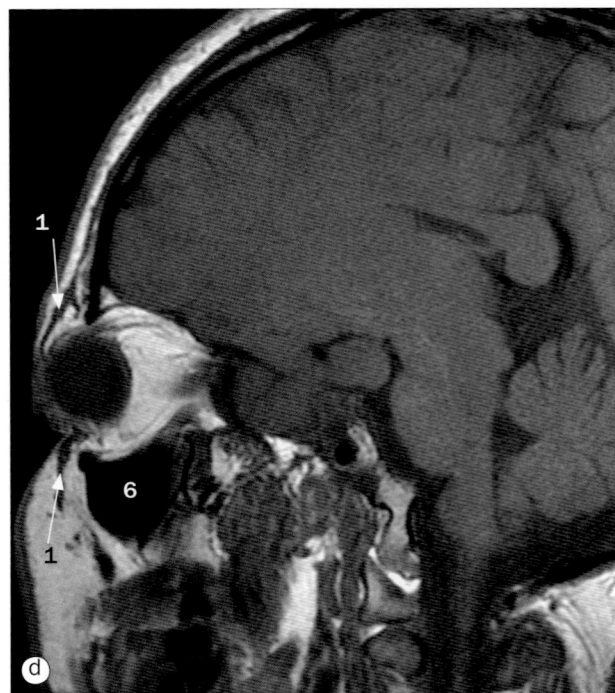

(a)–(d) Orbit, sagittal MR images, from medial to lateral.

1 Orbicularis oculi muscle
2 Globe
3 Optic nerve, intraocular segment
4 Levator palpebrae superioris
5 Superior rectus muscle
6 Maxillary sinus (antrum)
7 Dens (odontoid process)
8 Anterior arch of C1
9 Clivus
10 Internal carotid artery

11 Pons
12 Basilar artery
13 Inferior rectus muscle
14 Retrobulbar fat
15 Sella turcica/pituitary
16 Dorsum sellae
17 Optic nerve, intracranial segment
18 Pterygopalatine fossa
19 Inferior oblique muscle

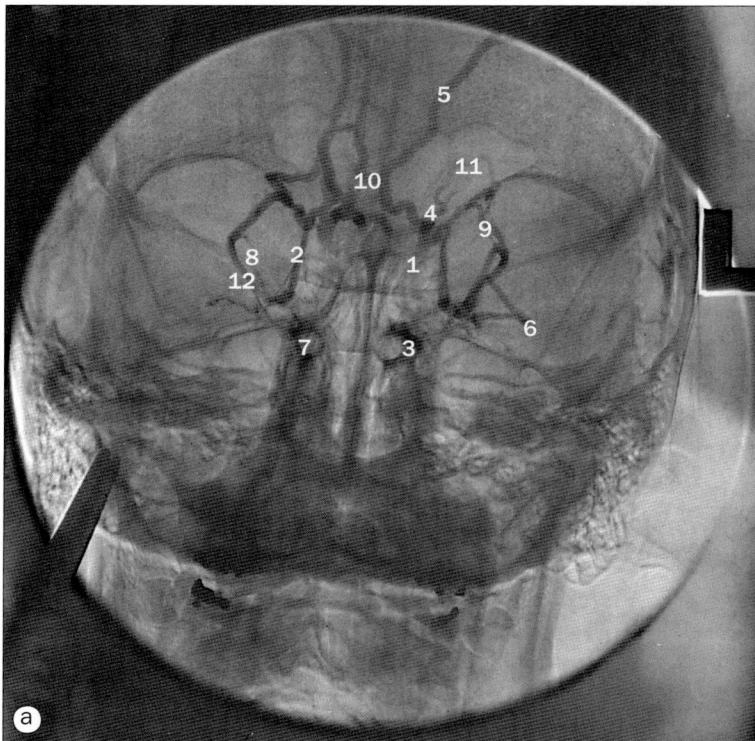

(a) Orbital venogram.

1 Angular veins
2 Anterior collateral vein
3 Cavernous sinus
4 First part of superior ophthalmic vein
5 Frontal veins
6 Inferior ophthalmic vein
7 Internal carotid artery
8 Medial collateral vein
9 Second part of superior ophthalmic vein
10 Superficial connecting vein
11 Supraorbital vein
12 Third part of superior ophthalmic vein

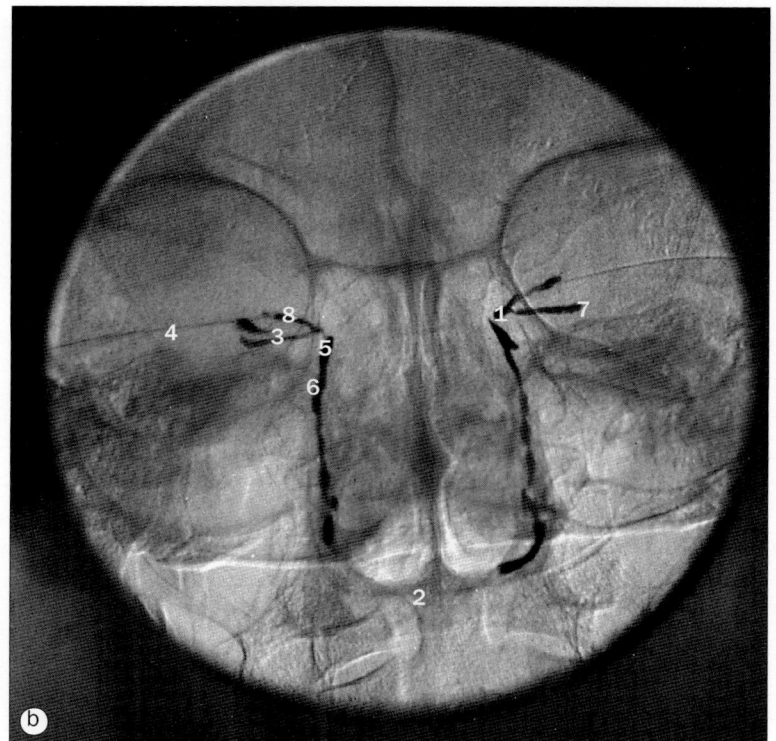

(b) Macrodacryocystogram.

1 Common canaliculus   5 Lacrimal sac
2 Hard palate   6 Nasolacrimal duct
3 Inferior canaliculus   7 Site of lacrimal punctum
4 Lacrimal catheters   8 Superior canaliculus

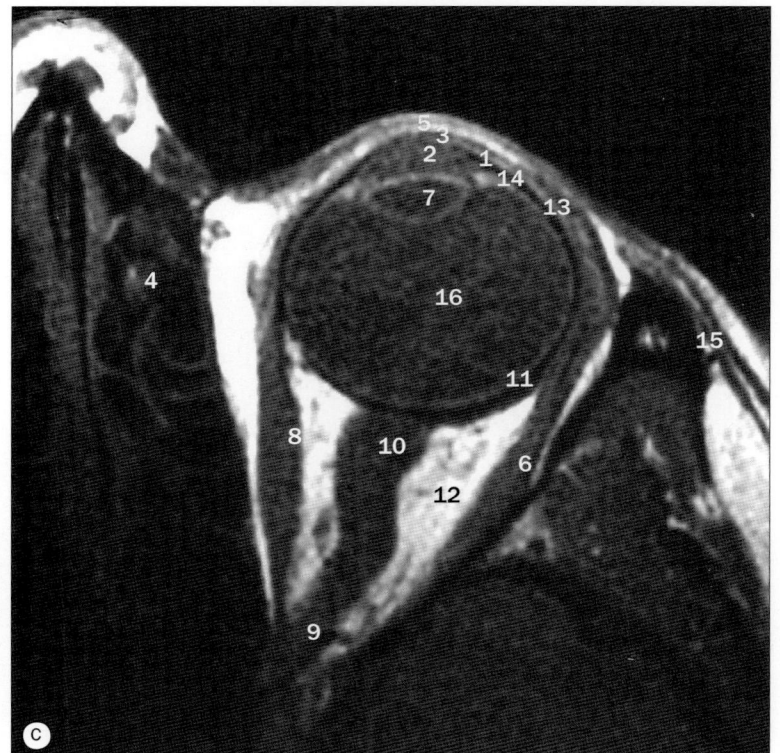

(c) Globe, axial MR image.

1 Anterior chamber   10 Optic nerve
2 Aqueous humour   11 Retina and choroid
3 Cornea   12 Retro-orbital fat
4 Ethmoidal sinuses   13 Sclera
5 Eyelid   14 Suspensory ligament of the
6 Lateral rectus muscle   lens
7 Lens   15 Temporalis muscle
8 Medial rectus muscle   16 Vitreous
9 Ophthalmic artery

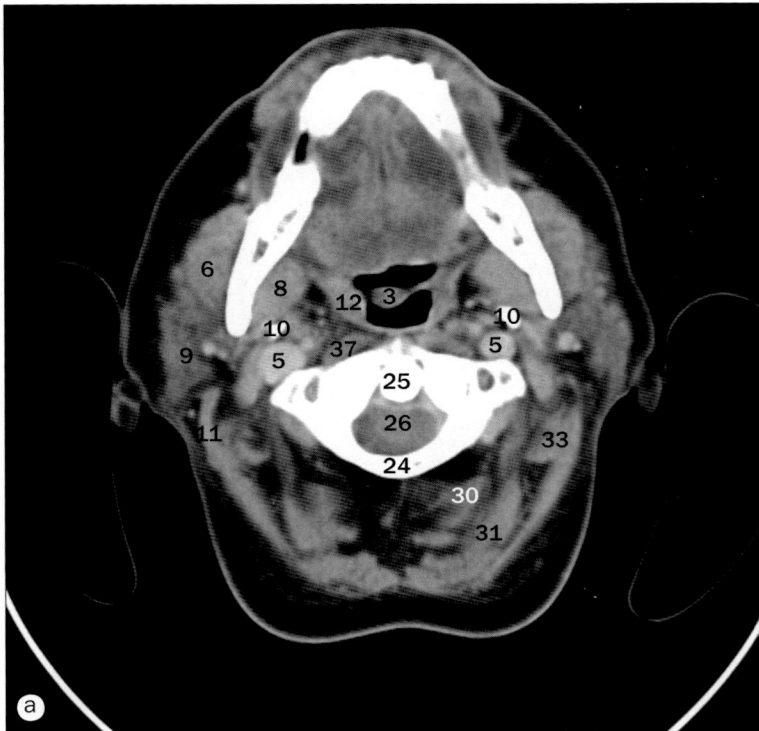

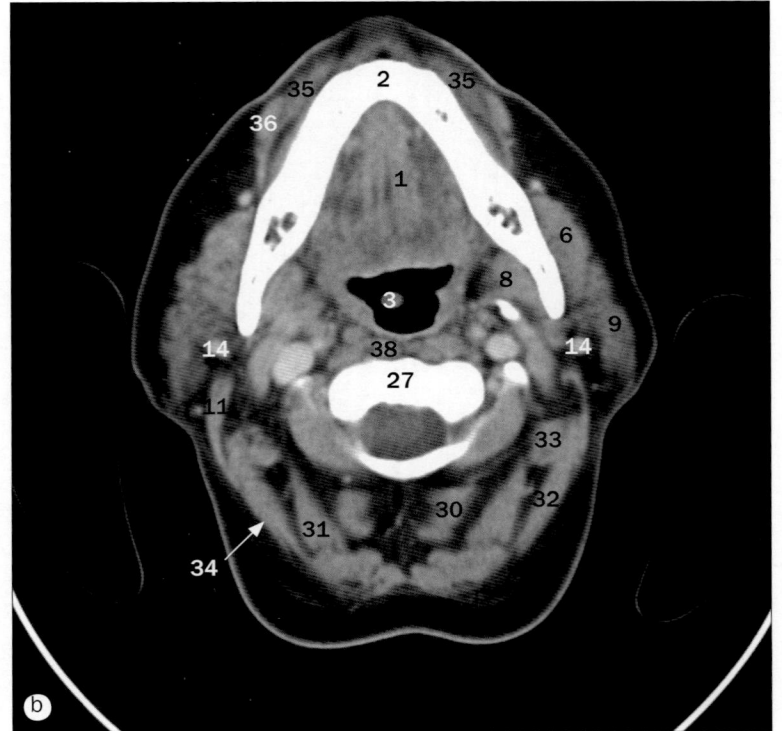

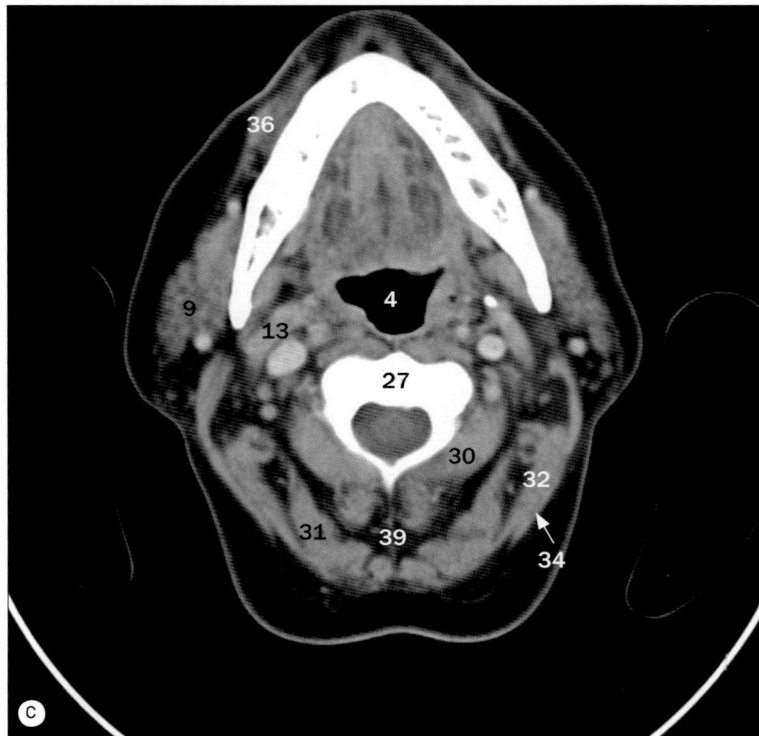

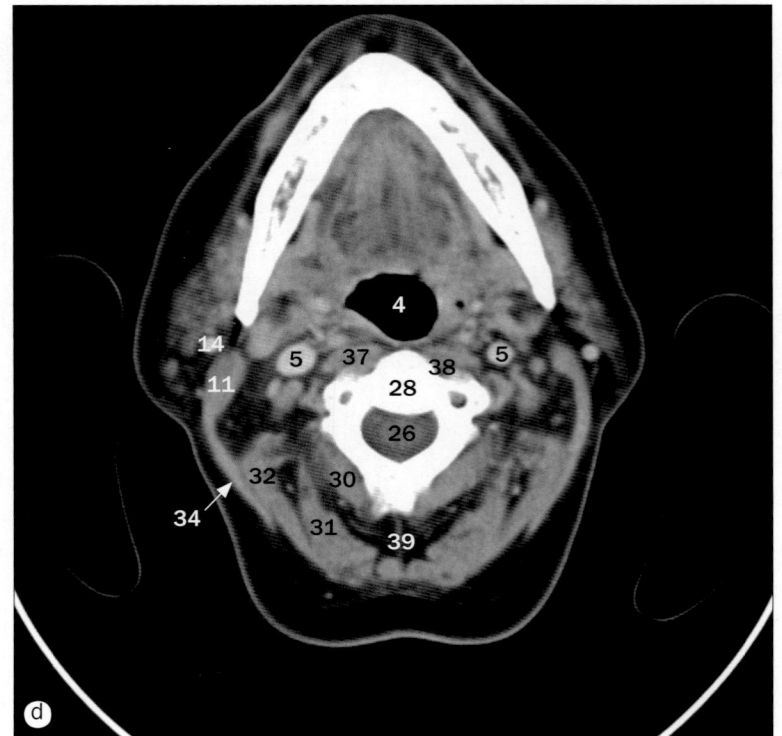

(a)–(h) Nasopharynx and oropharynx, axial CT images.

1 Genioglossus muscle	8 Medial pterygoid muscle	15 External jugular vein
2 Body of mandible	9 Parotid gland	16 Anterior belly of digastric muscle
3 Uvula	10 Styloid process	17 Epiglottis
4 Oropharynx	11 Sternocleidomastoid muscle	18 Vallecula
5 Internal jugular vein	12 Palatine tonsil	19 Hypopharynx
6 Masseter muscle	13 Posterior belly of digastric muscle	20 Mylohyoid muscle
7 Submandibular gland	14 Retromandioular vein	21 Platysma muscle

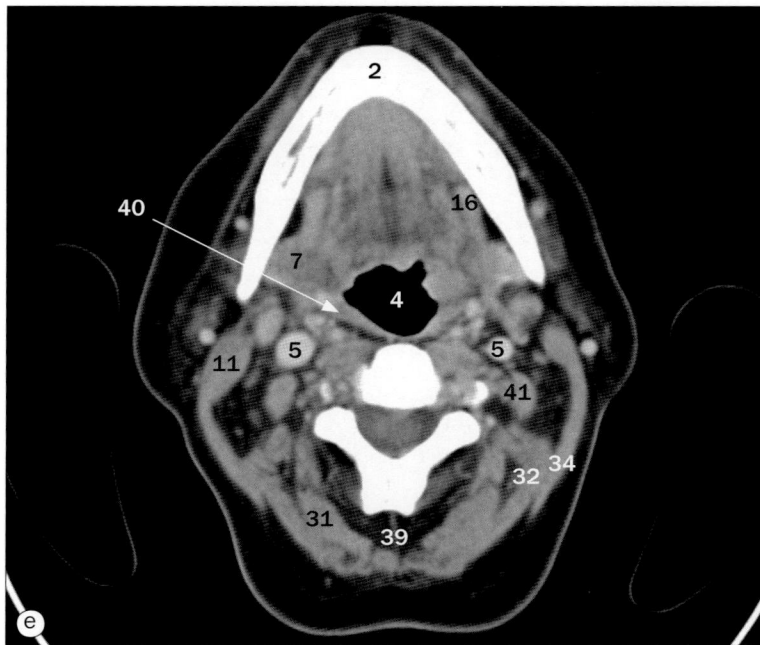

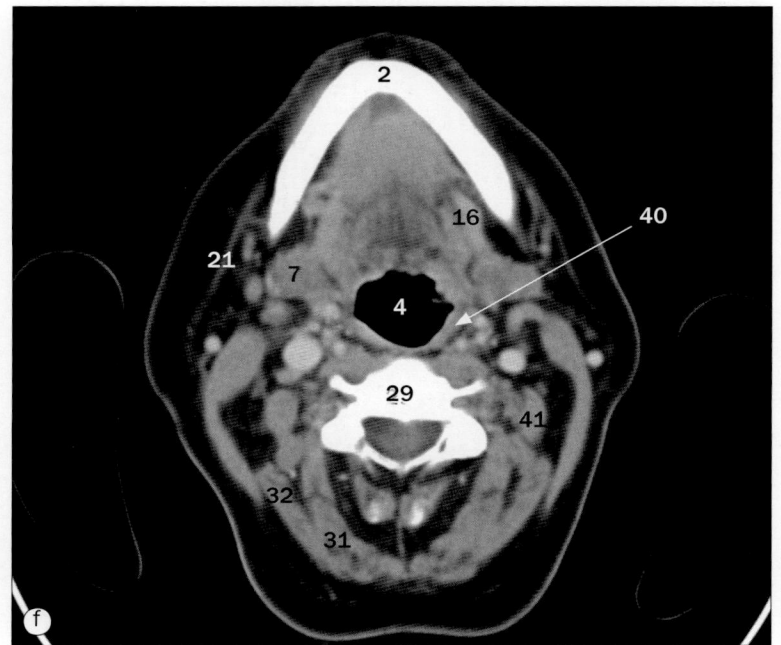

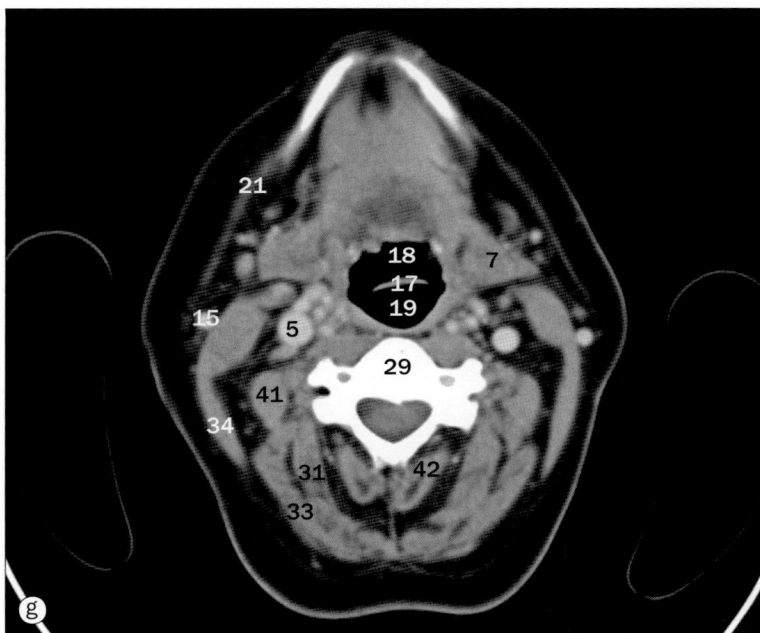

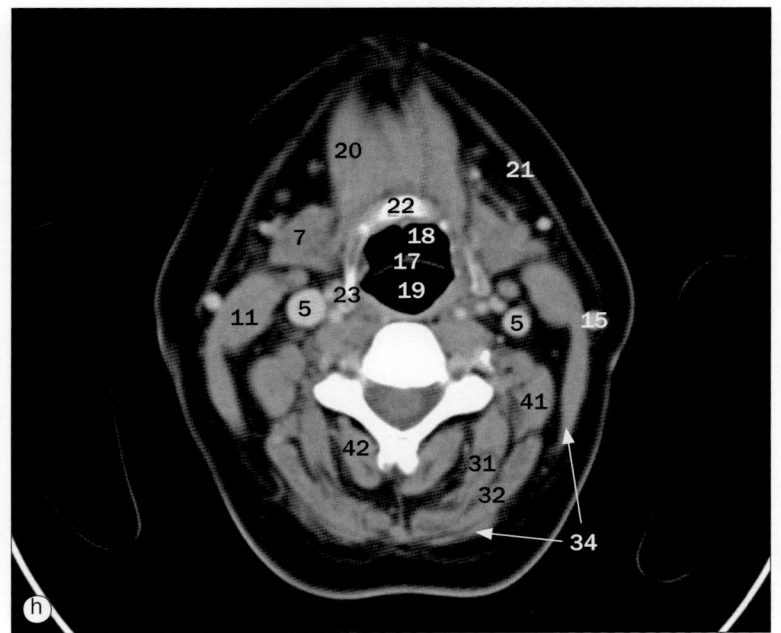

(a)–(h) Nasopharynx and oropharynx, axial CT images.

22 Hyoid body	30 Obliquus capitis inferior muscle	38 Longus colli muscle
23 Greater horn of hyoid	31 Semispinalis capitis muscle	39 Nuchal ligament
24 Posterior arch of C1	32 Splenius capitis muscle	40 Superior constrictor muscle of pharynx
25 Dens (odontoid process)	33 Longissimus capitis muscle	41 Levator scapulae muscle
26 Spinal cord	34 Trapezius muscle	42 Spinalis capitis muscle and multifidus muscle
27 Body of C2	35 Orbicularis oris muscle	
28 Body of C3	36 Levator anguli oris muscle	
29 Body of C4	37 Longus capitis muscle	

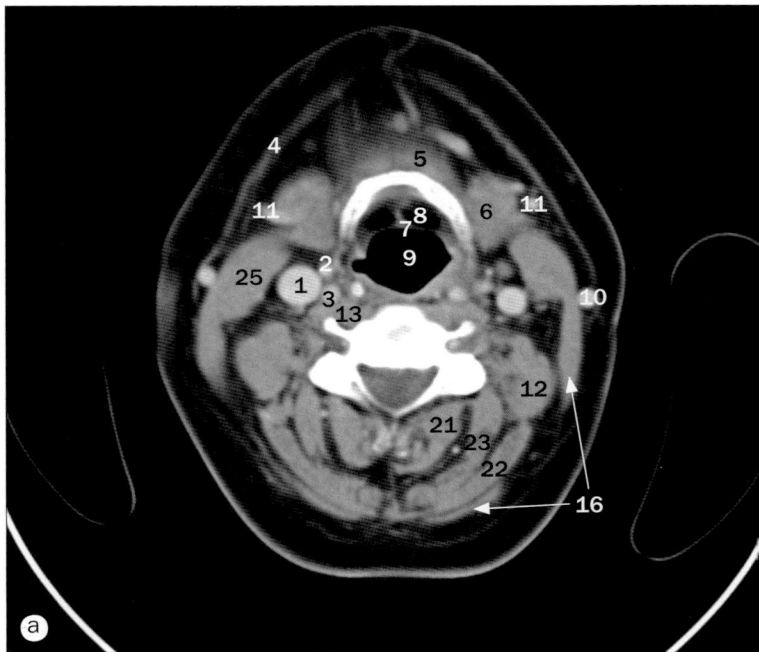

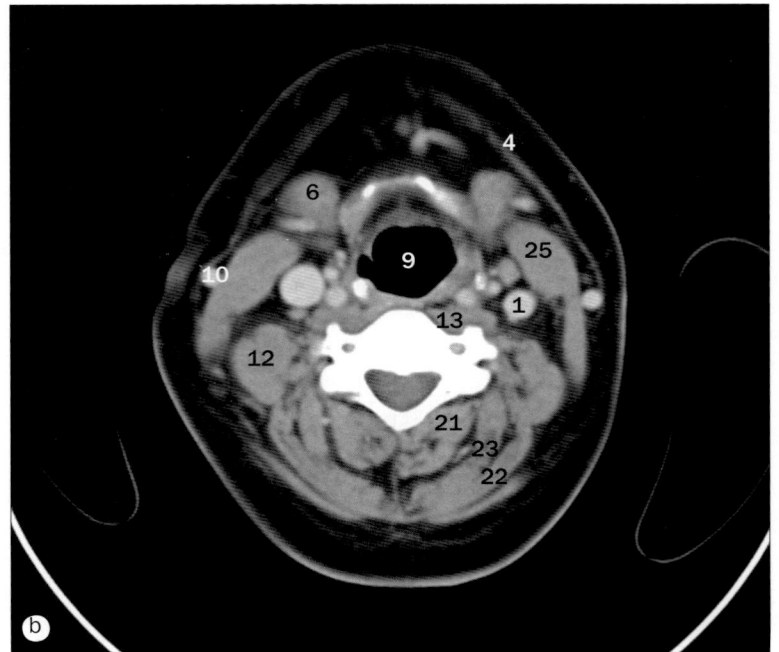

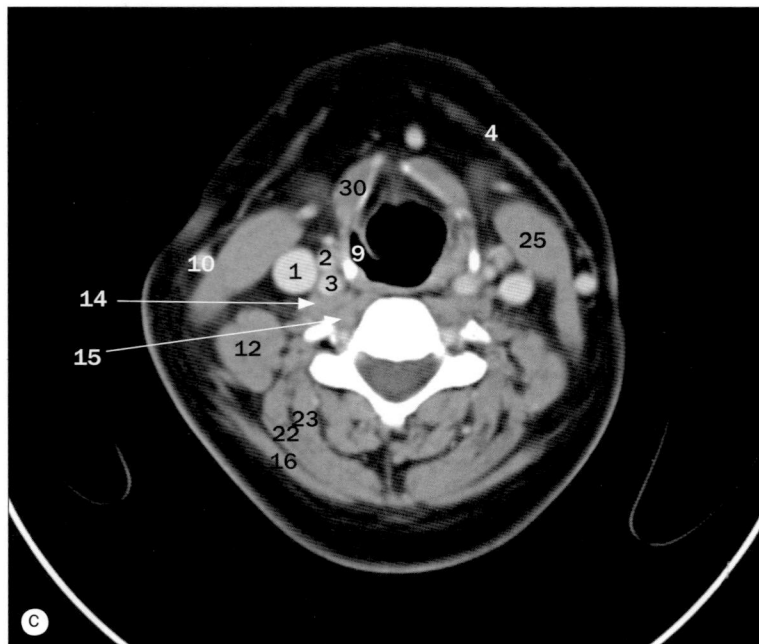

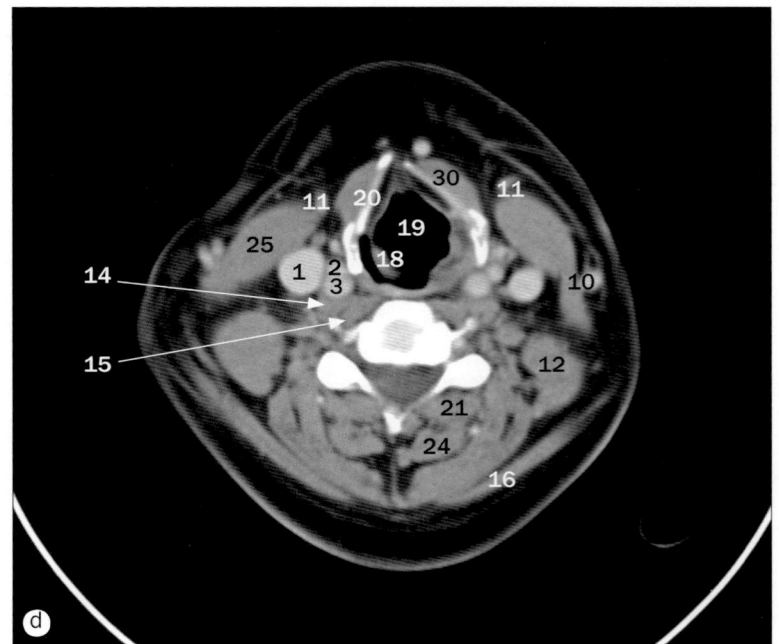

(a)–(I) Larynx and hypopharynx, axial CT images.

1 Internal jugular vein	**8** Vallecula
2 External carotid artery	**9** Hypopharynx
3 Internal carotid artery	**10** External jugular vein
4 Platysma muscle	**11** Anterior jugular vein
5 Geniohyoid muscle	**12** Levator scapulae muscle
6 Submandibular gland	**13** Longus capitus and colli muscles
7 Epiglottis	**14** Longus capitus muscle

The legends for pages 26–28 are common for all 3 pages.

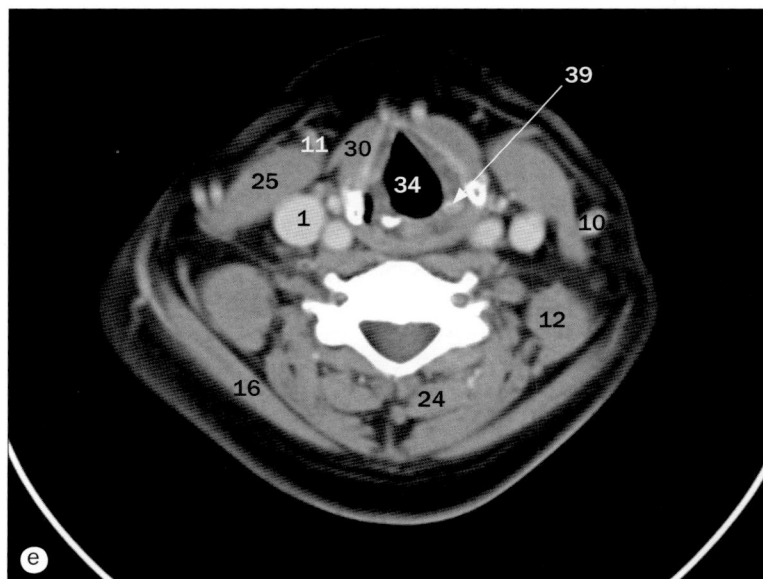

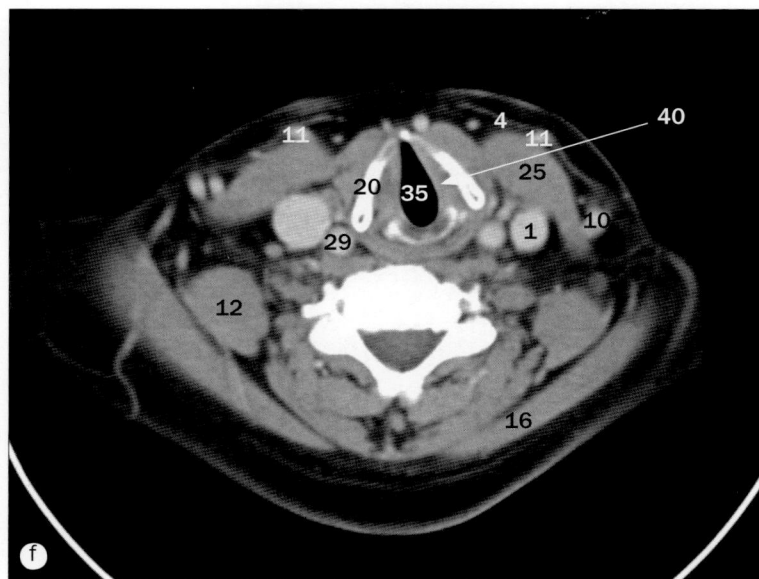

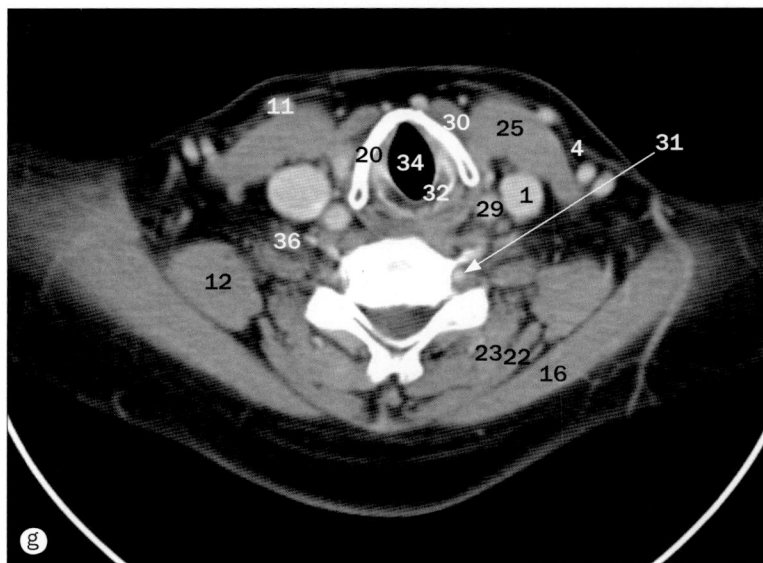

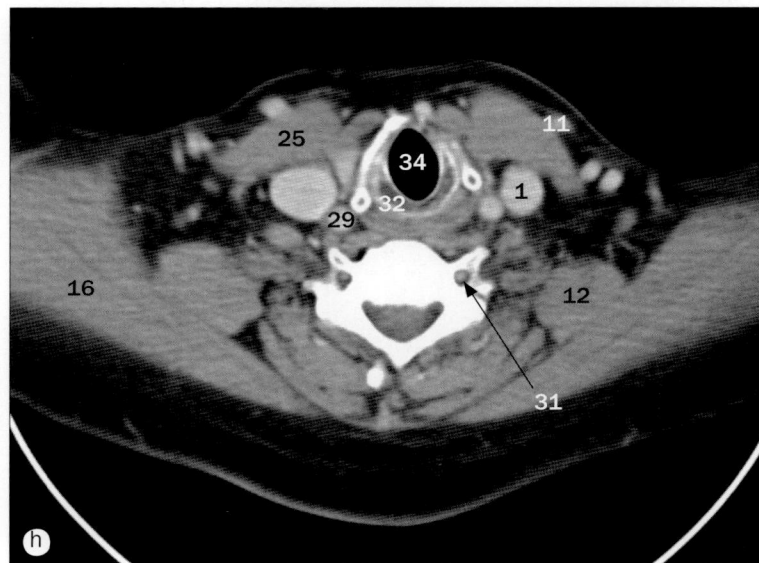

(a)–(l) Larynx and hypopharynx, axial CT images.

15 Longus colli muscle	**22** Splenius capitis muscle
16 Trapezius muscle	**23** Semispinalis capitis muscle
17 Clavicle	**24** Semispinalis cervicis muscle
18 Aryepiglottic fold	**25** Sternocleidomastoid muscle
19 Laryngeal vestibule	**26** Sternohyoid muscle
20 Thyroid cartilage lamina	**27** Thyroid gland
21 Spinalis cervicis muscle	**28** Oesophagus

The legends for pages 26–28 are common for all 3 pages.

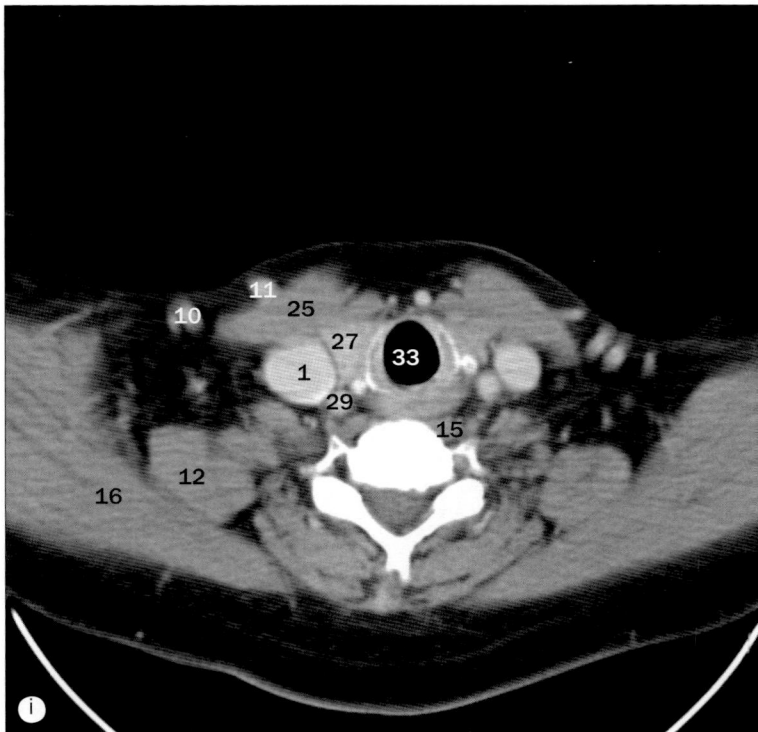

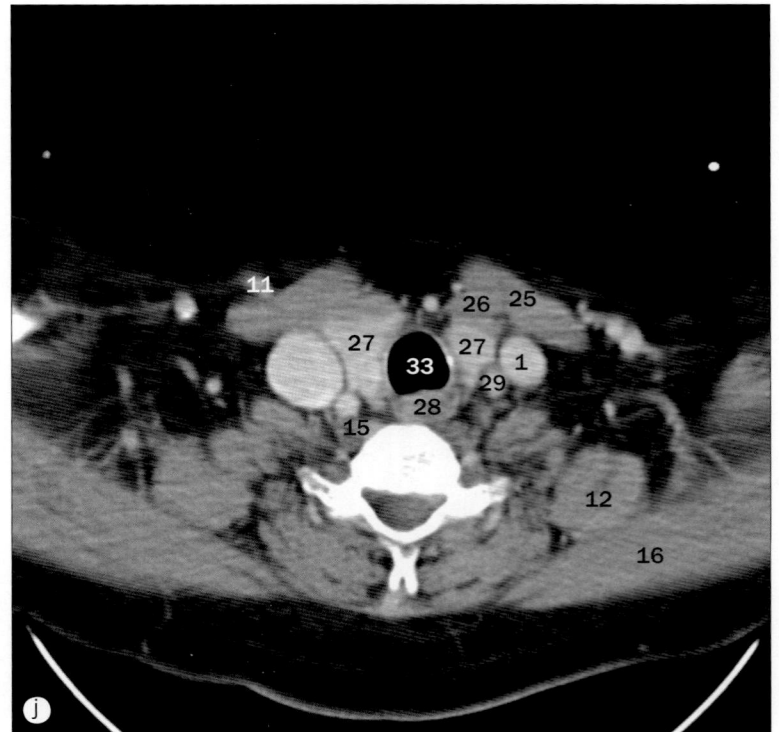

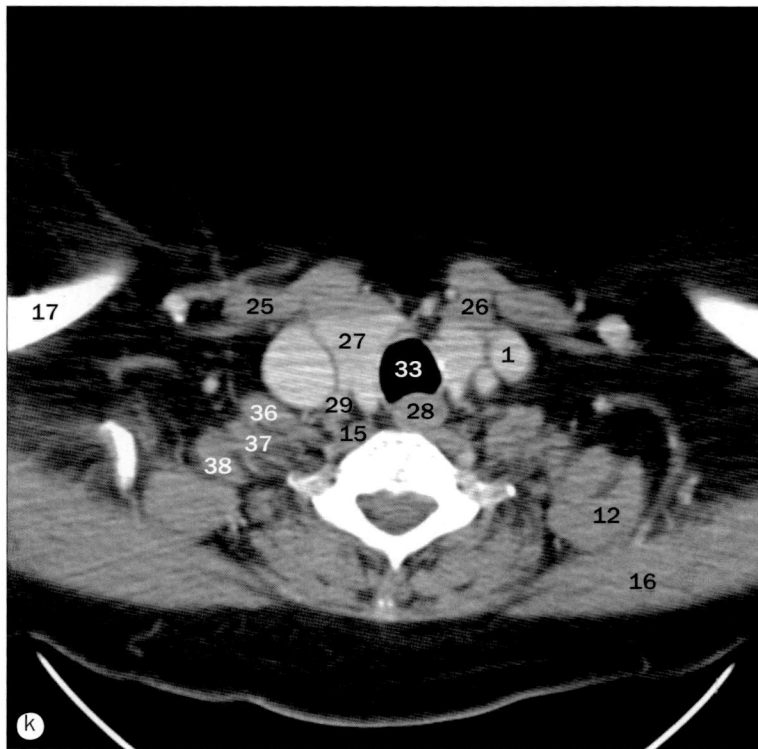

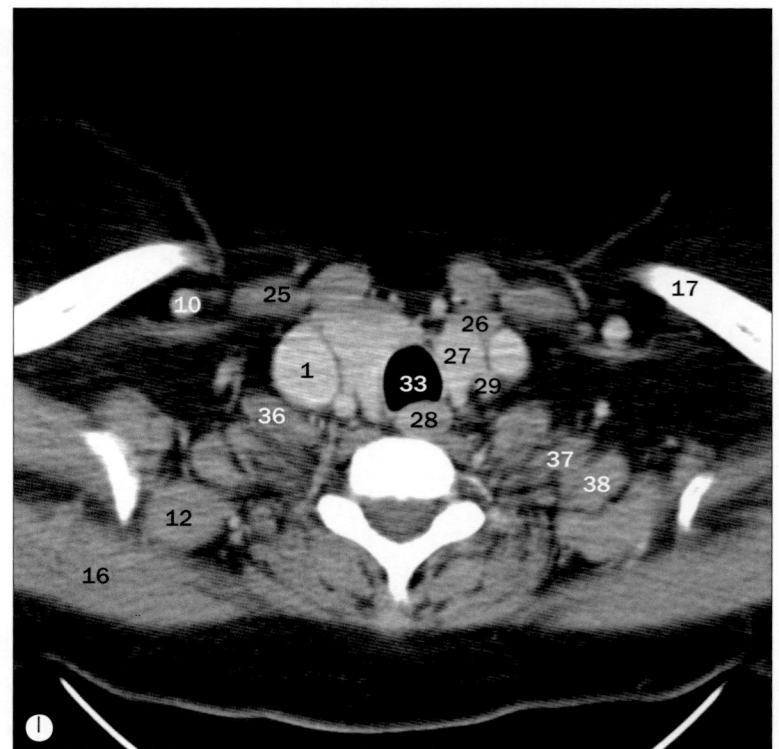

(a)–(l) Larynx and hypopharynx, axial CT images.

29 Common carotid artery	35 Glottis
30 Infrahyoid strap muscle	36 Anterior scalene muscle
31 Vertebral artery	37 Middle scalene muscle
32 Cricoid cartilage	38 Posterior scalene muscle
33 Trachea	39 Arytenoid cartilage
34 Larynx	40 Vocalis muscle

The legends for pages 26–28 are common for all 3 pages.

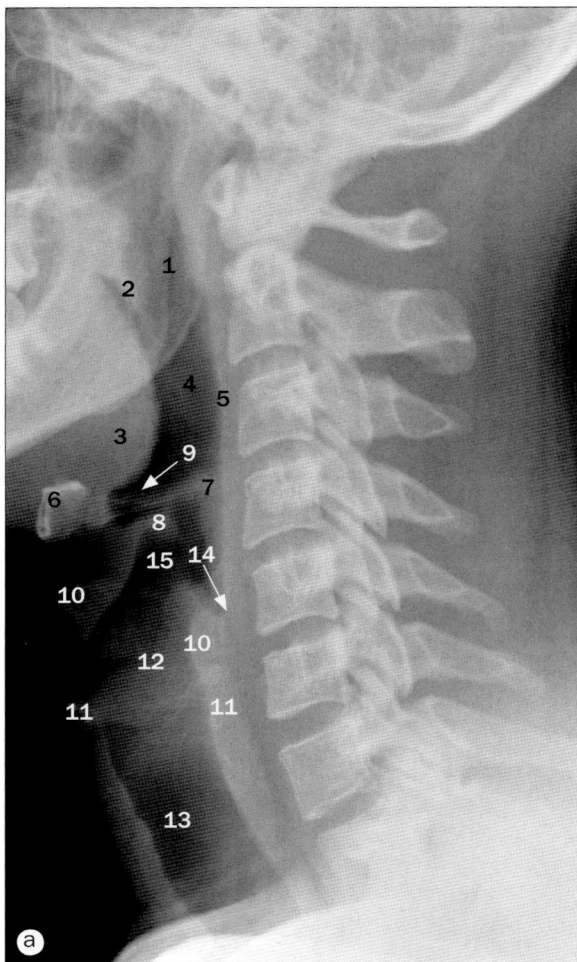

1 Nasopharynx   9 Vallecula
2 Soft palate   10 Thyroid cartilage
3 Base of tongue   11 Cricoid cartilage
4 Oropharynx   12 Larygneal space
5 Retropharyngeal soft tissues 13 Trachea
6 Body of hyoid   14 Entrance to oesophagus
7 Greater horn of hyoid   15 Hypopharynx
8 Epiglottis

(a) Soft tissues of the neck, lateral projection.

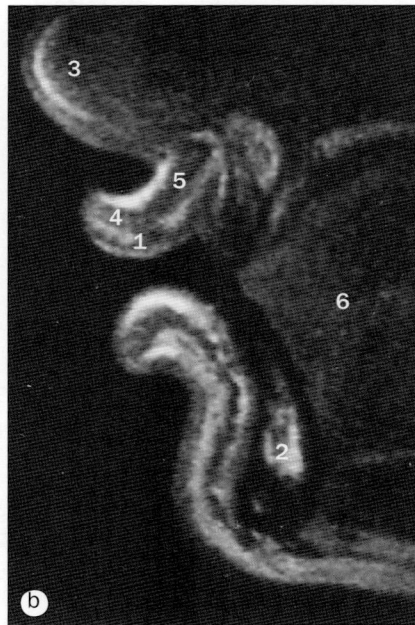

1 Deltoid insertion of levator muscle
2 Mandible
3 Nose
4 Pars marginalis of orbicularis oris
   muscle
5 Pars peripheralis of orbicularis oris
   muscle
6 Tongue

(b) The kiss, sagittal MR image.

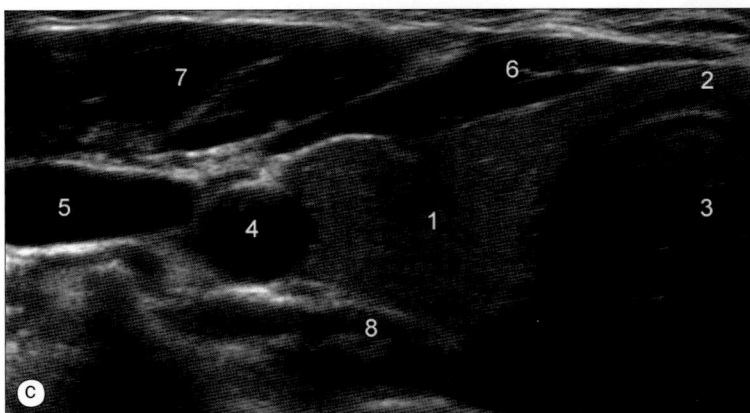

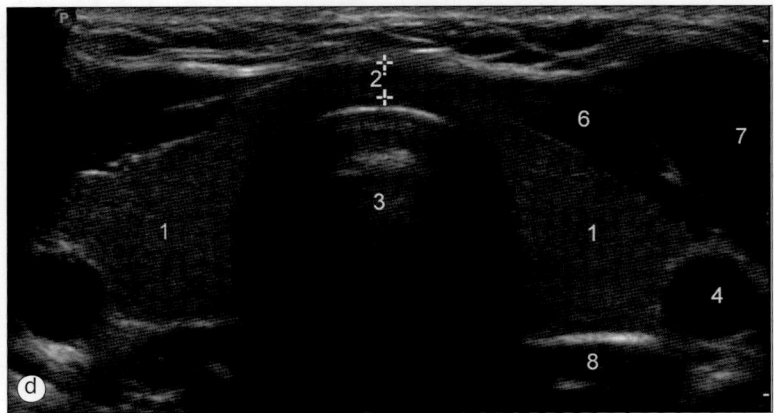

(c) and (d) Thyroid ultrasound, axial projection.

1 Thyroid gland lobe
2 Thyroid gland isthmus
3 Trachea
4 Common carotid artery
5 Internal jugular vein
6 Infrahyoid strap muscle
7 Sternocleidomastoid muscle
8 Prevertebral muscle

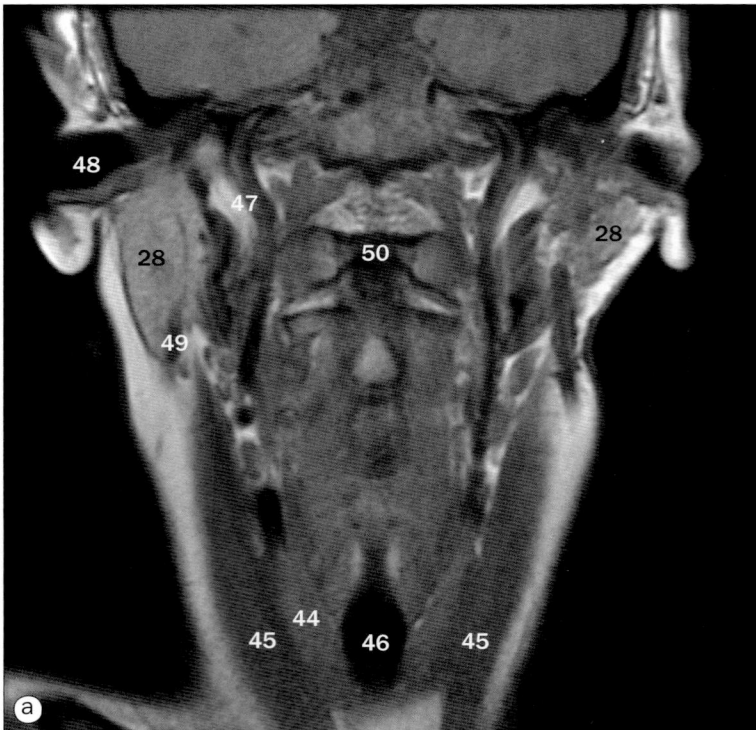

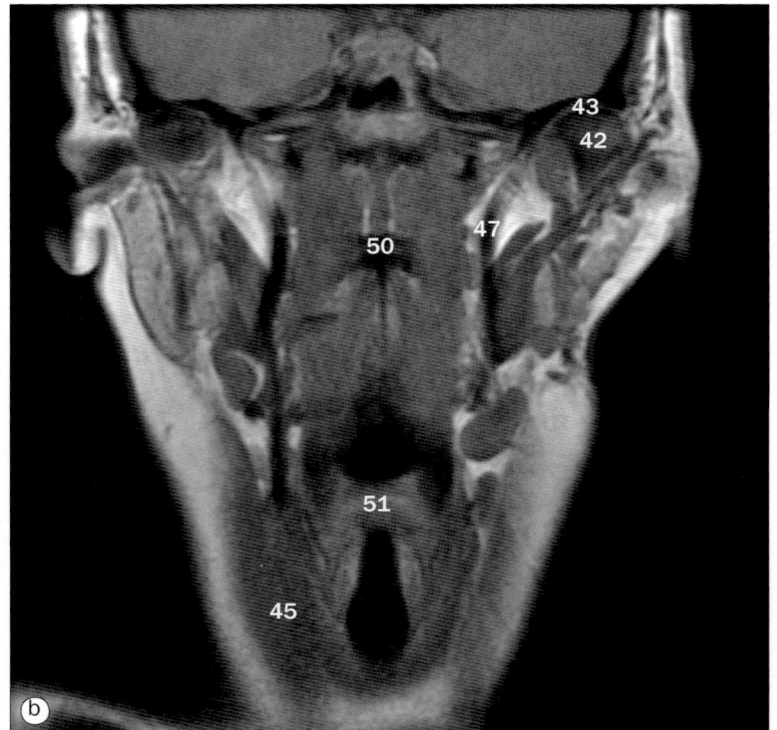

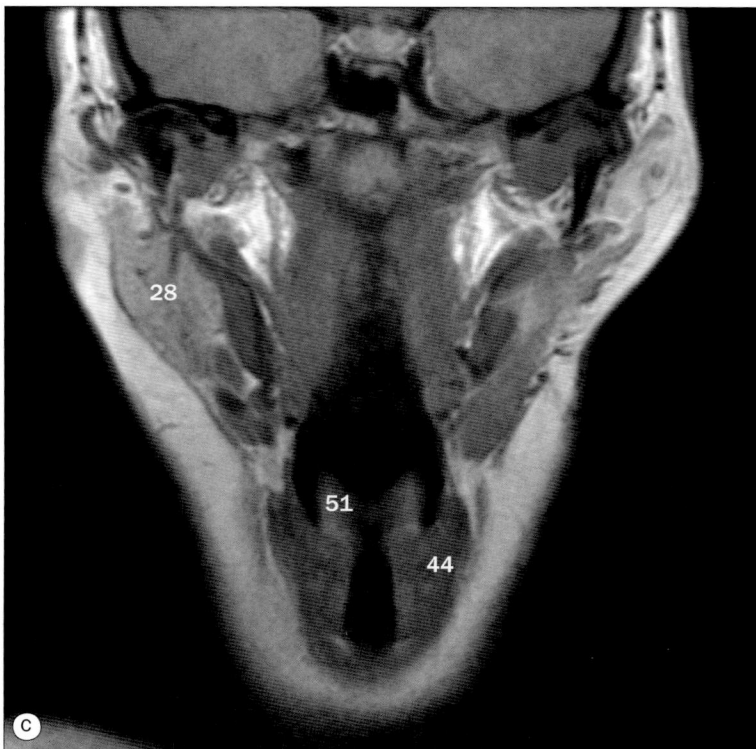

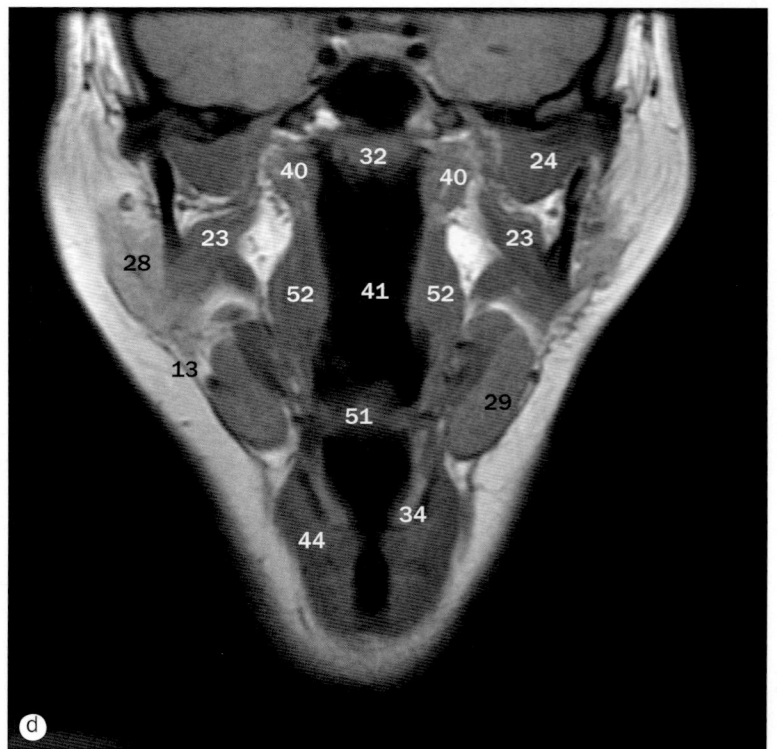

(a)–(l) Coronal MR images of pharynx, from posterior to anterior.

1 Maxillary sinus (antrum)	8 Nasal septum
2 Hard palate	9 Genioglossus muscle
3 Mandible	10 Geniohyoid muscle
4 Alveolar ridge of maxilla	11 Anterior belly of digastric muscle
5 Oral cavity	12 Lingual septum
6 Inferior turbinate	13 Platysmus muscle
7 Middle turbinate	14 Hypoglossus muscle

The legends for pages 30–32 are common for all 3 pages.

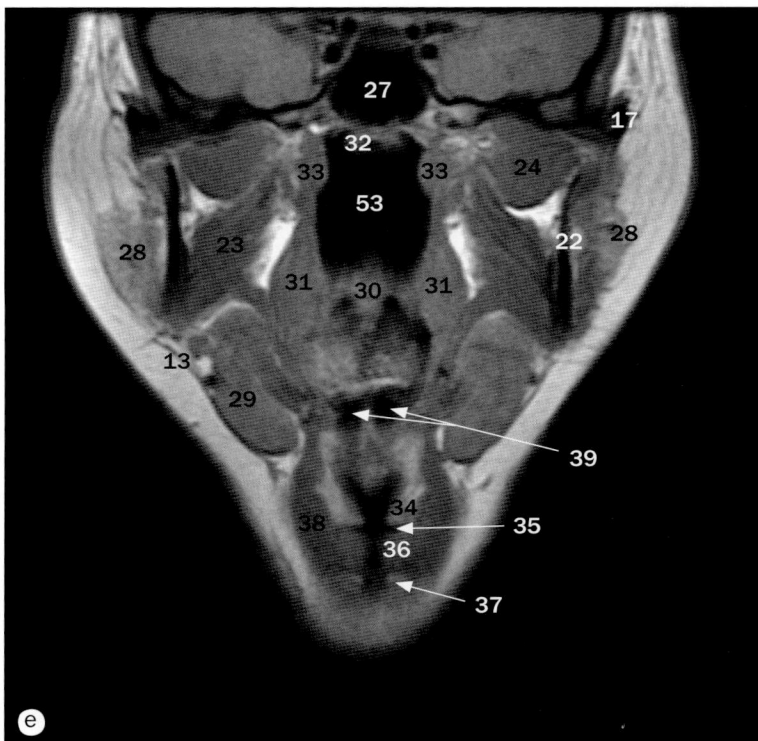

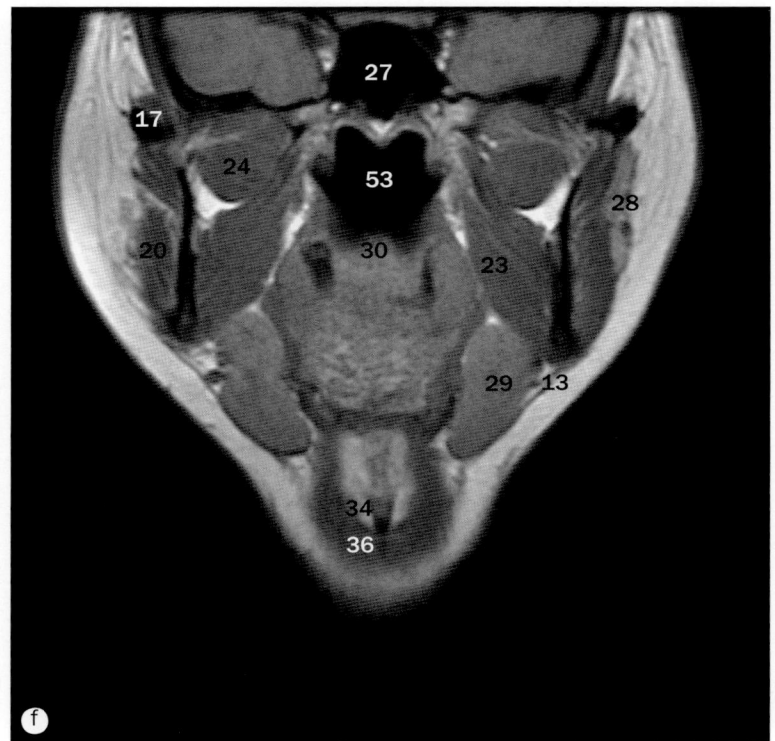

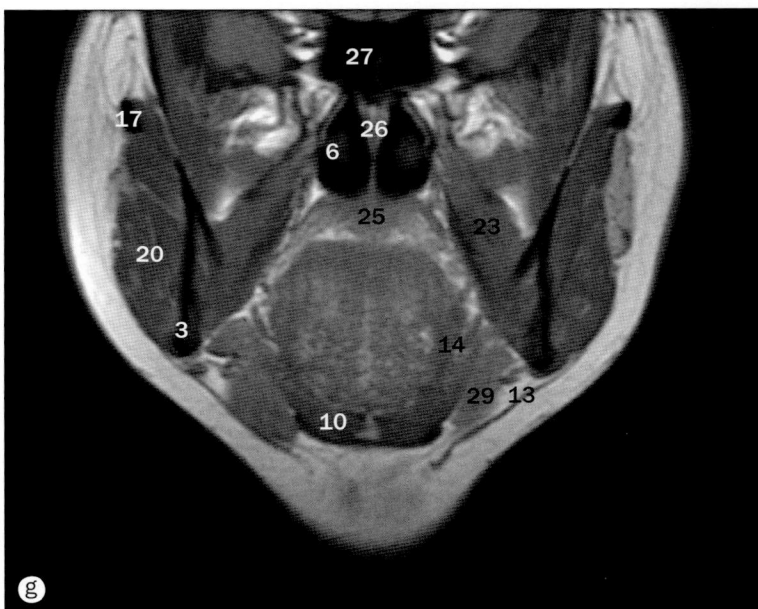

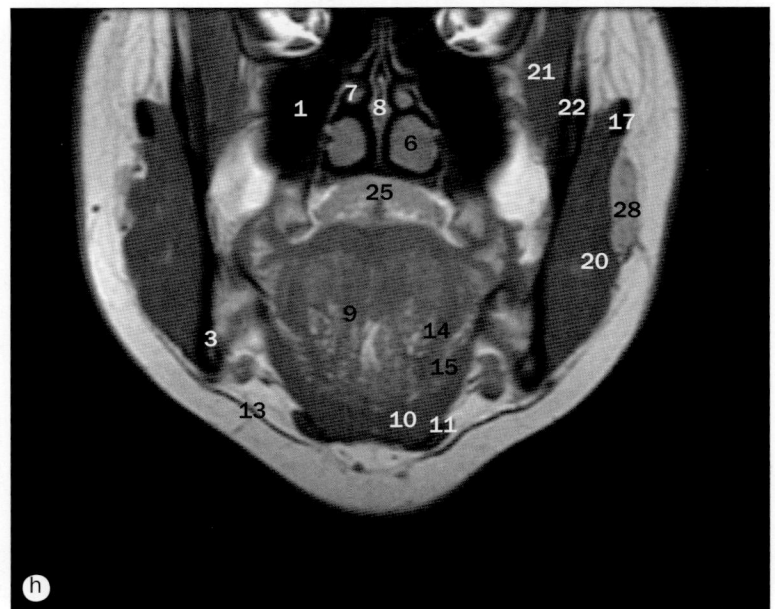

(a)–(l) Coronal MR images of pharynx, from posterior to anterior.

15 Mylohyoid muscle
16 Zygomatic bone
17 Zygomatic arch
18 Transverse muscle of tongue
19 Longitudinal muscle of tongue
20 Masseter muscle
21 Temporal muscle
22 Ramus of mandible
23 Medial pterygoid muscle

24 Lateral pterygoid muscle
25 Soft palate
26 Vomer
27 Sphenoid sinus (antrum)
28 Parotid gland
29 Submandibular gland
30 Uvula
31 Palatopharyngeus muscle
32 Pharyngeal tonsils

The legends for pages 30–32 are common for all 3 pages.

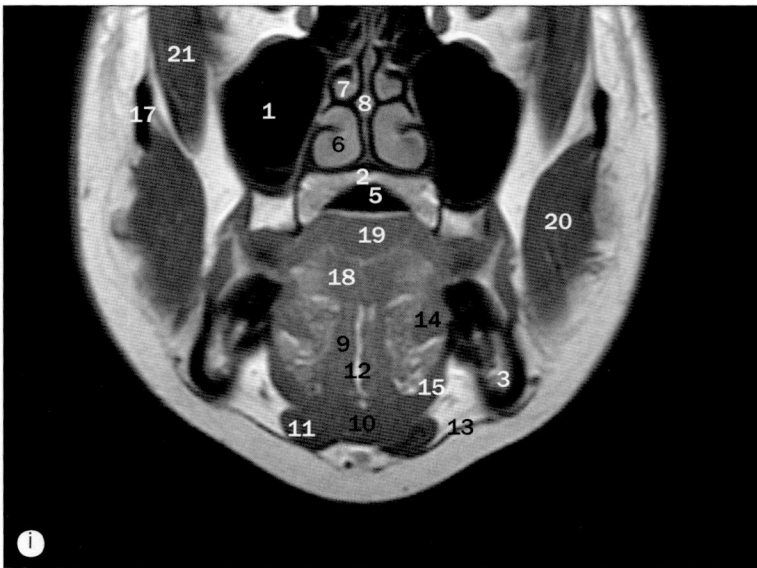

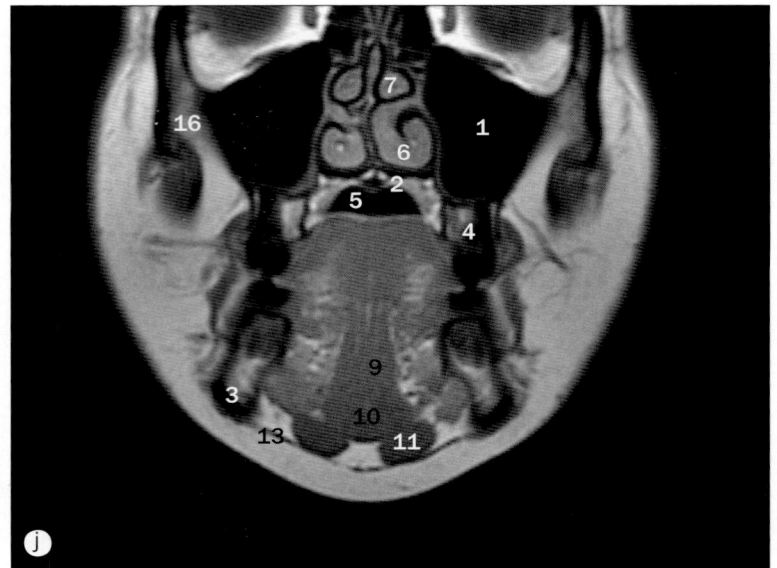

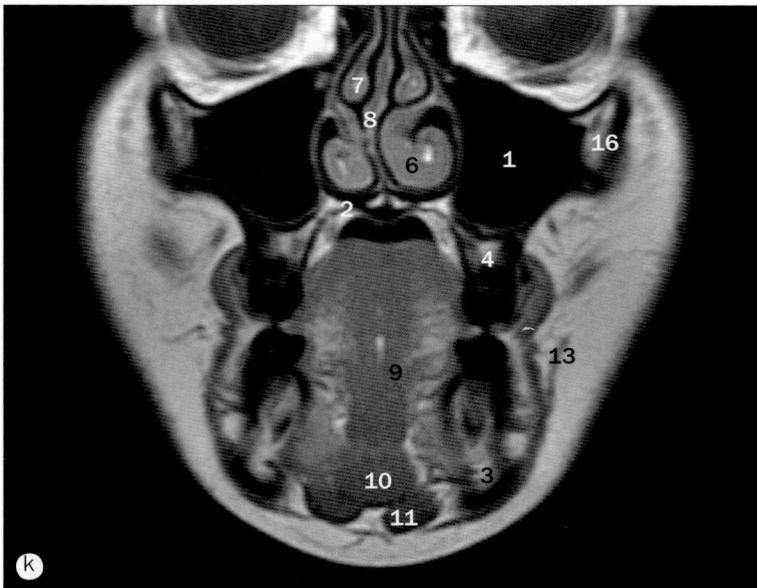

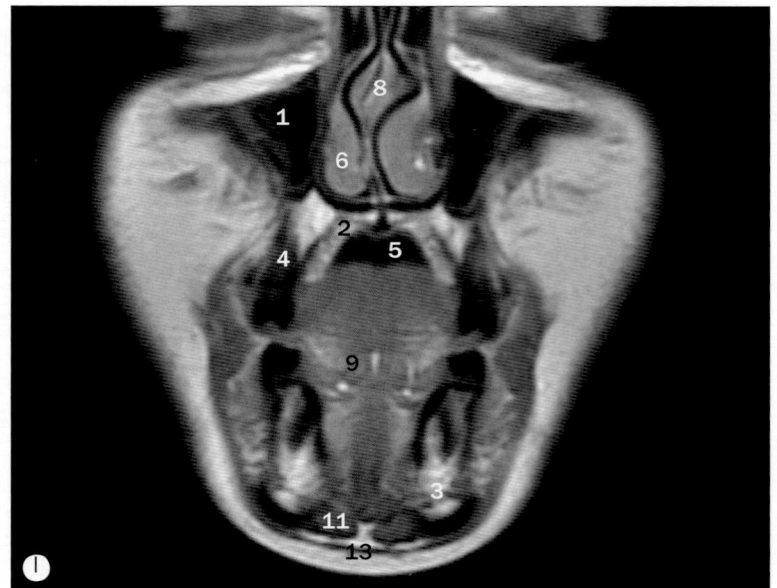

(a)–(l) Coronal MR images of pharynx, from posterior to anterior.

33 Levator veli palatini muscle
34 Vestibular fold
35 Laryngeal ventricle
36 Vocalis muscle
37 Cricoid cartilage
38 Thyrohyoid muscle
39 Vallecula
40 Eustachian tubes
41 Oropharynx
42 Mandibular condyles
43 Temporomandibular joint

44 Thyroid gland
45 Sternocleidomastoid muscle
46 Trachea
47 Internal carotid artery
48 External auditory canal
49 Retromandibular vein
50 Anterior arch of C1
51 Epiglottis
52 Palatine tonsils
53 Nasopharynx

The legends for pages 30–32 are common for all 3 pages.

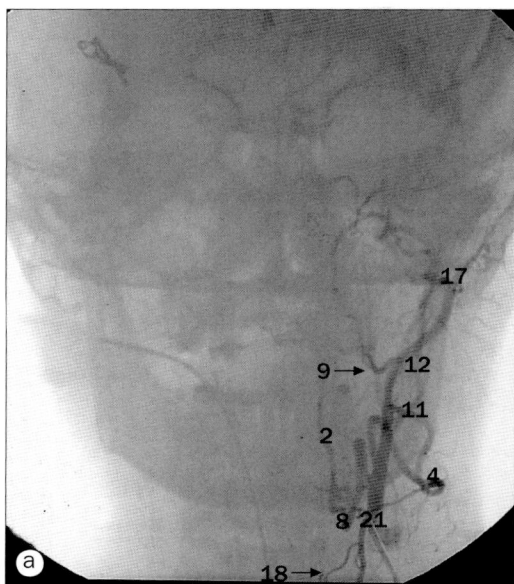
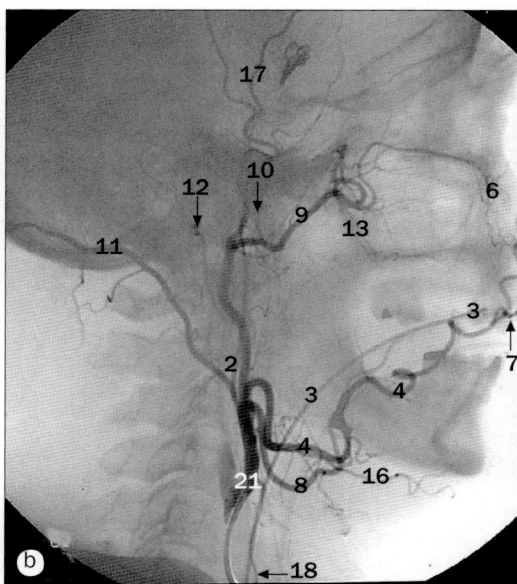
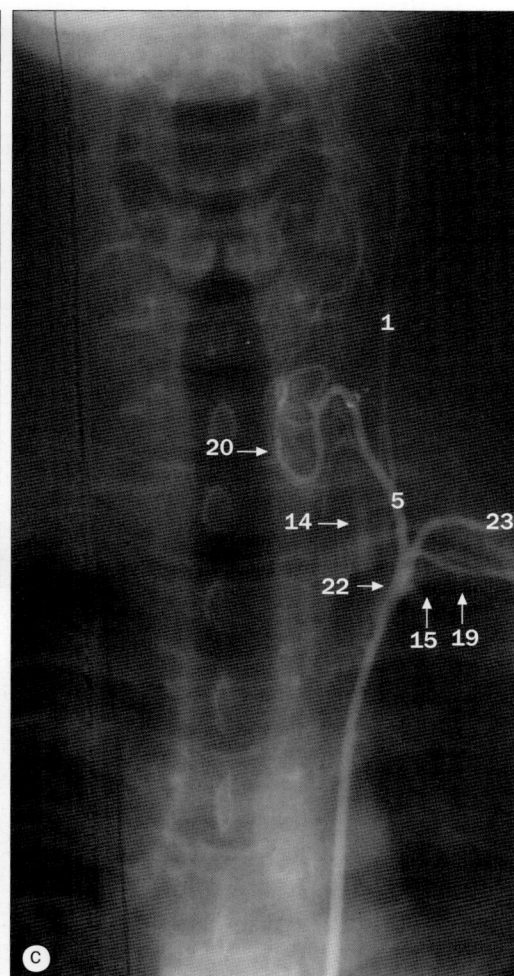

Digitally subtracted arteriograms of the external carotid artery, (a) anteroposterior projection, (b) lateral projection. (c) Thyroid arteriogram.

1 Ascending cervical artery	10 Middle meningeal artery	18 Superior thyroid artery
2 Ascending pharyngeal artery	11 Occipital artery	19 Suprascapular artery
3 Endotracheal tube	12 Posterior auricular artery	20 Thyroid branches of inferior thyroid artery
4 Facial artery	13 Posterior superior alveolar artery	21 Tip of catheter in external carotid artery
5 Inferior thyroid artery	14 Reflux of contrast into vertebral artery	22 Tip of catheter in thyrocervical trunk
6 Infra-orbital artery	15 Subclavian artery	23 Transverse cervical artery
7 Labial branch of facial artery	16 Submental artery	
8 Lingual artery	17 Superficial temporal artery	
9 Maxillary artery		

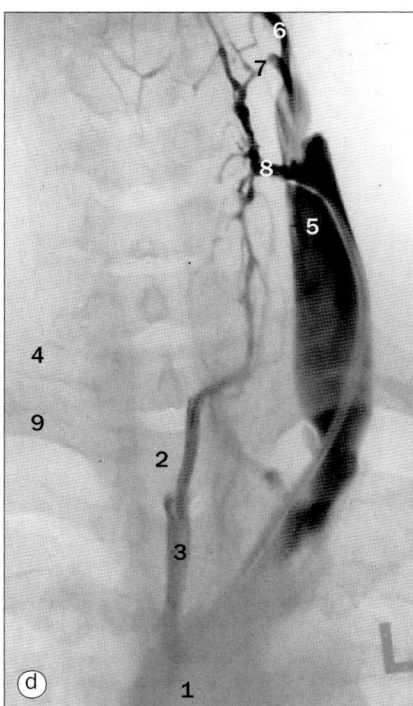
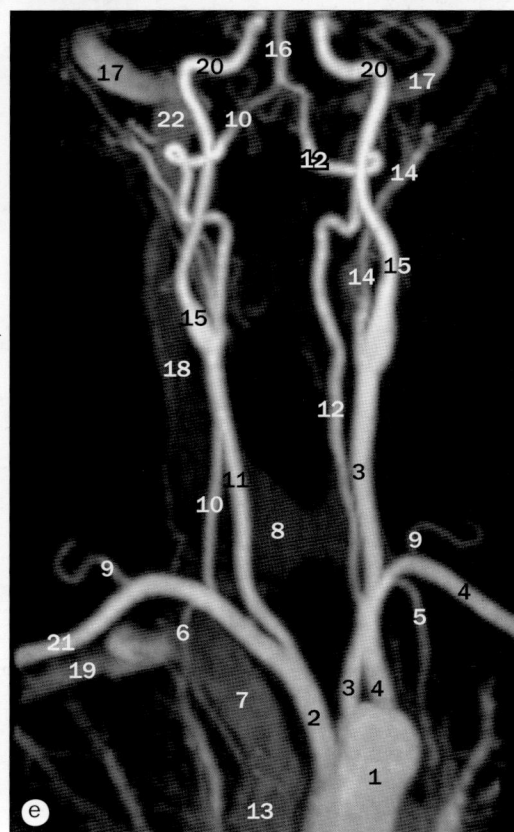

(d) Neck venogram.
(e) MR angiogram of neck vessels.

1 Left brachiocephalic vein	5 Internal jugular vein
2 Trachea	6 Lingual vein
3 Inferior thyroid vein	7 Superior thyroid vein
4 Transverse process of C7	8 Tip of catheter in middle thyroid vein
	9 Right first rib

1 Aortic arch	11 Right common carotid artery
2 Brachiocephalic artery	12 Left vertebral artery
3 Left common carotid artery	13 Superior vena cava
4 Left subclavian artery	14 External carotid artery
5 Left internal thoracic artery	15 Internal carotid artery
6 Right internal thoracic artery	16 Basilar artery
7 Right brachio-cephalic vein	17 Sigmoid sinus
8 Right lobe of the thyroid gland	18 Internal jugular vein
9 Costocervical trunk	19 Right subclavian vein
10 Right vertebral artery	20 Petrous portion of the internal carotid artery
	21 Right subclavian artery
	22 Jugular bulb

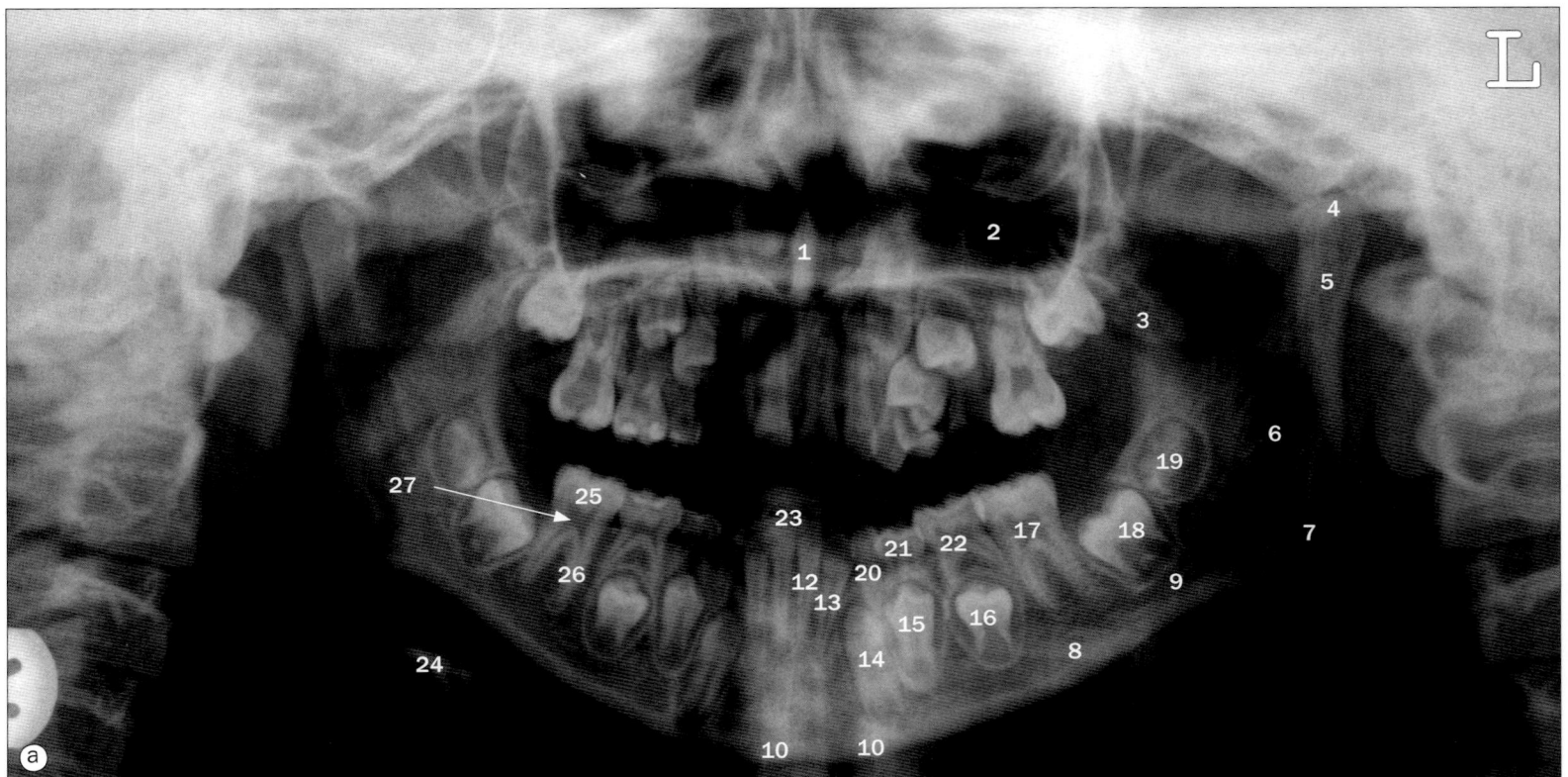

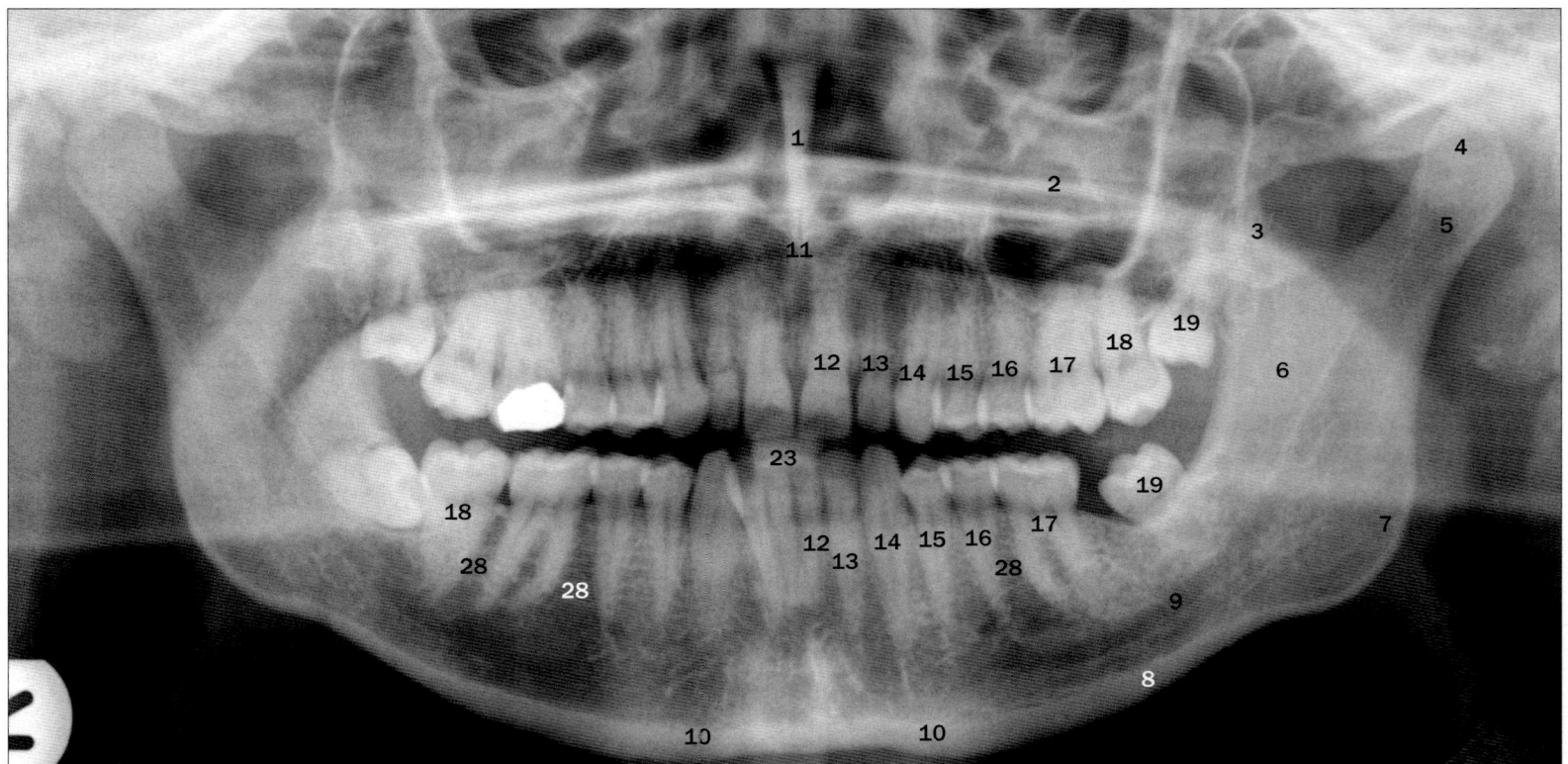

Dental panoramic tomogram (orthopantomogram) of **(a)** a 6-year-old child, **(b)** an adult.

1 Nasal septum	8 Mandibular body	15 Anterior premolar	22 Deciduous posterior premolar
2 Maxillary sinus (antrum)	9 Mandibular canal	16 Posterior premolar	23 Bite block
3 Coronoid process of mandible	10 Mental tubercle	17 First molar	24 Hyoid bone
4 Mandibular condylar head	11 Anterior nasal spine	18 Second molar	25 Crown of tooth
5 Mandibular condylar neck	12 Medial incisor	19 Third molar (wisdom tooth)	26 Root of tooth
6 Mandibular ramus	13 Lateral incisor	20 Deciduous canine tooth	27 Pulp chamber of tooth
7 Angle of mandible	14 Canine tooth	21 Deciduous anterior premolar	28 Alveolar bone

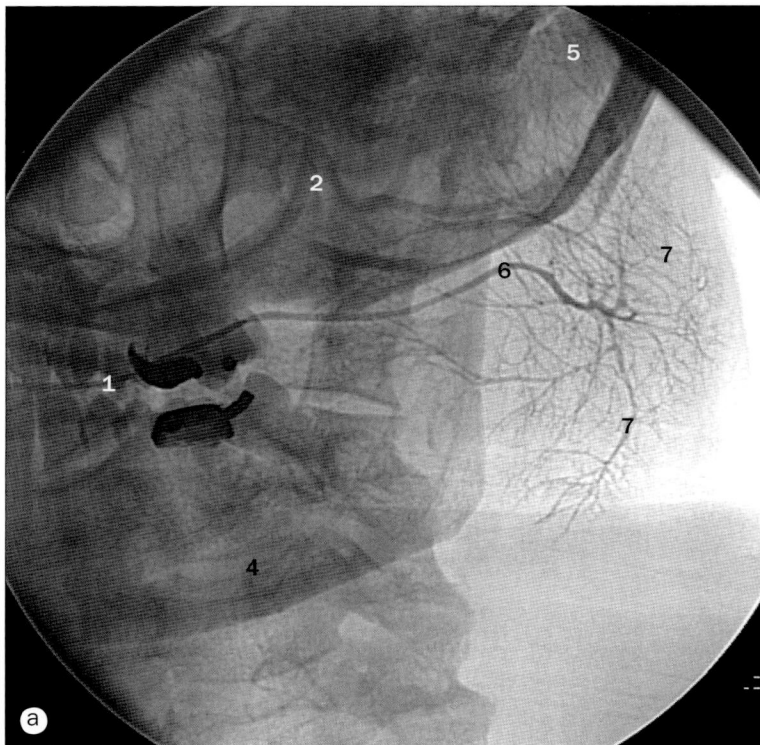

(a) Parotid sialogram.

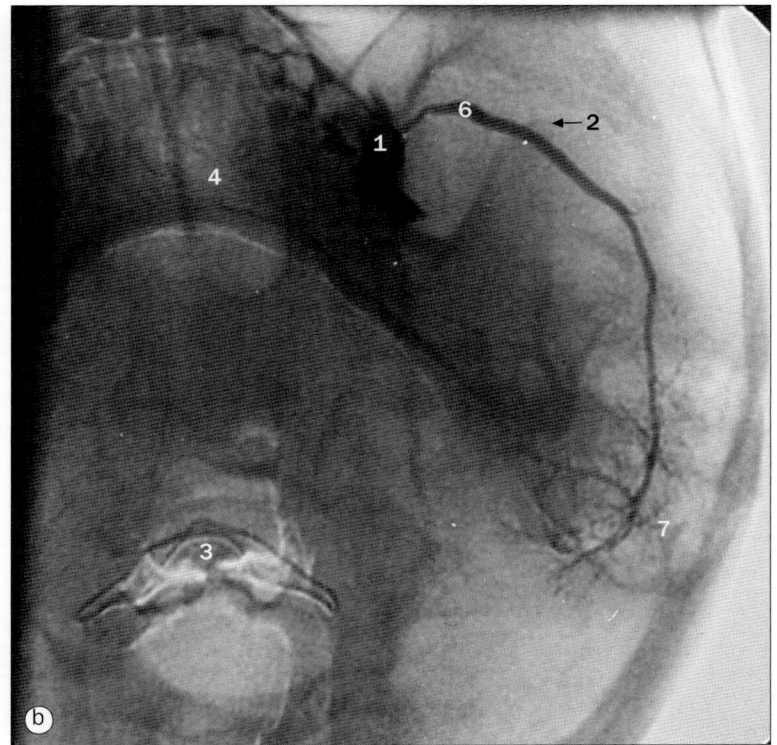

(b) Parotid sialogram, submentovertical projection.

1 Catheter
2 Coronoid process of mandible
3 Hyoid bone
4 Mandible
5 Mastoid process
6 Parotid (Stensen's) duct
7 Secondary ductules

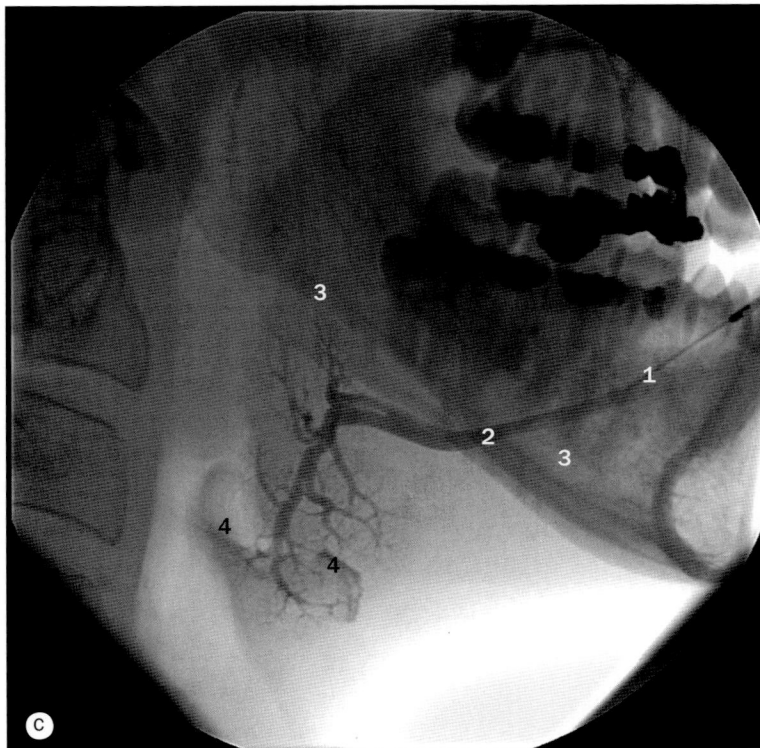

(c) Submandibular sialogram.

1 Catheter
2 Main submandibular (Wharton's) duct
3 Mandible
4 Secondary ductules

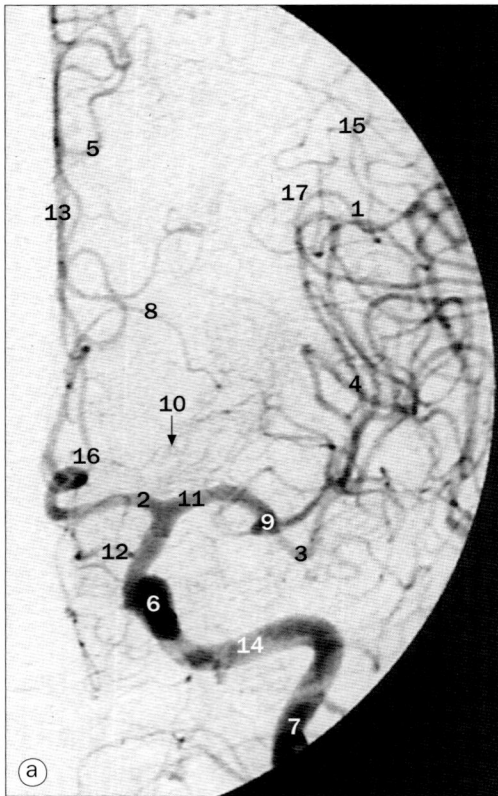

1 Angular branches of middle cerebral artery
2 Anterior cerebral artery
3 Anterior temporal branches of middle cerebral artery
4 Branches (in insula) of middle cerebral artery
5 Callosomarginal artery
6 Cavernous portion of internal carotid artery
7 Cervical portion of internal carotid artery
8 Frontopolar artery
9 Genu of middle cerebral artery
10 Lenticulostriate arteries
11 Middle cerebral artery
12 Orbitofrontal branch of pericallosal artery
13 Pericallosal artery
14 Petrous portion of internal carotid artery
15 Posterior parietal branches of middle cerebral artery
16 Recurrent artery of Heubner
17 Sylvian point

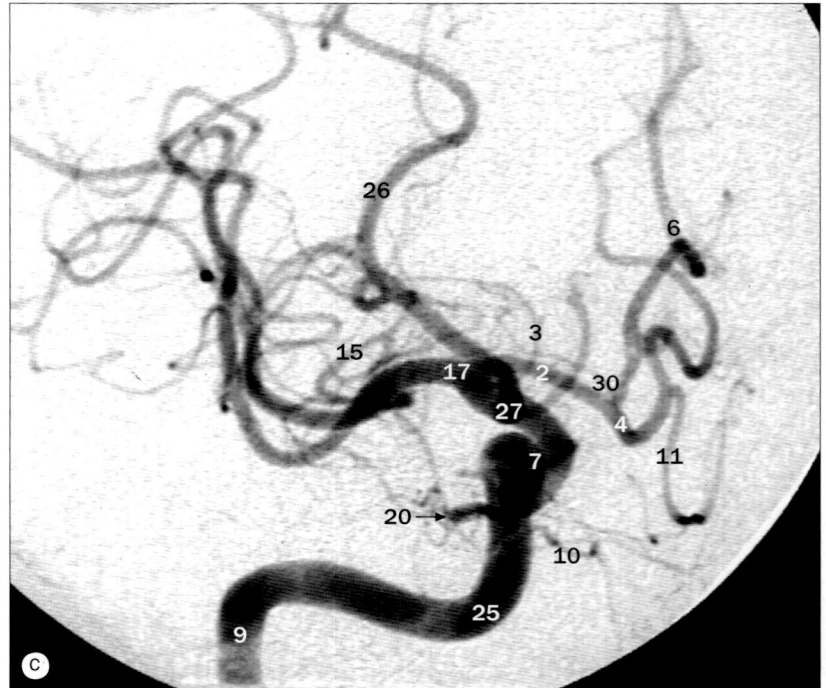

Digitally subtracted arterial phase of carotid arteriograms,
(a) anteroposterior projection, (b) lateral projection, (c) oblique
projection.

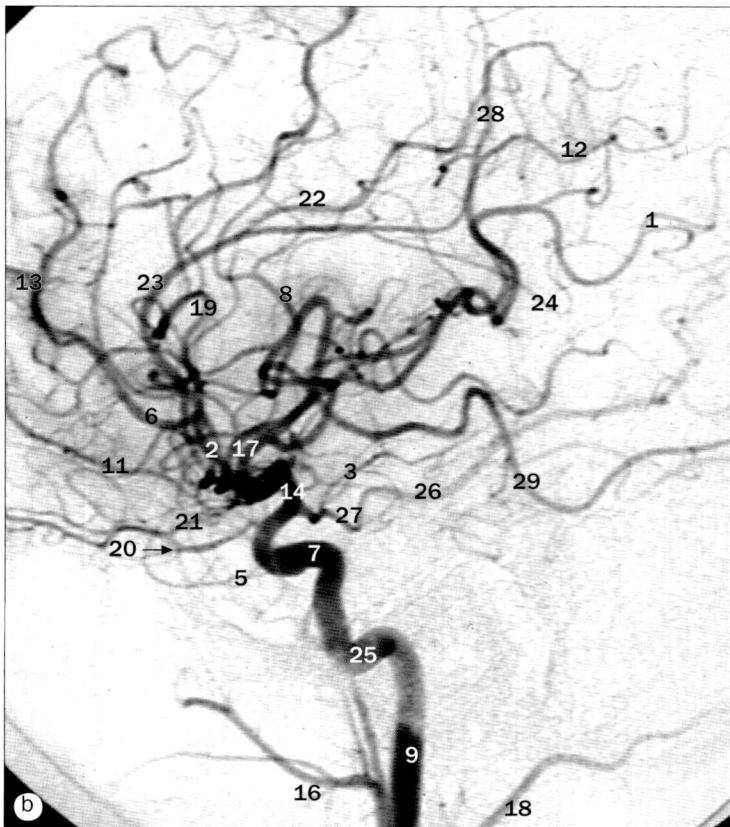

1 Angular artery
2 Anterior cerebral artery
3 Anterior choroidal artery
4 Anterior communicating artery
5 Anterior temporal artery
6 Callosomarginal artery
7 Cavernous portion of internal carotid artery
8 Central sulcus artery
9 Cervical portion of internal carotid artery
10 Ethmoidal branch of ophthalmic artery
11 Frontopolar artery
12 Inferior internal parietal artery
13 Internal frontal branch of anterior cerebral artery
14 Intracranial (supraclinoid) internal carotid artery
15 Lenticulostriate artery
16 Maxillary artery
17 Middle cerebral artery
18 Occipital artery
19 Operculofrontal artery
20 Ophthalmic artery
21 Orbitofrontal artery
22 Paracentral artery
23 Pericallosal artery
24 Pericallosal artery extending around corpus callosum
25 Petrous portion of internal carotid artery
26 Posterior cerebral artery
27 Posterior communicating artery
28 Posterior parietal artery
29 Posterior temporal artery
30 Recurrent artery of Heubner

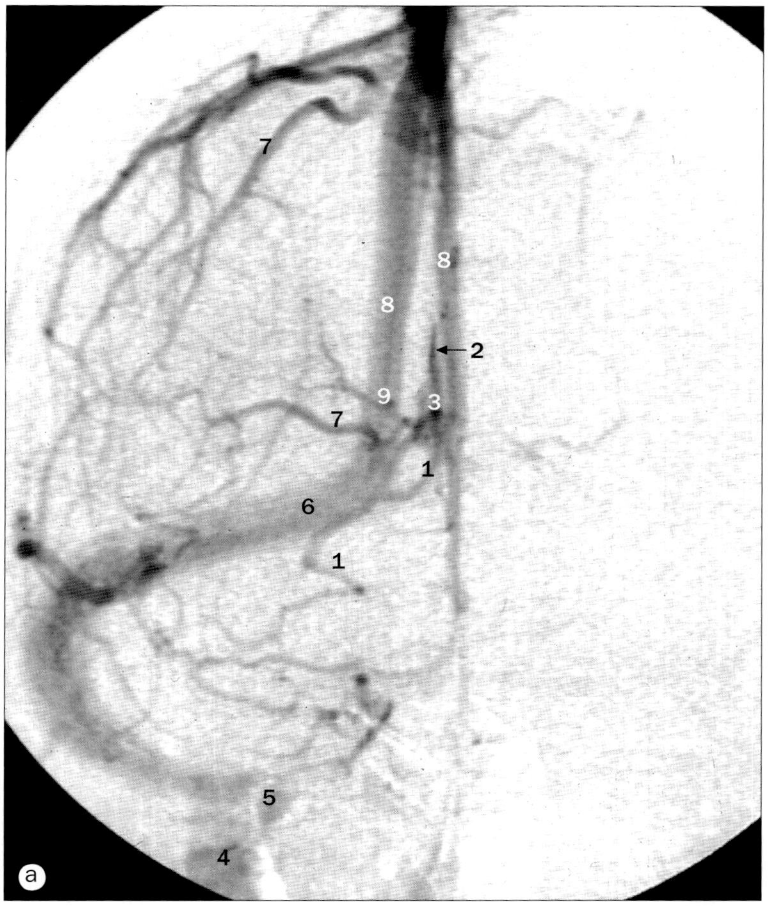

(**a**) Digitally subtracted venous phase of carotid arteriogram, anteroposterior projection.

1 Basal vein of Rosenthal
2 Inferior sagittal sinus
3 Internal cerebral vein
4 Internal jugular vein
5 Jugular bulb
6 Right transverse sinus
7 Superficial cortical veins
8 Superior sagittal sinus
9 Thalamostriate vein

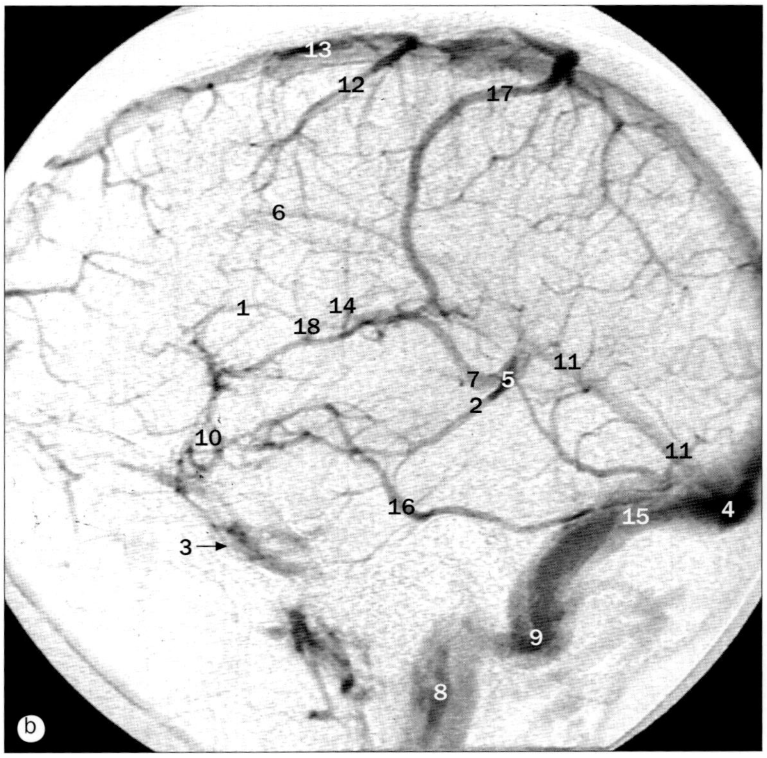

(**b**) Digitally subtracted venous phase of carotid arteriogram, lateral projection.

1 Anterior caudate vein
2 Basal vein of Rosenthal
3 Cavernous sinus
4 Confluence of venous sinuses (torcular Herophili)
5 Great cerebral vein of Galen
6 Inferior sagittal sinus
7 Internal cerebral vein
8 Internal jugular vein
9 Sigmoid sinus
10 Sphenoparietal sinus
11 Straight sinus
12 Superficial cerebral veins
13 Superior sagittal sinus
14 Thalamostriate vein
15 Transverse sinus
16 Vein of Labbé
17 Vein of Trolard
18 Venous angle

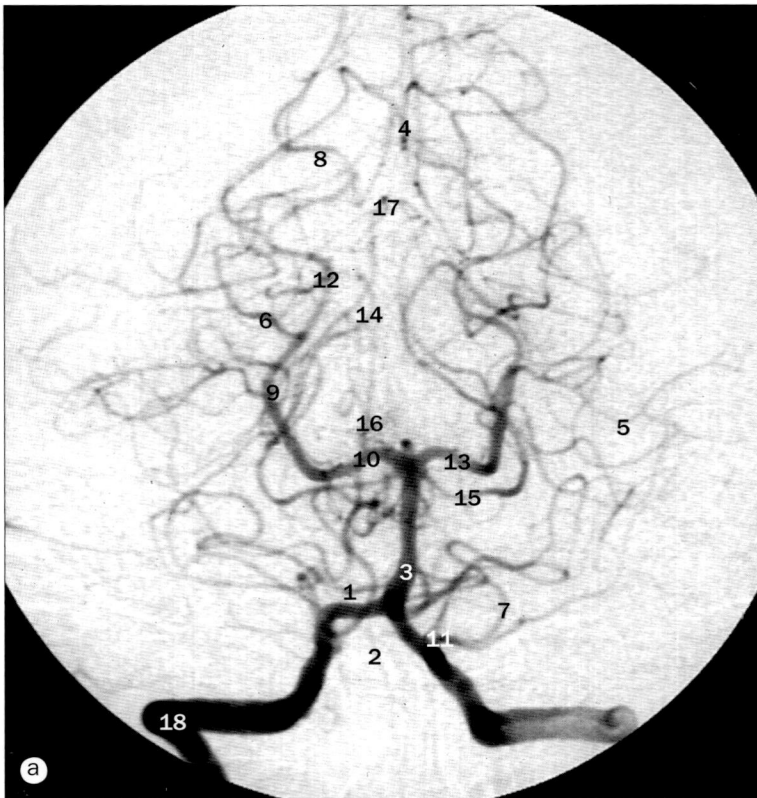

(a) Digitally subtracted arterial phase of vertebral arteriogram, anteroposterior projection.

1 Anterior inferior cerebellar artery
2 Anterior spinal artery
3 Basilar artery
4 Calcarine artery
5 Hemispheric branch of superior cerebellar artery
6 Inferior temporal artery
7 Medullary segment of posterior inferior cerebellar artery
8 Parieto-occipital artery
9 Posterior cerebral artery in ambient cistern
10 Posterior cerebral artery in interpeduncular cistern
11 Posterior inferior cerebellar artery
12 Quadrigeminal portion of posterior cerebral artery
13 Site of junction with posterior communicating artery
14 Superior cerebellar arteries behind brainstem
15 Superior cerebellar artery
16 Thalamoperforating branches of superior cerebellar artery
17 Vermian branch of superior cerebellar artery
18 Vertebral artery exiting transverse foramen of atlas
   (first cervical vertebra)

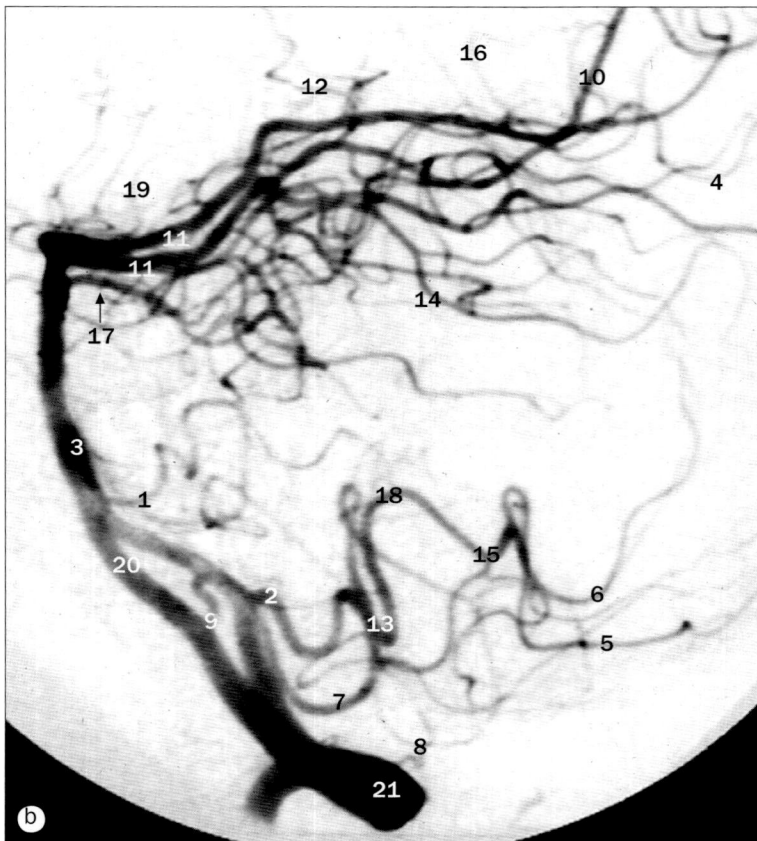

(b) Digitally subtracted arterial phase of vertebral arteriogram, lateral projection.

1 Anterior inferior cerebellar artery
2 Anterior medullary segment of posterior inferior cerebellar artery
3 Basilar artery
4 Calcarine artery
5 Hemispheric branches of posterior inferior cerebellar artery
6 Inferior vermian segment of posterior inferior cerebellar artery
7 Lateral medullary segment of posterior inferior cerebellar artery
8 Meningeal branch of vertebral artery
9 Origin of posterior inferior cerebellar artery
10 Parieto-occipital artery
11 Posterior cerebral artery
12 Posterior choroidal branches of posterior cerebral artery
13 Posterior medullary segment of posterior inferior cerebellar artery
14 Posterior temporal artery
15 Retrotonsillar segment of posterior inferior cerebellar artery
16 Splenial branches of posterior cerebral artery
17 Superior cerebellar artery
18 Supratonsillar segment of posterior inferior cerebellar artery
19 Thalamoperforate branches of posterior cerebral artery
20 Vertebral artery
21 Vertebral artery exiting transverse foramen of atlas
   (first cervical vertebra)

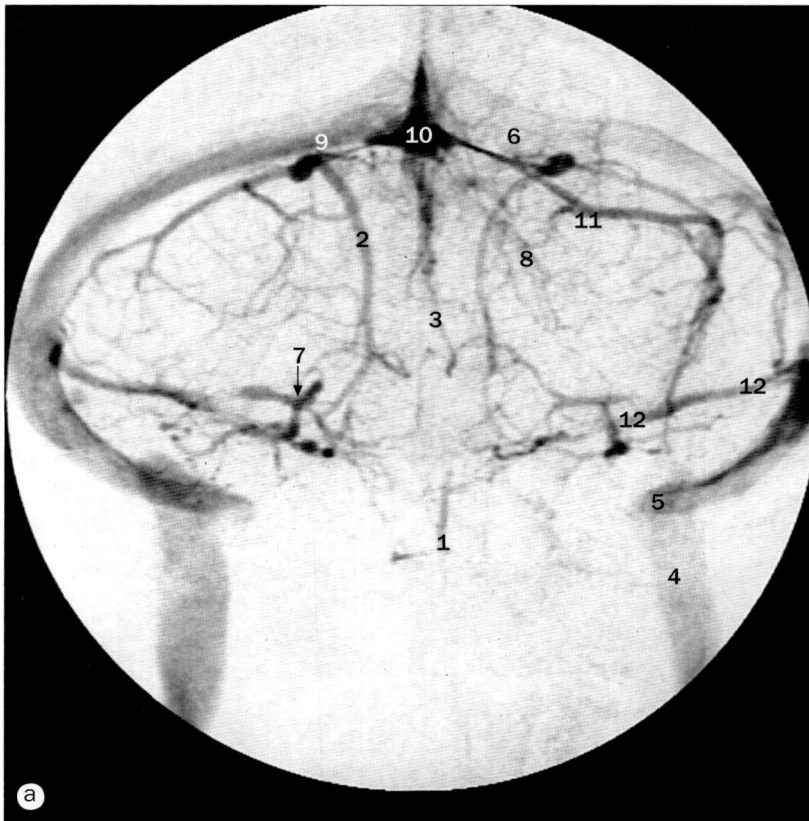

(a) Digitally subtracted venous phase of vertebral arteriogram, anteroposterior projection.

1 Anterior pontomesencephalic vein
2 Inferior hemispheric vein
3 Inferior vermian vein
4 Internal jugular vein
5 Jugular bulb
6 Left transverse sinus
7 Petrosal vein
8 Posterior mesencephalic vein
9 Right transverse sinus
10 Straight sinus
11 Superior hemispheric vein
12 Superior petrosal sinus

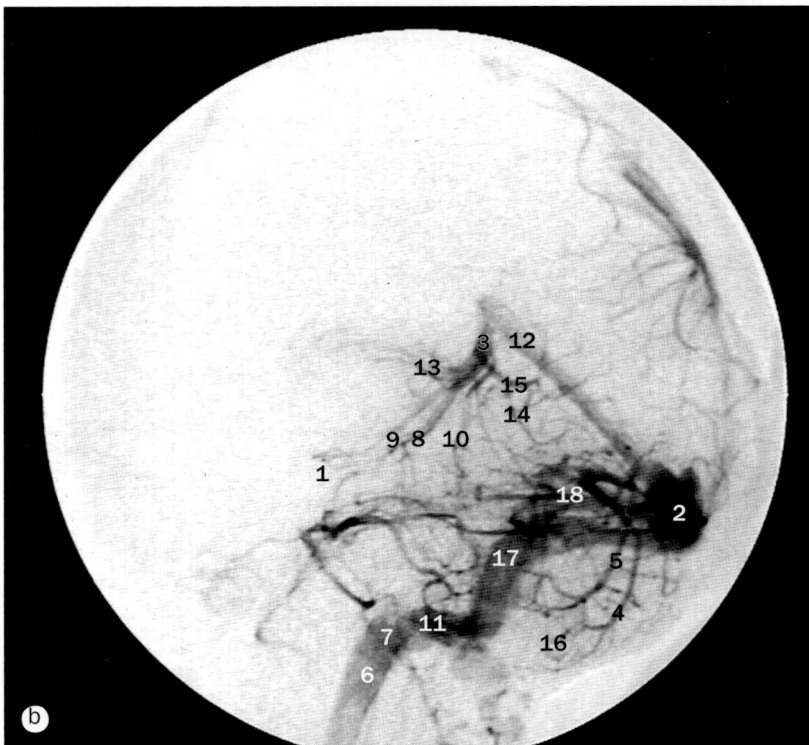

(b) Digitally subtracted venous phase of vertebral arteriogram, lateral projection.

1 Anterior pontomesencephalic vein
2 Confluence of venous sinuses (torcular Herophili)
3 Great cerebral vein of Galen
4 Inferior hemispheric vein
5 Inferior vermian vein
6 Internal jugular vein
7 Jugular bulb
8 Lateral mesencephalic vein
9 Posterior mesencephalic vein
10 Precentral cerebellar vein
11 Sigmoid sinus
12 Straight sinus
13 Superior choroidal vein
14 Superior hemispheric vein
15 Superior vermian vein
16 Tonsillar vein
17 Transverse sinus
18 Vein of the great horizontal fissure

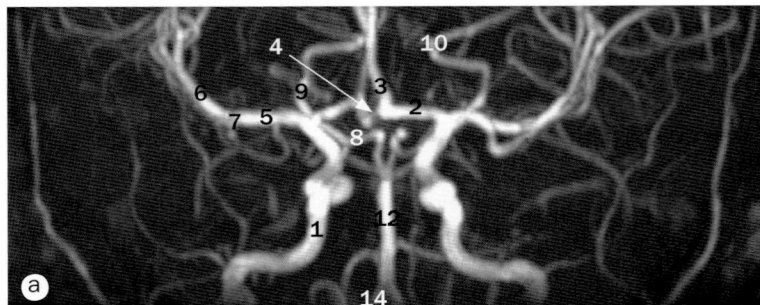

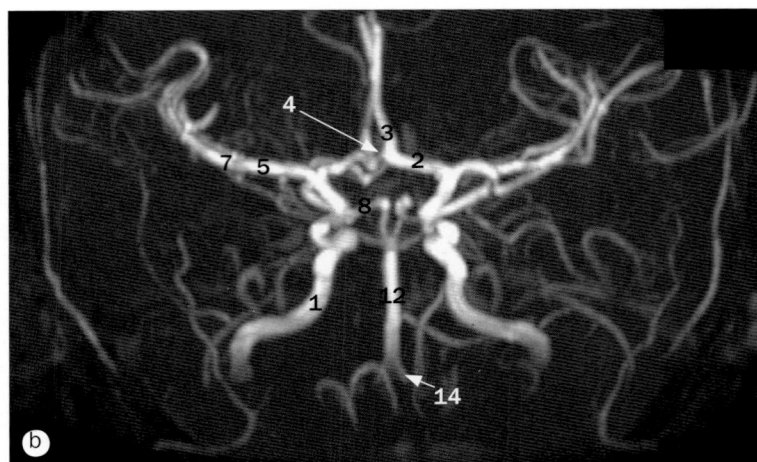

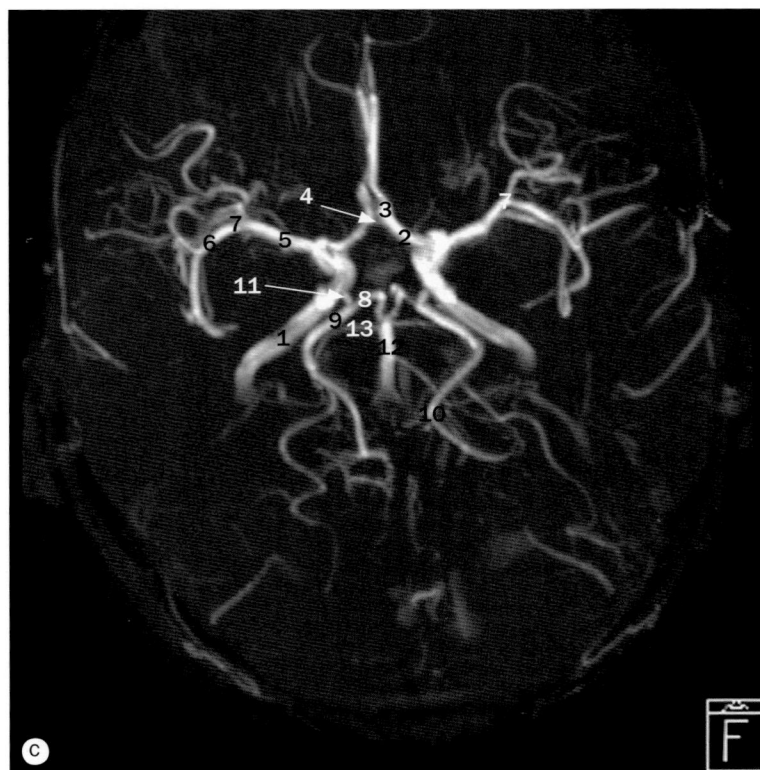

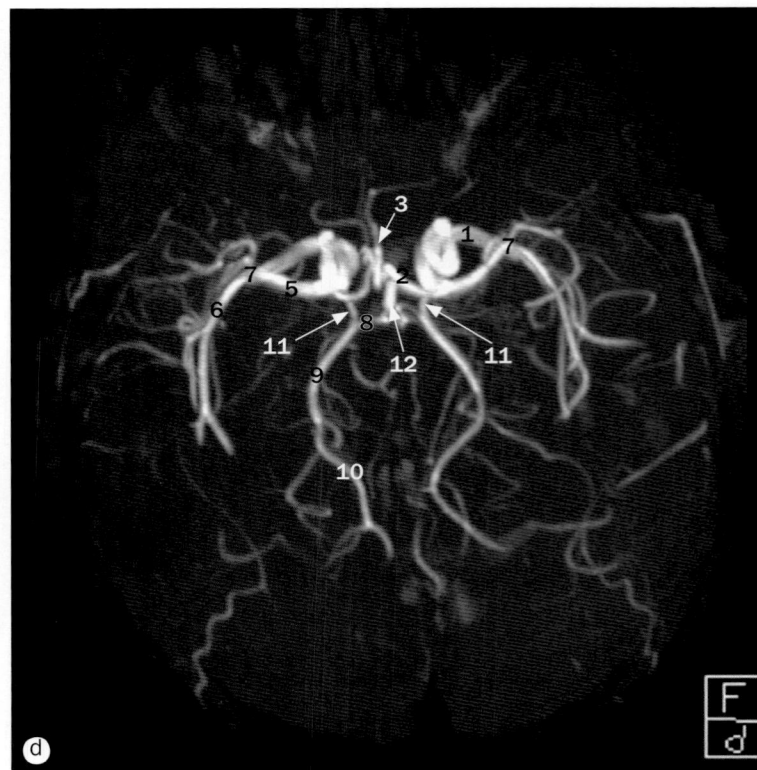

MR angiograms of the Circle of Willis, (a) and (b) coronal, (c) and (d) axial.

1 Internal carotid artery
2 Horizontal (A1) anterior cerebral artery (ACA) segment
3 Vertical (A2) ACA segment
4 Anterior communicating artery
5 Horizontal (M1) middle cerebral artery (MCA) segment
6 Insular (M2) MCA segment
7 MCA genu (bifurcation)
8 Precommunicating (P1) posterior cerebral artery (PCA) segment
9 Ambient (P2) PCA segment
10 Quadrigeminal (P3) PCA segment
11 Posterior communicating artery
12 Basilar artery
13 Superior cerebellar artery
14 Vertebral artery

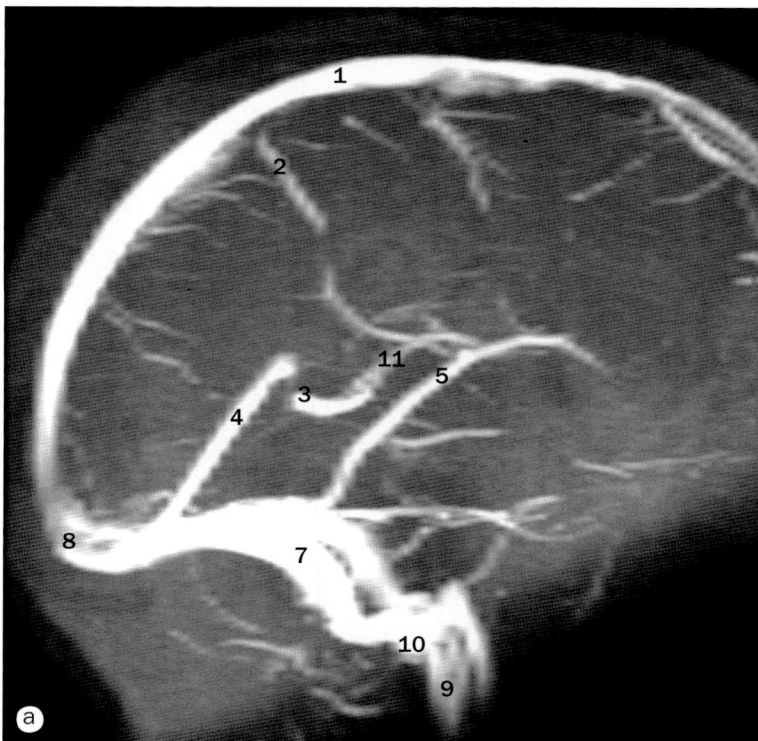

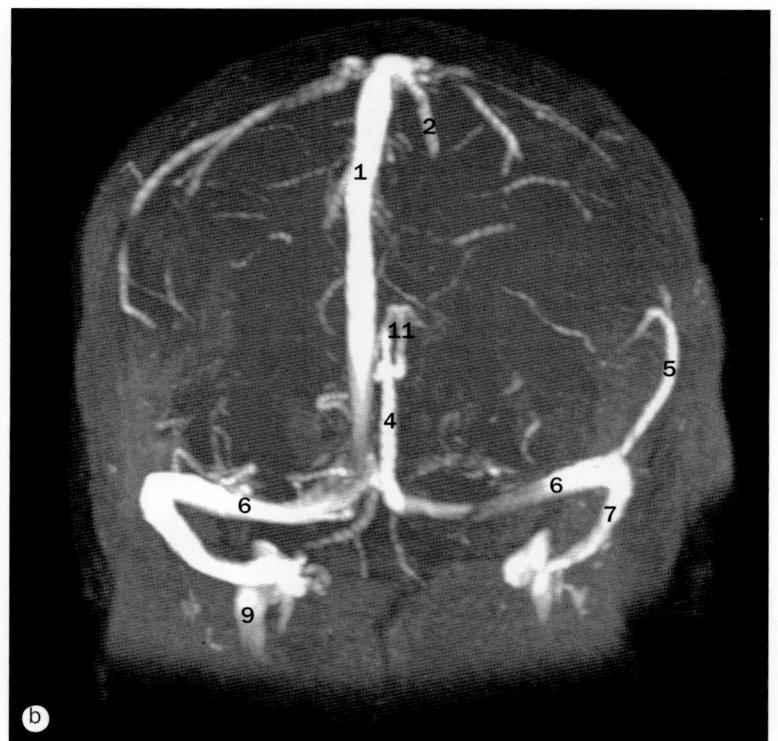

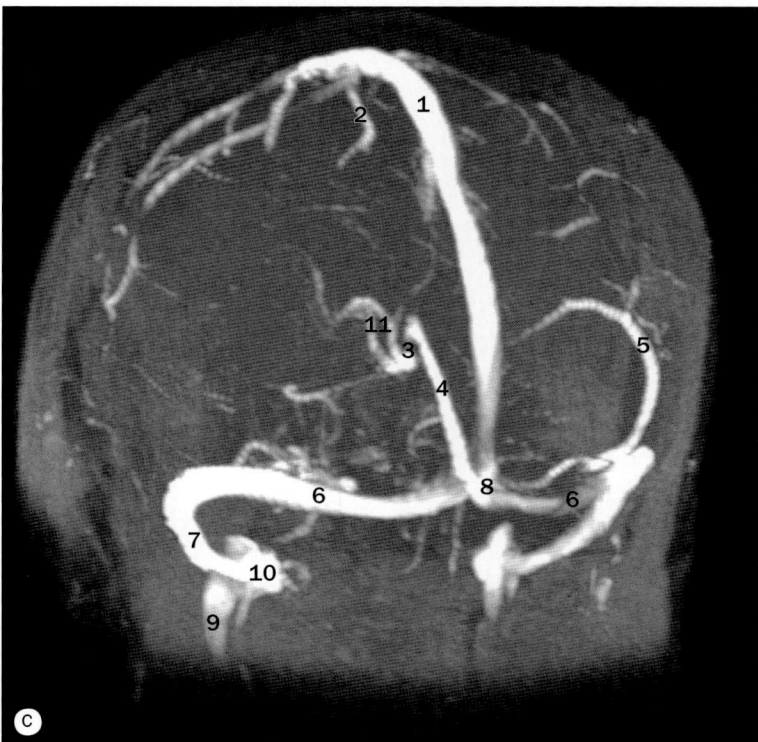

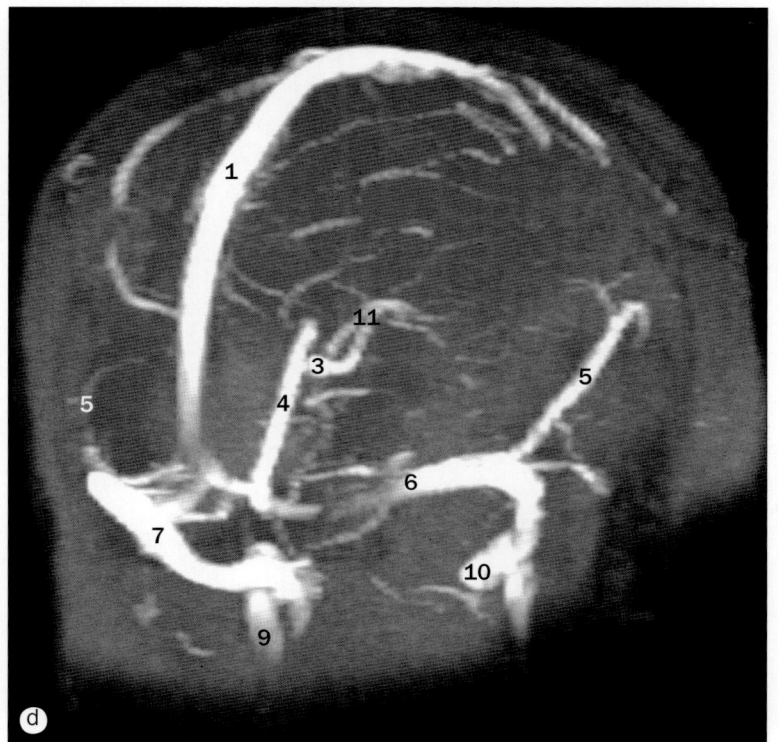

MR images of the venous circulation, (a) lateral view, (b) frontal view, (c) left posterior oblique view, (d) right posterior oblique view.

1 Superior sagittal sinus
2 Superficial cerebral veins
3 Vein of Galen
4 Straight sinus
5 Vein of Labbe'
6 Transverse sinus
7 Sigmoid sinus
8 Sinus confluence (torcular Herophilli)
9 Internal jugular vein
10 Jugular bulb
11 Internal cerebral vein

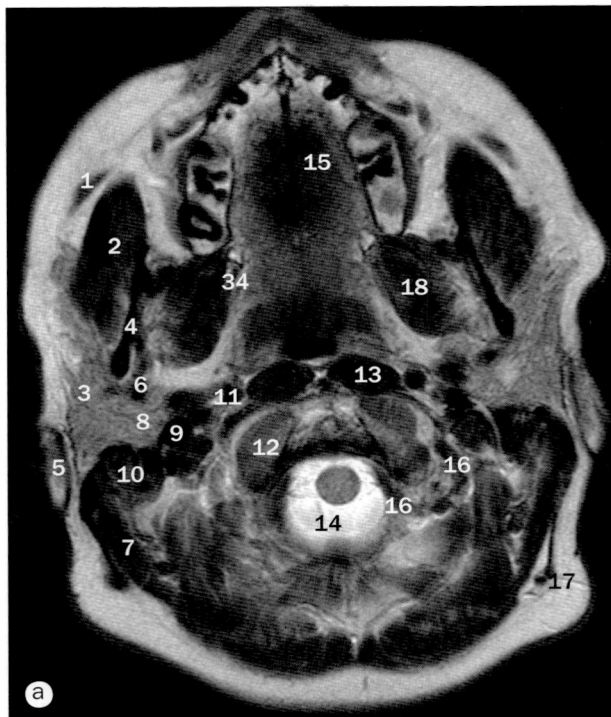

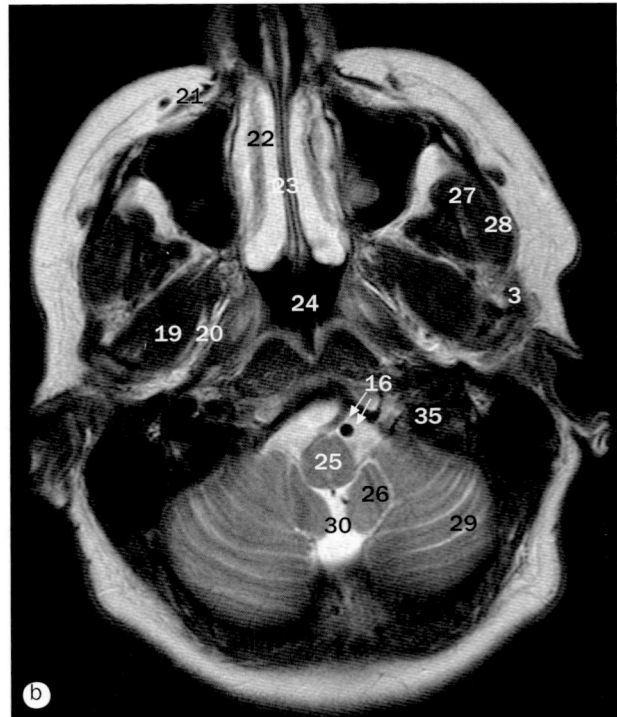

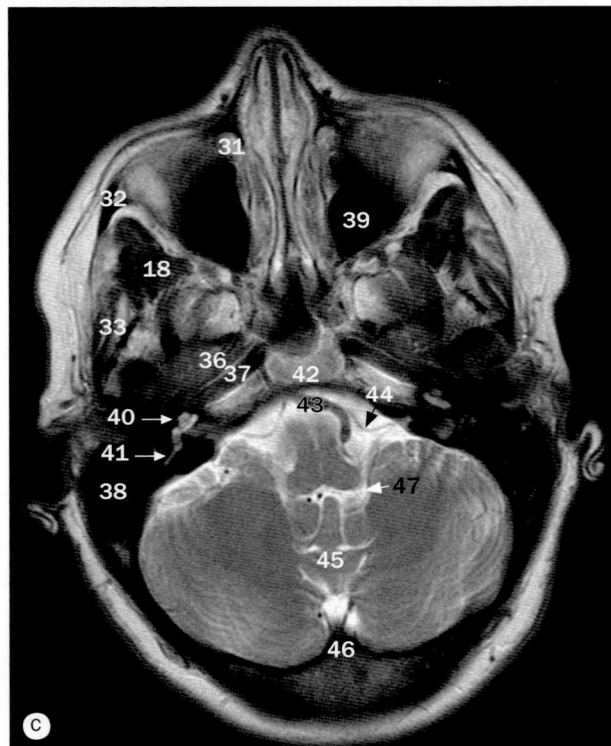

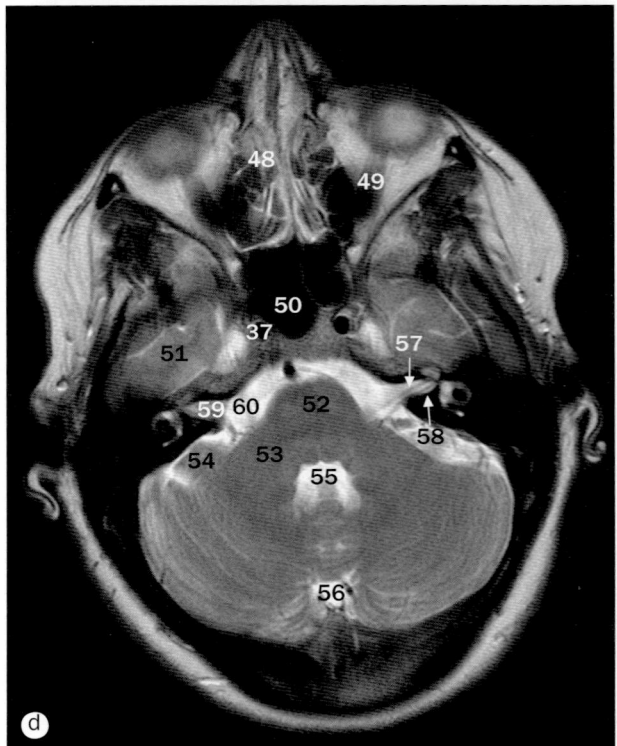

(a)–(n) Brain axial T2 images, from inferior to superior.

1 Parotid duct	9 Internal jugular vein	17 Occipital vessels	24 Nasopharynx
2 Masseter muscle	10 Mastoid process	18 Medial pterygoid muscle	25 Medulla oblongata
3 Parotid gland (superficial lobe)	11 Internal carotid artery	19 Lateral pterygoid muscle	26 Cerebellar tonsil
4 Ramus of mandible	12 Occipital condyle	20 Lateral pterygoid plate	27 Coronoid process of mandible
5 Pinna of ear	13 Longus capitis muscle	21 Levator labii superioris	28 Temporalis muscle
6 Retromandibular vein	14 Foramen magnum	alaeque nasi muscle	29 Folia of cerebellar hemisphere
7 Sternocleidomastoid muscle	15 Hard palate	22 Inferior turbinate	30 Foramen of Magendie
8 Parotid gland (deep lobe)	16 Vertebral artery	23 Nasal septum	

Numbers 1–161 are common to pages 42–45.

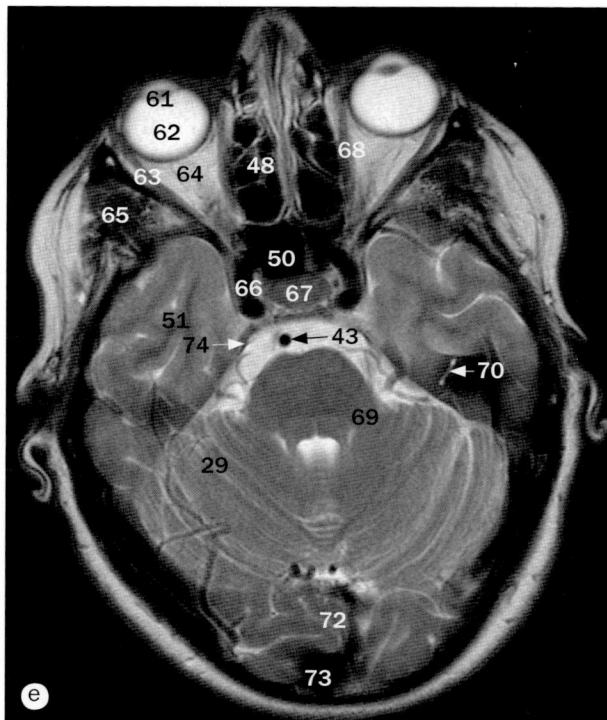

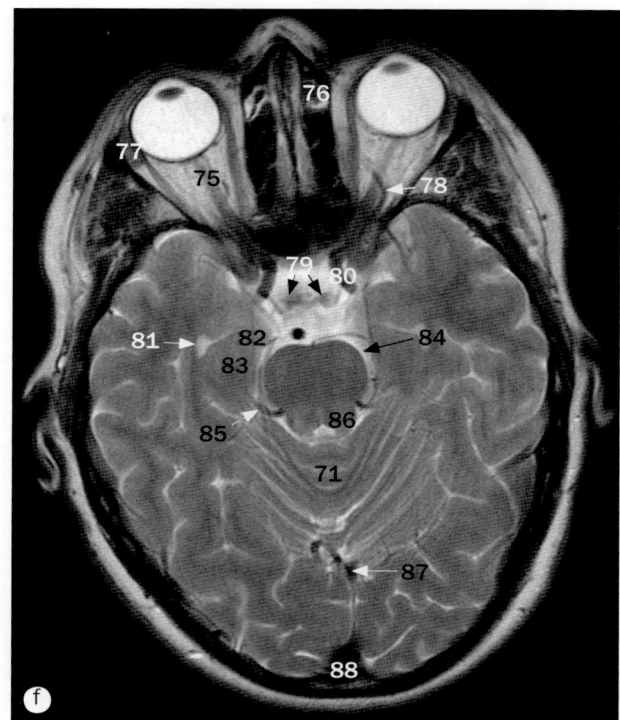

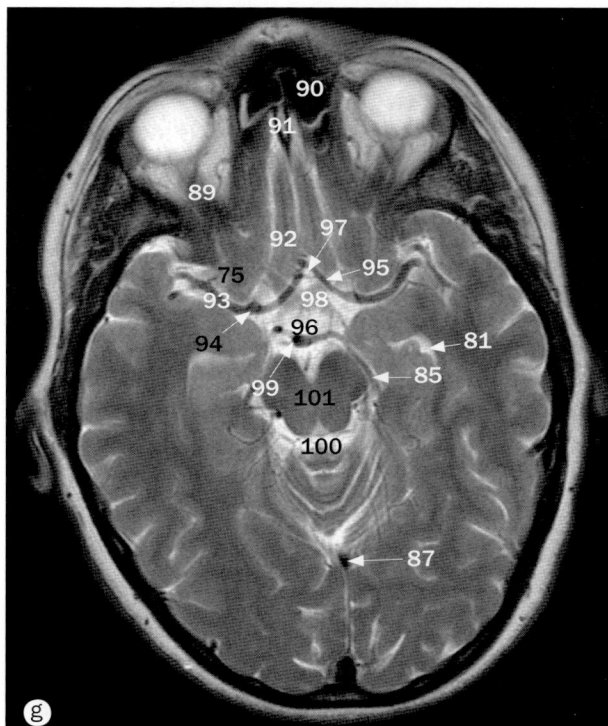

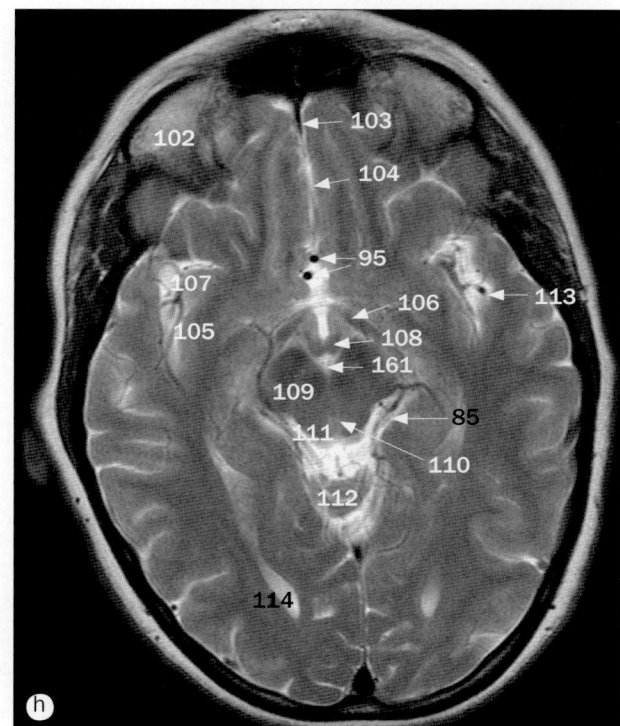

(a)–(n) Brain axial T2 images, from inferior to superior.

31 Nasolacrimal duct	**40** Cochlear	**48** Ethmoid air cells	**56** Cisterna magna
32 Zygomatic arch	**41** Posterior semicircular canal	**49** Inferior rectus muscle	**57** Facial nerve (seventh cranial nerve)
33 Head of mandible	**42** Clivus	**50** Sphenoid sinus	
34 Medial pterygoid plate	**43** Basilar artery	**51** Temporal lobe	**58** Vestibulocochlear nerve (eighth cranial nerve)
35 Jugular foramen	**44** Labyrinthine artery	**52** Pons	
36 Petrous temporal bone	**45** Inferior cerebellar vermis	**53** Middle cerebellar peduncle	**59** Internal auditory meatus
37 Internal carotid artery	**46** Inion (internal occipital protuberance)	**54** Flocculonodular lobe of cerebellum	**60** Cerebellopontine angle
38 Mastoid air cells			
39 Maxillary sinus (antrum)	**47** Foramen of Lushka	**55** Fourth ventricle	

Numbers 1–161 are common to pages 42–45.

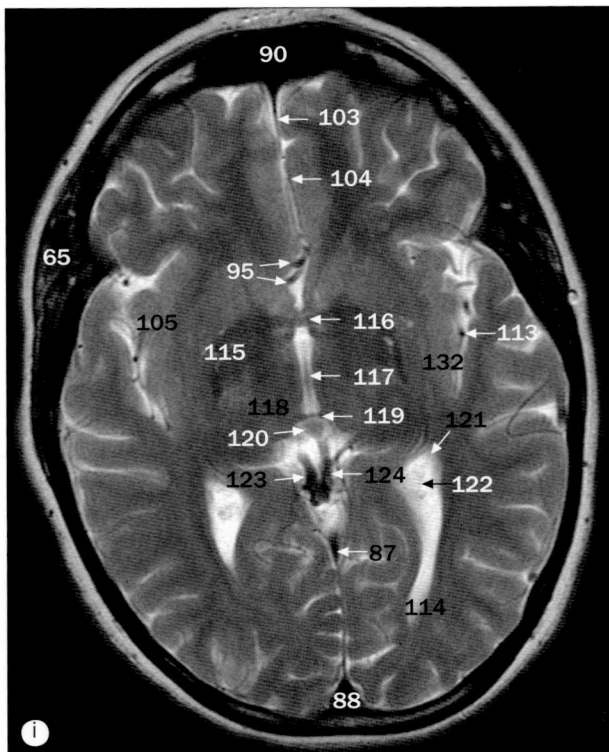

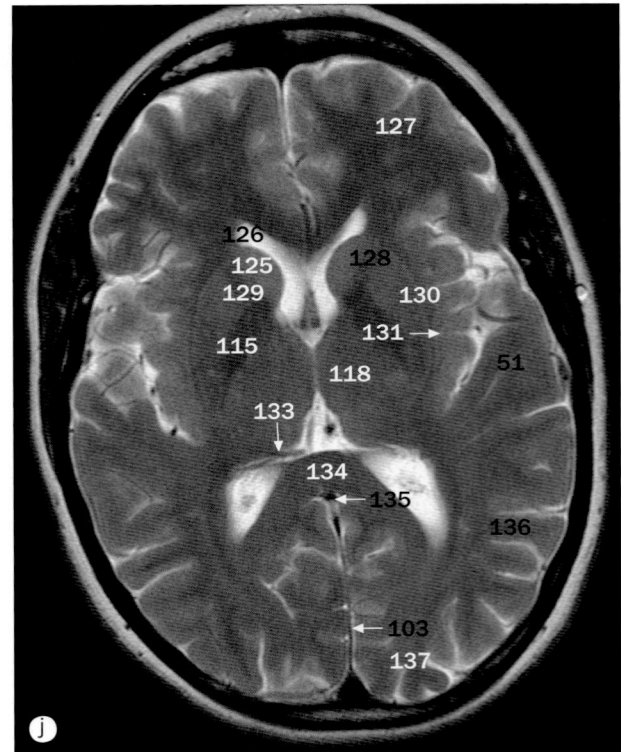

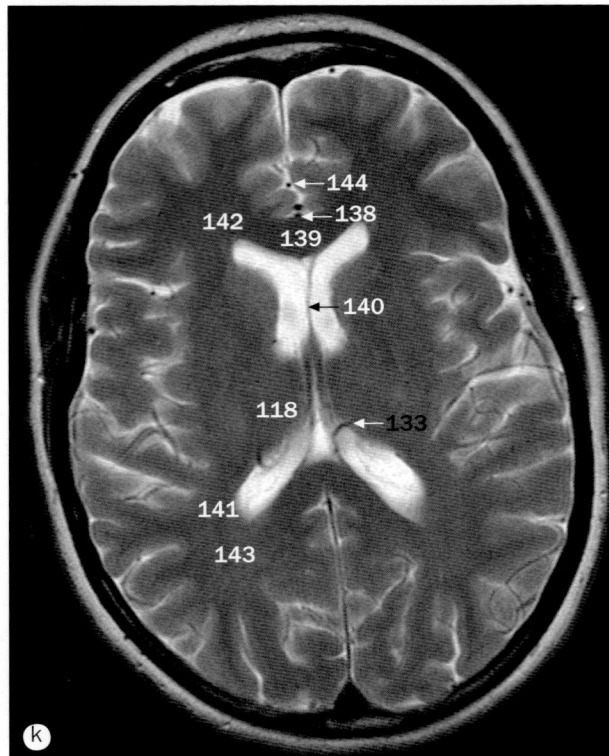

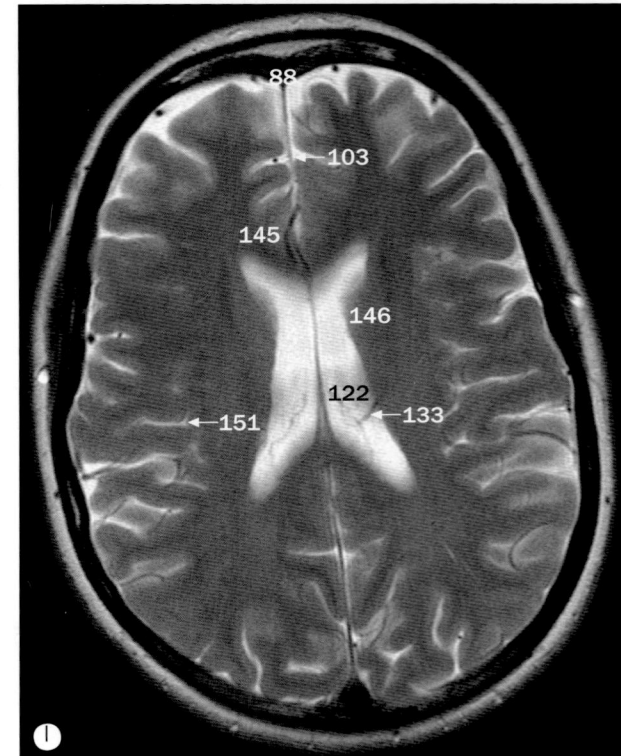

(a)–(n) Brain axial T2 images, from inferior to superior.

61 Lens	67 Body of sphenoid	73 Torcula herophili (confluence of venous sinuses)	78 Superior ophthalmic vein
62 Vitreous humour	68 Medial rectus muscle		79 Pituitary gland
63 Lateral rectus muscle	69 Superior cerebellar peduncle	74 Petroclinoid ligament	80 Internal carotid artery (supraclinoid part)
64 Retro-orbital fat	70 Superior semicircular canal	75 Optic nerve (second cranial nerve)	
65 Temporalis muscle	71 Superior cerebellar vermis		81 Temporal horn of lateral ventricle
66 Internal carotid artery (cavernous part)	72 Calcarine cortex of occipital lobe	76 Infundibulum of frontal sinus	
		77 Lacrimal gland	82 Uncus of temporal lobe

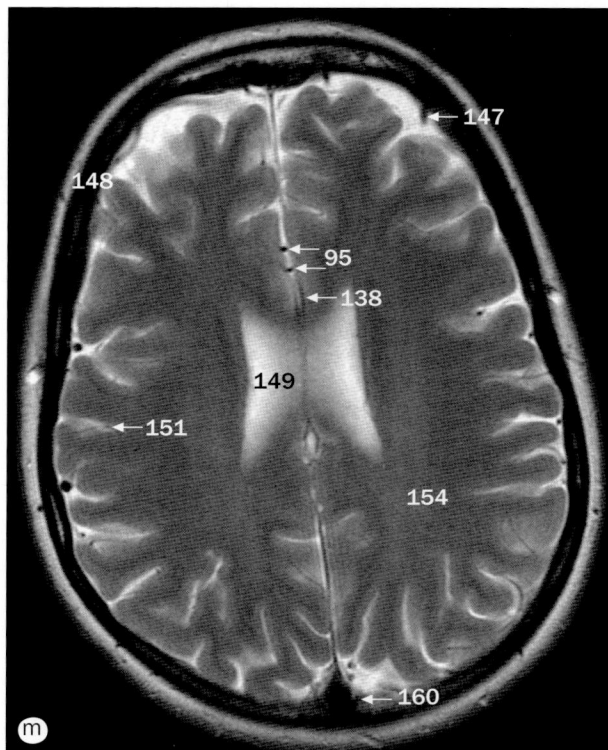

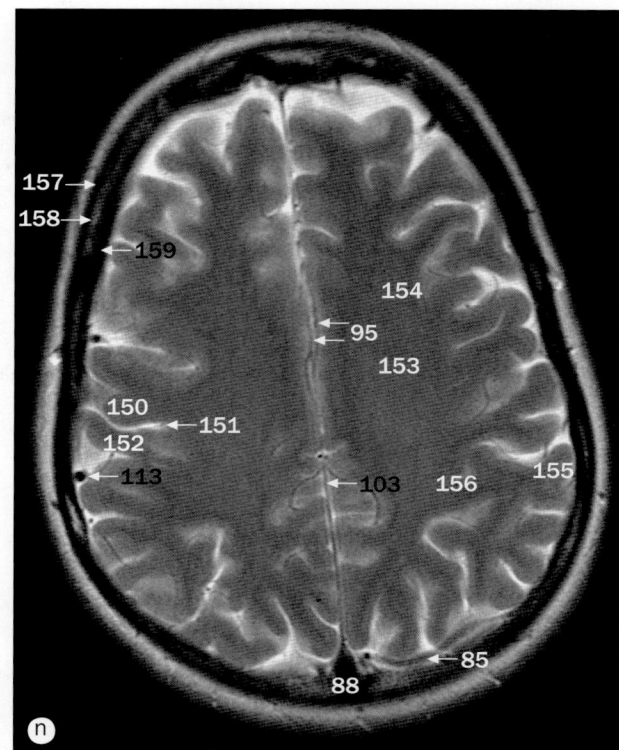

(a)–(n) Brain axial T2 images, from inferior to superior.

83 Hippocampus	103 Falx cerebri	121 Trigone of lateral ventricle	140 Septum pellucidum
84 Ambient cistern	104 Interhemispheric fissure	122 Choroid plexus	141 Optic radiation
85 Posterior cerebral artery	105 Insular gyri	123 Basal vein (of Rosenthal)	142 Forceps minor
86 Inferior colliculus	106 Optic tract	124 Internal cerebral vein (of Galen)	143 Forceps major
87 Straight sinus	107 Sylvian fissure (lateral sulcus)	125 Head of caudate nucleus	144 Frontopolar artery
88 Superior sagittal sinus	108 Mamillary body (of hypothalamus)	126 Frontal horn of lateral ventricle	145 Cingulate gyrus
89 Superior rectus muscle	109 Cerebral peduncle	127 Frontal lobe	146 Body of caudate nucleus
90 Frontal sinus	110 Aqueduct of Sylvius	128 Anterior limb of internal capsule	147 Cortical vein
91 Crista gali	111 Superior colliculus	129 Globus pallidus	148 Calvarium of skull
92 Olfactory nerve (first cranial nerve)	112 Folia of cerebellum	130 Putamen	149 Body (atrium) of lateral ventricle
93 Middle cerebral artery	113 Middle cerebral artery (second order branch)	131 External capsule	150 Precentral gyrus
94 Bifurcation of internal carotid artery	114 Occipital horn of lateral ventricle	132 Claustrum	151 Central sulcus of Rolando
95 Anterior cerebral artery	115 Posterior limb of internal capsule	133 Choroidal vessels	152 Post central gyrus
96 Suprasellar cistern	116 Anterior commisure	134 Splenium of corpus callosum	153 Centrum semiovale
97 Anterior communicating artery	117 Third ventricle	135 Inferior sagittal sinus	154 Corona radiata
98 Optic chiasma	118 Thalamus	136 Parietal lobe	155 Grey matter
99 Basilar artery bifurcation	119 Posterior commisure	137 Occipital lobe	156 White matter
100 Quadrigeminal cistern	120 Pineal gland	138 Callosomarginal artery	157 Outer table of calvarium
101 Midbrain (mesencephalon)		139 Genu of corpus callosum	158 Diploe
102 Orbital plate of frontal bone			159 Inner table of calvarium
			160 Arachnoid granulation
			161 Interpeduncular cistern

Numbers 1–161 are common to pages 42–45.

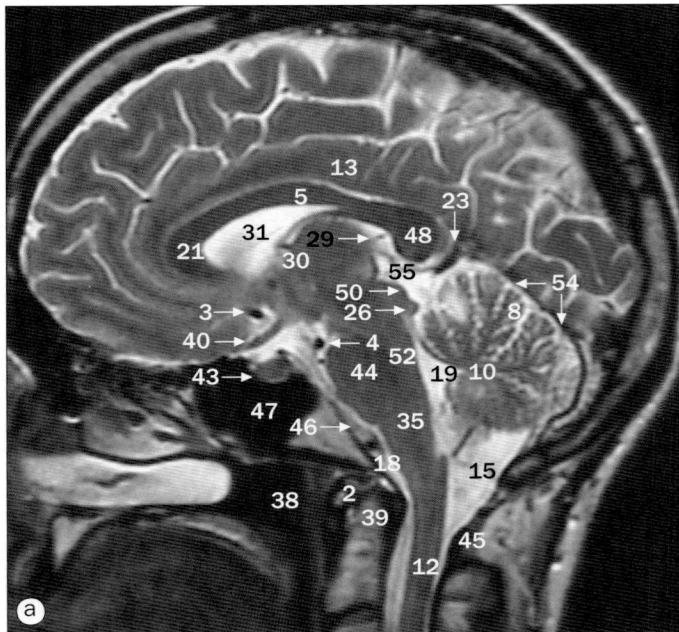

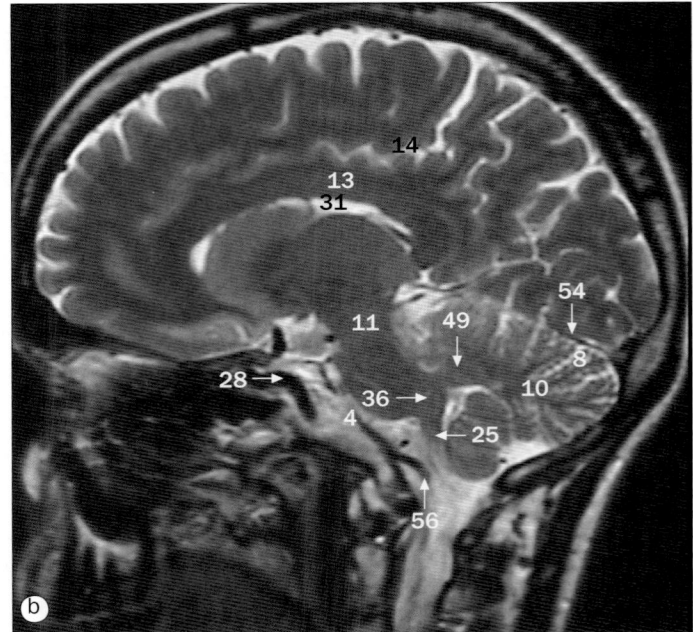

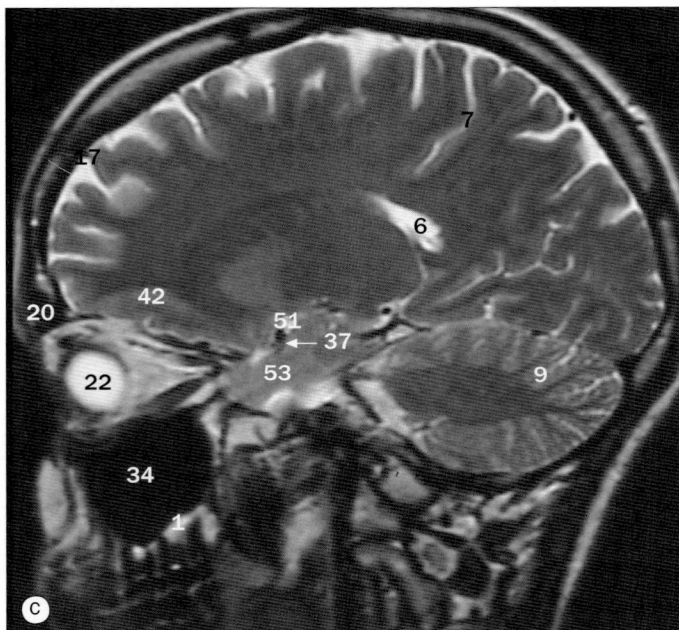

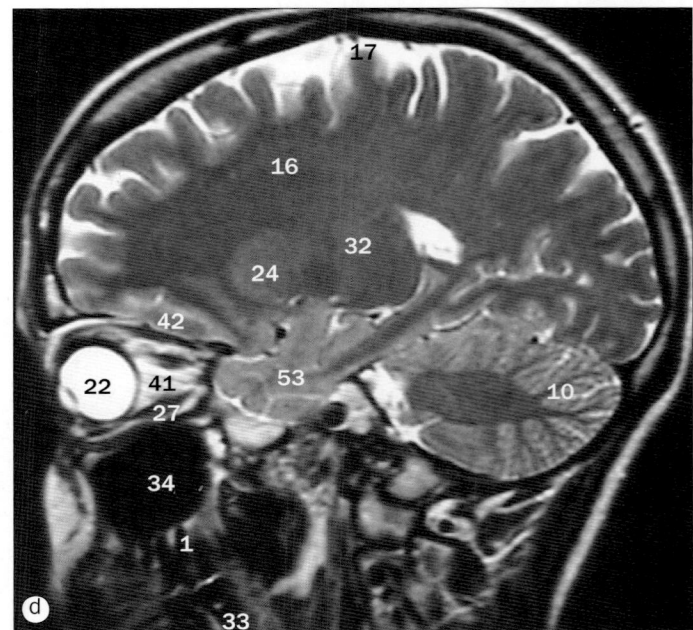

(a)–(d) Brain, sagittal MR images.

1 Alveolar ridge	15 Cisterna magna (cerebellomedullary cistern)	29 Internal cerebral vein	42 Orbital cortex of frontal lobe
2 Anterior arch of atlas (first cervical vertebra)	16 Corona radiata	30 Interventricular foramen of Monro	43 Pituitary gland
3 Anterior cerebral artery	17 Cortical vein	31 Lateral ventricle	44 Pons
4 Basilar artery	18 Foramen magnum	32 Lentiform nucleus	45 Posterior arch of atlas
5 Body of corpus callosum	19 Fourth ventricle	33 Mandible	46 Prepontine cistern
6 Body of lateral ventricle	20 Frontal sinus	34 Maxillary sinus (antrum)	47 Sphenoidal sinus
7 Central sulcus of Rolando	21 Genu of corpus callosum	35 Medulla oblongata	48 Splenium of corpus callosum
8 Cerebellar folia	22 Globe	36 Middle cerebellar peduncle	49 Superior cerebellar peduncle
9 Cerebellar hemisphere	23 Great cerebral vein of Galen	37 Middle cerebral artery	50 Superior colliculus
10 Cerebellum	24 Head of caudate nucleus	38 Nasopharynx	51 Sylvian fissure
11 Cerebral peduncle	25 Inferior cerebellar peduncle	39 Odontoid process (dens)	52 Tegmentum of pons
12 Cervical spinal cord	26 Inferior colliculus	40 Optic chiasma in suprasellar cistern	53 Temporal lobe of brain
13 Cingulate gyrus	27 Inferior rectus muscle	41 Optic nerve	54 Tentorium cerebelli
14 Cingulate sulcus	28 Internal carotid artery (in cavernous sinus)		55 Pineal gland
			56 Vertebral artery

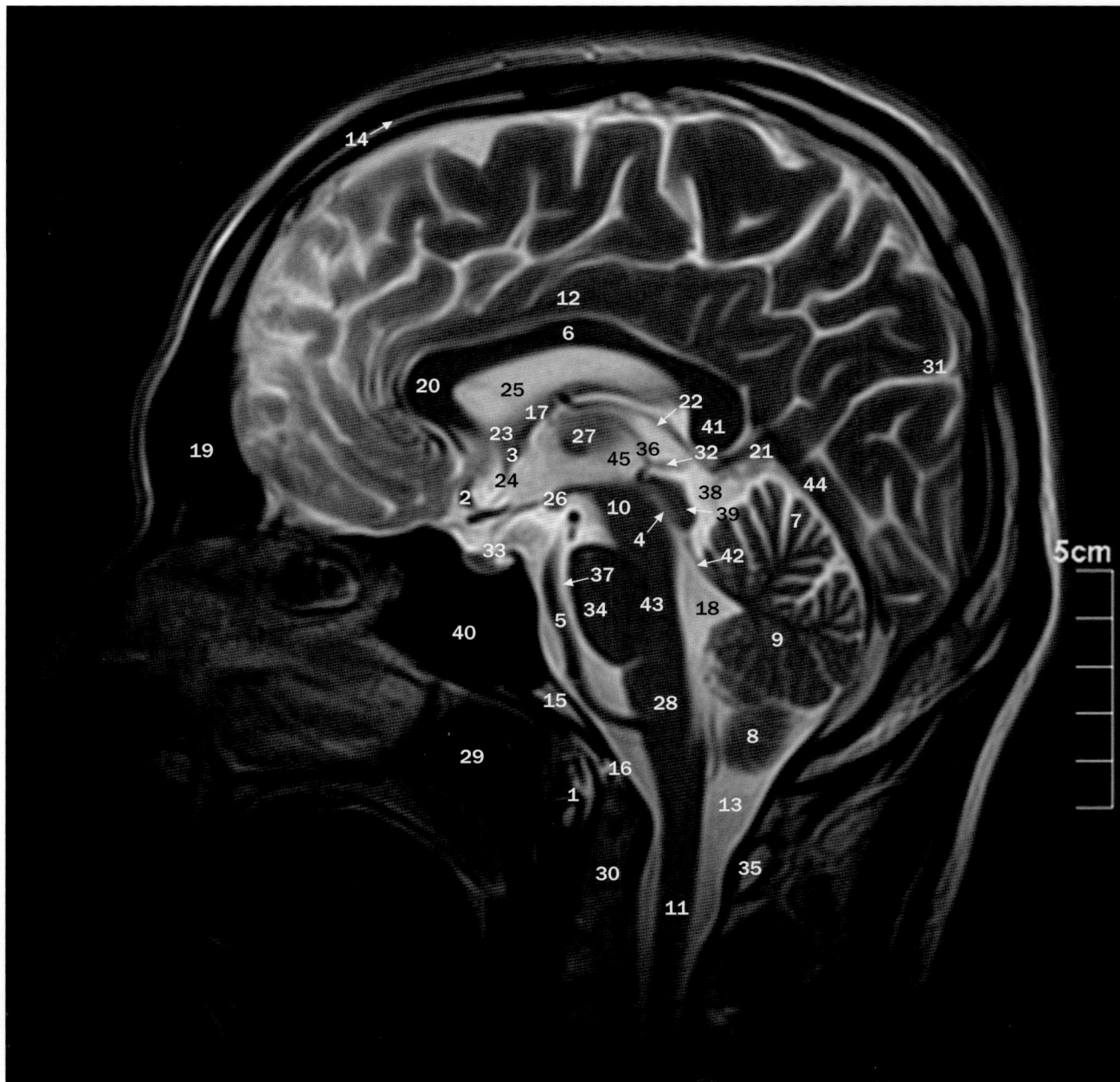

Brain, sagittal MR midline image.

1 Anterior arch of atlas (first cervical vertebra)	15 Fat in marrow of clivus	31 Parieto-occipital fissure
2 Anterior cerebral artery	16 Foramen magnum	32 Pineal gland
3 Anterior commissure	17 Fornix	33 Pituitary gland
4 Aqueduct of Sylvius	18 Fourth ventricle	34 Pons
5 Basilar artery	19 Frontal sinus	35 Posterior arch of atlas
6 Body of corpus callosum	20 Genu of corpus callosum	36 Posterior commissure
7 Cerebellar folia	21 Great cerebral vein of Galen	37 Prepontine cistern
8 Cerebellar tonsil	22 Internal cerebral vein	38 Quadrigeminal cistern
9 Cerebellum	23 Interventricular foramen of Monro	39 Quadrigeminal plate (tectum) of midbrain
10 Cerebral peduncle of midbrain	24 Lamina terminalis	40 Spheroidal sinus
11 Cervical spinal cord	25 Lateral ventricle	41 Splenium of corpus callosum
12 Cingulate gyrus	26 Mammillary body	42 Superior medullary velum
13 Cisterna magna (cerebellomedullary cistern)	27 Massa intermedia of thalamus	43 Tegmentum of pons
14 Diploe of calvarium	28 Medulla oblongata	44 Tentorium cerebelli
	29 Nasopharynx	45 Third ventricle
	30 Odontoid process (dens)	

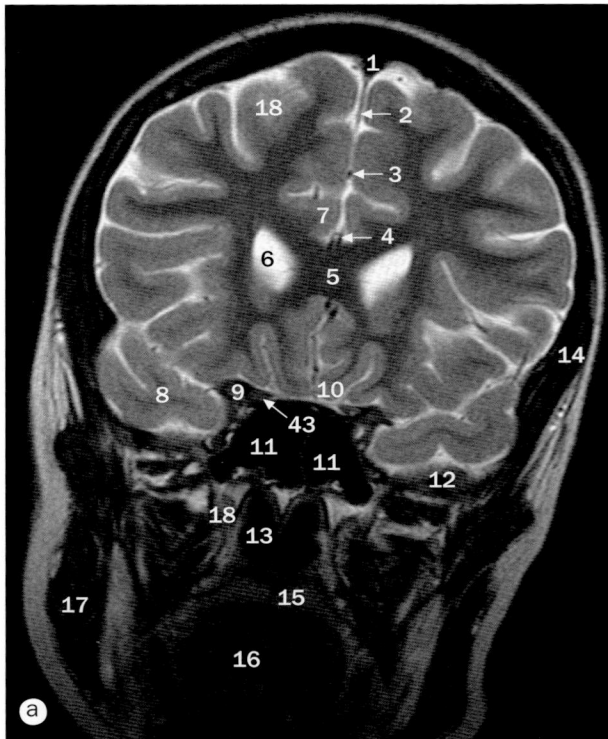

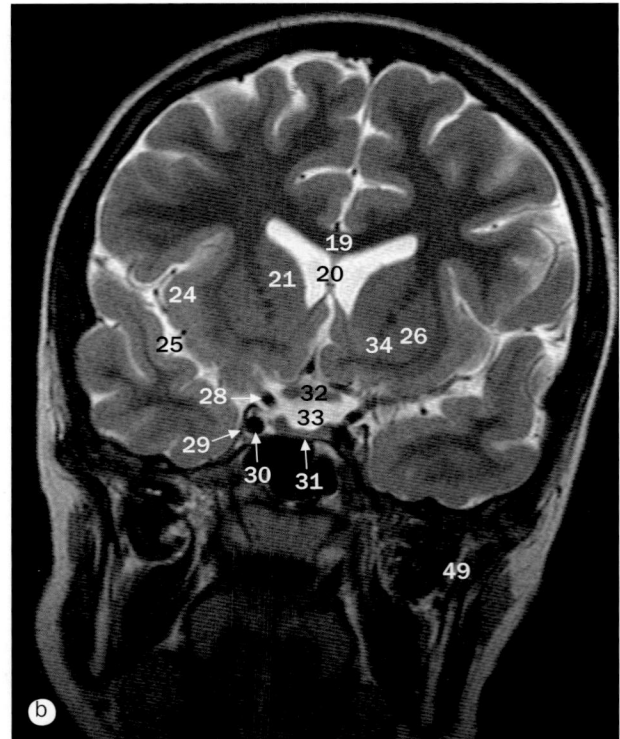

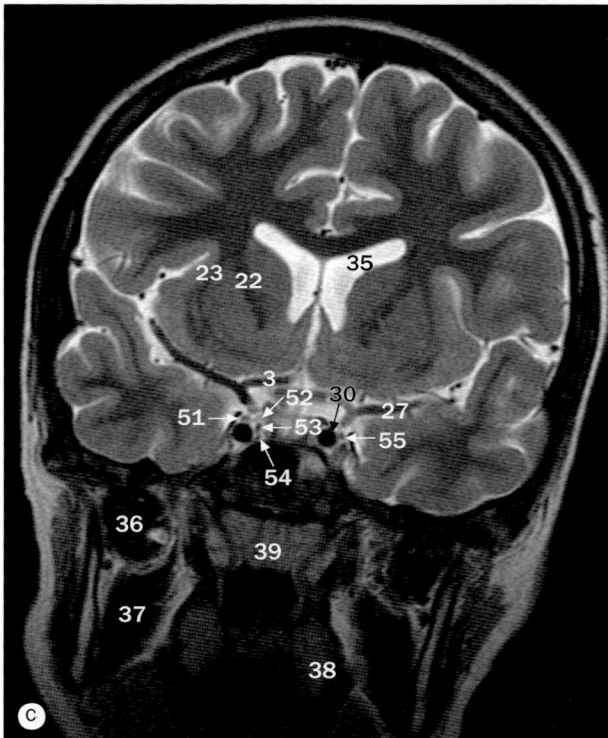

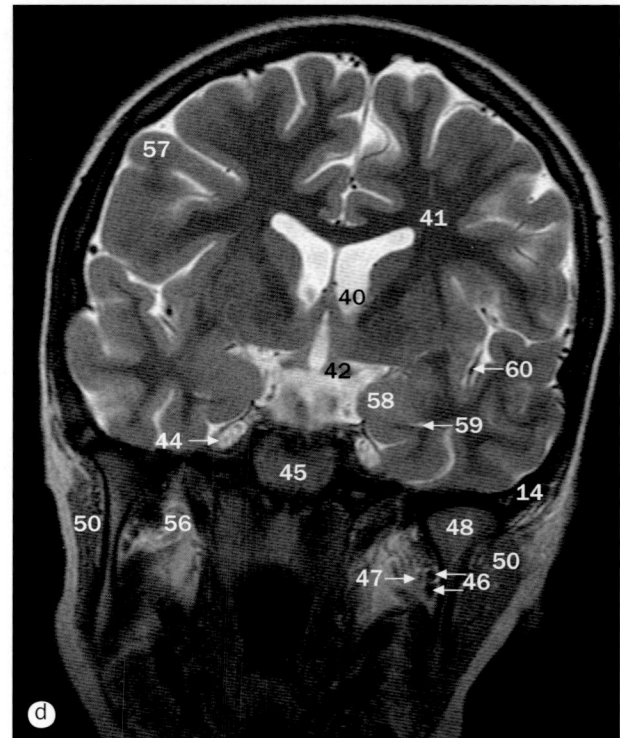

(a)–(p) Brain, coronal T2w MR images, from anterior to posterior.

1 Superior sagittal sinus	9 Anterior clinoid process	18 Frontal lobe	26 Putamen
2 Falx cerebri	10 Olfactory cortex	19 Body of corpus callosum	27 Middle cerebral artery
3 Anterior cerebral artery	11 Sphenoidal sinus	20 Septum pellucidum	28 Supraclinoid part of internal
4 Callosomarginal artery	12 Greater wing of sphenoid	21 Head of caudate nucleus	carotid artery
5 Genu of corpus callosum	13 Nasopharynx	22 Anterior limb of internal	29 Dural lateral wall of
6 Frontal horn of lateral	14 Temporalis muscle	capsule	cavernous sinus
ventricle	15 Hard palate	23 External capsule	30 Internal carotid artery
7 Cingulate gyrus	16 Oropharynx	24 Insula gyrus	31 Pituitary gland
8 Temporal lobe	17 Masseter muscle	25 Sylvian fissure (lateral sulcus)	32 Optic chiasma

Numbers 1–130 are common to pages 48–51.

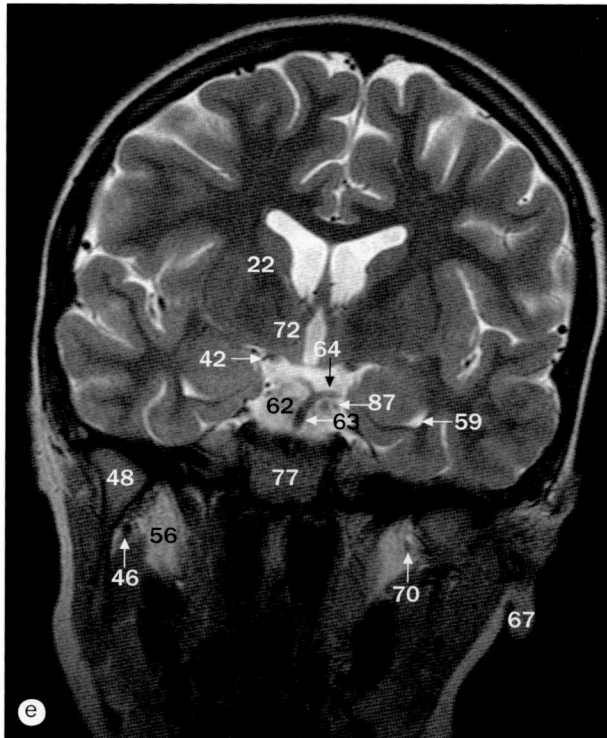

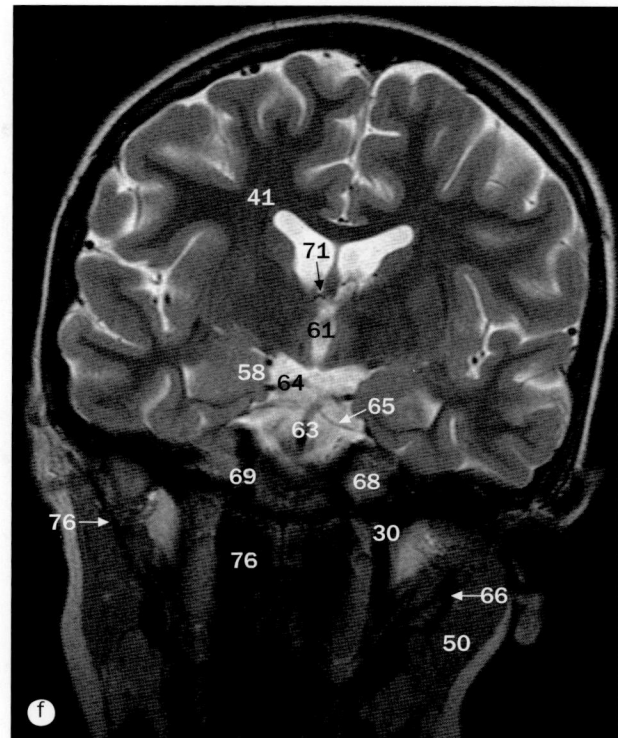

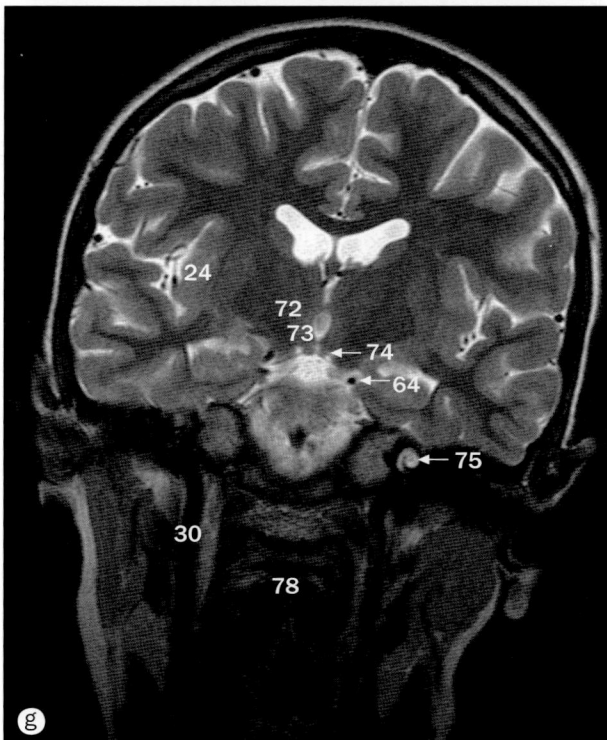

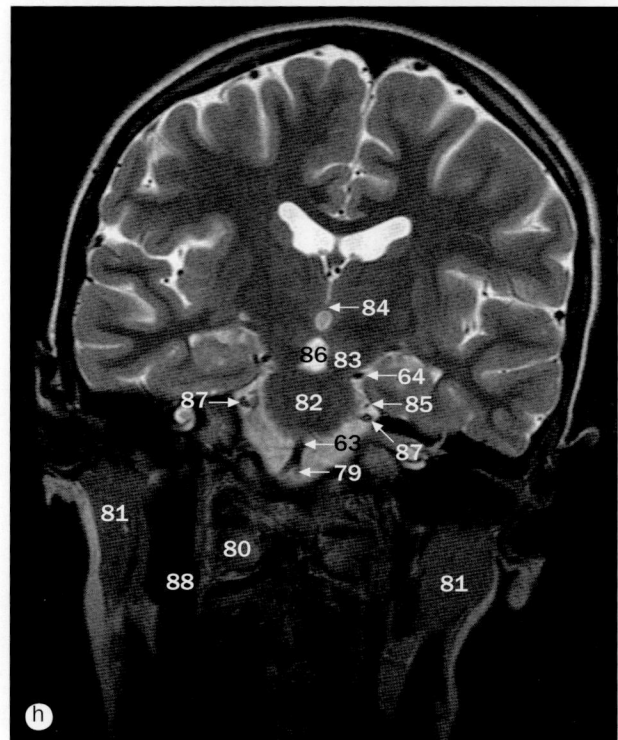

(a)–(p) Brain, coronal T2w MR images, from anterior to posterior.

33 Suprasellar cistern	**42** Optic tract
34 Globus pallidus	**43** Optic nerve (second cranial nerve)
35 Body (atrium) of lateral ventricle	**44** Trigeminal ganglion in Meckel's cave
36 Lateral pterygoid muscle	**45** Body of sphenoid
37 Medial pterygoid muscle	**46** Inferior alveolar vessels
38 Tongue	**47** Inferior alveolar nerve
39 Soft palate	**48** Head of mandible
40 Choroid plexus	**49** Coronoid process of mandible
41 Corona radiata	

50 Parotid gland	**55** Abducens nerve (sixth cranial nerve)
51 Occulomotor nerve (third cranial nerve)	**56** Infratemporal fossa
52 Trochlear nerve (fourth cranial nerve)	**57** Parietal lobe
53 Ophthalmic nerve (fifth cranial nerve, first division)	**58** Hippocampus
54 Maxillary nerve (fifth cranial nerve, second division)	**59** Temporal horn of lateral ventricle
	60 Middle cerebral artery (second order branch)
	61 Third ventricle

Numbers 1–130 are common to pages 48–51.

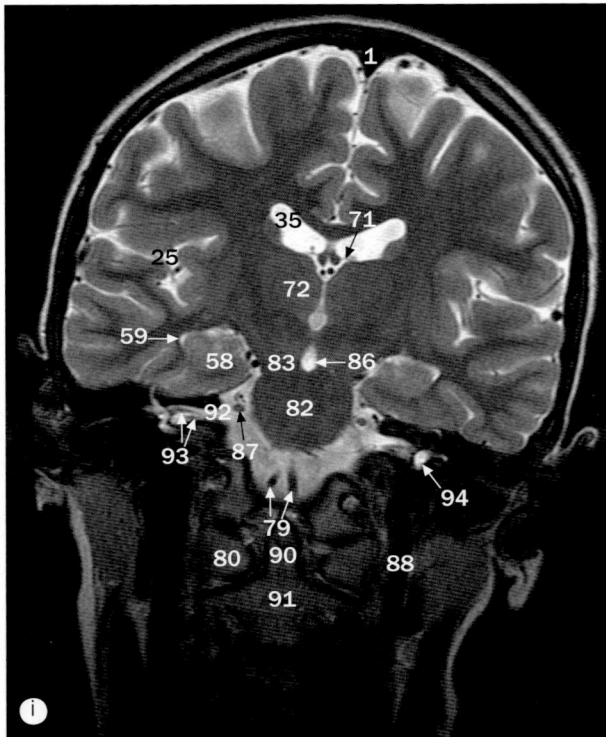

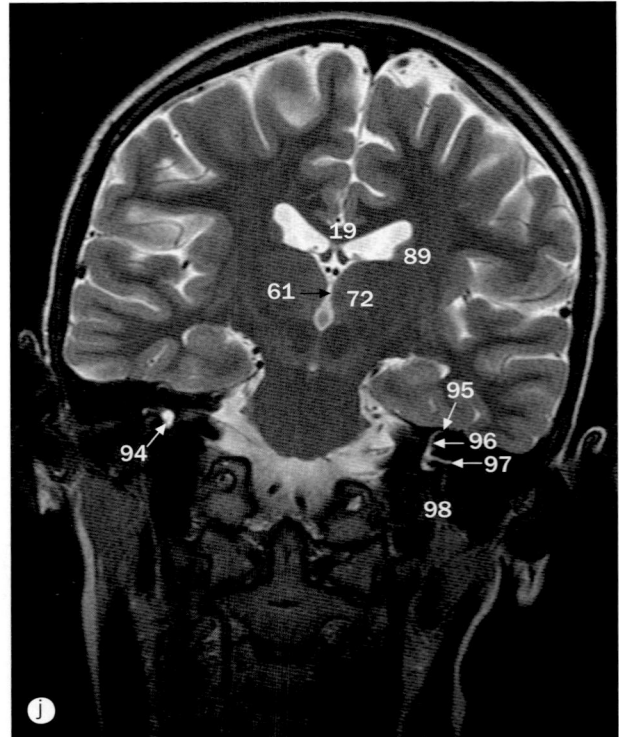

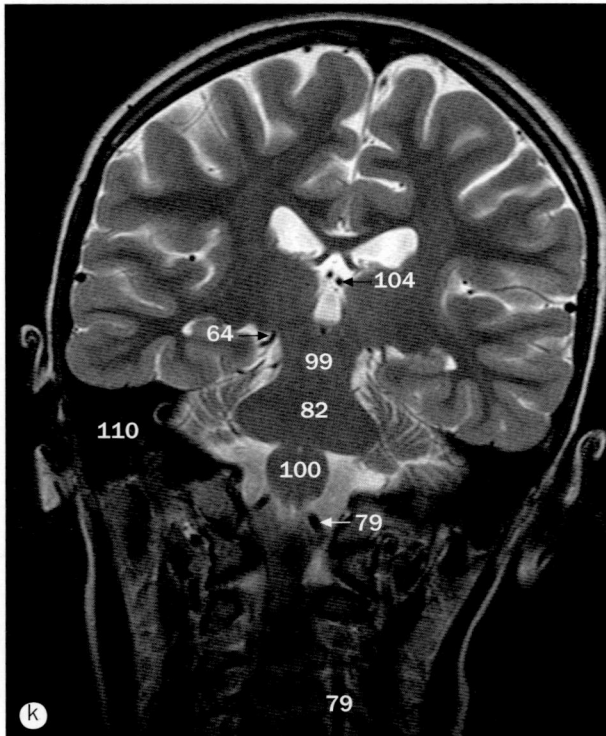

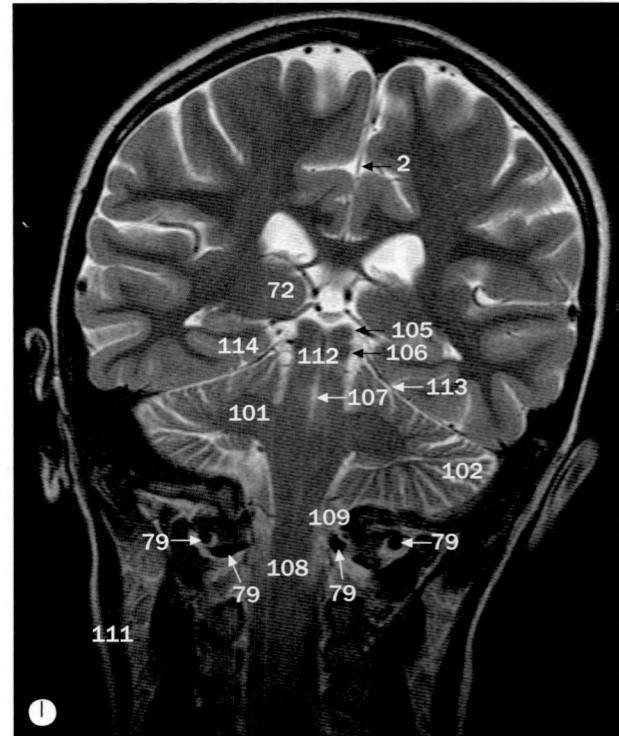

(a)–(p) Brain, coronal T2w MR images, from anterior to posterior.

62 Prepontine cistern	72 Thalamus	82 Pons	90 Odontoid peg of C2
63 Basilar artery	73 Hypothalamus	83 Cerebral peduncle	91 Body of C2
64 Posterior cerebral artery	74 Mamillary body (of	84 Massa intermedia of	92 Internal auditory meatus
65 Superior cerebellar artery	hypothalamus)	thalamus	93 Facial (seventh) and
66 Retromandibular vein	75 Cochlea	85 Abducens nerve (sixth cranial	vestibulocochlear (eighth)
67 Tragus of external ear	76 Pharyngobasilar raphe	nerve) in ambient cistern	nerves
68 Basiocciput	77 Basisphenoid	86 Interpeduncular cistern	94 Vestibule of vestibular
69 Spheno-occipital	78 Anterior arch of C1	87 Trigeminal nerve (fifth cranial	apparatus
synchondrosis	79 Vertebral artery	nerve)	95 Arcuate eminence of petrous
70 Auriculotemporal nerve	80 Lateral mass of C1	88 Internal jugular vein	temporal bone
71 Foramen of Monro	81 Sternocleidomastoid muscle	89 Body of caudate nucleus	96 Superior semicircular canal

Numbers 1–130 are common to pages 48–51.

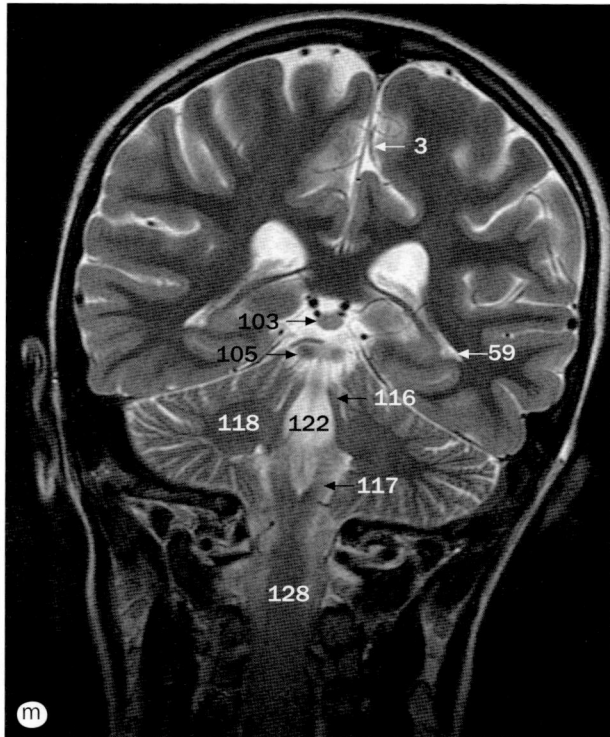

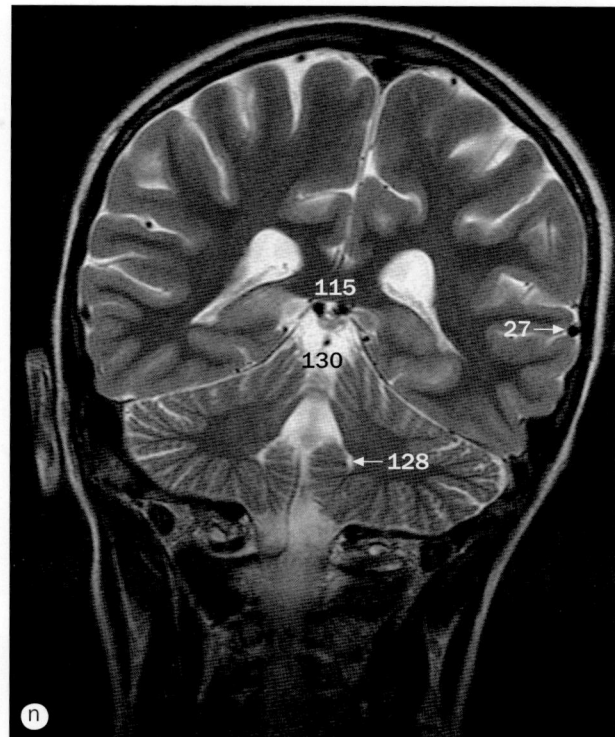

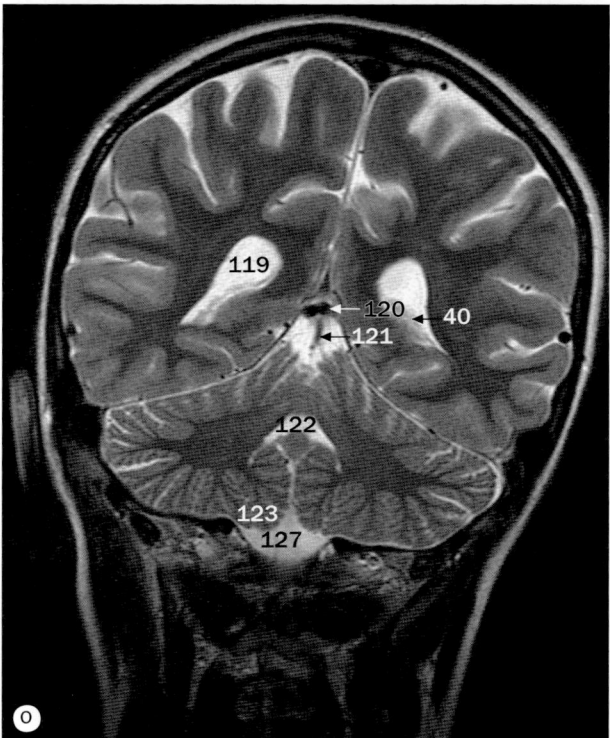

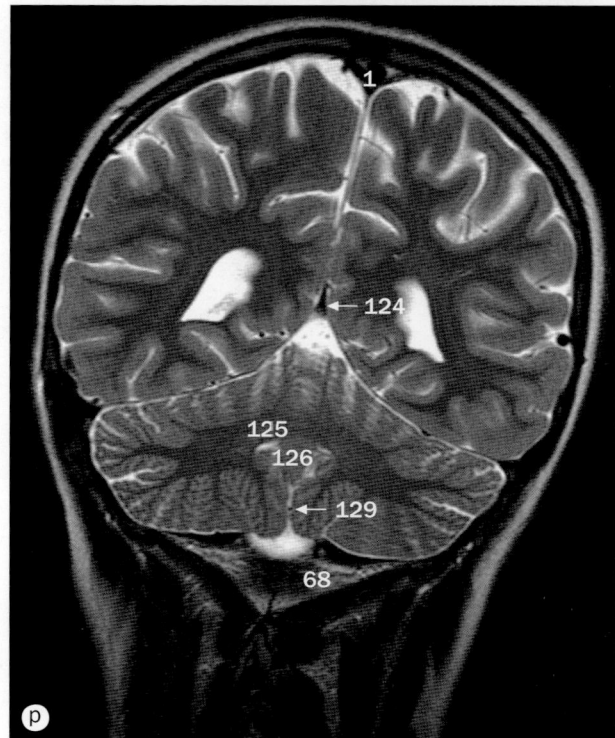

(a)–(p) Brain, coronal T2w MR images, from anterior to posterior.

97 Horizontal (lateral) semicircular canal	106 Inferior colliculus	115 Splenium of corpus callosum	123 Cerebellar tonsil
98 Posterior semicircular canal	107 Aqueduct of Sylvius	116 Superior cerebellar peduncle	124 Inferior sagittal sinus
99 Midbrain (mesencephalon)	108 Spinal cord	117 Inferior cerebellar peduncle	125 Dentate nucleus of cerebellum
100 Medulla oblongata	109 Foramen magnum	118 Cerebellar hemisphere	126 Nodule of cerebellum
101 Middle cerebellar peduncle	110 Mastoid air cells	119 Trigone of lateral ventricle	127 Cisterna magna
102 Cerebellar folia	111 Trapezius muscle	120 Internal cerebral vein (of Galen)	128 Lateral foramen (of Lushka)
103 Pineal gland	112 Tectum (quadrigeminal plate) of midbrain	121 Basal vein (of Rosenthal)	129 Medial foramen (of Magendie)
104 Internal cerebral veins	113 Tentorium cerebelli	122 Fourth ventricle	130 Quadrigeminal cistern
105 Superior colliculus	114 Uncus of temporal lobe		

Numbers 1–130 are common to pages 48–51.

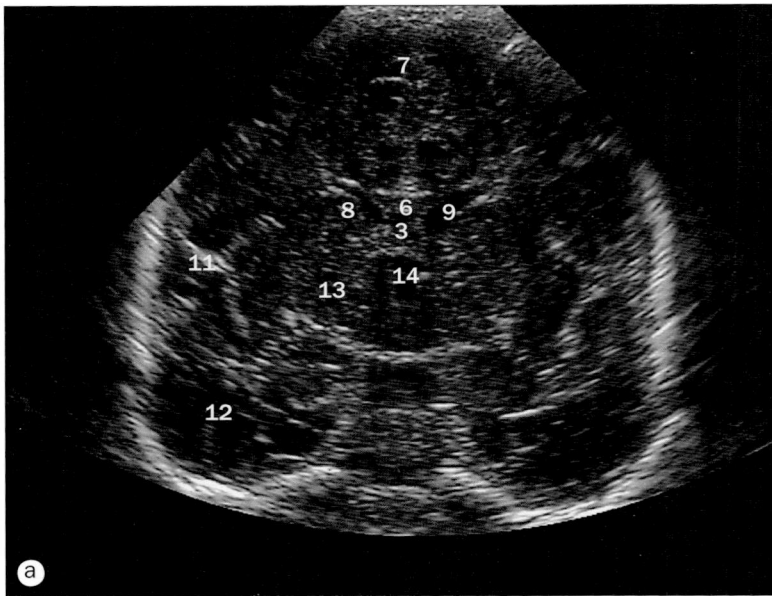

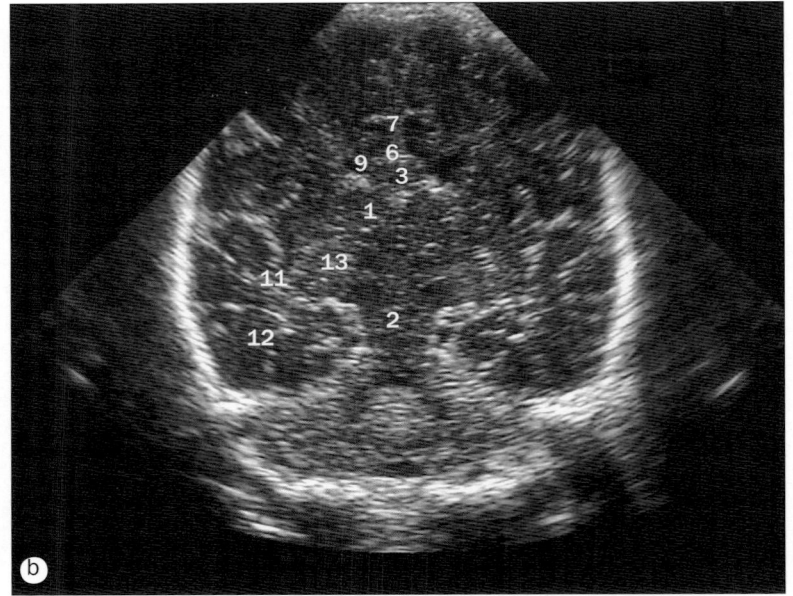

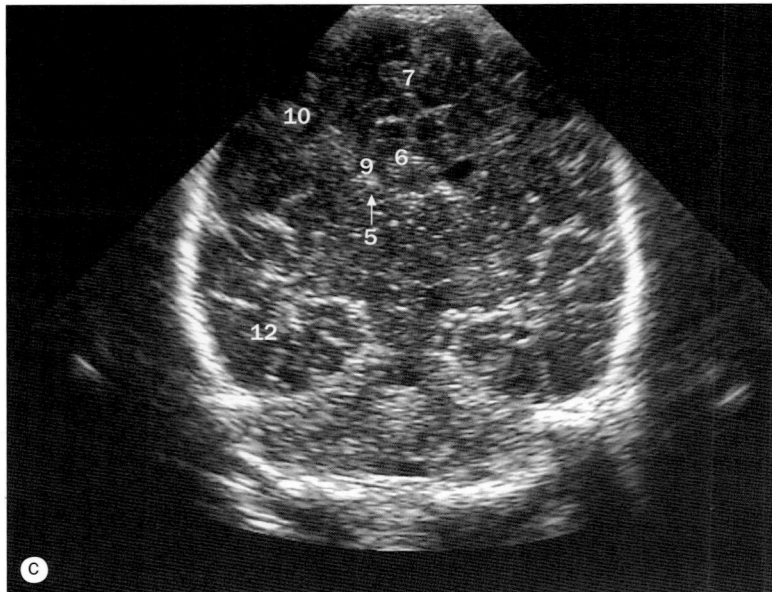

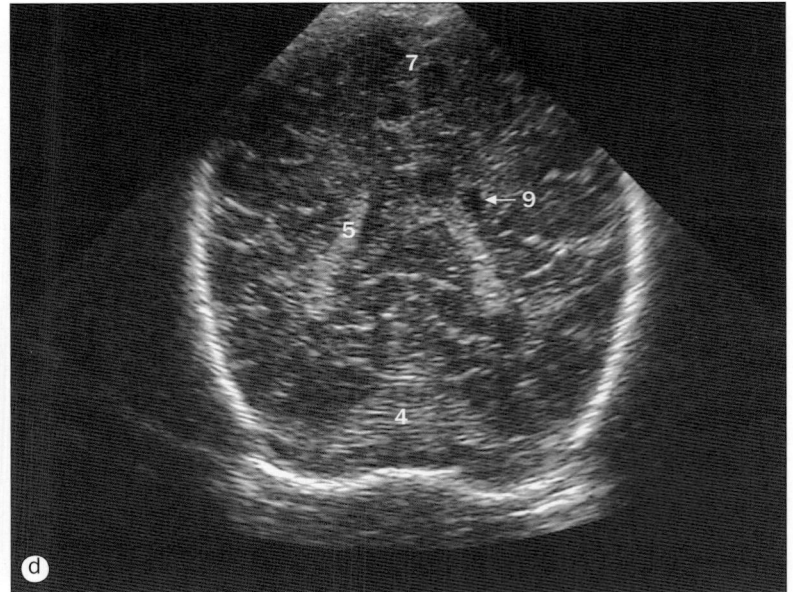

(a)–(d) Neonatal brain, coronal ultrasound images.

1 Body of caudate nucleus
2 Brainstem
3 Cavum septum pellucidum
4 Cerebellum
5 Choroid plexus
6 Corpus callosum
7 Falx cerebri
8 Head of caudate nucleus
9 Lateral ventricle
10 Parietal lobe of brain
11 Sylvian fissure
12 Temporal lobe
13 Thalamus
14 Third ventricle

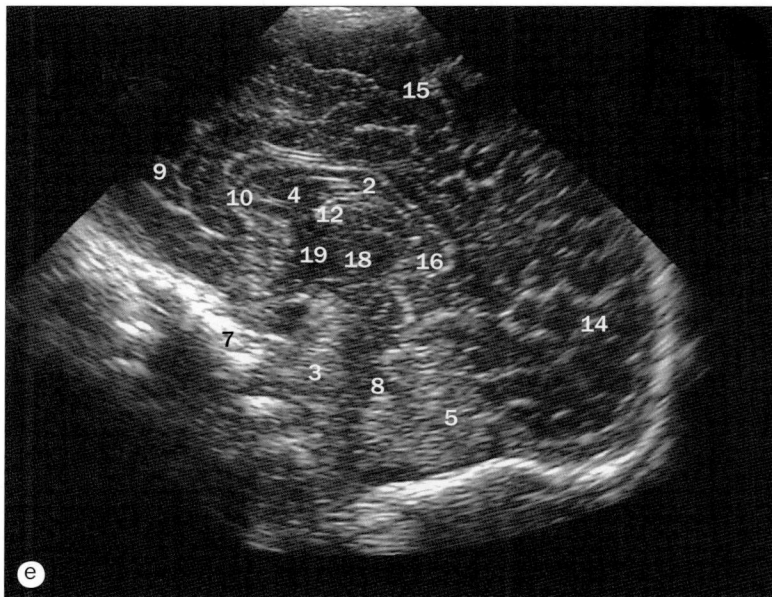

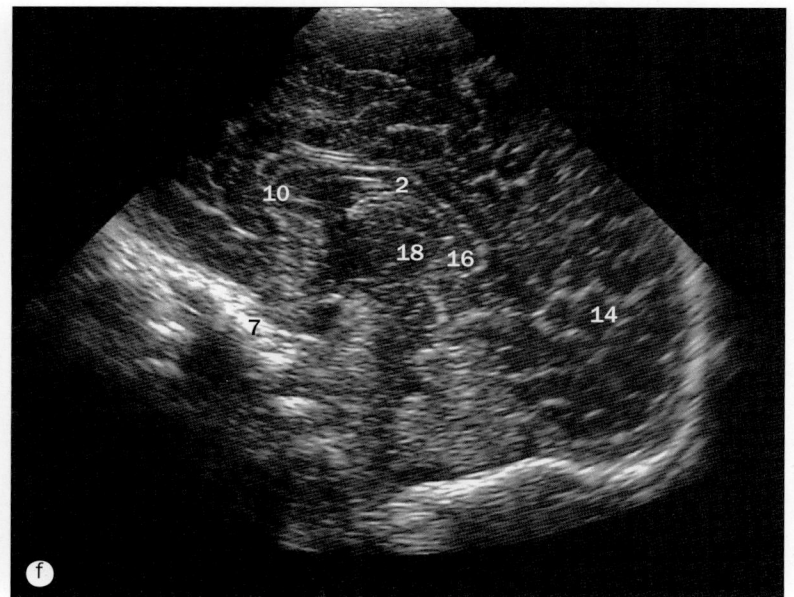

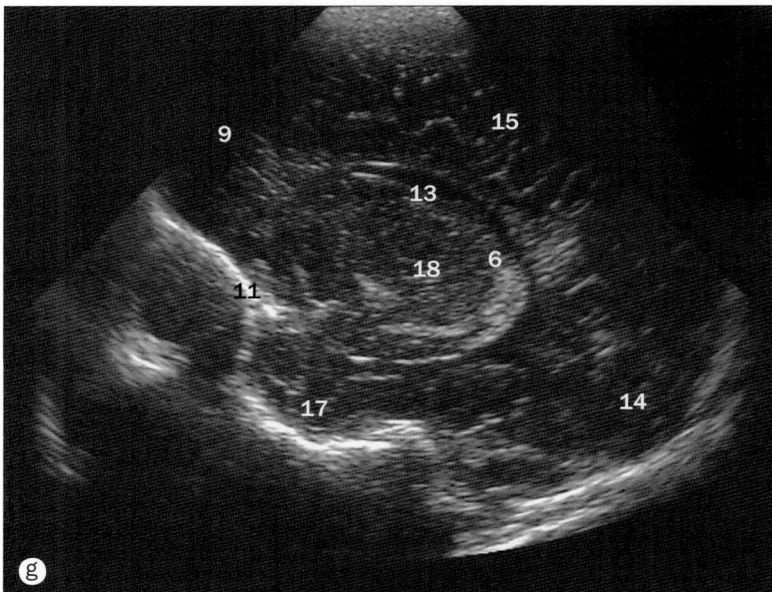

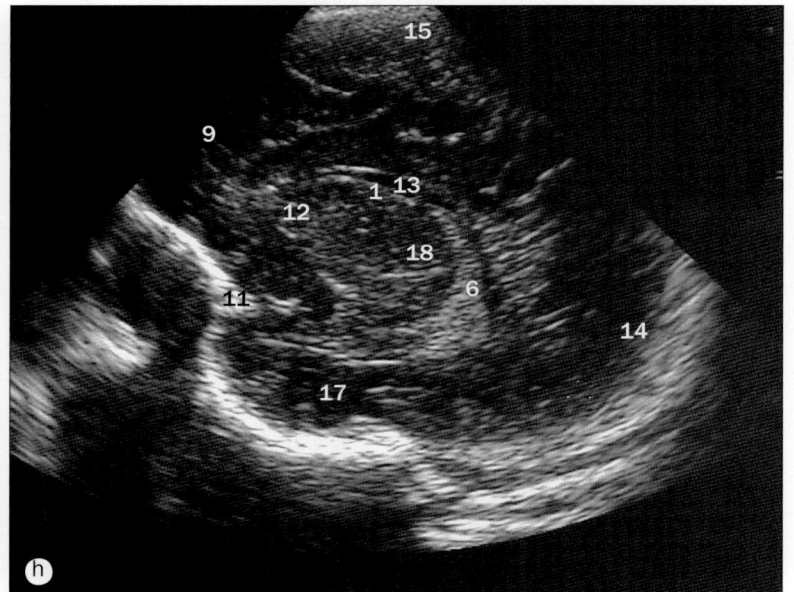

(e)–(h) Neonatal brain, sagittal ultrasound images.

1 Body of caudate nucleus	11 Greater wing of sphenoid
2 Body of corpus callosum	12 Head of caudate nucleus
3 Brainstem	13 Lateral ventricle
4 Cavum septum pellucidum	14 Occipital lobe
5 Cerebellum	15 Parietal lobe of brain
6 Choroid plexus	16 Splenium of corpus callosum
7 Clivus	17 Temporal lobe
8 Fourth ventricle	18 Thalamus
9 Frontal lobe	19 Third ventricle
10 Genu of corpus callosum	

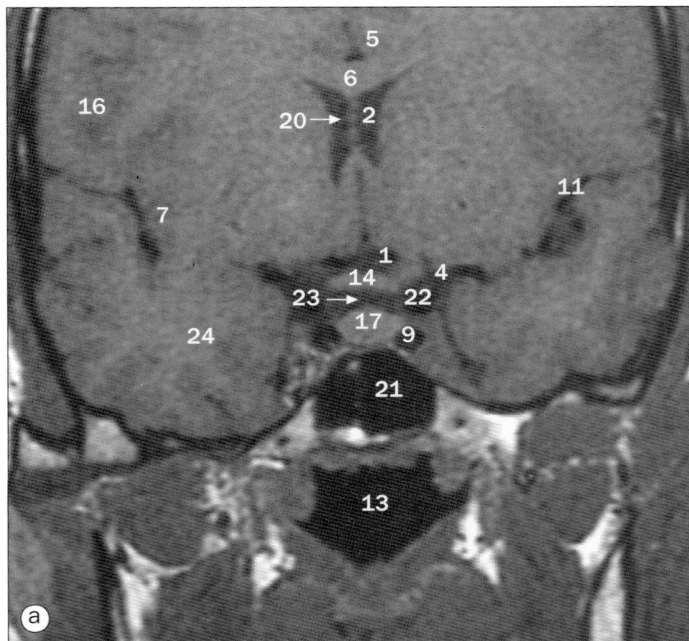

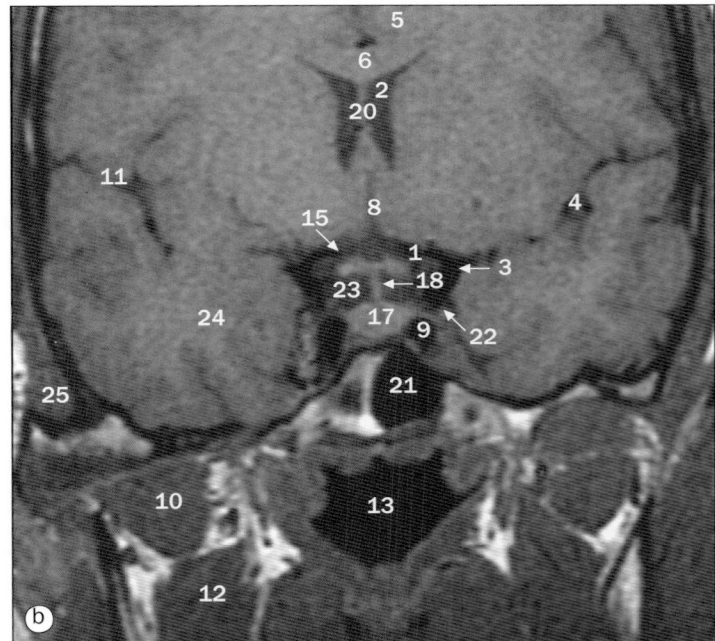

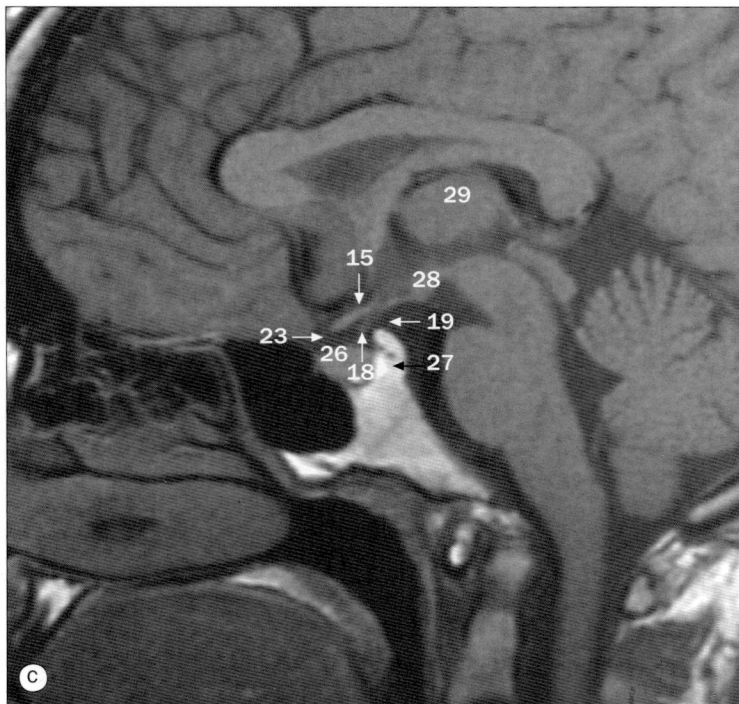

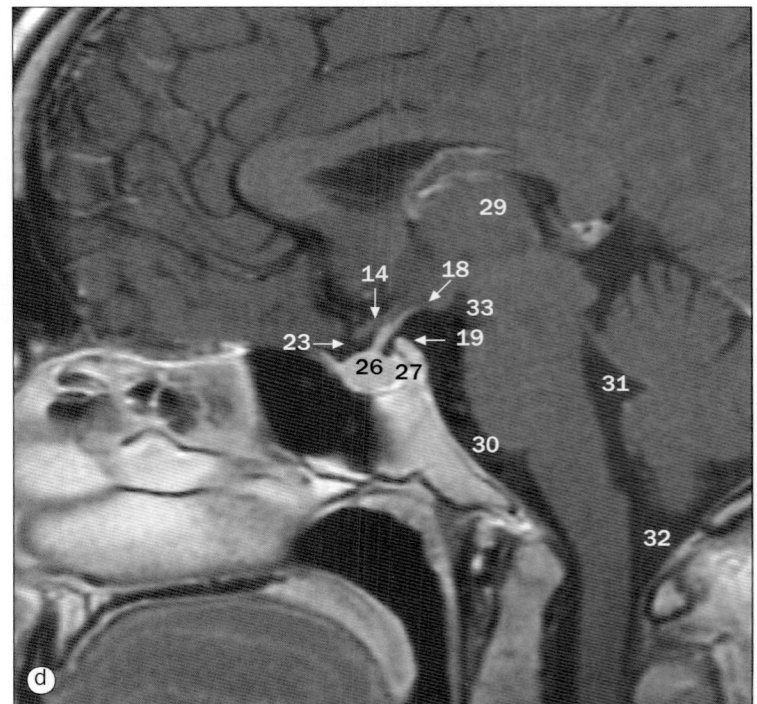

T1w MR images of pituitary fossa (a) and (b) coronal, (c) sagittal, (d) sagittal post gadolinium.

1 Anterior cerebral artery	7 Insula	15 Optic tract	25 Temporalis muscle
2 Anterior horn of lateral ventricle	8 Interhemispheric fissure	16 Parietal lobe of brain	26 Anterior pituitary gland
3 Bifurcation of internal carotid artery	9 Internal carotid artery in cavernous sinus	17 Pituitary gland	27 Posterior pituitary gland
		18 Pituitary stalk	28 Mammillary body
4 Branch of middle cerebral artery in lateral sulcus (Sylvian fissure)	10 Lateral pterygoid muscle	19 Posterior clinoid process	29 Thalamus
	11 Lateral sulcus (Sylvian fissure)	20 Septum pellucidum	30 Prepontine cistern
	12 Medial pterygoid muscle	21 Sphenoidal sinus	31 Fourth ventricle
5 Cingulate gyrus	13 Nasopharynx	22 Supraclinoid carotid artery	32 Cisterna magna
6 Corpus callosum	14 Optic chiasma	23 Suprasellar cistern	33 Interpeduncular cistern
		24 Temporal lobe of brain	

2 Vertebral column and spinal cord

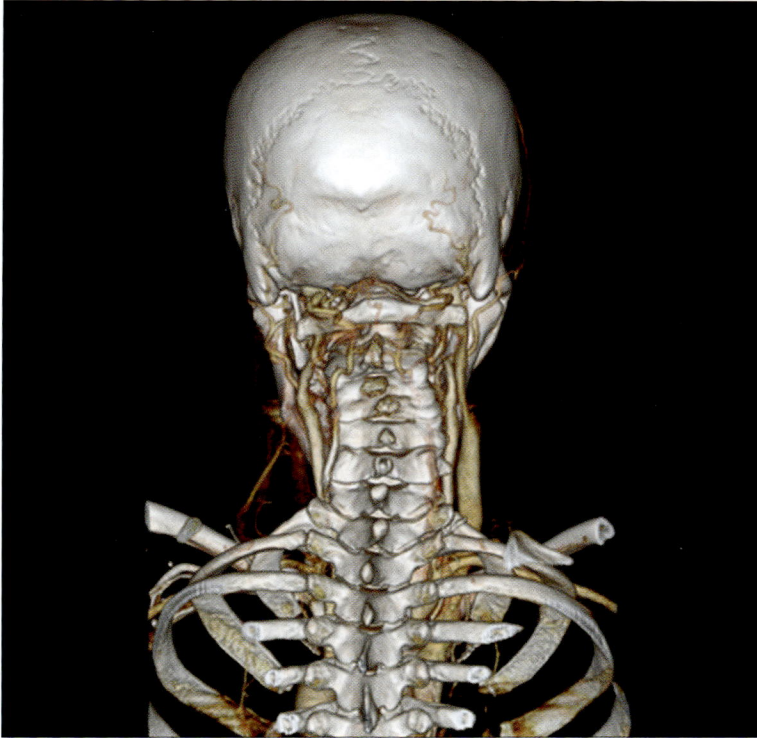

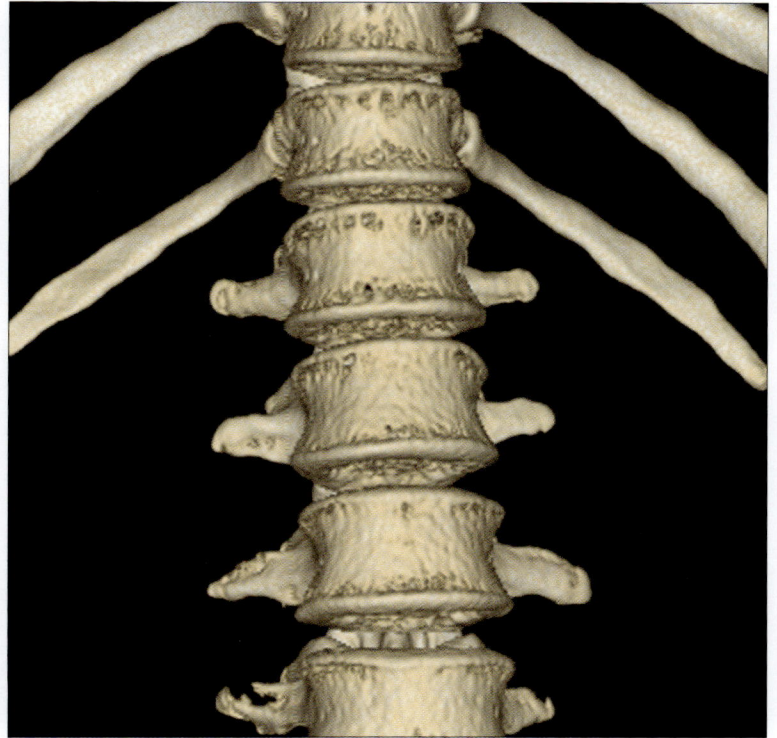

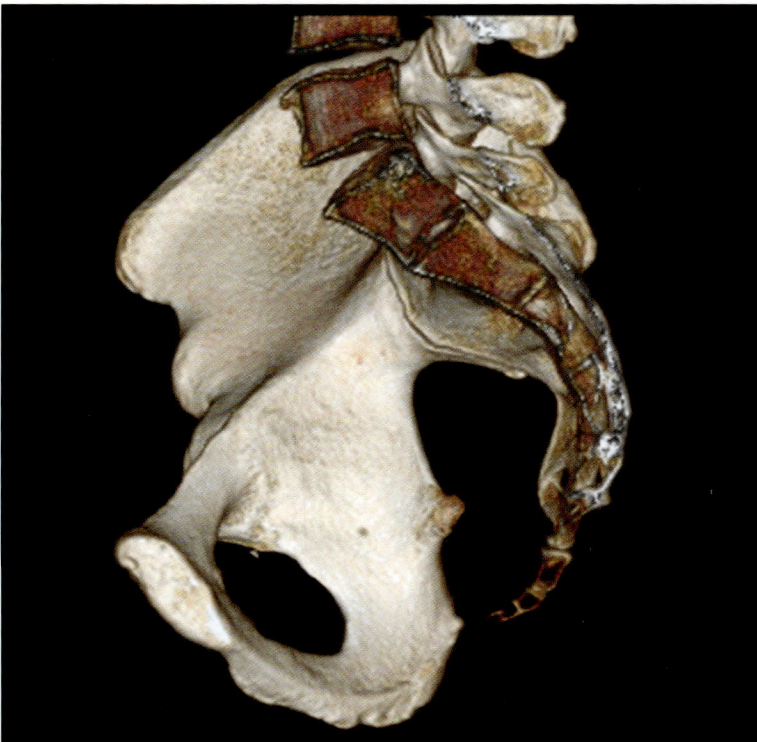

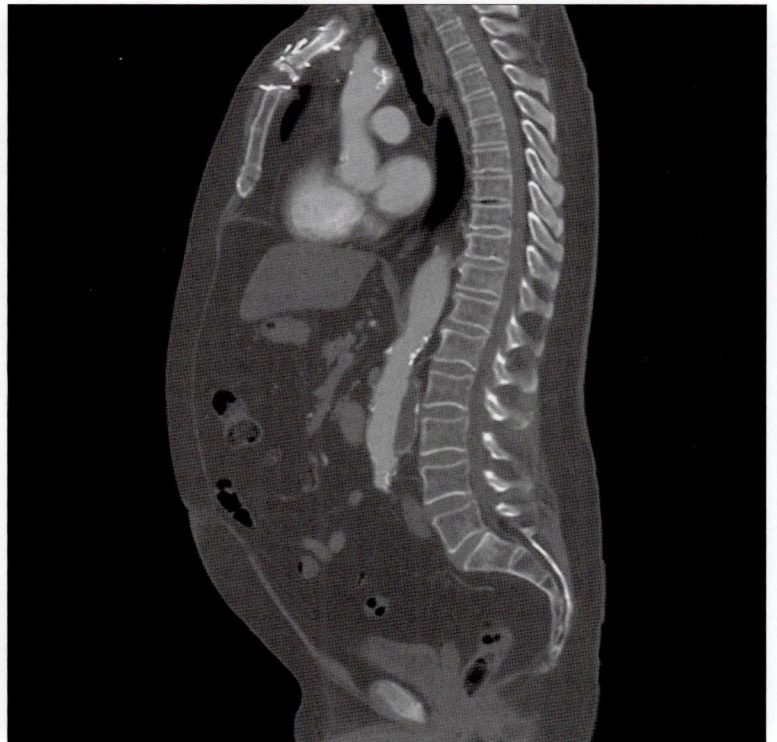

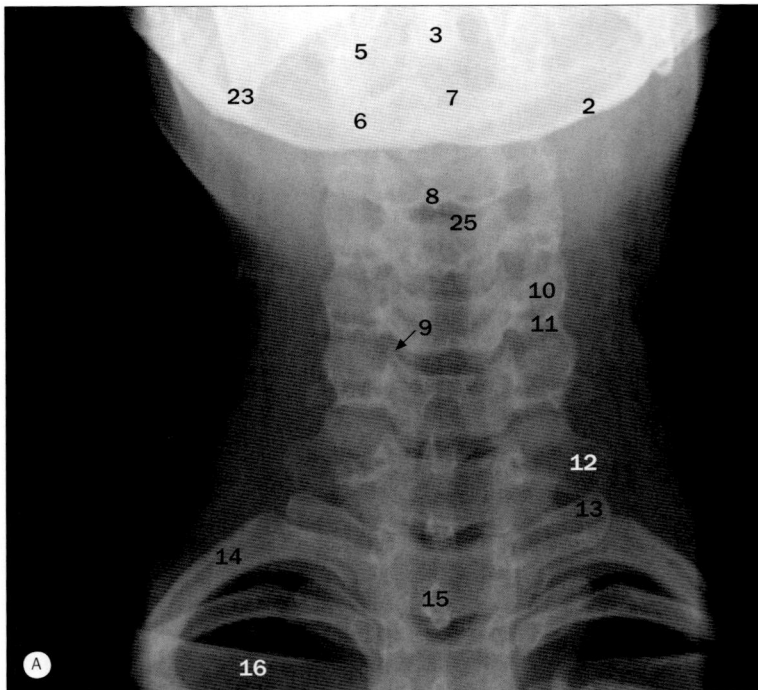

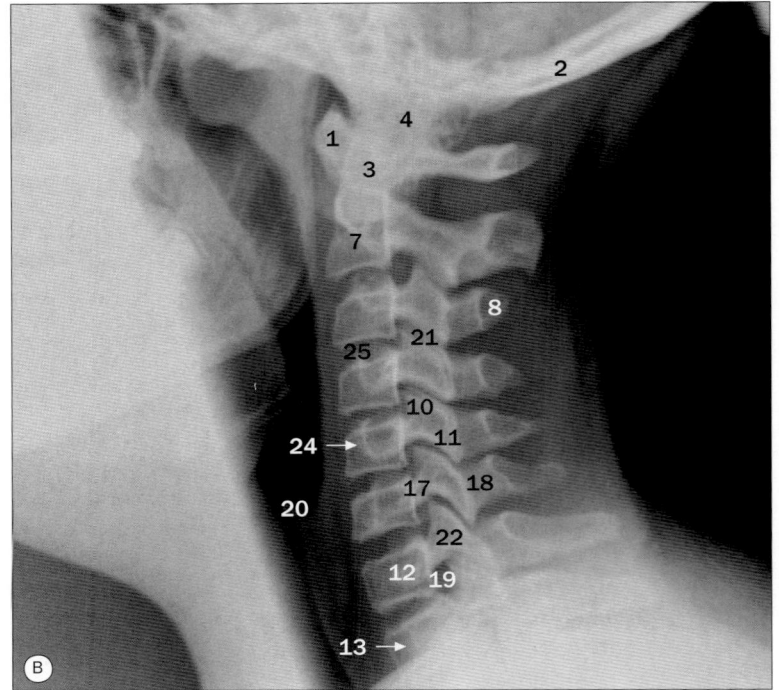

(a) Cervical spine, anteroposterior projection, (b) cervical spine, lateral projection.

1 Anterior arch of atlas	9 Uncovertebral joint (Lushka) of C5/6	15 Spinous process of T1	21 Facet (zygaphophyseal joint) of C3/4
2 Basiocciput	10 Superior articular process of C5	16 Clavicle	22 Pars interarticularis of C7
3 Odontoid peg (of axis)	11 Inferior articular process of C5	17 Pedicle of C6	23 Angle of mandible
4 Occipital condyle	12 Transverse process of C7	18 Lamina of C6	24 Transverse process of C5
5 Lateral mass of atlas (C1)	13 Transverse process of T1	19 Intervertebral foramen of C7/T1 (for C8 root)	25 Intervertebral disc at C3/4
6 Lateral mass of axis (C2)	14 First rib	20 Epig ottis	
7 Body of axis (C2)			
8 Spinous process of C3			

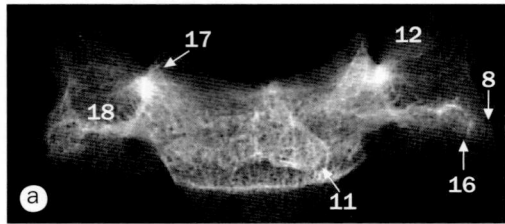

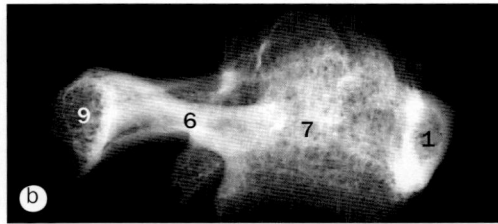

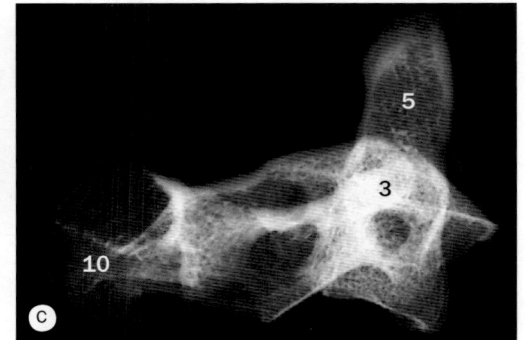

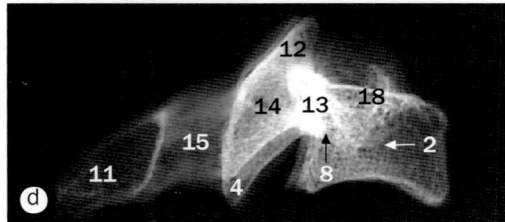

X-ray films of dessicated cervical vertebrae.
(a) AP view C4.
(b) Lateral view C1.
(c) Lateral view C2.
(d) Lateral view C4.

1 Anterior arch of atlas (first cervical vertebra)	vertebra)	12 Superior articular process (facet) of fourth cervical vertebra
2 Anterior tubercle of transverse process of fourth cervical vertebra	7 Body of atlas (first cervical vertebra)	13 Pedicle of C4
3 Body of axis (second cervical vertebra)	8 Posterior tubercle of transverse process of fourth cervical vertebra	14 Pars interarticularis of C4
4 Inferior articular process (facet) of fourth cervical vertebra	9 Posterior tubercle of atlas (first cervical vertebra)	15 Lamina of C4
5 Odontoid process (dens) of axis (second cervical vertebra)	10 Spinous process of axis (second cervical vertebra)	16 Intertubercular lamella of C4 transverse process
6 Posterior arch of atlas (first cervical	11 Spinous process of fourth cervical vertebra	17 Posterolateral lip (uncus) of C4
		18 Body of transverse process of C4

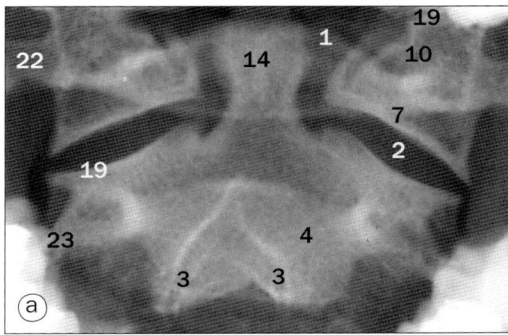

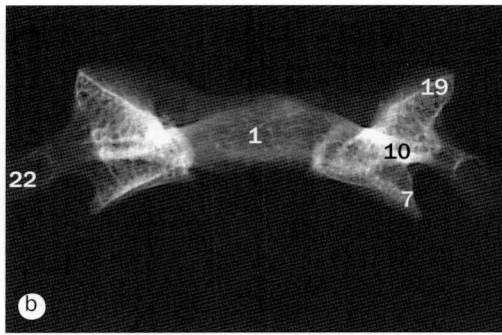

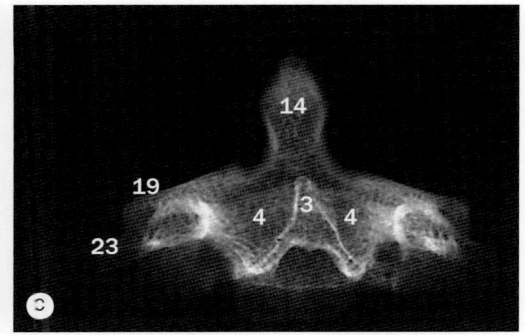

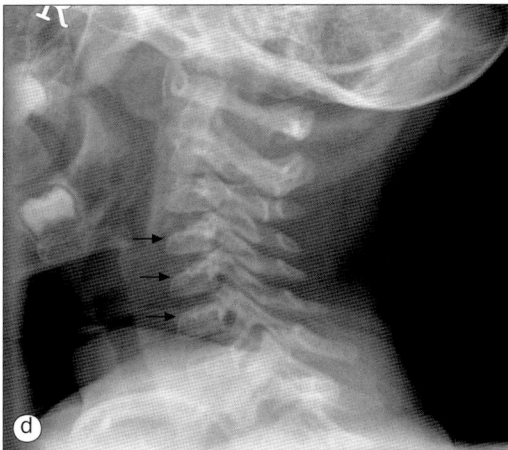

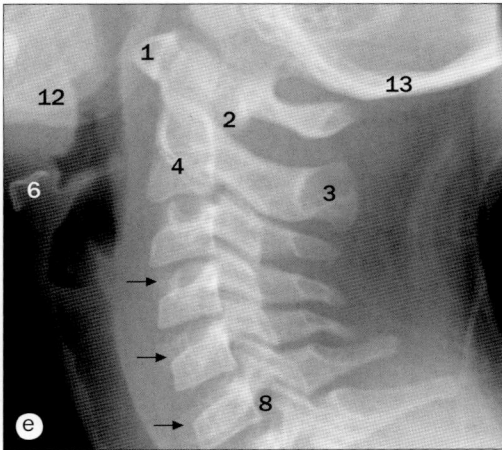

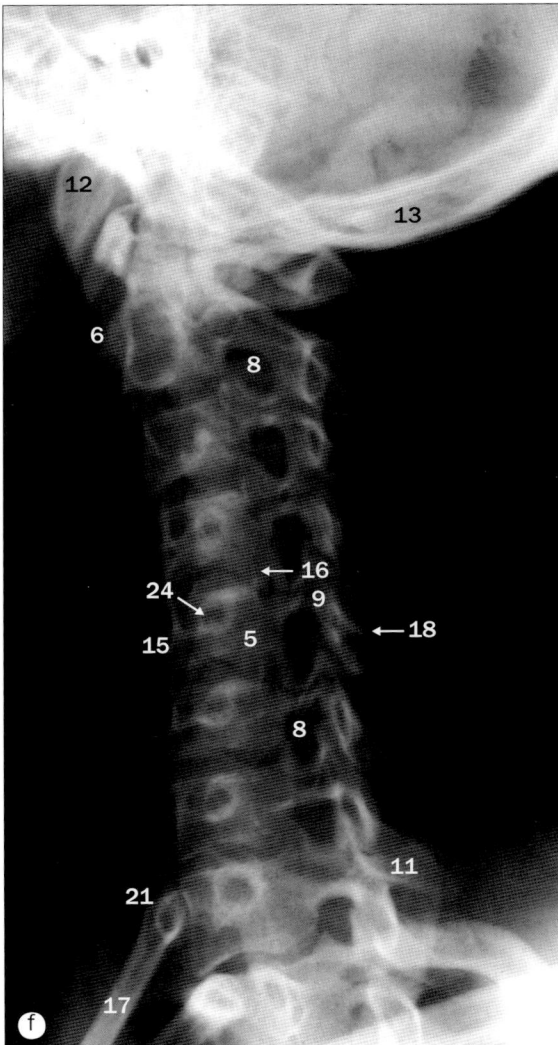

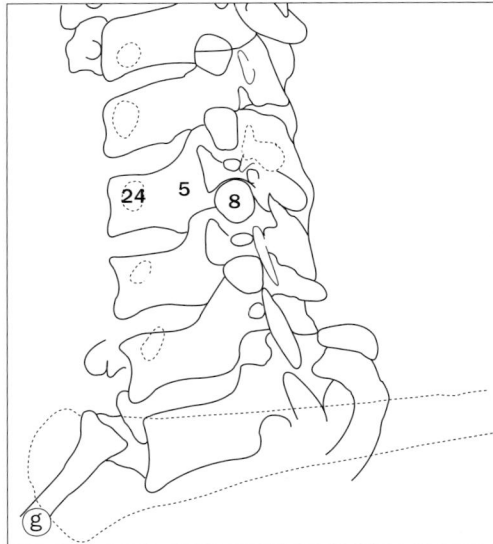

1 Anterior arch of atlas (first cervical
  vertebra)
2 Atlanto-axial joint
3 Bifid spinous process of axis
  (second cervical vertebra)
4 Body of axis (second cervical
  vertebra)
5 Body of fifth cervical vertebra
6 Hyoid bone
7 Inferior articular process (facet) of
  atlas (first cervical vertebra)
8 Intervertebral foramen
9 Lamina of fifth cervical vertebra
10 Lateral mass of atlas (first cervical
   vertebra)
11 Left first rib
12 Mandible
13 Occipital bone
14 Odontoid process (dens) of axis
   (second cervical vertebra)
15 Posterior tubercle of transverse
   process of fifth cervical vertebra
16 Posterolateral lip (uncus) of fifth
   cervical vertebra
17 Right first rib
18 Spinous process of fifth cervical
   vertebra
19 Superior articular process (facet) of
   atlas (first cervical vertebra)
20 Superior articular process (facet) of
   axis (second cervical vertebra)
21 Trachea
22 Transverse process of atlas (first
   cervical vertebra)
23 Transverse process of axis (second
   cervical vertebra)
24 Transverse process of fifth cervical
   vertebra

(a) Atlas (first cervical vertebra) and axis
(second cervical vertebra), 'open mouth'
anteroposterior projection.
(b) Dried atlas (first cervical vertebra), anteroposterior projection.
(c) Dried axis (second cervical vertebra), anteroposterior projection.
(d) Cervical spine X-ray of a 3 year old, lateral projection. The atlanto-axial joint
can normally be up to 5 mm (up to 3 mm in adults).
(e) Cervical spine X-ray of a 9 year old, lateral projection. Note normal
physiological wedging of the vertebral bodies (arrows) due to unossified superior
endplate apophyses.
(f) Oblique X-ray of adult cervical spine.
(g) Line drawing of (f).

(a) Thoracic spine, anteroposterior projection.

(b) Thoracic spine, lateral projection.

(c) Dried thoracic vertebra, anteroposterior projection.

(d) Dried sixth thoracic vertebra, lateral projection.

Thoracic spine, (e) of a 7-day-old neonate, (f) of a 12-year-old child, lateral projections.

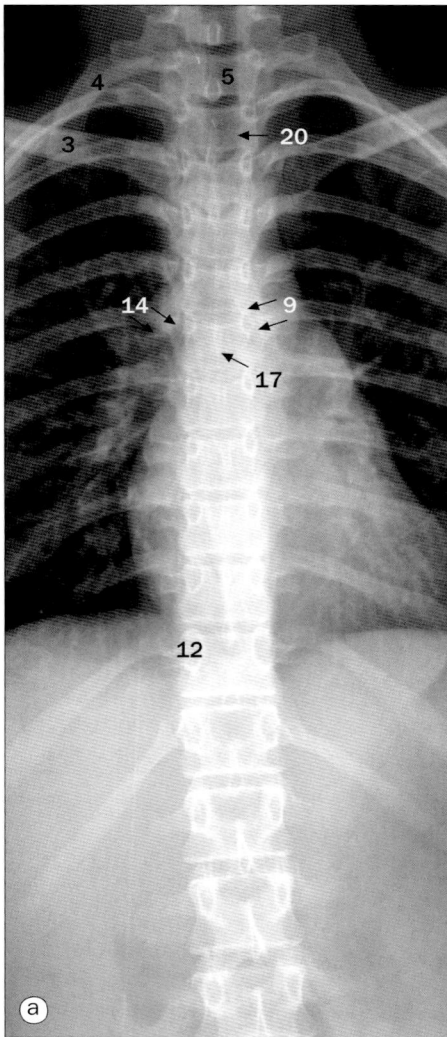

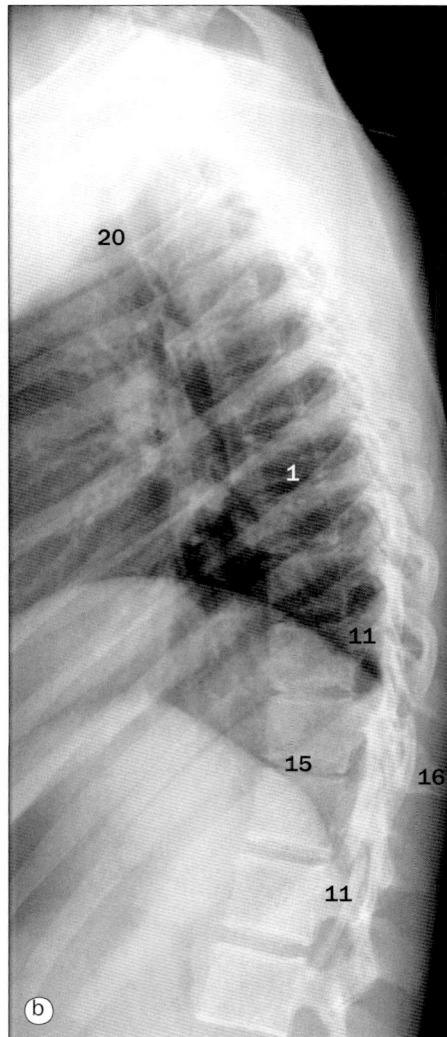

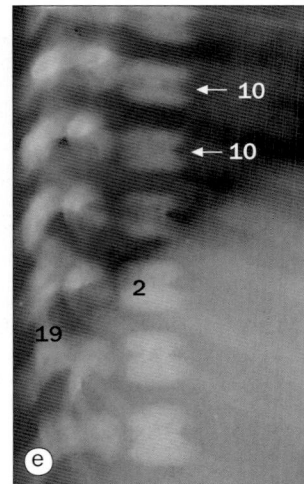

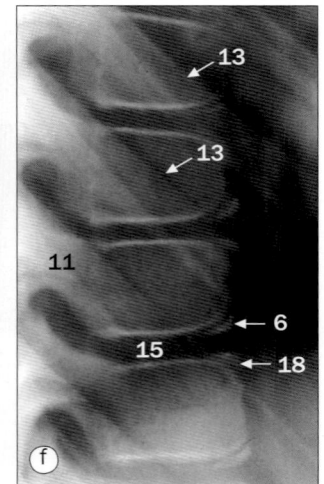

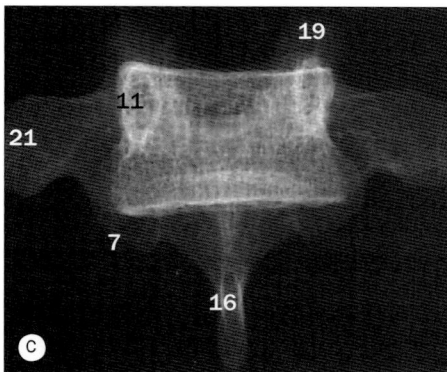

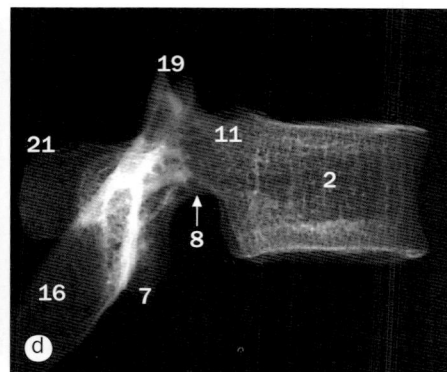

1 Body of sixth thoracic vertebra
2 Body of vertebra
3 Clavicle
4 First rib
5 First thoracic vertebra
6 Inferior annular epiphysial discs for vertebral body
7 Inferior articular process (facet)
8 Inferior vertebral notch
9 Left main bronchus
10 Natal cleft
11 Pedicle
12 Pedicle of eleventh thoracic vertebra
13 Ribs
14 Right main bronchus
15 Site of intervertebral disc
16 Spinous process
17 Spinous process of sixth thoracic vertebra
18 Superior annular epiphysial discs for vertebral body
19 Superior articular process (facet)
20 Trachea
21 Transverse process

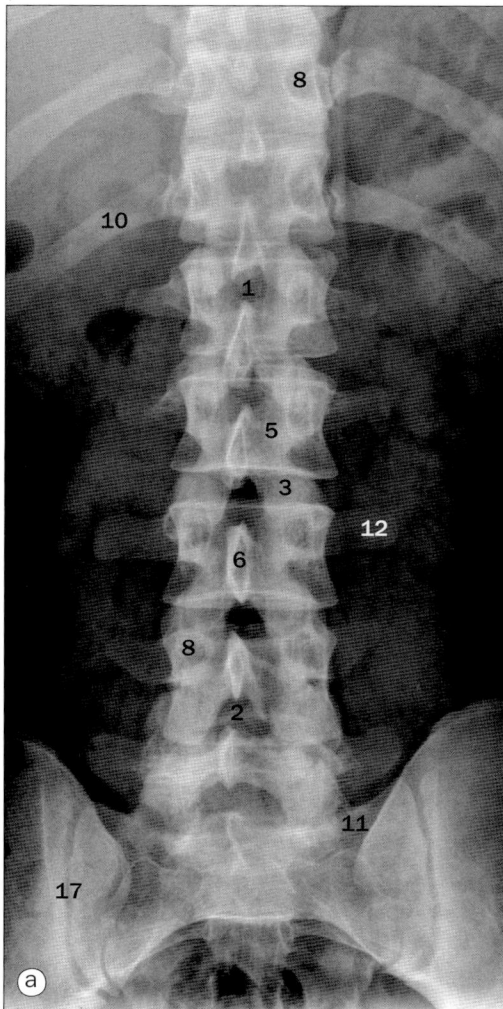

(a) Lumbar spine, anteroposterior radiograph.

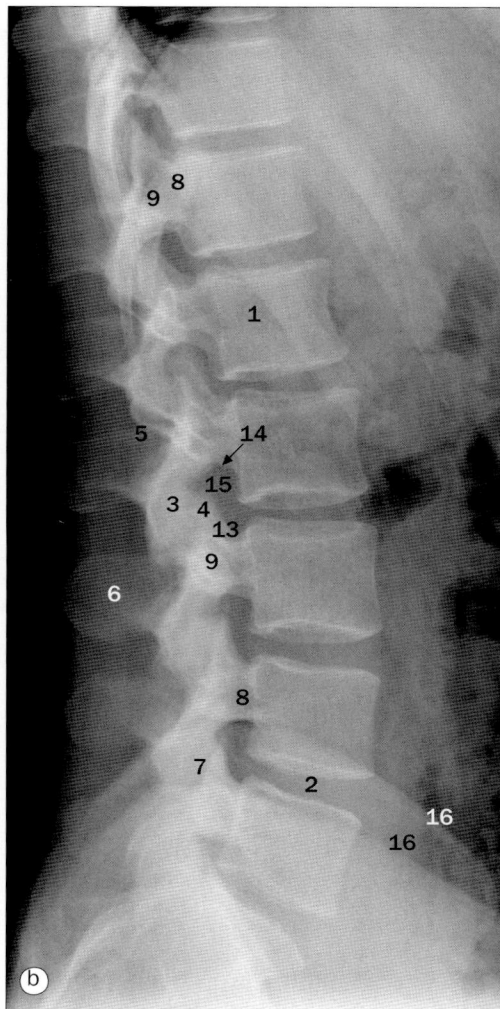

(b) Lumbar spine, lateral projection.

(c) Dried second lumbar vertebra, anteroposterior projection.

(c) Dried second lumbar vertebra, lateral projection.

(e) Lumbar spine, oblique projection.

1 Body of first lumbar vertebra
2 Intervertebral disc L4/5
3 Inferior articular process (facet) of L2
4 Superior articular process (facet) L3
5 Lamina of L2
6 Spinous process of L3
7 Facet (zygapophyseal joint) of L4/5
8 Pedicle
9 Pars interarticularis
10 Right twelfth rib
11 Sacral promontory
12 Transverse process of L3
13 Mamillary process
14 Inferior vertebral notch of L2
15 Neural foramen of L2/3 (for L2 root)
16 Iliac crest
17 Sacroiliac joint

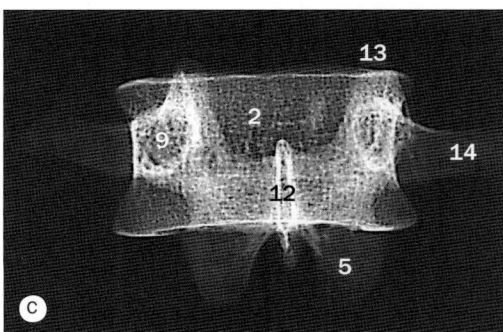

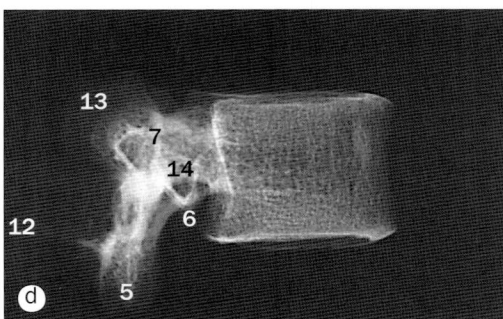

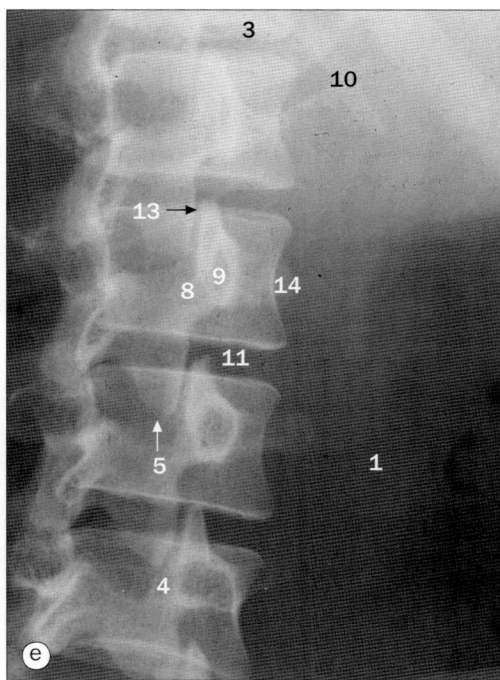

1 Psoas muscle outline
2 Body of second lumbar vertebra
3 Body of twelfth thoracic vertebra
4 Body of fourth lumbar vertebra
5 Inferior articular process (facet) of second lumbar vertebra
6 Inferior vertebral notch of second lumbar vertebra
7 Mamillary process of second lumbar vertebra
8 Pars interarticularis
9 Pedicle of second lumbar vertebra
10 Twelfth rib
11 Intervertebral disc space between L2 and L3
12 Spinous process of second lumbar vertebra
13 Superior articular process (facet) of second lumbar vertebra
14 Transverse process of second lumbar vertebra

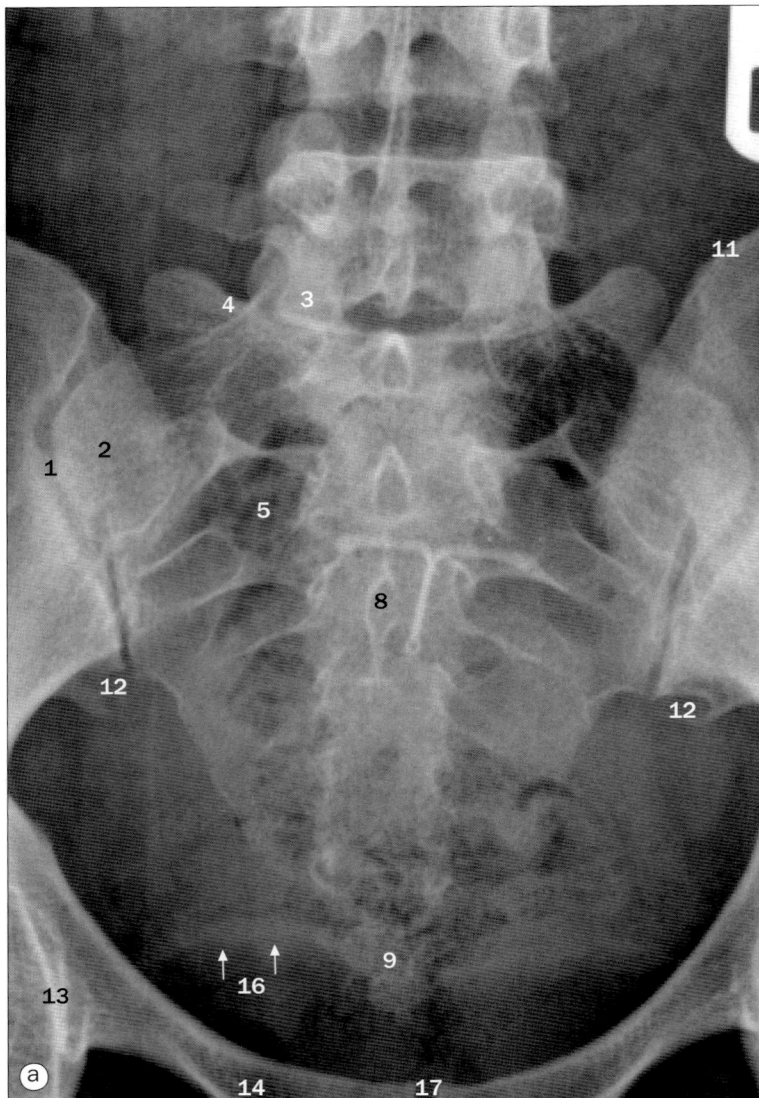

(a) Sacrum, anteroposterior projection.

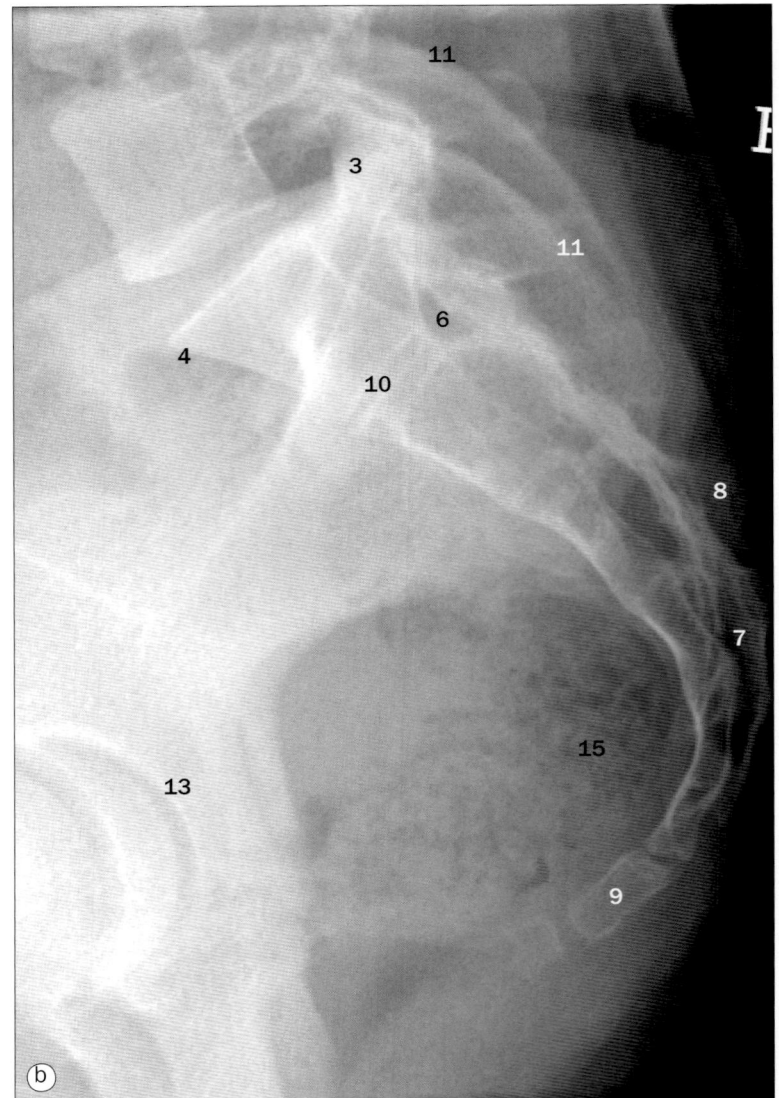

(b) Sacrum and coccyx, lateral projection.

1 Sacroiliac joint
2 Ala of sacrum
3 Superior articular process of sacrum
4 Sacral promontory
5 Sacral foramen (S1/2 for right S1 root)
6 Upper part of sacral canal
7 Lower part of sacral canal
8 Spinous tubercle on median sacral crest
9 Coccyx
10 Rudimentary S1/2 disc space
11 Iliac crest
12 Preauricular (paraglenoid) sulcus
13 Acetabular roof
14 Superior pubic ramus
15 Rectum
16 Levator ani (outlined by fat in ischioanal fossa)
17 Symphysis pubis

The preauricular (paraglenoid) sulcus is a characteristic of the female pelvis and is due to bone resorption at the insertion of the anterior sacroiliac ligament. It is prominent in parous women.

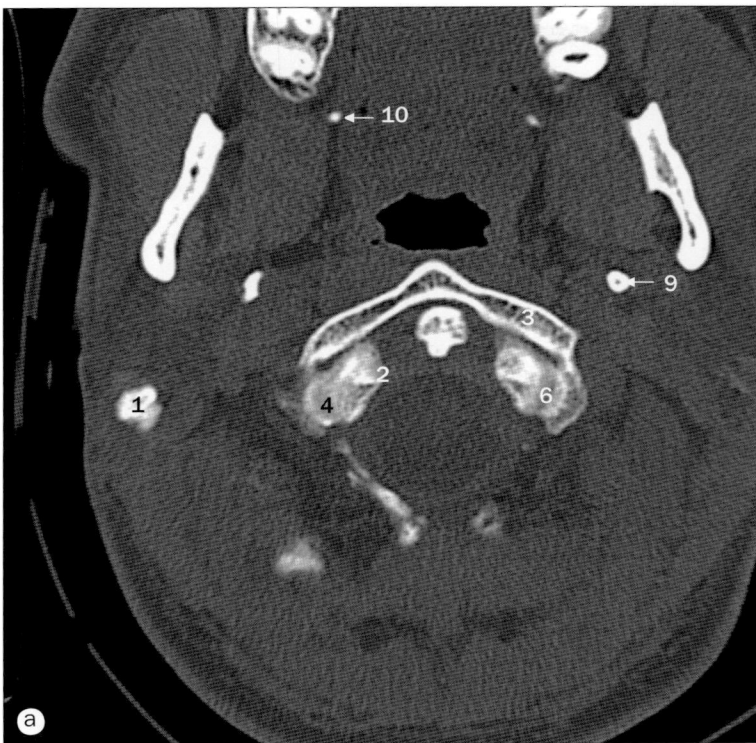

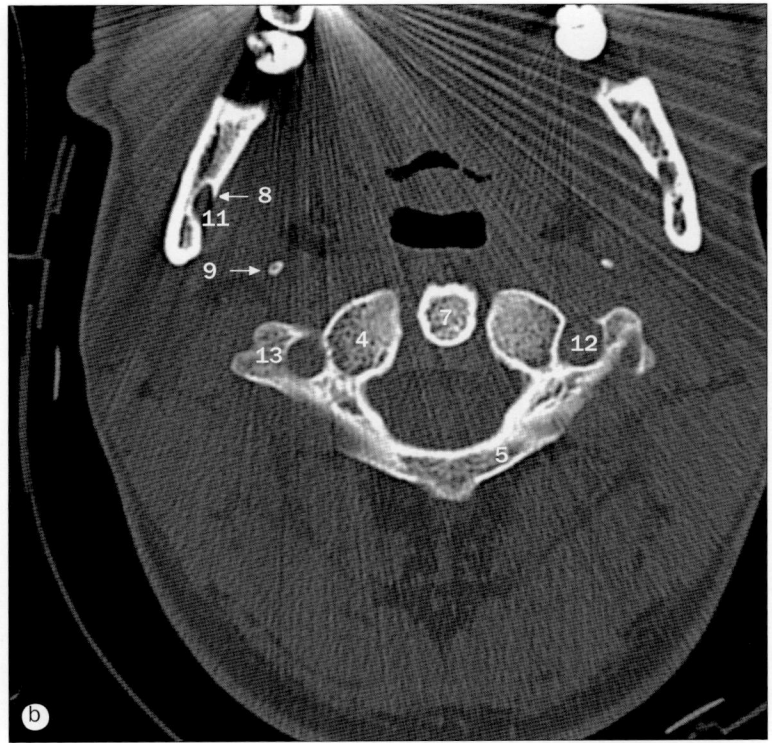

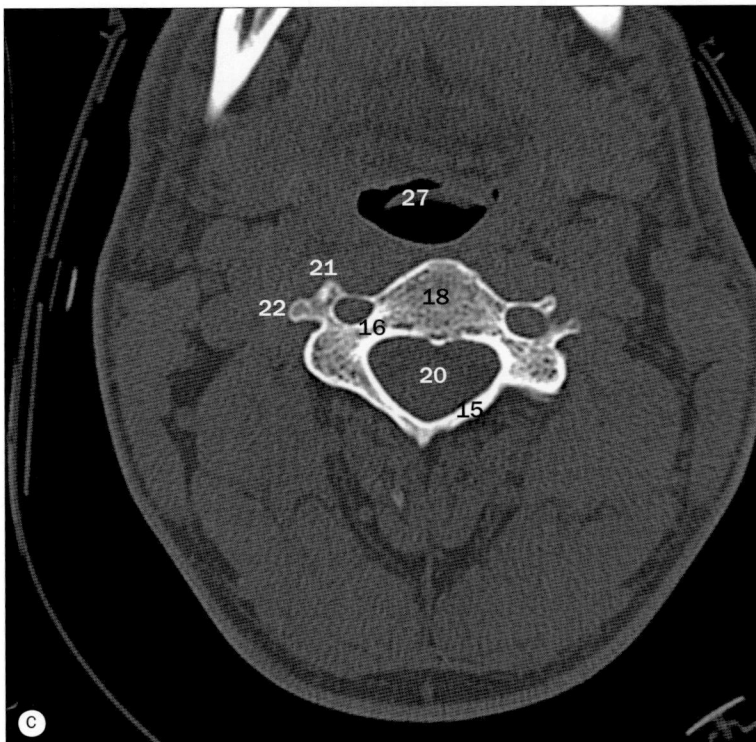

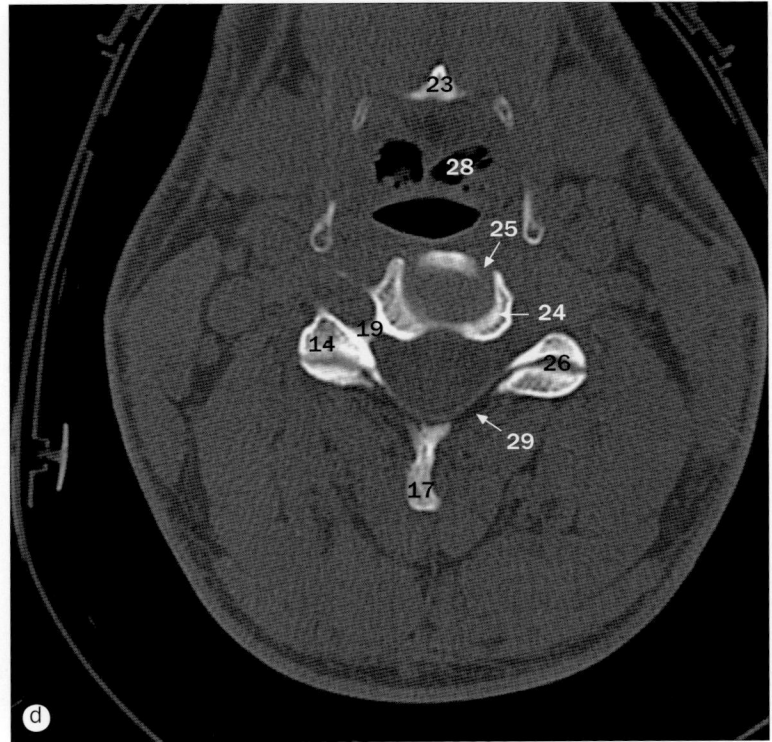

Axial CT images of the upper cervical spine at C1/2 (**a,b**), C2 (**c**) and C2/3 level (**d**).

1 Mastoid process (tip)	11 Inferior alveolar foramen of mandibular ramus	21 Anterior tubercle of transverse process of C2
2 Transverse ligament (attachment)		22 Posterior tubercle of transverse process of C2
3 Anterior arch of atlas (C1)	12 Foramen transversarium of C1	
4 Lateral mass of atlas	13 Transverse process of C1	23 Thyroid cartilage
5 Posterior arch of C1	14 Inferior articular process of C2	24 Uncus of C3 vertebral body
6 Groove for vertebral artery	15 Lamina of C2	25 Uncovertebral joint (of Luschka) at C2/3
7 Odontoid process (dens) of axis (C2)	16 Pedicle of C2	26 Facet (zygapophyseal) joint at C2/3
8 Lingula of mandible	17 Spinous process of C2	27 Epiglottis
9 Styloid process	18 Body of C2	28 Vallecula
10 Hamulus of medial pterygoid plate	19 Intervertebral foramen of C2/3	29 Ligamentum flavum
	20 Spinal cord	

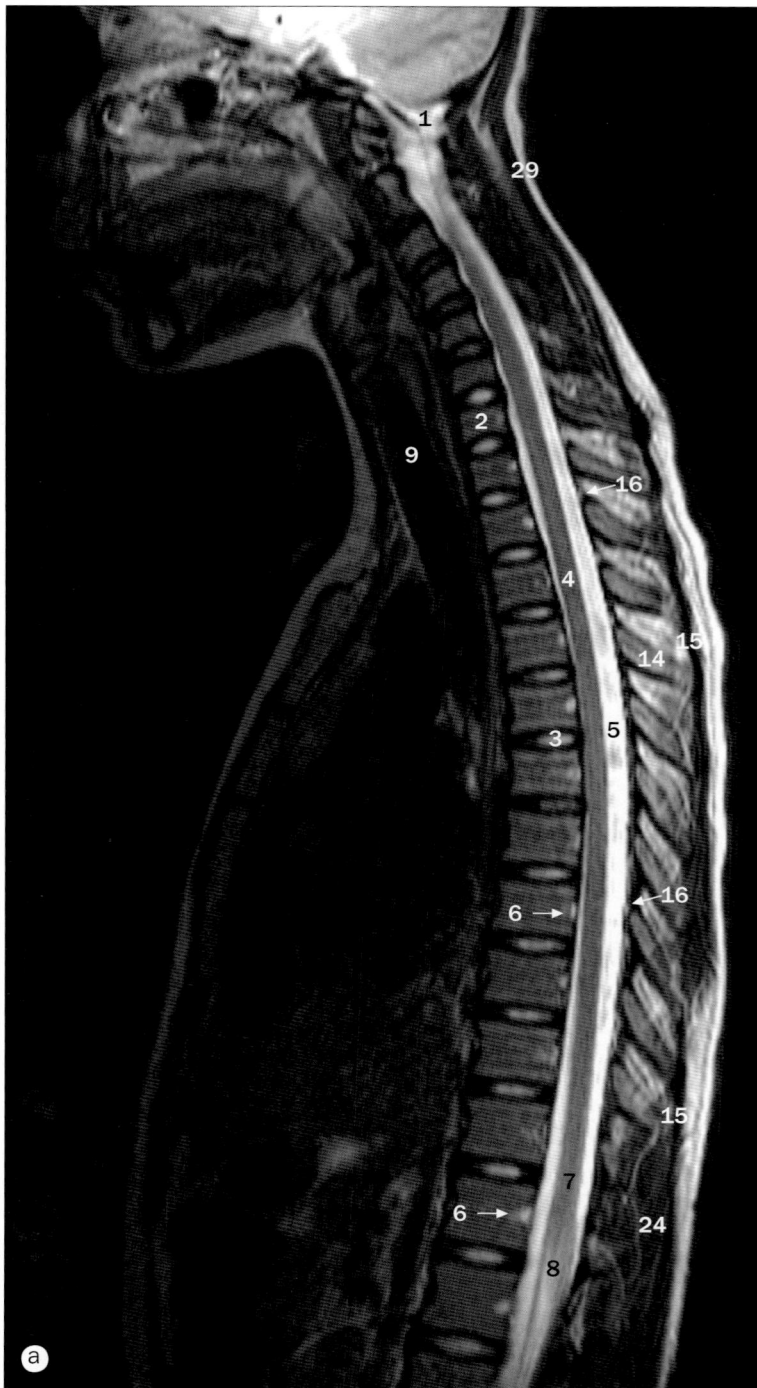

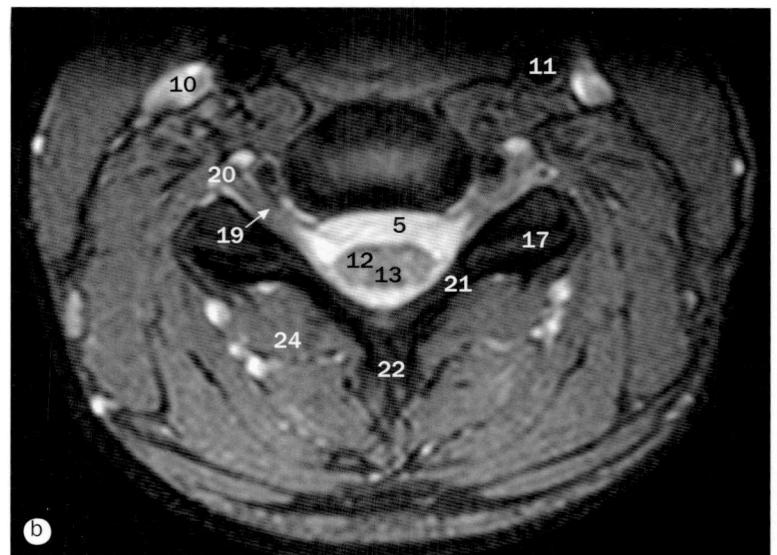

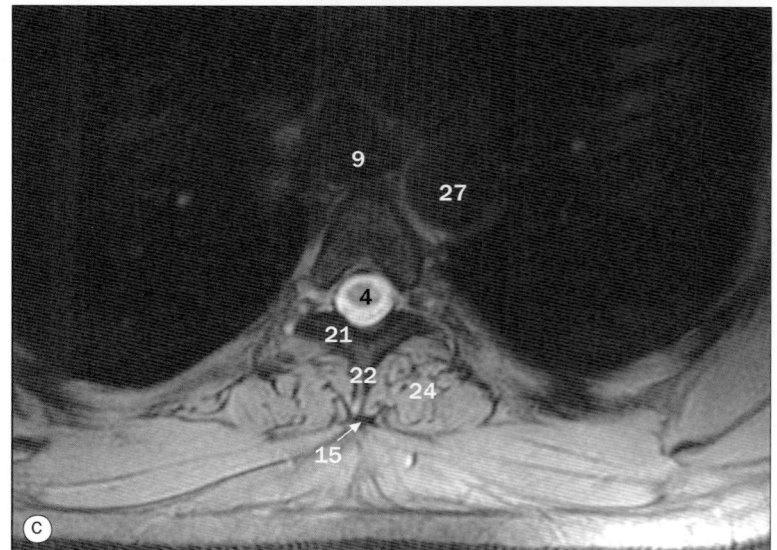

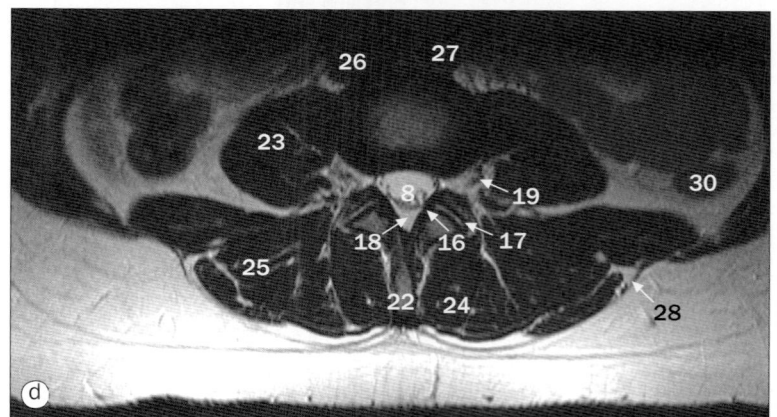

MR images of the spine, (a) sagittal T2 wide field of view and axial T2 sections from the (b) cervical, (c) thoracic and (d) lumbar regions.

1 Foramen magnum
2 Body of C7
3 Nucleus pulposus of T5/6 intervertebral disc
4 Spinal cord
5 CSF in subarachnoid space (flow void artefact)
6 Basivertebral vein
7 Conus medullaris
8 Cauda equina
9 Trachea
10 Internal jugular vein
11 Common carotid artery
12 Grey matter of spinal cord
13 White matter of spinal cord
14 Spinous process of T4
15 Supraspinous ligament
16 Ligamentum flavum
17 Facet (zygapophyseal) joint
18 Epidural fat
19 Dorsal root ganglion
20 Spinal nerve root
21 Lamina
22 Spinous process
23 Psoas major muscle
24 Erector spinae muscle
25 Multifidus muscle
26 Inferior vena cava
27 Aorta
28 Thoracolumbar fascia
29 Ligamentum nuchae
30 Descending colon

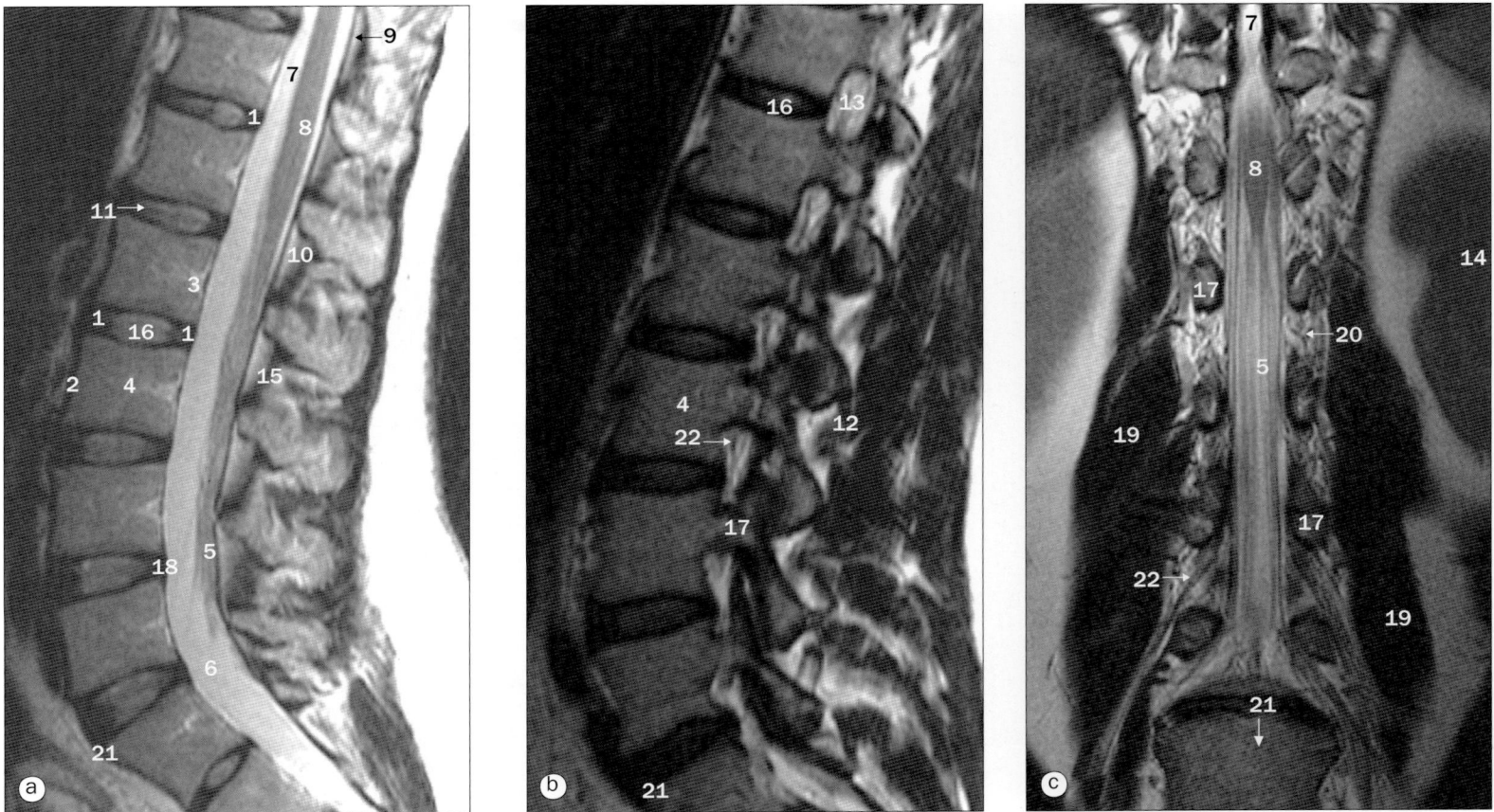

Lumbosacral spine, (a) sagittal MR image, (b) parasagittal MR image, (c) coronal MR image.

1 Annulus fibrosus	9 Dural sac	17 Pedicle
2 Anterior longitudinal ligament	10 Epidural space (fat filled)	18 Posterior longitudinal ligament and
3 Basivertebral vein	11 Internuclear cleft	annulus fibrosus
4 Body of third lumbar vertebra	12 Interspinous ligament	19 Psoas muscle
5 Cauda equina	13 Intervertebral foramen	20 Radicular vessels
6 Caudal lumbar thecal sac	14 Kidney	21 Sacral promontory
7 Cerebrospinal fluid	15 Ligamentum flavum	22 Spinal nerve root in intervertebral
8 Conus medullaris	16 Nucleus pulposus	foramen

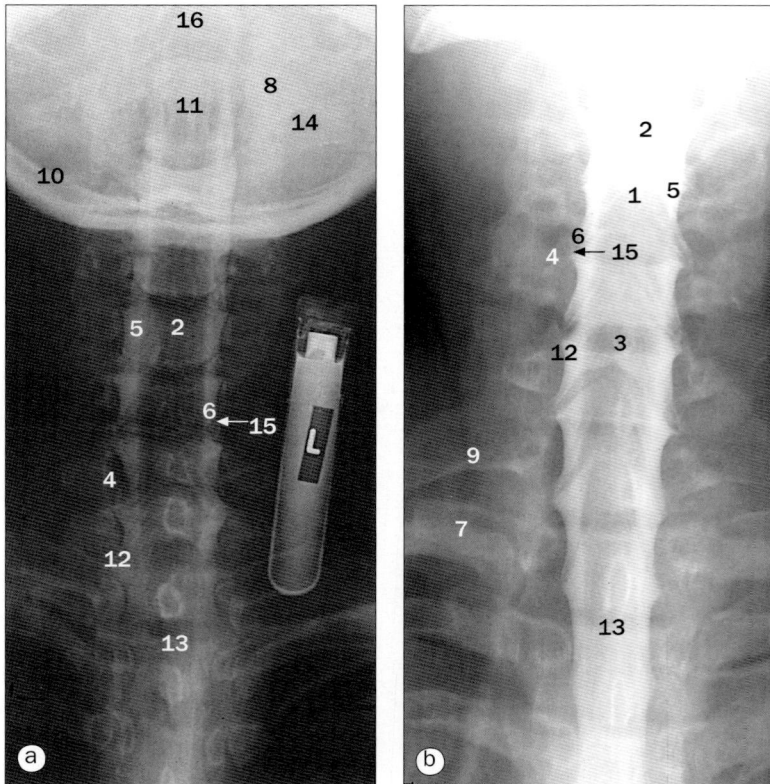

Cervical myelogram, (a) with the neck extended, (b) with the neck slightly flexed, anteroposterior projections.

Non-ionic water-soluble contrast medium is introduced into the lumbar subarachnoid space via a lumbar puncture. The patient is positioned prone, with the neck hyperextended, and strapped onto a tilting table. The contrast medium is then run up into the cervical region to demonstrate the cervical spinal cord and exiting nerve roots. There are eight cervical nerve roots: the roots of the eighth cervical nerve exit through the intervertebral foramina between the seventh cervical vertebra and the first thoracic vertebra. The normal cervical cord enlargement (3) (for the brachial plexus) extends from the third cervical vertebra to the second thoracic vertebra. It is maximal at the fifth cervical vertebra and should not be mistaken for an intramedullary lesion.

 1 Anterior spinal artery
 2 Cervical cord
 3 Cervical cord enlargement
 4 Cervical spinal nerve exiting through intervertebral foramen
 5 Contrast medium in cervical subarachnoid space
 6 Dorsal root of spinal nerve
 7 First rib
 8 Lateral mass of atlas (first cervical vertebra)
 9 Normal large transverse process of seventh cervical vertebra
10 Occiput
11 Odontoid process (dens)
12 Root of eighth cervical nerve
13 Thoracic cord
14 Transverse foramen
15 Ventral root of spinal nerve
16 Vertebral artery

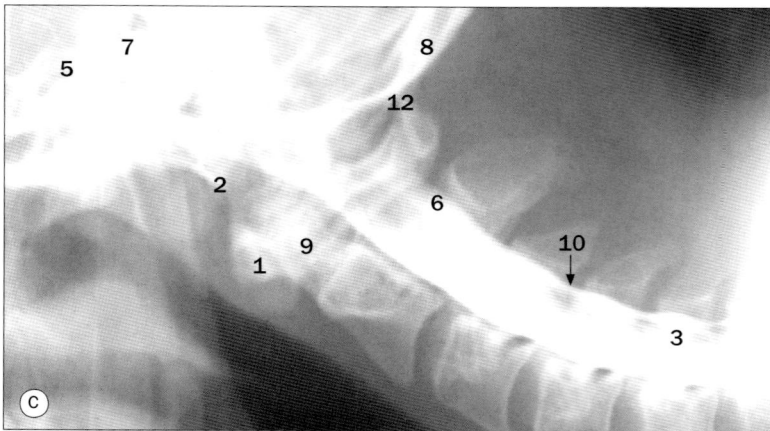

Cervical myelogram, (c) with the patient prone, (d) with the patient supine, lateral projections.

 1 Anterior arch of atlas (first cervical vertebra)
 2 Anterior rim of foramen magnum
 3 Cervical cord
 4 Cisterna magna (cerebellomedullary cistern)
 5 Clivus
 6 Contrast medium in cervical subarachnoid space
 7 External acoustic meatus
 8 Occiput
 9 Odontoid (process) dens
10 Posterior indentation on theca from ligamentum flavum
11 Posterior inferior cerebellar artery
12 Posterior rim of foramen magnum
13 Posterior tubercle of atlas (first cervical vertebra)

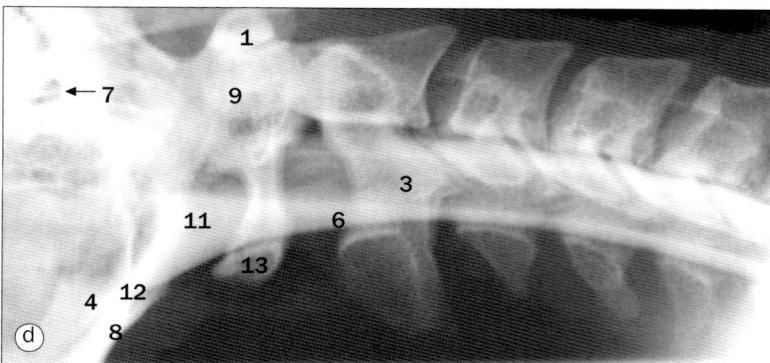

Lumbar radiculogram, (a) lateral projection, (b) oblique projection, (c) anteroposterior projection.

Non-ionic water-soluble contrast medium is introduced into the lumbar subarachnoid space via a lumbar puncture. The nerve roots of the cauda equina are well demonstrated and exit through the intervertebral foramina. The nerve roots extending from the conus to the terminal thecal sac pass below the pedicle of the corresponding vertebra. The thecal sac terminates at the level of the first/second sacral vertebrae. The filum terminale may be seen. Tilting the prone patient slightly head down allows the contrast to flow cranially and outlines the conus and lower thoracic cord. The cord is uniform in size from the second to the tenth thoracic vertebra, at which point its second, smaller expansion (for the lumbosacral plexus) extends from the tenth thoracic vertebra to the level of the first lumbar vertebra. The conus medullaris usually terminates at the first/second lumbar vertebrae, but may be seen at a level above and below as a normal variant.

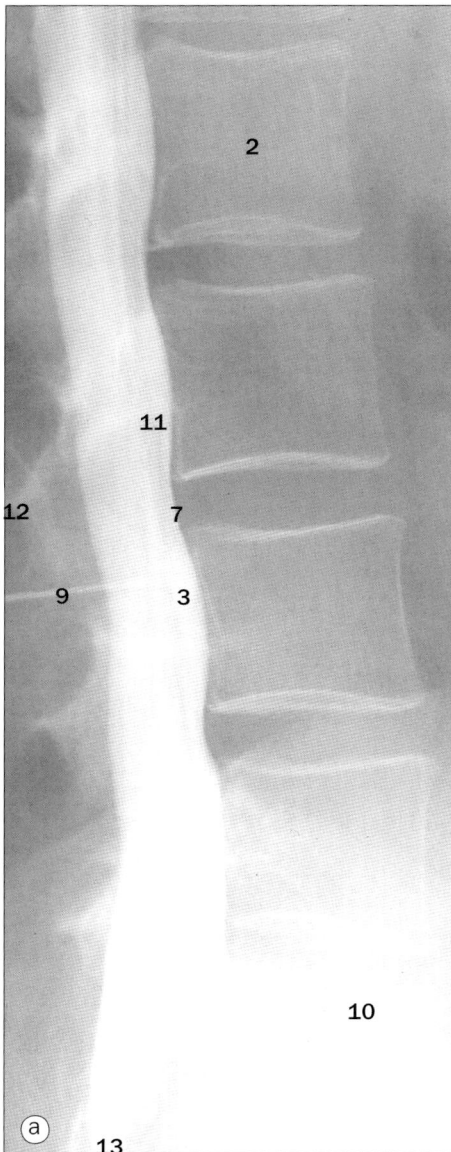

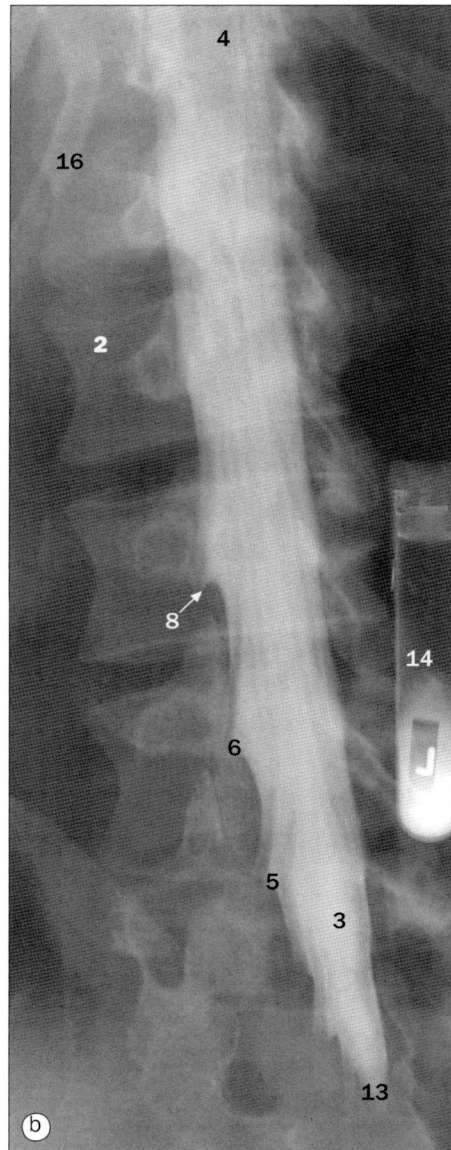

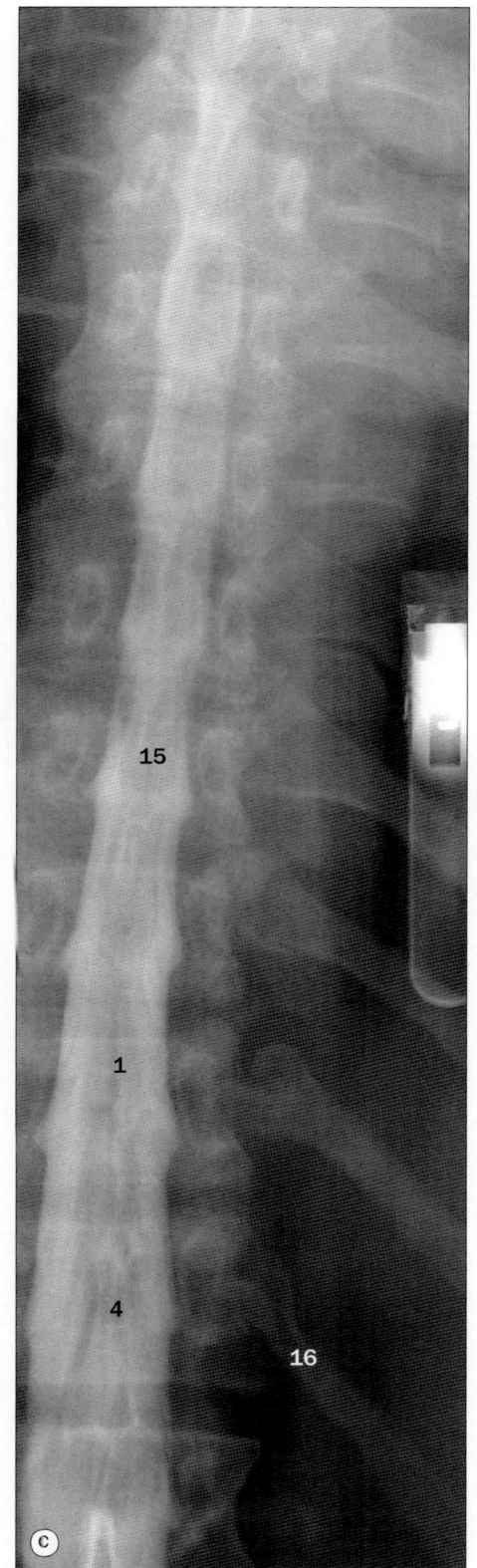

1 Anterior median fissure
2 Body of second lumbar vertebra
3 Contrast medium in subarachnoid space
4 Conus medullaris
5 Fifth lumbar spinal nerve
6 Fourth lumbar spinal nerve
7 Intervertebral disc indentations in anterior thecal margin
8 Lateral extension of subarachnoid space around spinal nerve roots
9 Lumbar puncture needle in space between third and fourth lumbar vertebrae
10 Sacral promontory
11 Spinal nerves within subarachnoid space (cauda equina)
12 Spinous process of third lumbar vertebra
13 Terminal theca at first/second sacral vertebra
14 Test tube containing contrast medium to indicate tilt of patient
15 Thoracic cord
16 Twelfth rib

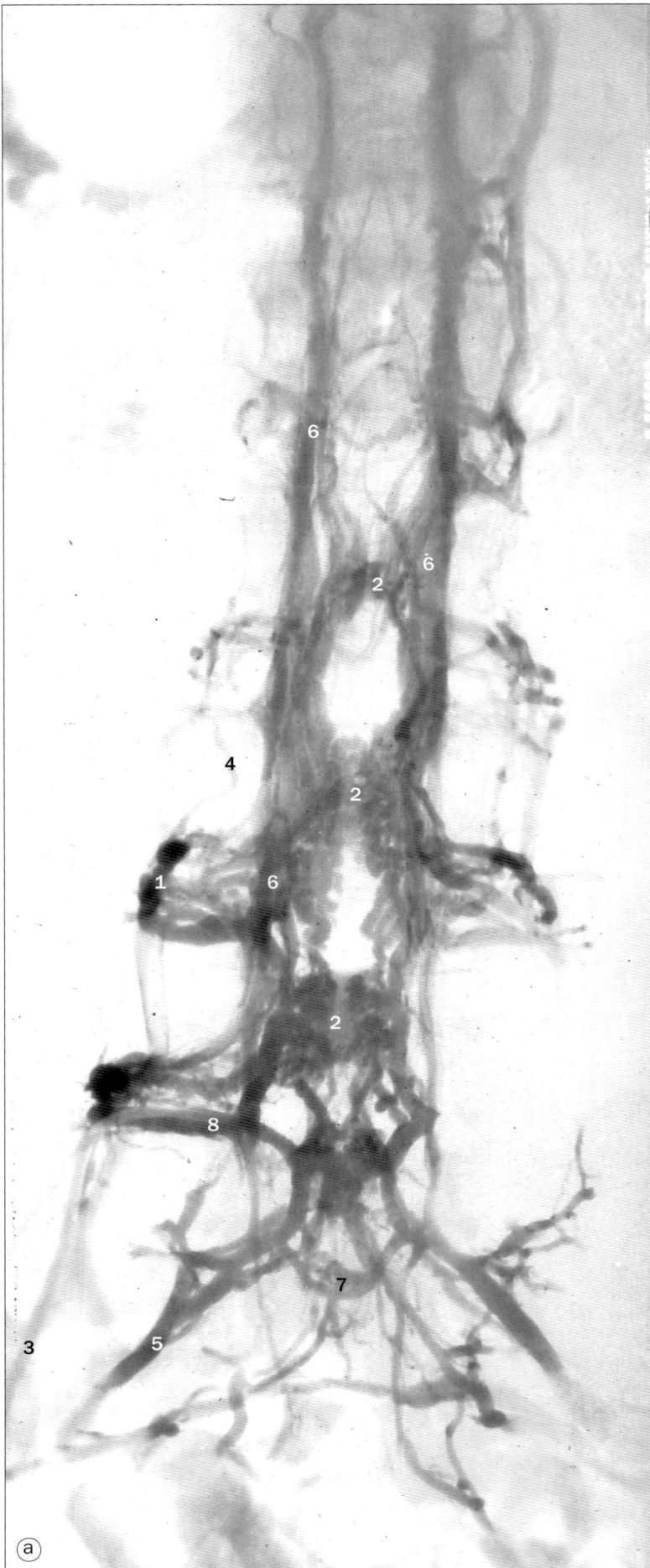

(a)

(a) Subtracted lumbar venogram.
Since the advent of CT and MR imaging techniques, lumbar venography is rarely performed. However, the anatomy of the vertebral veins is optimally demonstrated by this technique. Venous drainage of the spinal cord is longitudinally arranged via plexi, which anastomose freely with the internal (6) and external (1 and 4) vertebral venous plexi, which also communicate (4 and 2). Note how the internal veins bend laterally at the level of the disc interspace and medially at the level of pedicles, where they unite via a connecting vein (2).

1 Ascending lumbar veins
2 Basivertebral veins
3 Catheter in common iliac vein
4 Intervertebral veins
5 Lateral sacral veins
6 Longitudinal vertebral venous plexi
7 Sacral venous plexus
8 Tip of catheter in intravertebral vein

(b) Spinal arteriogram.

1 Anterior spinal artery
2 Arteria radicularis magna (Adamkiewicz)
3 Normal transdural stenosis of the arteria radicularis magna
4 Selective catheterisation of left eleventh intercostal artery

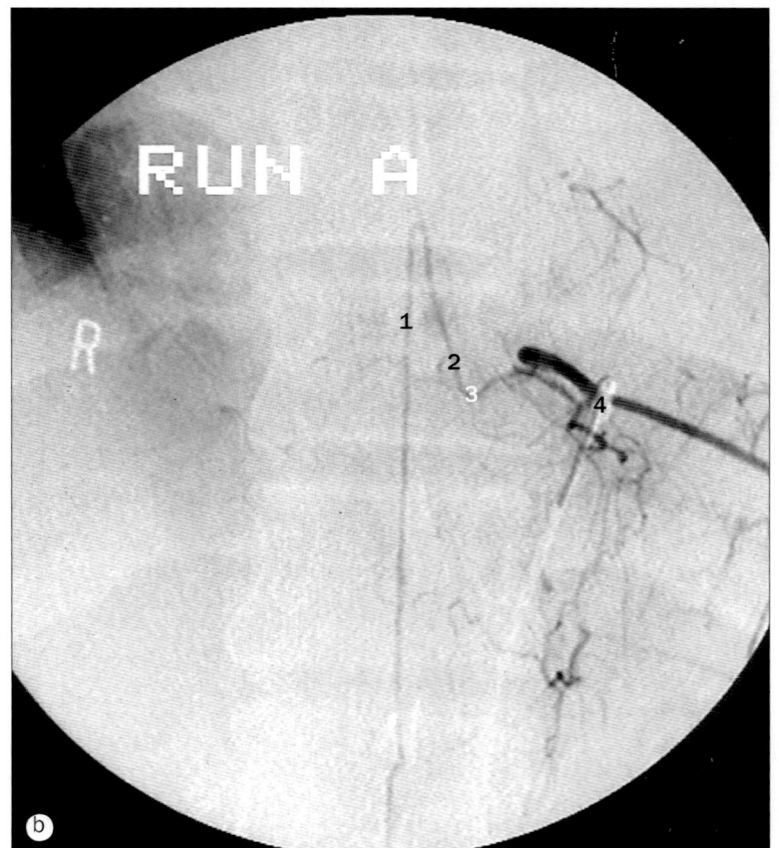

(b)

3 Upper limb

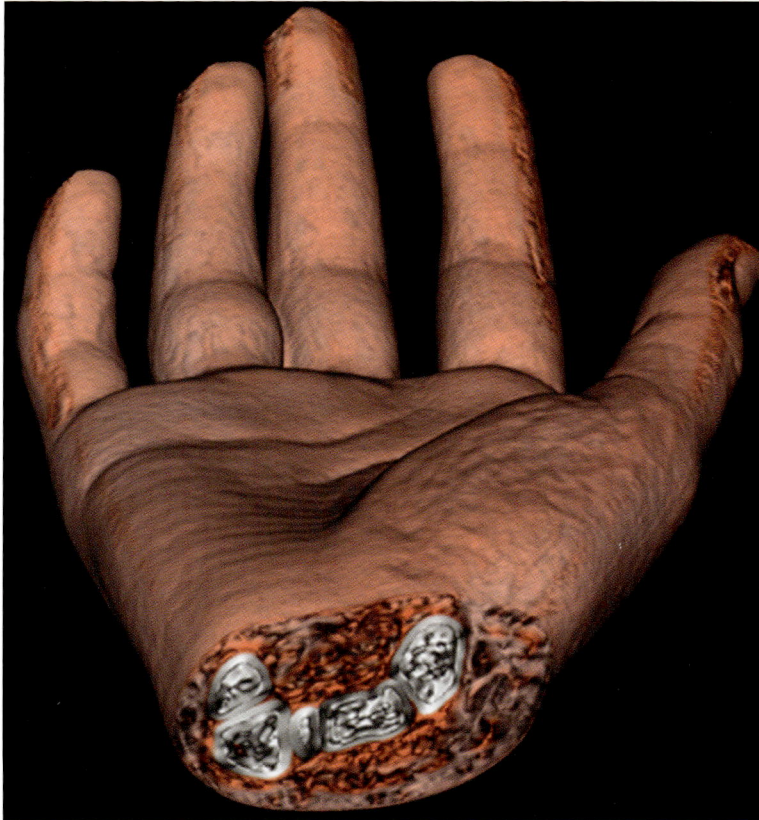

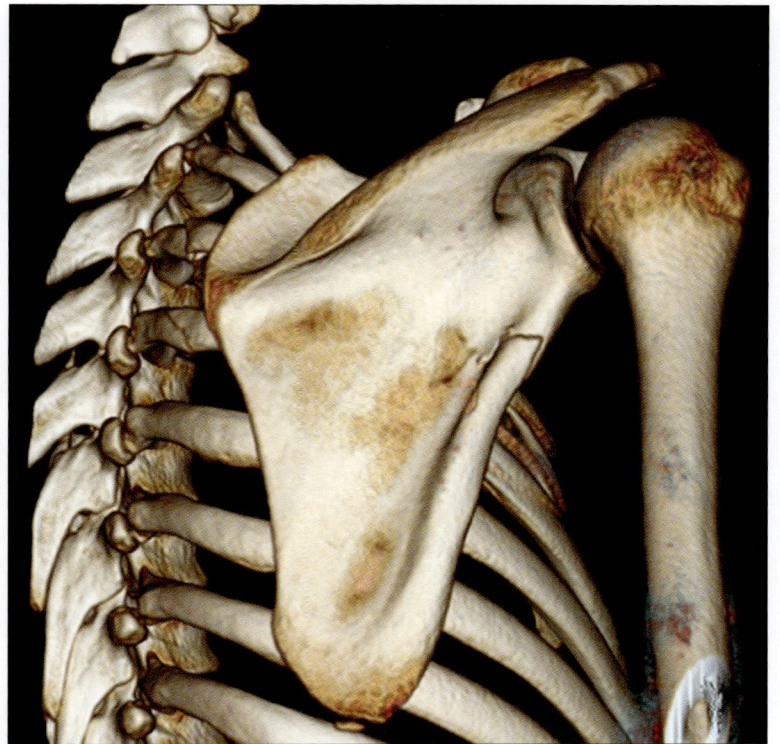

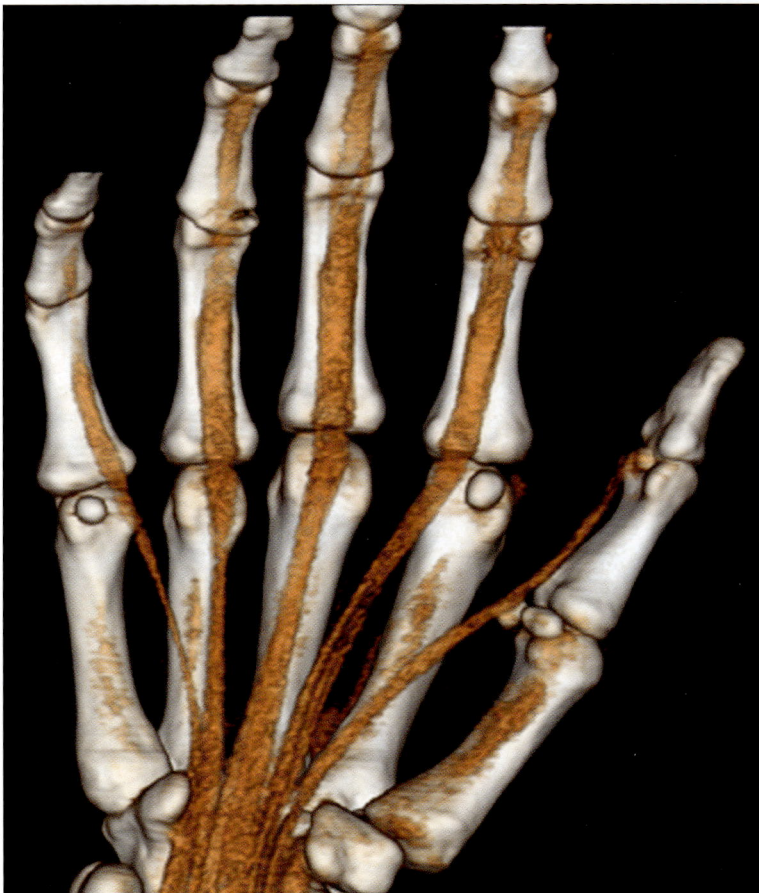

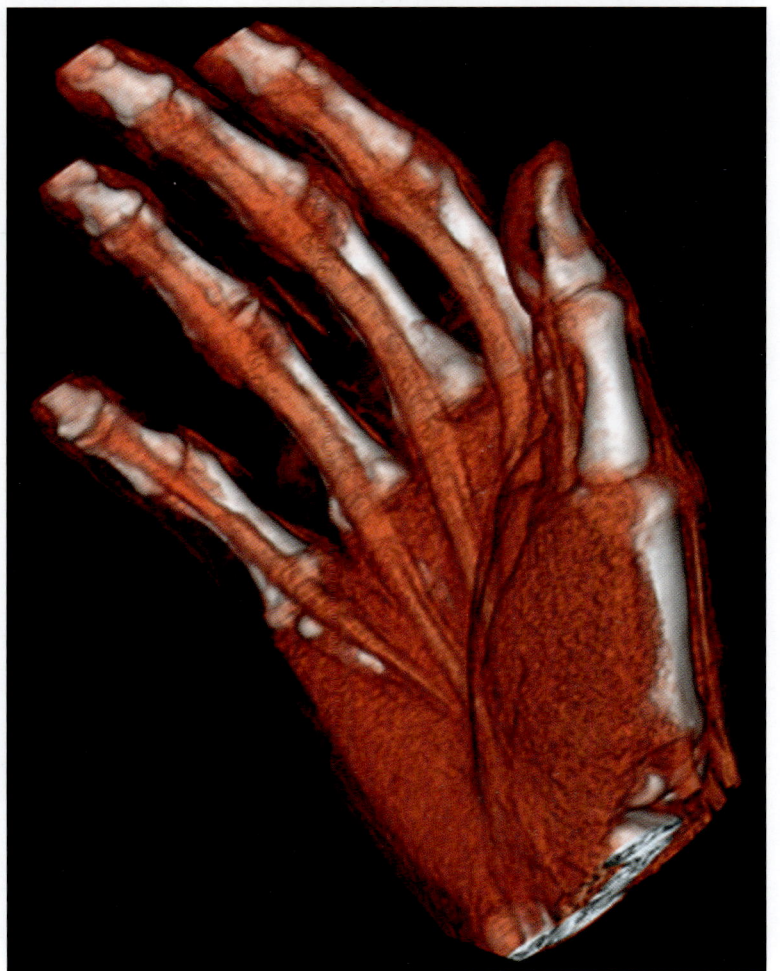

(a) Shoulder, anteroposterior radiograph.

1 Acromion of scapula
2 Anatomical neck
3 Clavicle
4 Coracoid process of scapula
5 Glenoid fossa of scapula
6 Greater tubercle (tuberosity) of
   humerus
7 Head of humerus
8 Lesser tubercle (tuberosity) of
   humerus
9 Scapula
10 Surgical neck

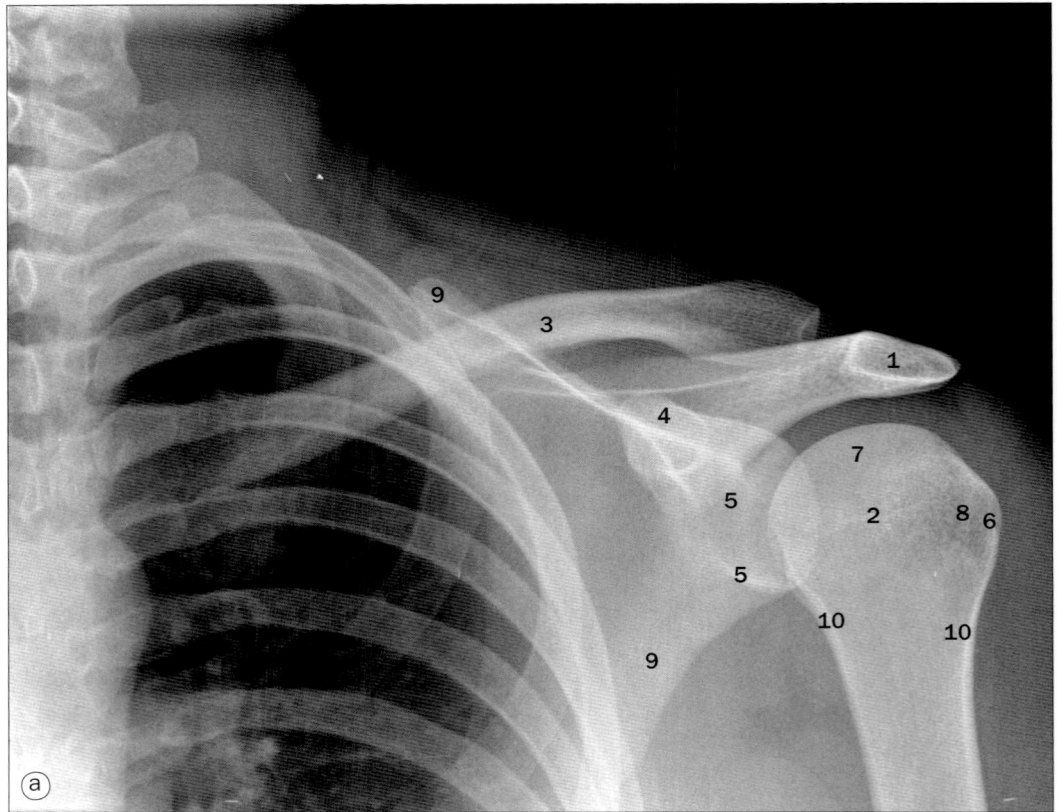

(b) Shoulder, axial (supero-inferior) projection.

1 Acromion of scapula
2 Clavicle
3 Coracoid process of scapula
4 Glenoid fossa of scapula
5 Greater tubercle (tuberosity) of
   humerus
6 Head of humerus
7 Intertubercular groove of humerus
8 Lesser tubercle (tuberosity) of
   humerus
9 Spine of scapula

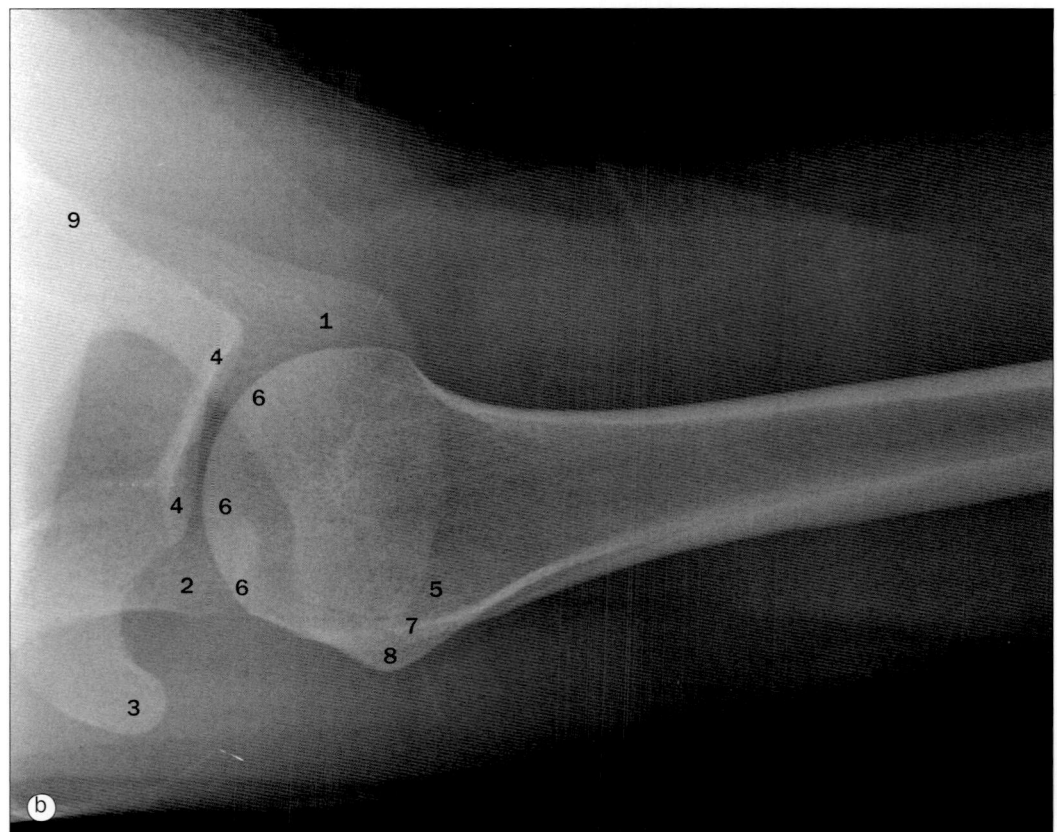

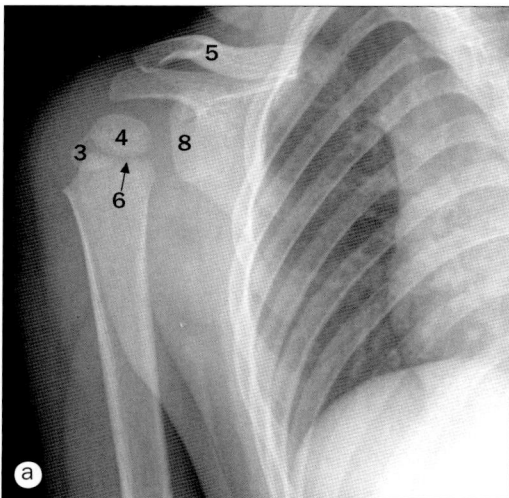

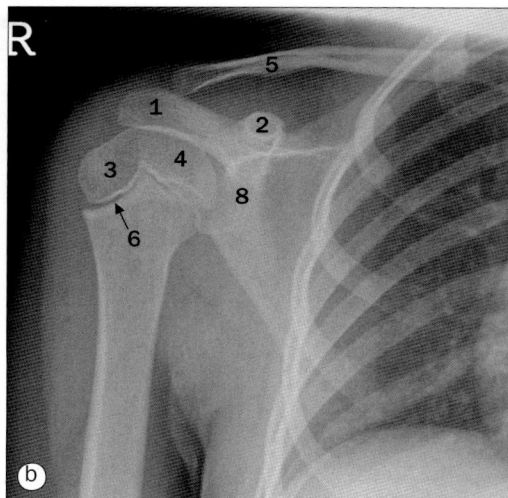

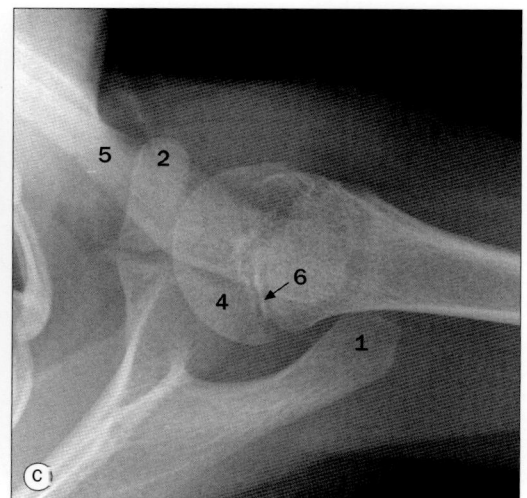

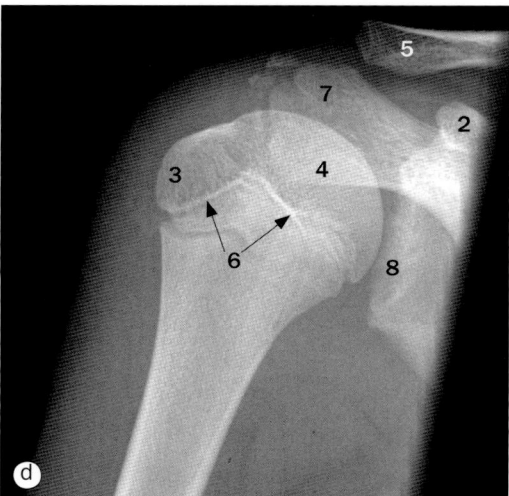

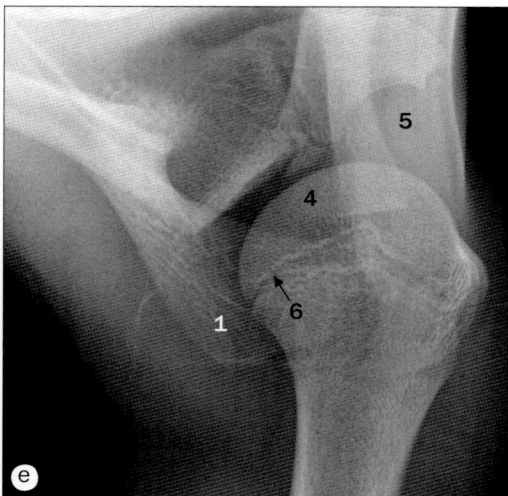

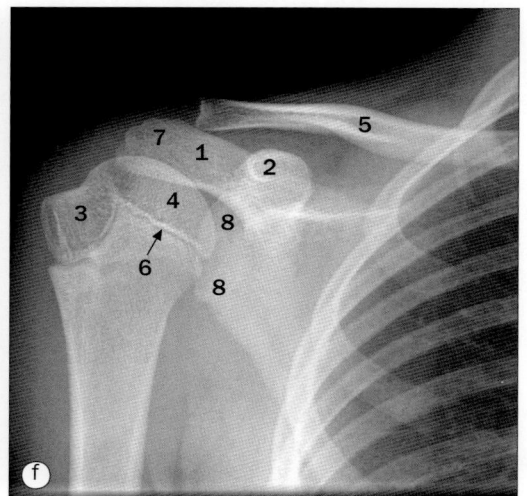

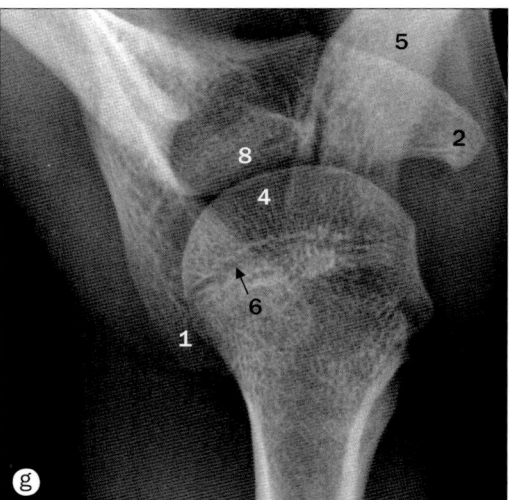

Shoulder, (a) (anteroposterior) of a 1-year-old child, (b) (anteroposterior) and (c) (axial) of a 6-year-old child, (d) (anteroposterior) and (e) (axial) of a 12-year-old child (f) (anteroposterior) and (g) (axial) of a 14-year-old child.

1 Acromion of scapula
2 Centre for coracoid process
3 Centre for greater tubercle (tuberosity) of humerus
4 Centre for head of humerus
5 Clavicle
6 Epiphysial line
7 Centre for acromion
8 Glenoid fossa of scapula

CLAVICLE (m)	Appears	Fused
Lateral end	5 wiu	20+ yrs
Medial end	15 yrs	20+ yrs
SCAPULA (c)		
Body	8 wiu	15 yrs
Coracoid	<1 yr	20 yrs
Coracoid base	Puberty	15–20 yrs
Acromion	Puberty	15–20 yrs

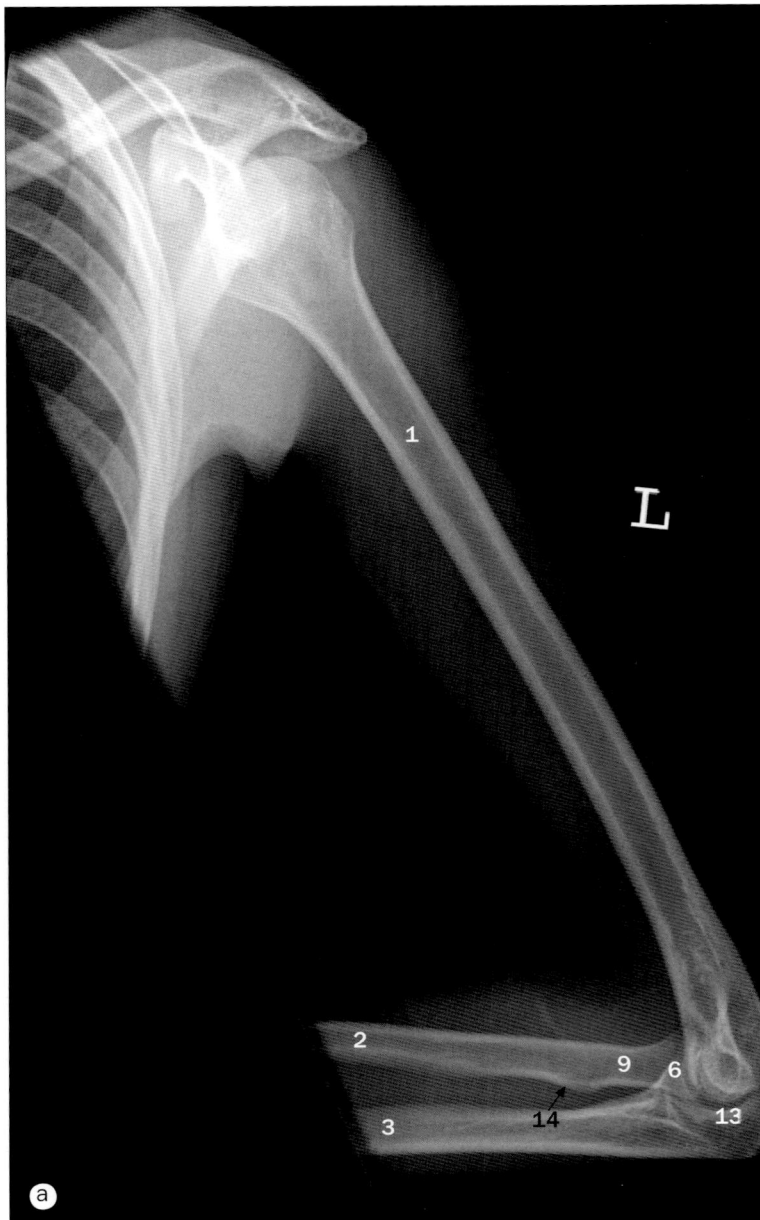

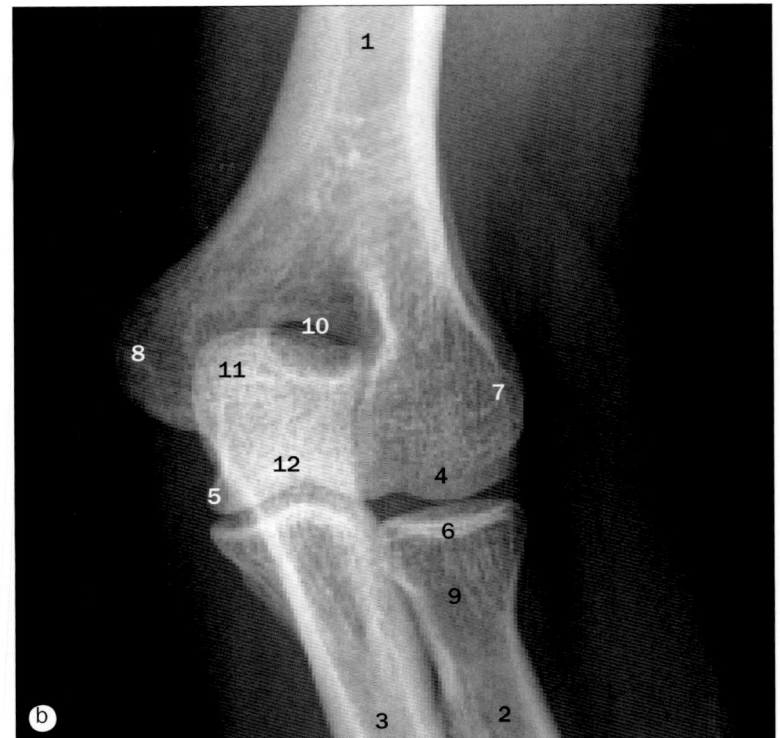

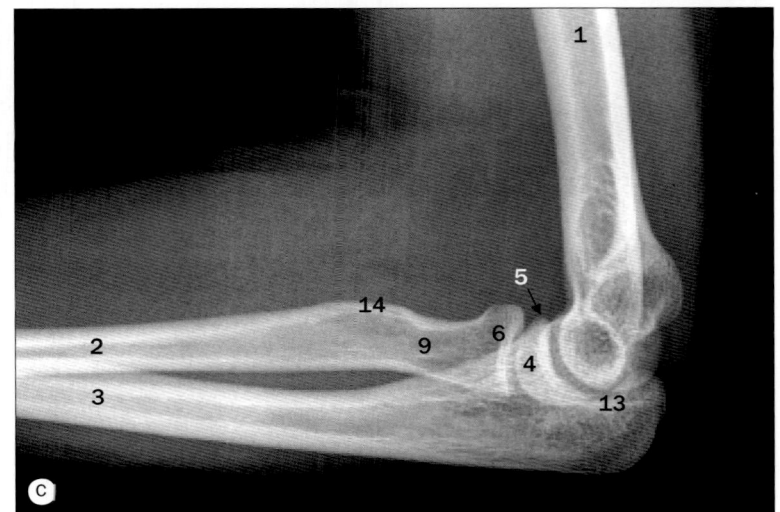

(a) Humerus, lateral projection, (b) elbow, anteroposterior projection, (c) elbow, lateral projection.

1 Humerus	8 Medial epicondyle of humerus
2 Radius	9 Neck of radius
3 Ulna	10 Olecranon fossa of humerus
4 Capitulum of humerus	11 Olecranon of ulna
5 Coronoid process of ulna	12 Trochlea of humerus
6 Head of radius	13 Trochlear notch of ulna
7 Lateral epicondyle of humerus	14 Tuberosity of radius

HUMERUS (c)	Appears	Fused
Shaft	8 wiu	15–20 yrs
Head	1–6 mths	15–20 yrs
Greater tubercle	6 mths–1 yr	15–20 yrs
Lesser tubercle	3–5 yrs	18–20 yrs
Capitulum	4 mths–1 yr	13–16 yrs
Medial trochlea	10 yrs	13–16 yrs
Medial epicondyle	3–6 yrs	13–16 yrs
Lateral epicondyle	9–12 yrs	13–16 yrs

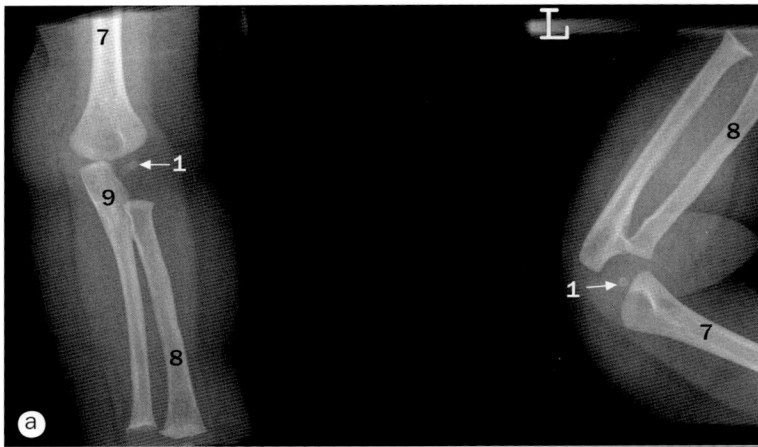

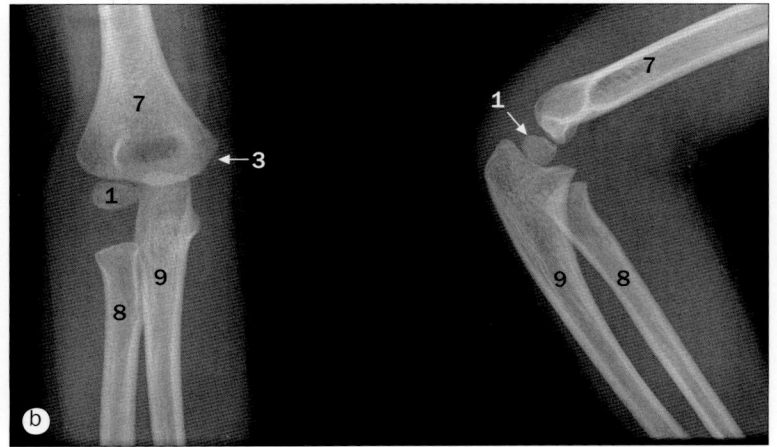

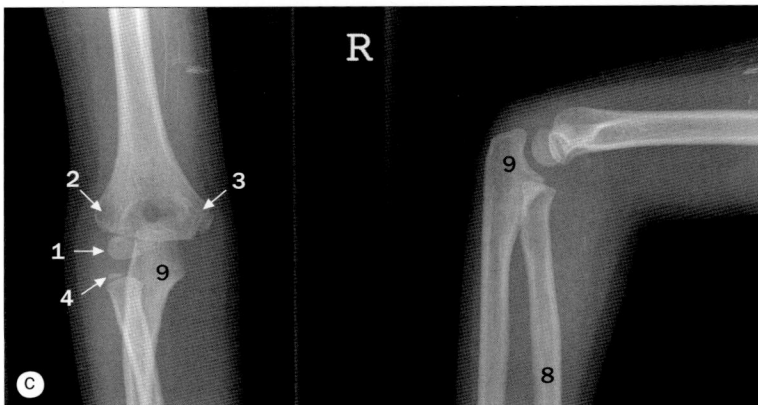

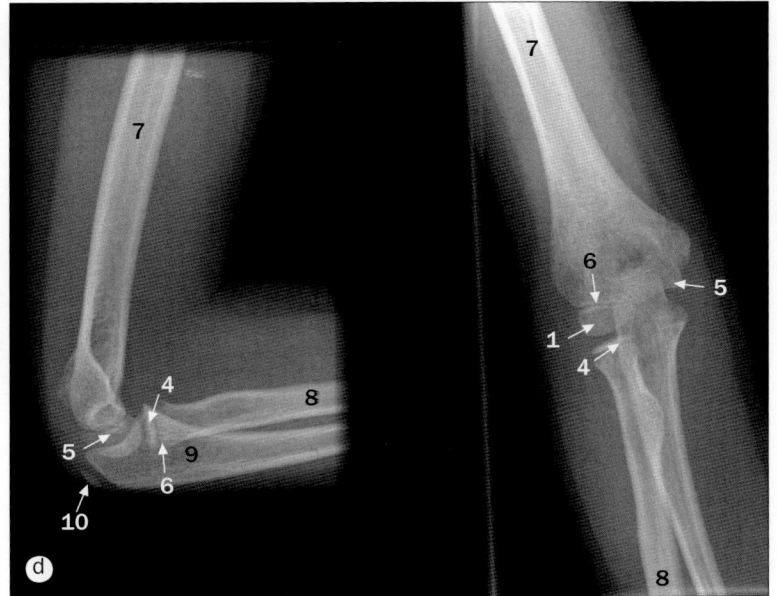

Elbow images, (a) 7-month-old child, (b) 3-year-old child, (c) 6-year-old child, (d) 9-year-old child.

RADIUS (c)		
Shaft	8 wiu	
Proximal	4–6 yrs	13–16 yrs
Distal	1 yr	16–18 yrs

ULNA (c)		
Shaft	8 wiu	
Proximal	8–10 yrs	13–15 yrs
Distal	5–7 yrs	16–18 yrs

1 Centre for capitulum
2 Centre for lateral epicondyle
3 Centre for medial epicondyle
4 Centre for radial head
5 Centre for trochlea
6 Epiphysial line
7 Humerus
8 Radius
9 Ulna
10 Centre for olecranon

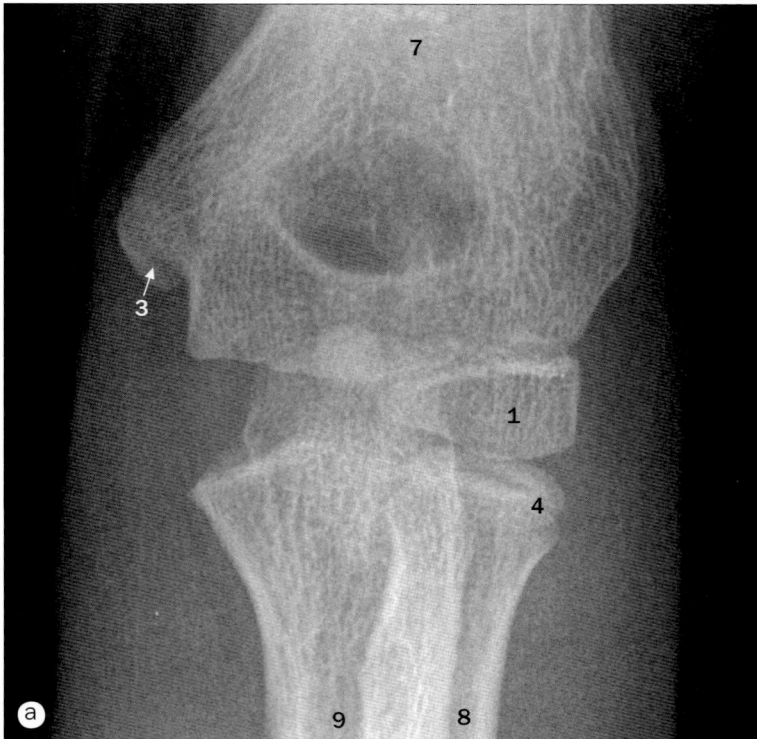

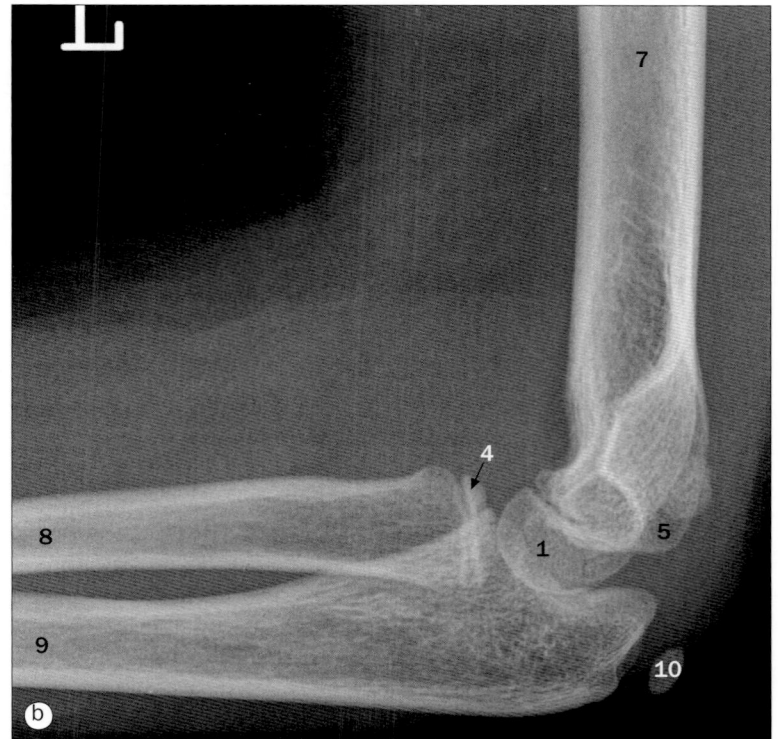

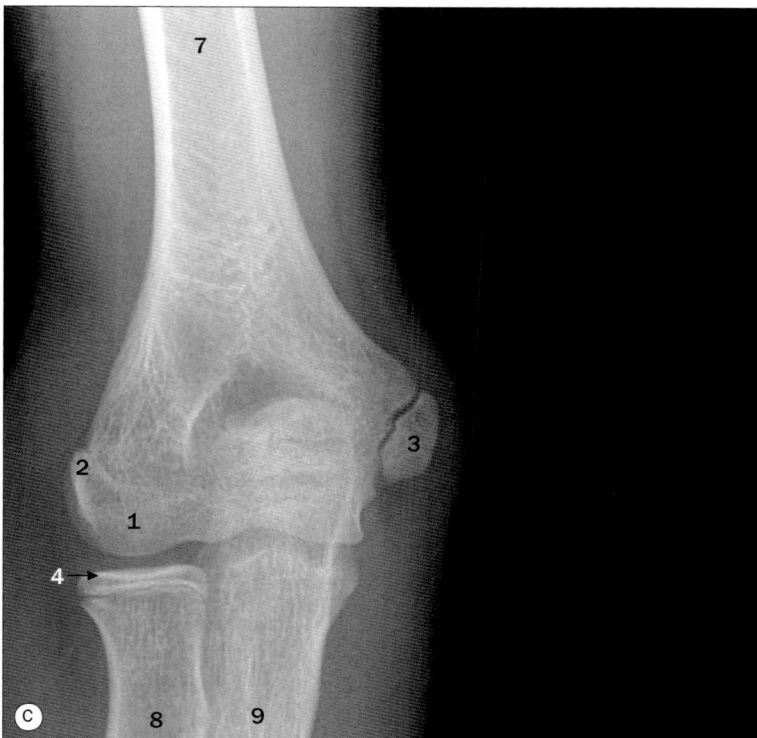

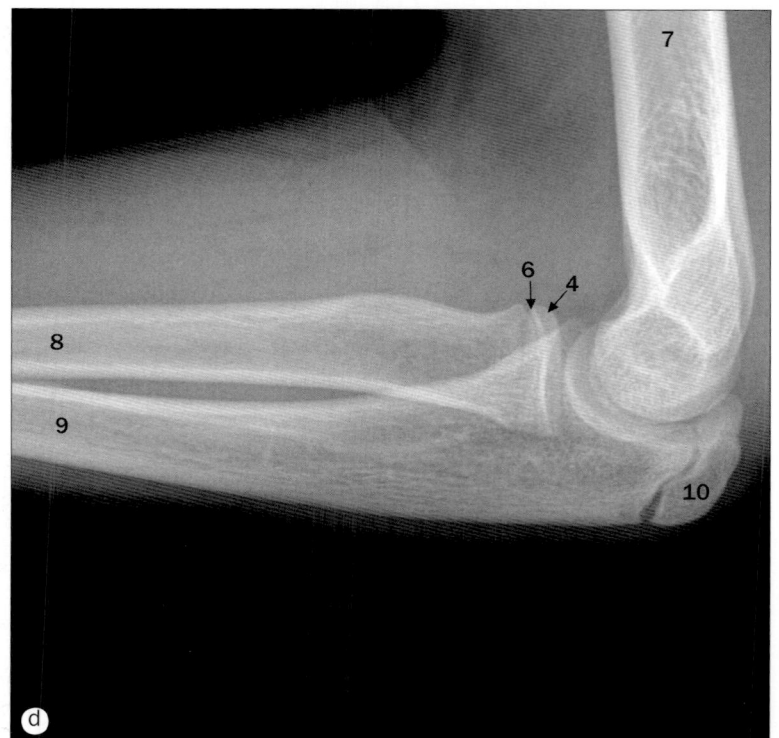

Elbow images, (a) and (b) 11-year-old child, (c) and (d) 14-year-old child.

1	Centre for capitulum	6	Epiphyseal line
2	Centre for lateral epicondyle	7	Humerus
3	Centre for medial epicondyle	8	Radius
4	Centre for radial head	9	Ulna
5	Centre for trochlea	10	Centre for olecranon

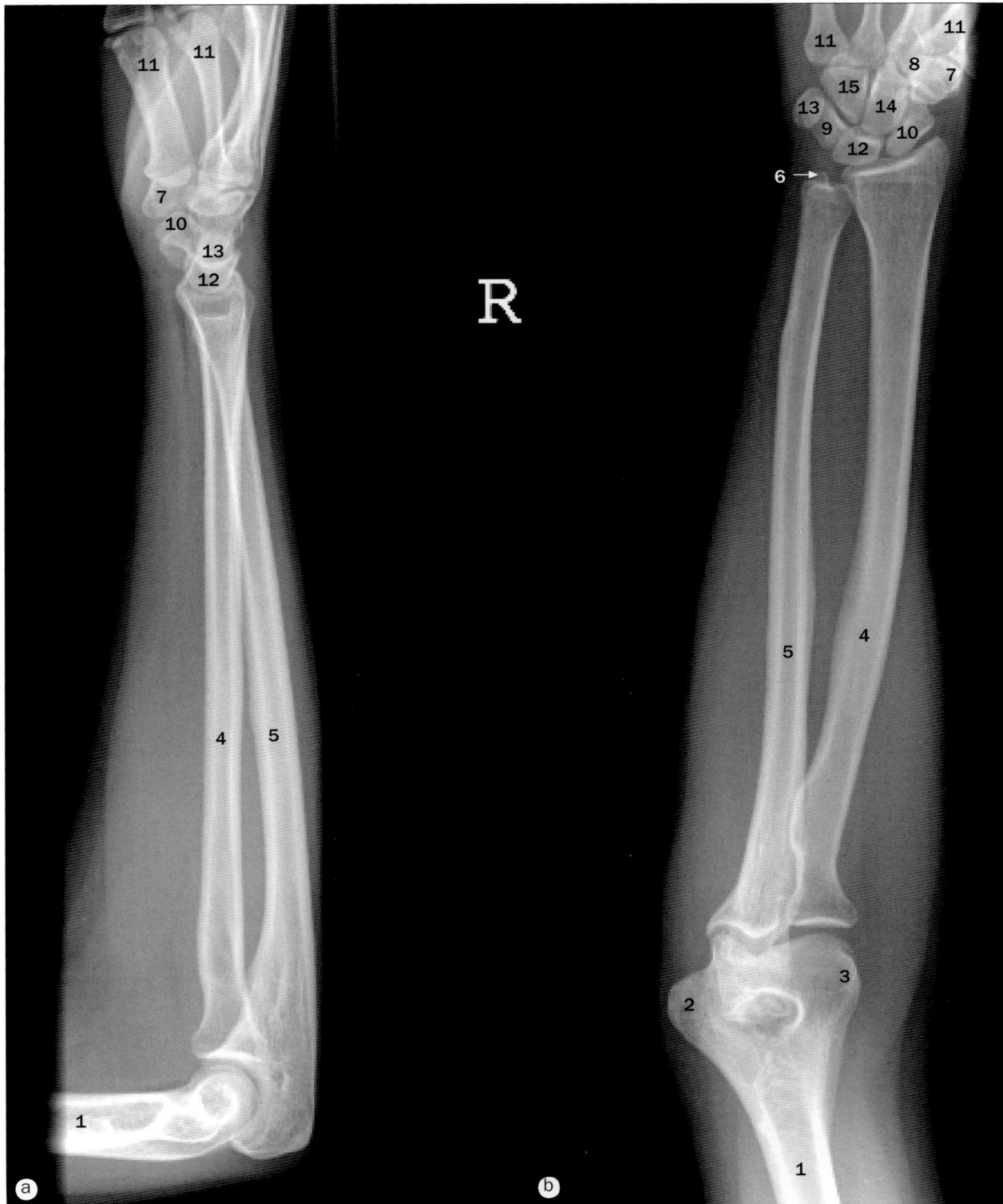

Forearm images, (a) lateral and (b) anteroposterior.

1 Humerus	5 Ulna	10 Scaphoid
2 Medial epicondyle of humerus	6 Styloid of ulna	11 Metacarpals
3 Lateral epicondyle of humerus	7 Trapezium	12 Lunate
4 Radius	8 Trapezoid	13 Pisiform
	9 Triquetral	14 Capitate
		15 Hamate

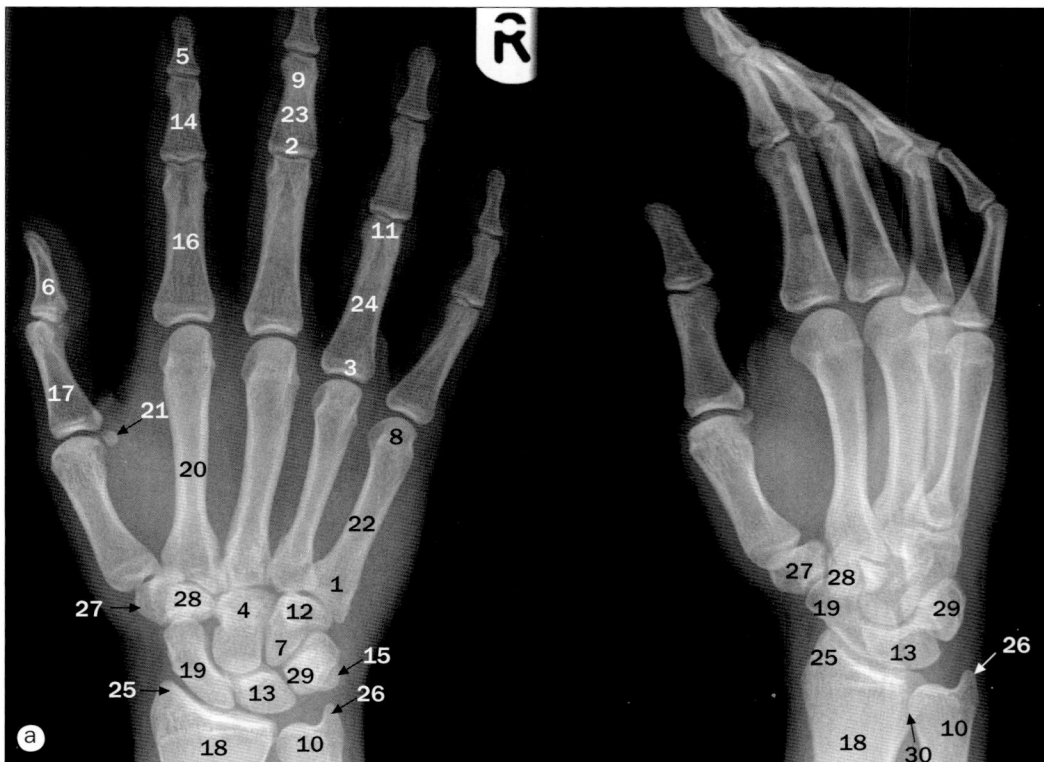

(a) Bones of the hand, dorsopalmar and oblique projection.

1 Base of fifth metacarpal	12 Hook of hamate	22 Shaft of fifth metacarpal
2 Base of middle phalanx of middle finger	13 Lunate	23 Shaft of middle phalanx of middle finger
3 Base of proximal phalanx of ring finger	14 Middle phalanx of index finger	24 Shaft of proximal phalanx of ring finger
4 Capitate	15 Pisiform	25 Styloid process of radius
5 Distal phalanx of index finger	16 Proximal phalanx of index finger	26 Styloid process of ulna
6 Distal phalanx of thumb	17 Proximal phalanx of thumb	27 Trapezium
7 Hamate	18 Radius	28 Trapezoid
8 Head of fifth metacarpal	19 Scaphoid	29 Triquetral
9 Head of middle phalanx of middle finger	20 Second metacarpal	30 Ulnar notch of radius
10 Head of ulna	21 Sesamoid bone	31 Base of metacarpal
11 Head of proximal phalanx of ring finger		

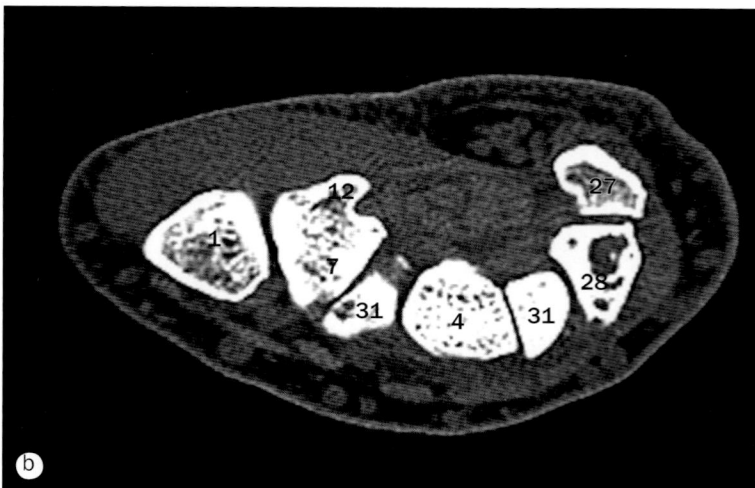

(b) Axial CT through carpal tunnel.

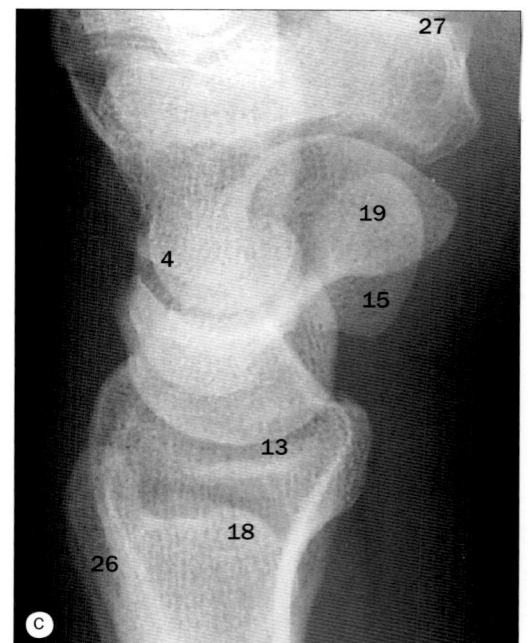

(c) Bones of the wrist, lateral projection.

Bones of the hand (dorsopalmar projections), (a) of a 10-month-old child, (b) of a 2-year-old child, (c) of a 6-year-old child, (d) of a 9-year-old child, to illustrate centres of ossification, (e) of an 11-year-old child.

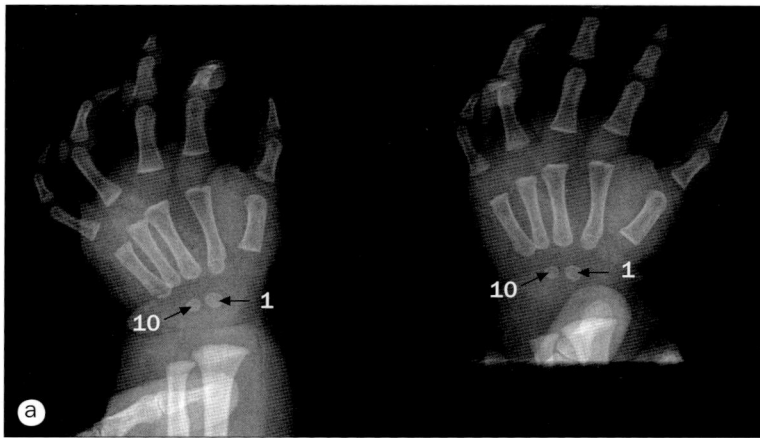

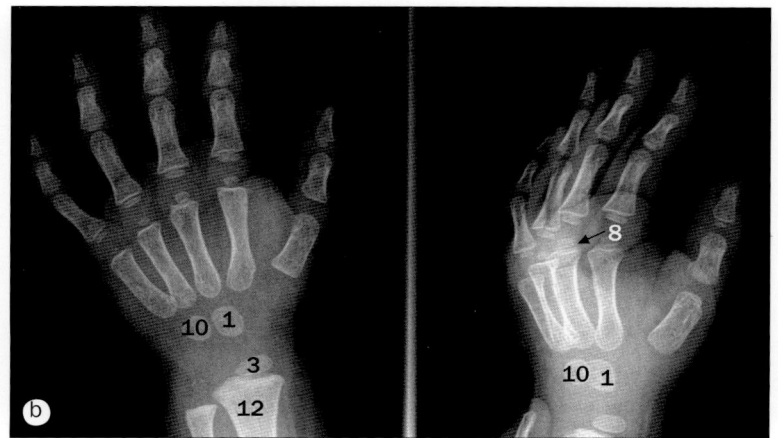

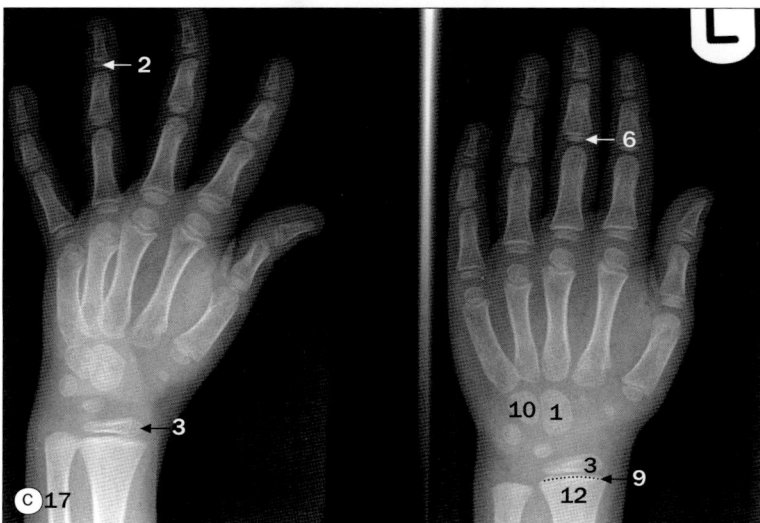

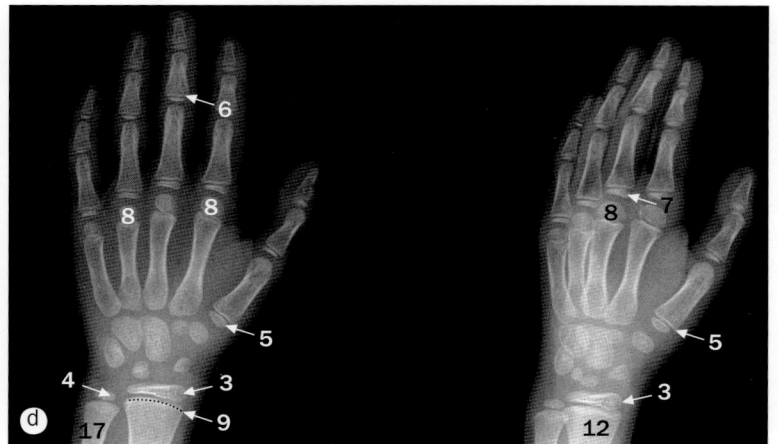

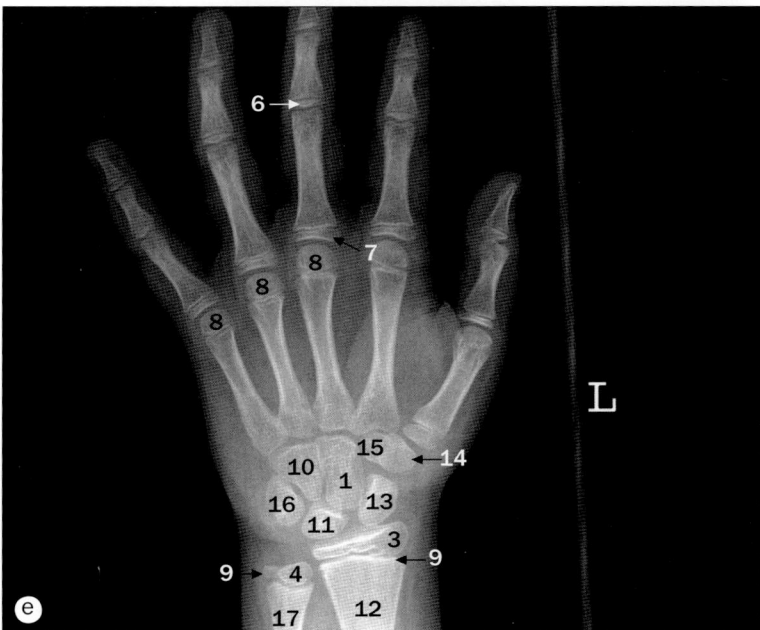

CARPUS (c)	Appears	Fused
Capitate	1–3 mths	
Hamate	2–4 mths	
Triquetral	2–3 yrs	
Lunate	2–4 yrs	
Scaphoid	4–6 yrs	
Trapezium	4–6 yrs	
Trapezoid	4–6 yrs	
Pisiform (sesamoid)	8–12 yrs	
METACARPALS (c)		
Shaft	9 wiu	
Head	1–2 yrs	14–19 yrs
PHALANGES (c)		
Shaft	8–12 wiu	
Base	1–3 yrs	14–18 yrs

1 Capitate
2 Centre for distal phalanx of ring finger
3 Centre for distal radius
4 Centre for distal ulna
5 Centre for first metacarpal
6 Centre for middle phalanx of middle finger
7 Centre for proximal phalanx of middle finger
8 Centre for second metacarpal (applies to second to fifth metacarpals)
9 Epiphysial line
10 Hamate
11 Lunate
12 Radius
13 Scaphoid
14 Trapezium
15 Trapezoid
16 Triquetral
17 Ulna

Axillary arteriograms, (**a**) subtracted, (**b**) digitally subtracted, (**c**) and (**d**) brachial arteriograms.

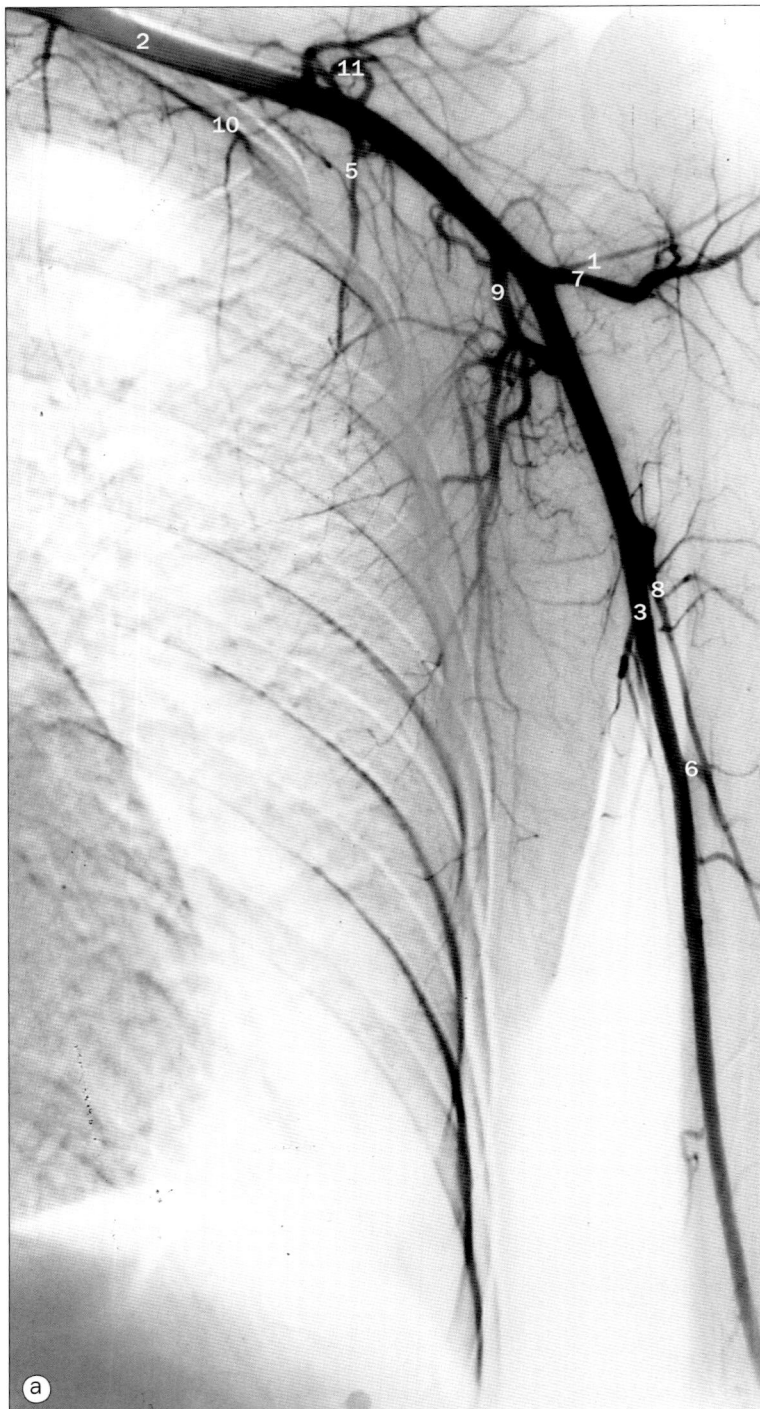

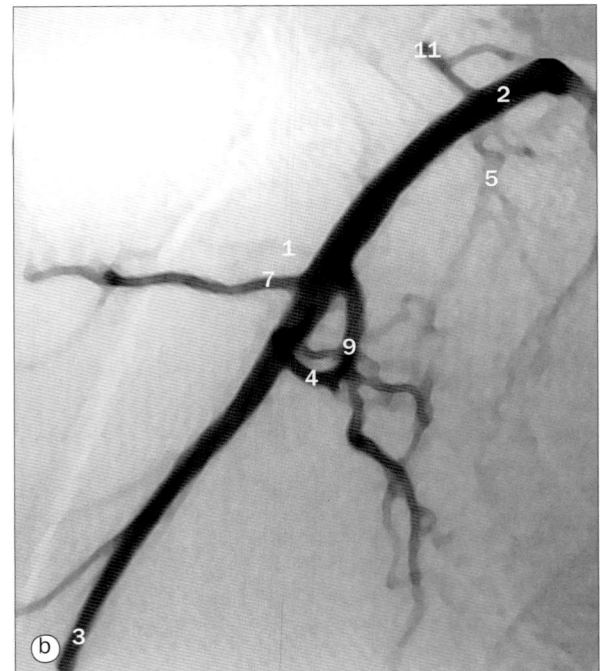

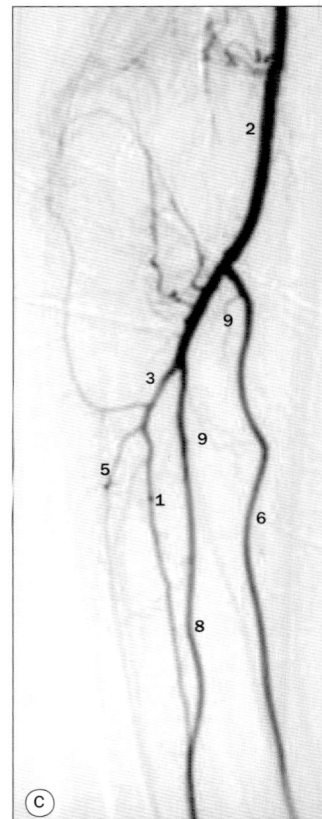

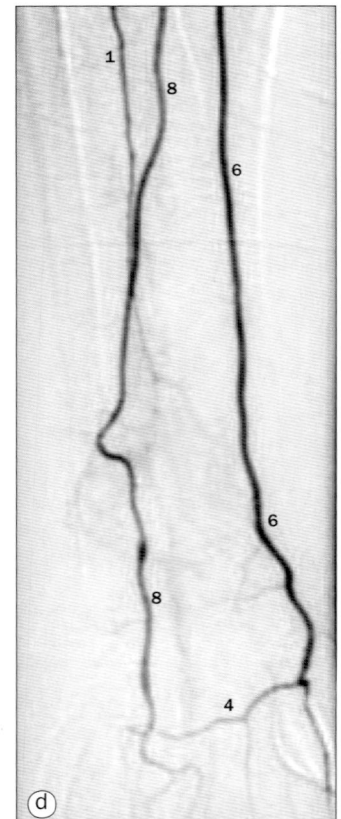

1 Anterior circumflex humeral artery	**7** Posterior circumflex humeral artery
2 Axillary artery	**8** Profunda brachii artery
3 Brachial artery	**9** Subscapular artery
4 Circumflex scapular artery	**10** Superior thoracic artery
5 Lateral thoracic artery	**11** Thoraco-acromial artery
6 Muscular branches of brachial artery	

1 Anterior interosseous artery	**5** Posterior interosseous artery
2 Brachial artery	**6** Radial artery
3 Common interosseous artery	**7** Radial recurrent artery
4 Deep palmar arch	**8** Ulnar artery
	9 Ulnar recurrent artery

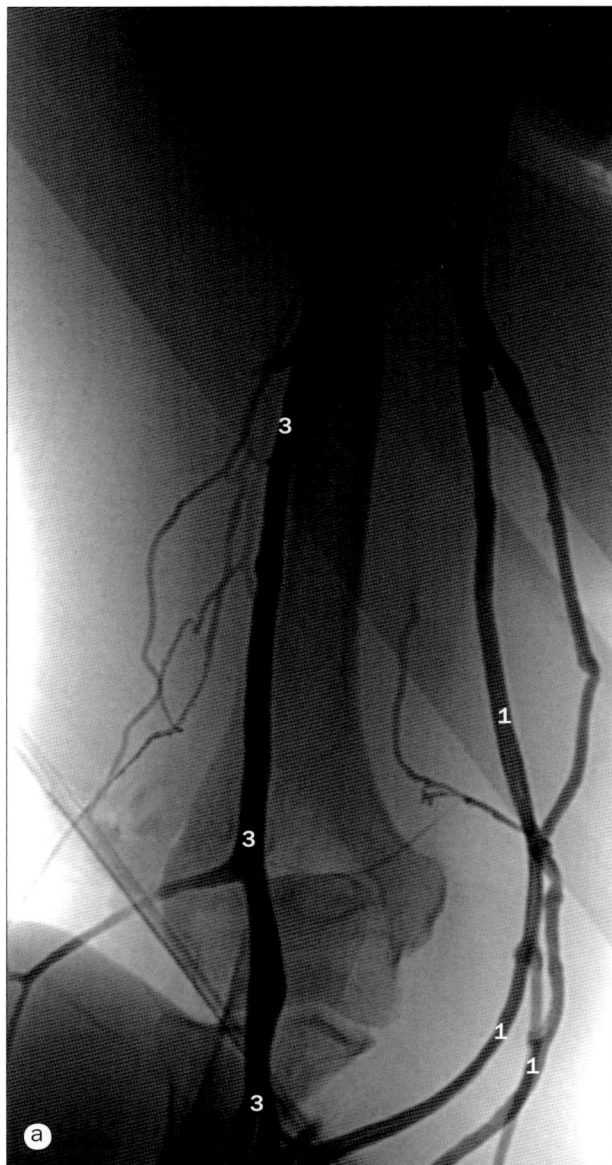

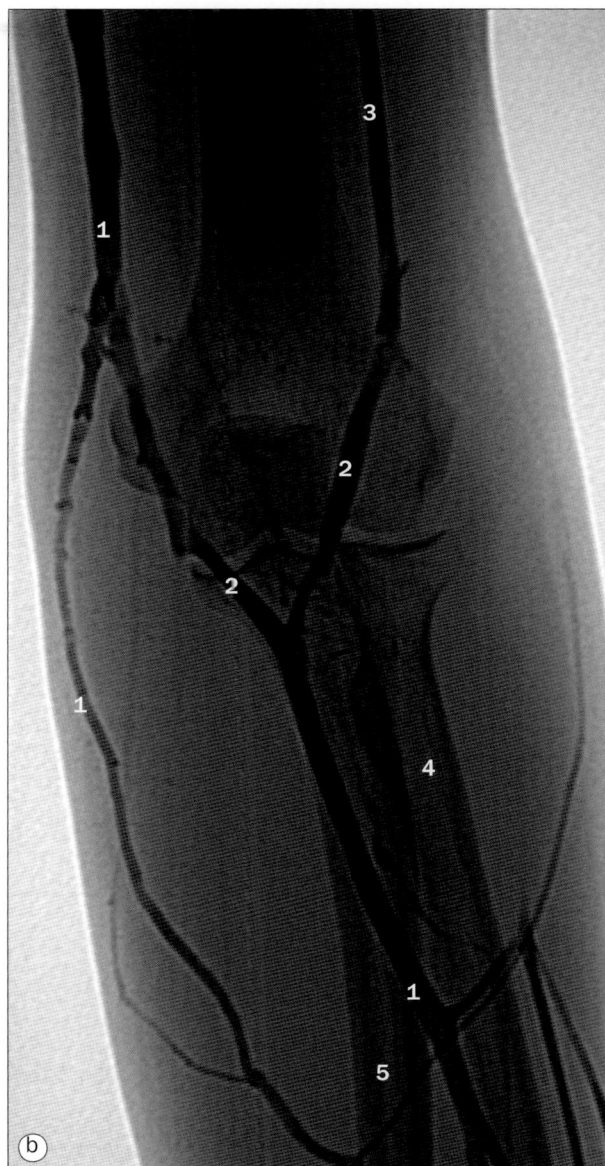

(a) and (b) Upper limbs venograms, (c) superior vena cavogram.

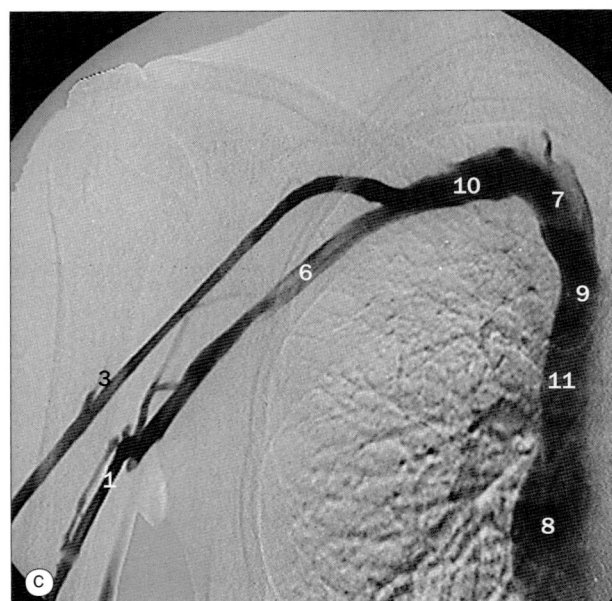

1 Basilic vein
2 Median cubital vein
3 Cephalic vein
4 Radius
5 Ulna
6 Axillary vein
7 Brachiocephalic vein
8 Right atrium
9 Site of entry of left brachiocephalic vein
10 Subclavian vein
11 Superior vena cava

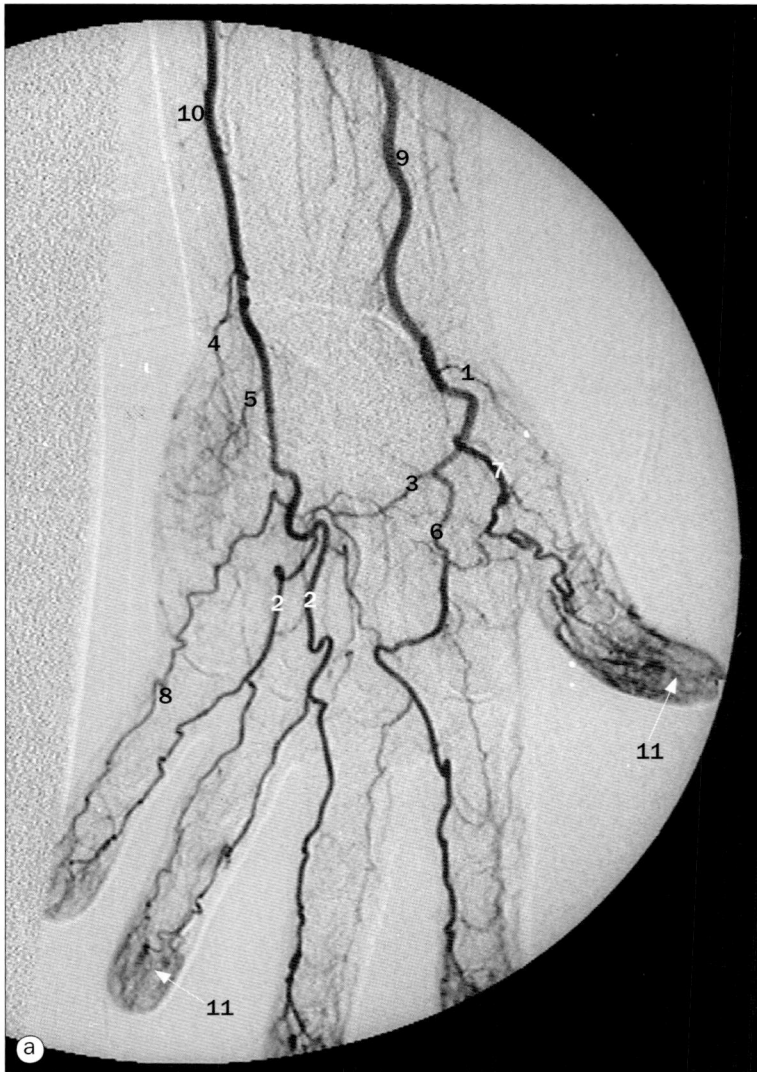

(a) Digitally subtracted hand arteriogram.
In this patient there is an incomplete superficial palmar arch.

(b) Venous phase of hand arteriogram.

1	Artery to radial aspects of thumb
2	Common palmar digital artery
3	Deep palmar arch
4	Deep palmar branch of ulnar artery
5	Palmar carpal branch of ulnar artery
6	Palmar metacarpal artery
7	Princeps pollicis artery
8	Proper palmar digital artery
9	Radial artery
10	Ulnar artery
11	Pulp anastomoses

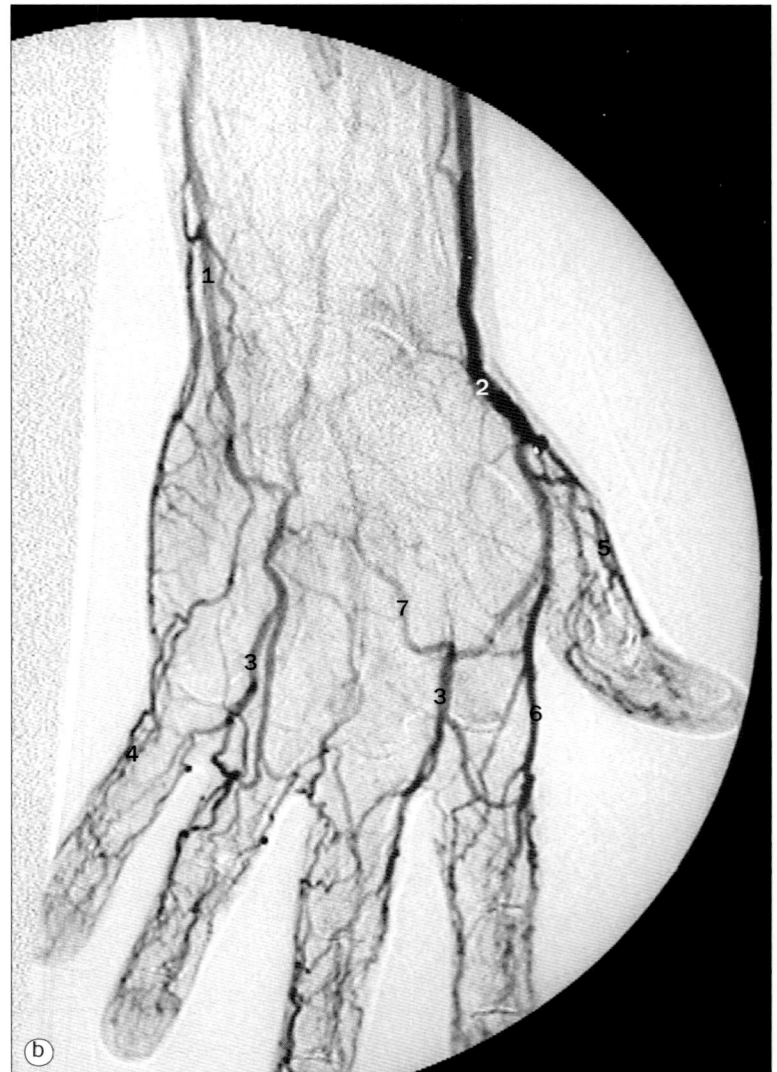

1	Basilic vein
2	Cephalic vein
3	Common palmar digital vein
4	Palmar digital vein
5	Princeps pollicis vein
6	Radialis indicis vein
7	Superficial palmar venous arch

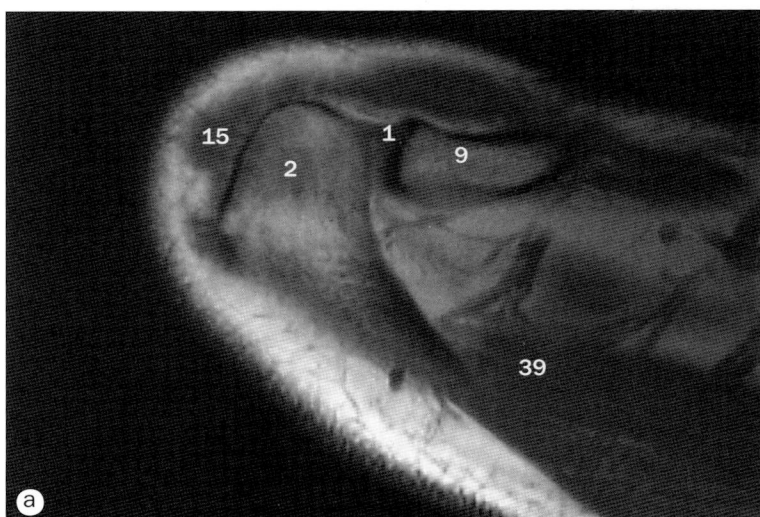

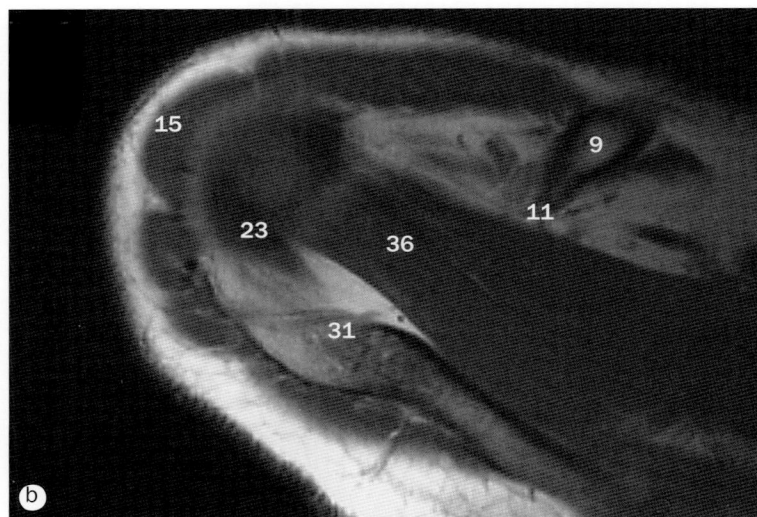

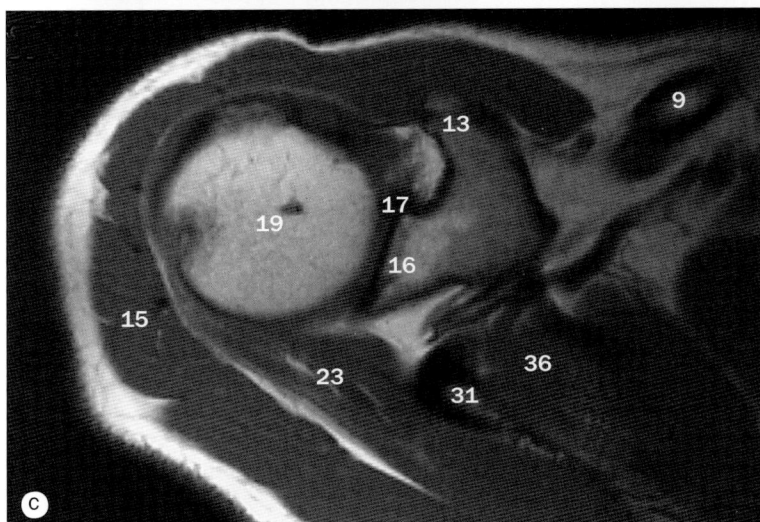

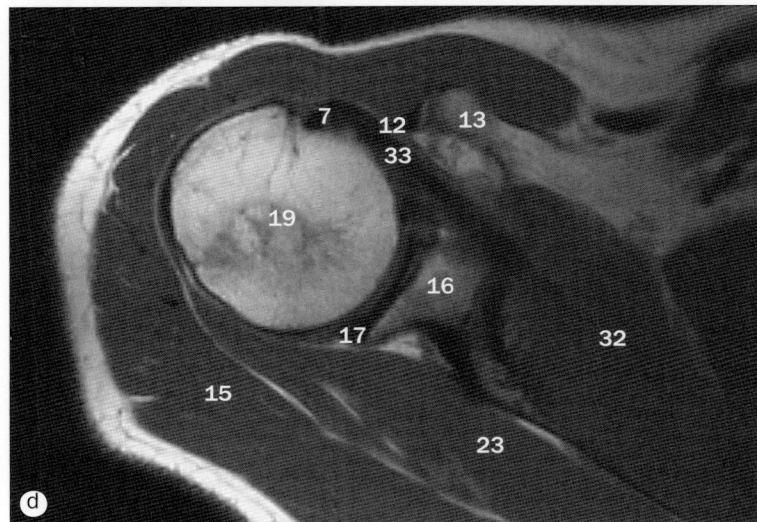

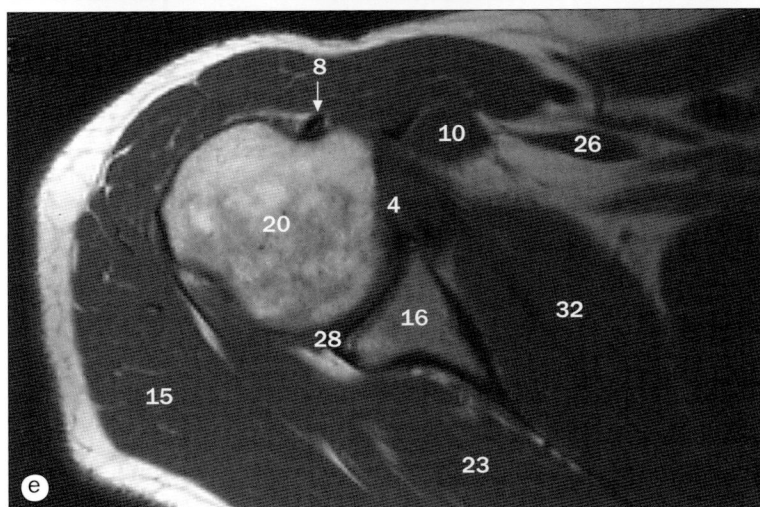

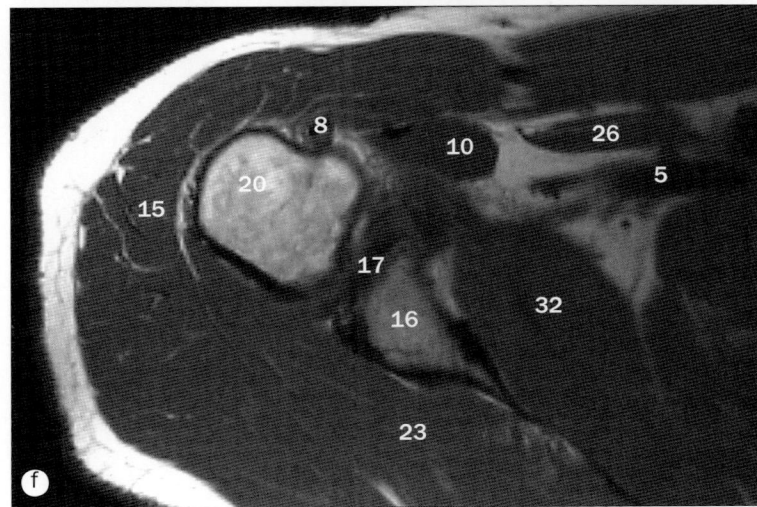

Shoulder, axial MR arthrography images.

1	Acromioclavicular joint	9	Clavicle	17	Glenoid labrum
2	Acromion	10	Coracobrachialis muscle	18	Greater tuberosity
3	Anterior capsule of shoulder joint	11	Coracoclavicular ligament	19	Head of humerus
4	Anterior labrum	12	Coracohumeral ligament	20	Humerus
5	Axillary artery and vein	13	Coracoid process	21	Inferior glenohumeral ligament
6	Axillary recess	14	Deltoid tendon	22	Inferior labrum
7	Biceps brachii tendon	15	Deltoid muscle	23	Infraspinatus muscle
8	Biceps brachii tendon (long head)	16	Glenoid	24	Infraspinatus tendon

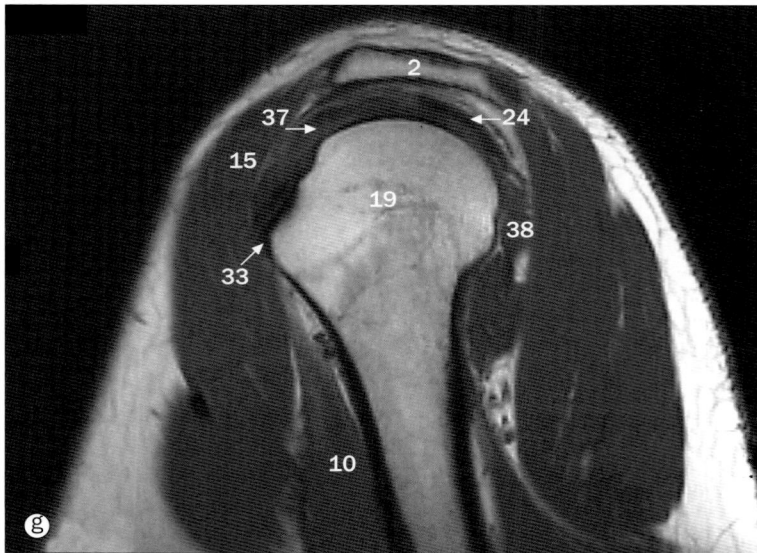

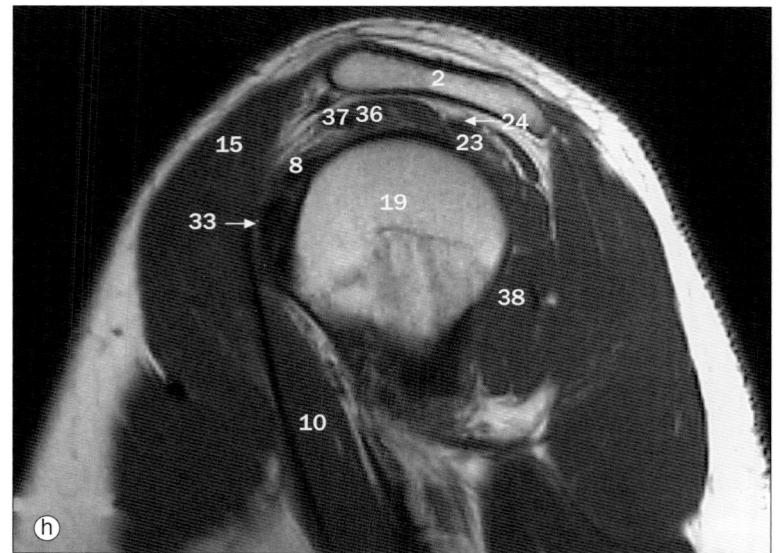

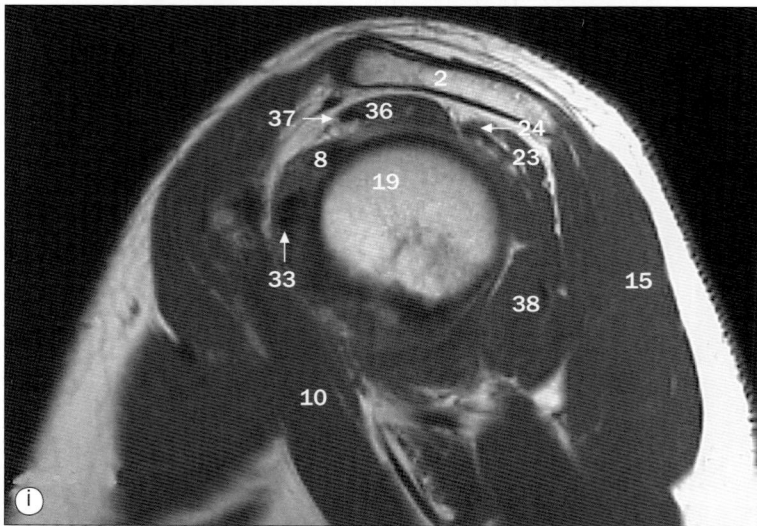

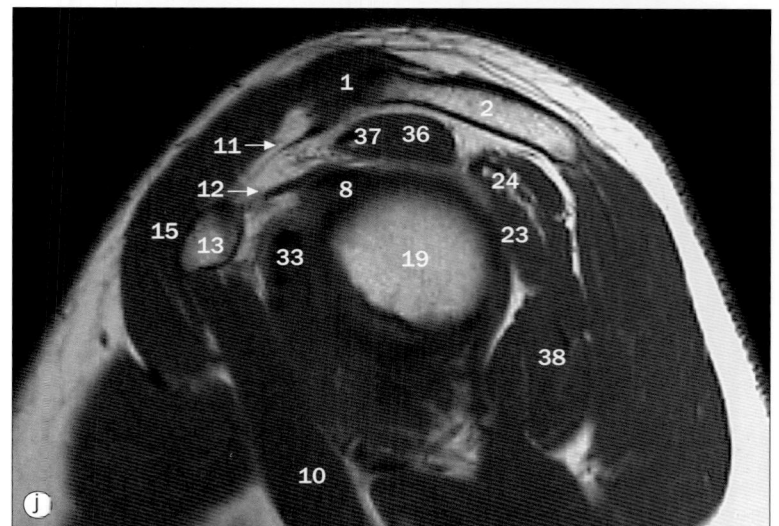

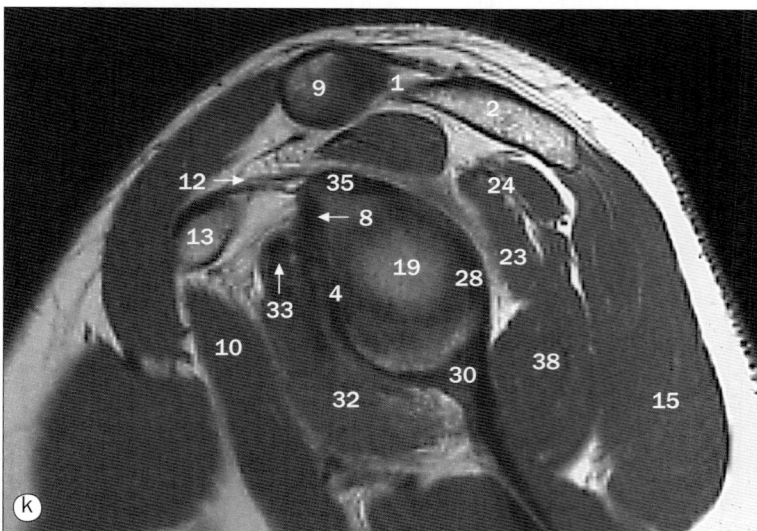

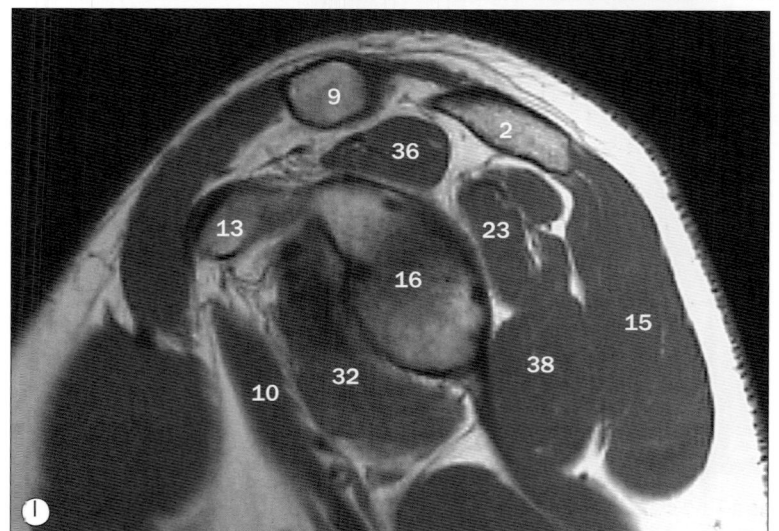

Shoulder, coronal MR arthrography images.

25 Middle glenohumeral ligament	30 Scapula	35 Superior labrum
26 Pectoralis minor muscle	31 Spine of scapula	36 Supraspinatus muscle
27 Posterior capsule of shoulder joint	32 Subscapularis muscle	37 Supraspinatus tendon
28 Posterior labrum	33 Subscapularis tendon	38 Teres minor muscle
29 Rotator cuff	34 Superior glenohumeral ligament	39 Trapezius muscle

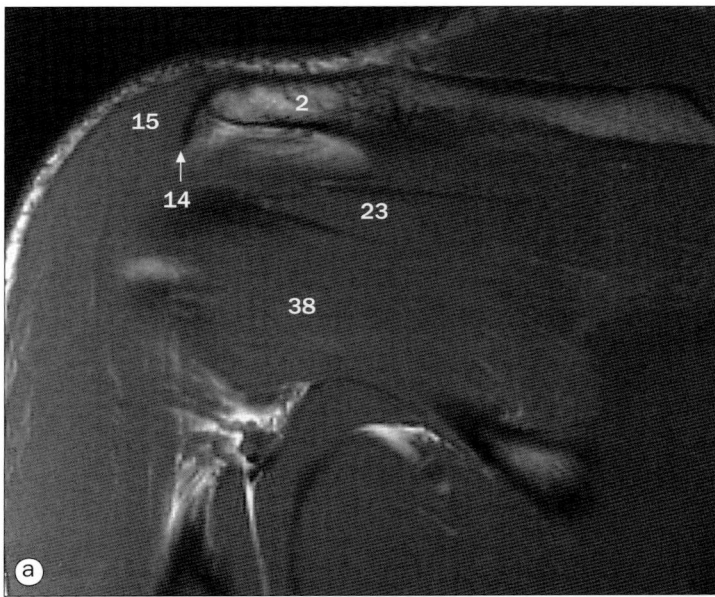

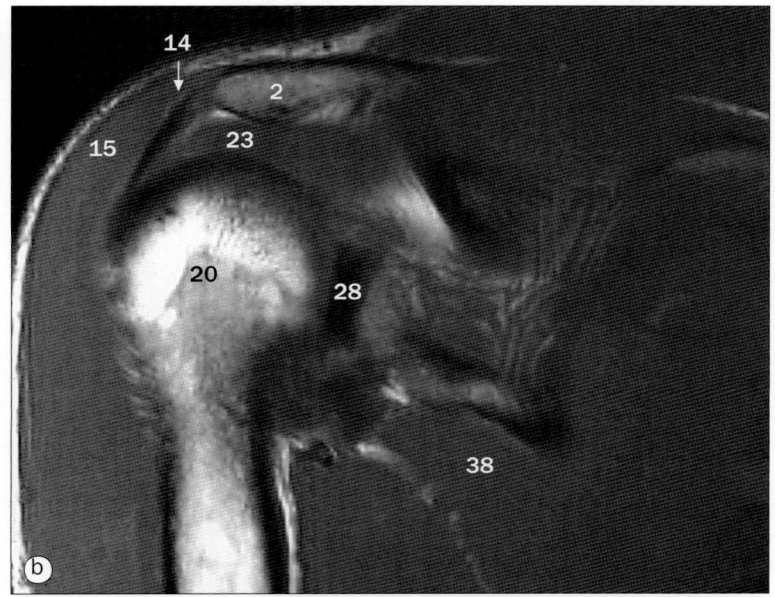

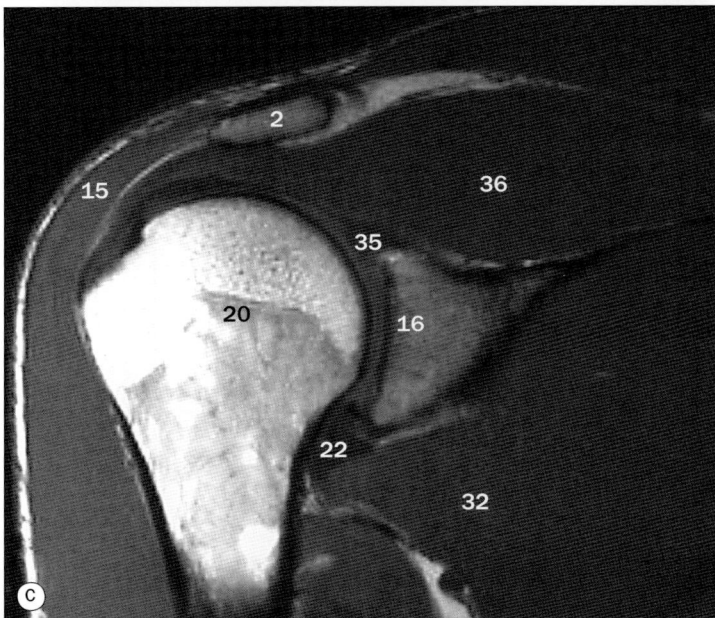

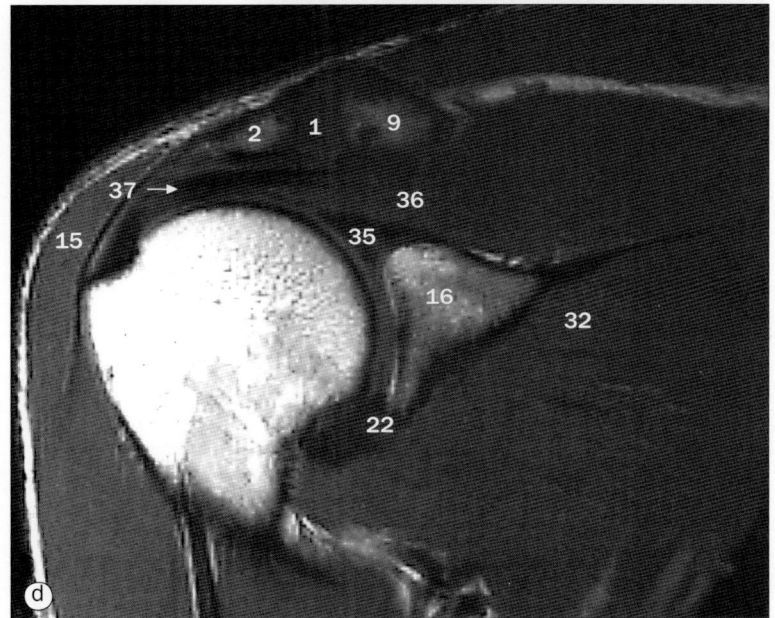

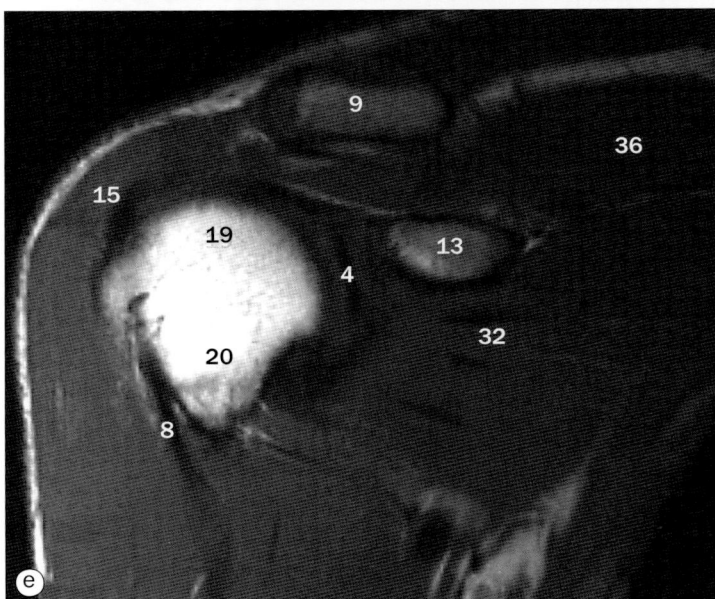

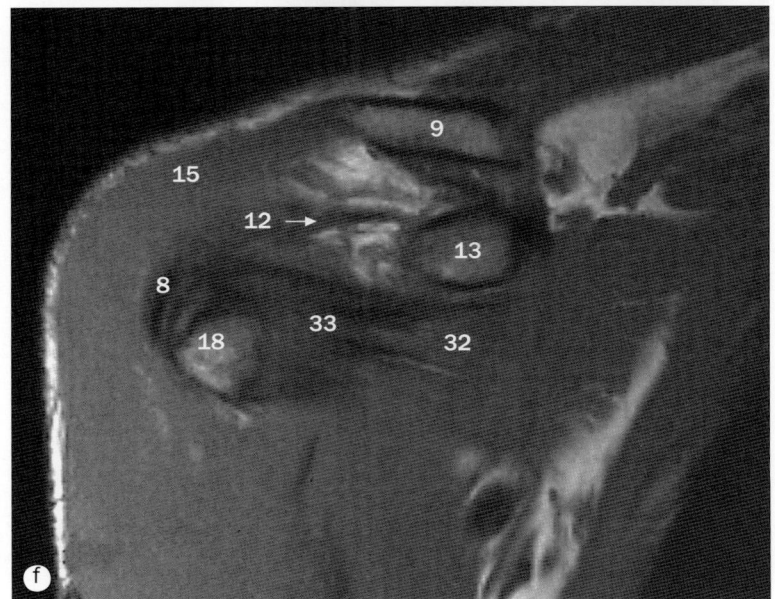

Shoulder, sagittal oblique MR arthrography images. See pages 79 and 80 for key to labels.

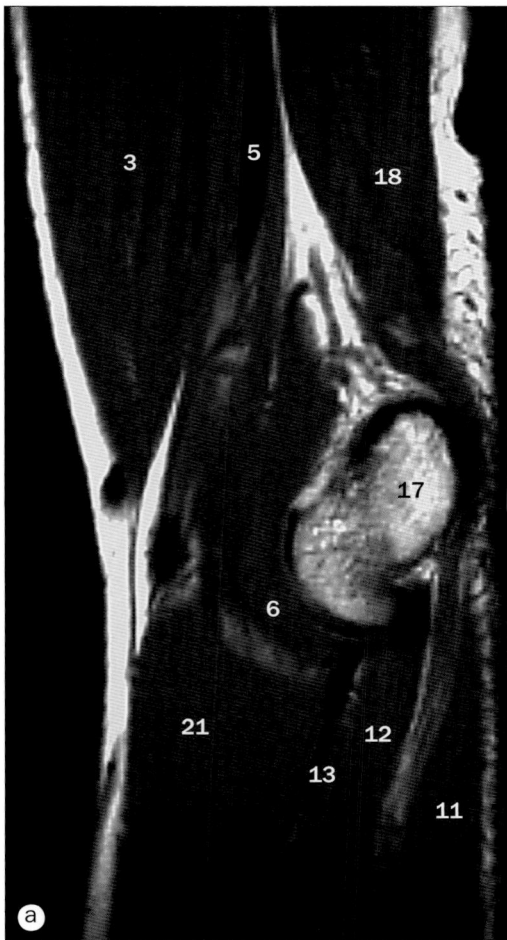

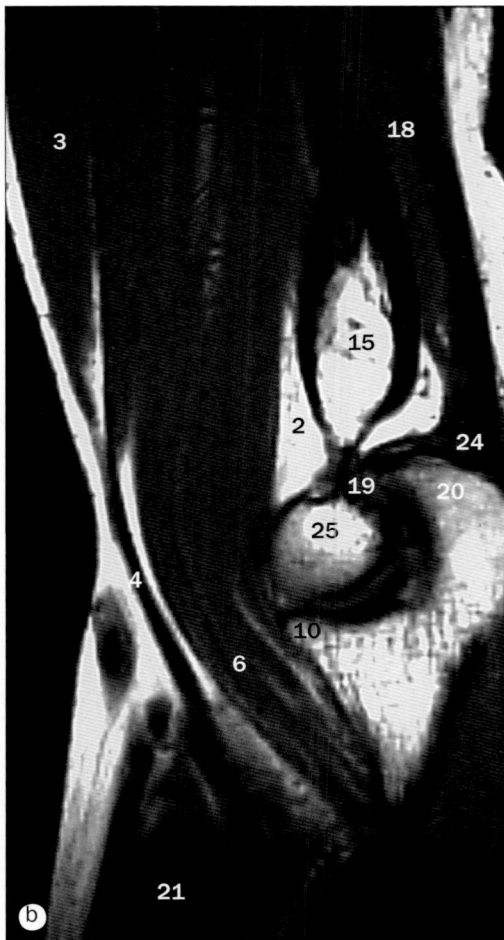

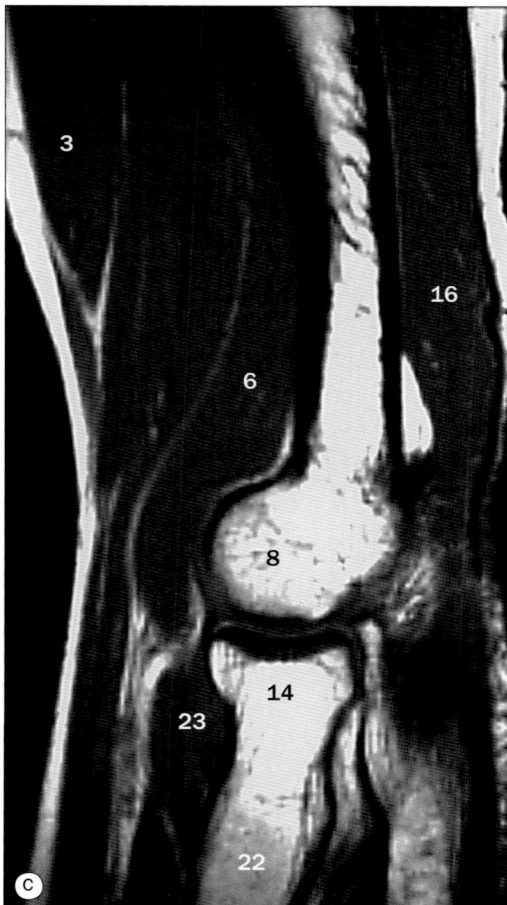

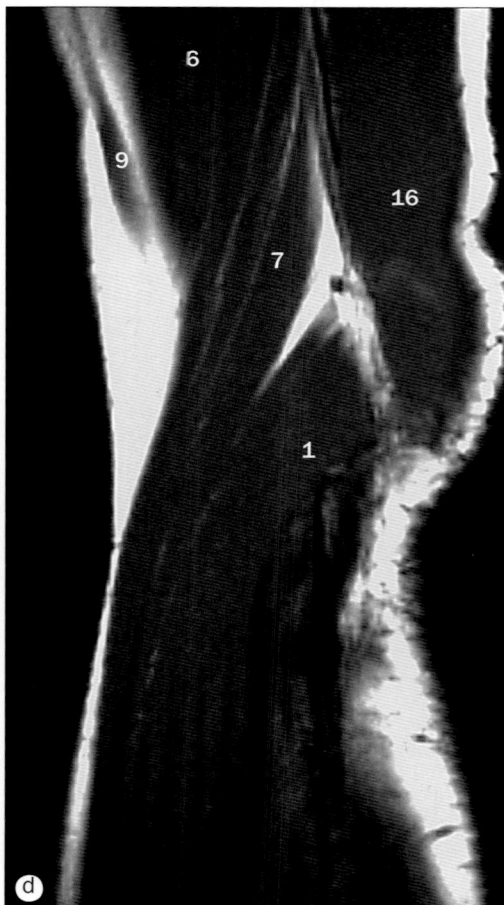

(a)–(d) Elbow, sagittal MR images.

1 Abductor pollicis longus muscle
2 Anterior fat pad
3 Biceps brachii muscle
4 Biceps brachii tendon
5 Brachial artery
6 Brachialis muscle
7 Brachioradialis muscle
8 Capitulum of humerus
9 Cephalic vein
10 Coronoid process of ulna
11 Flexor carpi ulnaris muscle
12 Flexor digitorum profundus muscle
13 Flexor digitorum superficialis muscle
14 Head of radius
15 Humerus
16 Lateral head of triceps muscle
17 Medial epicondyle
18 Medial head of triceps muscle
19 Olecranon fossa of humerus
20 Olecranon process of ulna
21 Pronator teres muscle
22 Radius
23 Supinator muscle
24 Tendon of triceps muscle
25 Trochlea of humerus

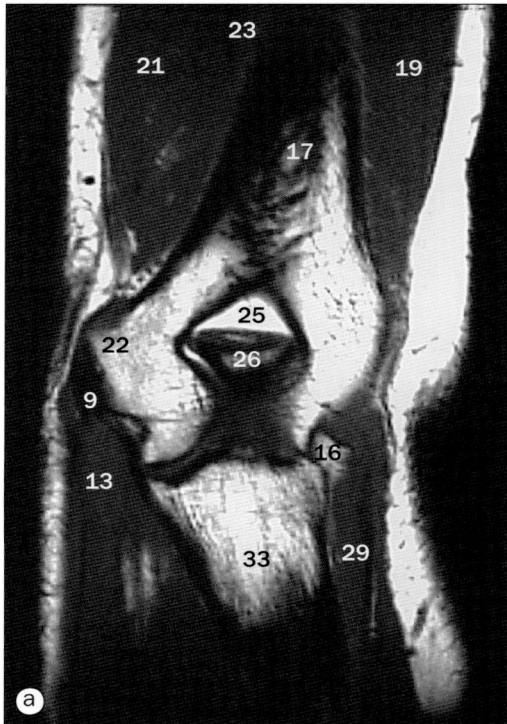

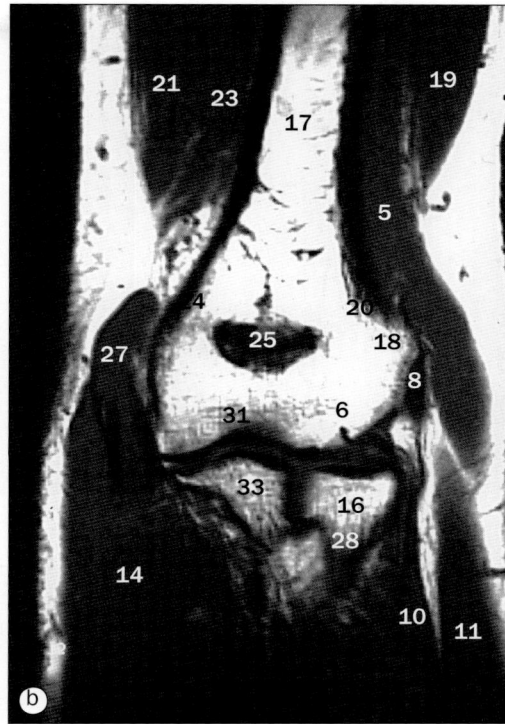

(a)–(d) Elbow, coronal MR images.

1 Basilic vein
2 Biceps brachii muscle
3 Brachial artery
4 Brachialis muscle
5 Brachioradialis muscle
6 Capitulum of humerus
7 Cephalic vein
8 Common extensor origin
9 Common flexor origin
10 Extensor carpi radialis brevis muscle
11 Extensor carpi radialis longus muscle
12 Flexor carpi radialis muscle
13 Flexor carpi ulnaris muscle
14 Flexor digitorum profundus muscle
15 Flexor digitorum superficialis muscle
16 Head of radius
17 Humerus
18 Lateral epicondyle
19 Lateral head of triceps muscle
20 Lateral supracondylar ridge
21 Long head of triceps muscle
22 Medial epicondyle
23 Medial head of triceps muscle
24 Medial supracondylar ridge
25 Olecranon fossa of humerus
26 Olecranon process of ulna
27 Pronator teres muscle
28 Radius
29 Supinator muscle
30 Tendon of biceps brachii muscle
31 Trochlea of humerus
32 Tuberosity of radius
33 Ulna

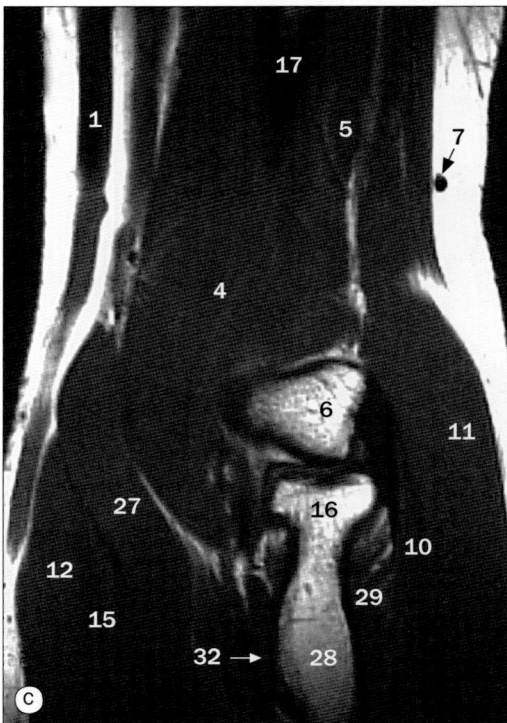

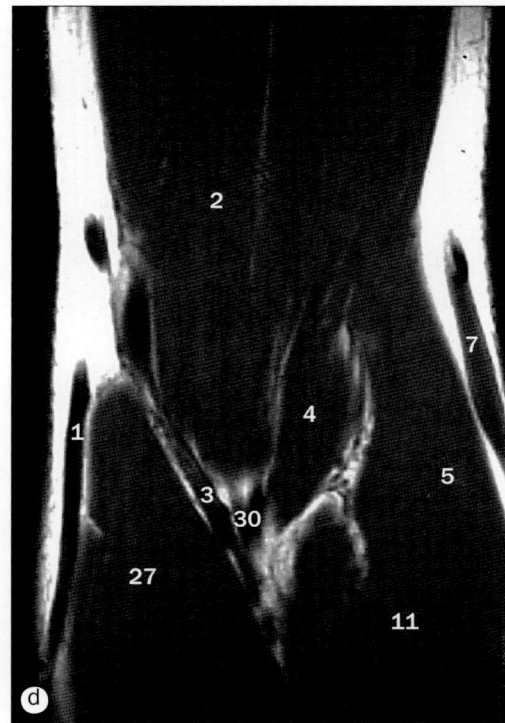

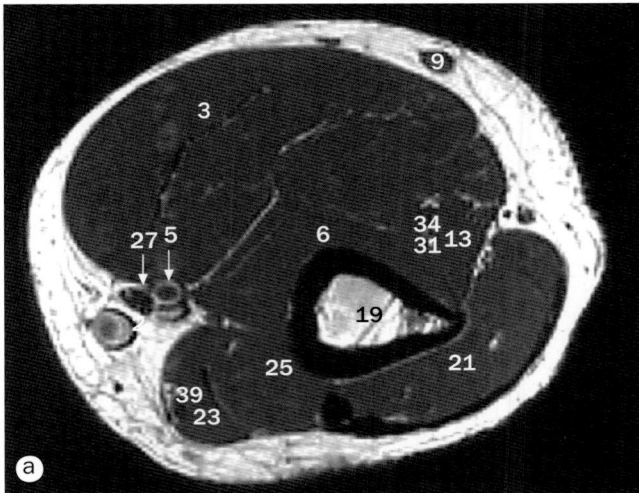

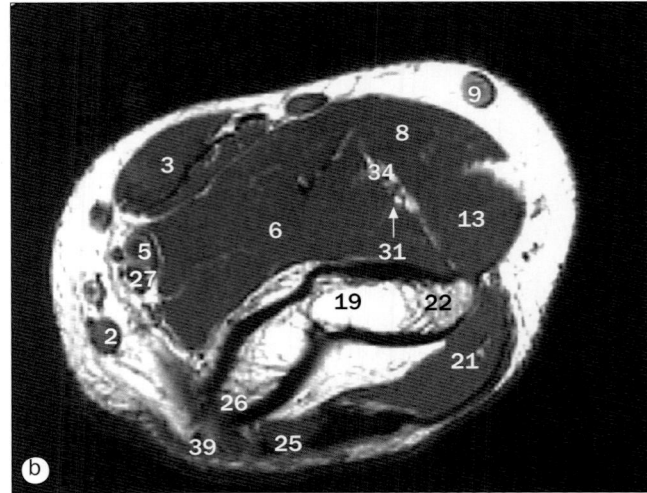

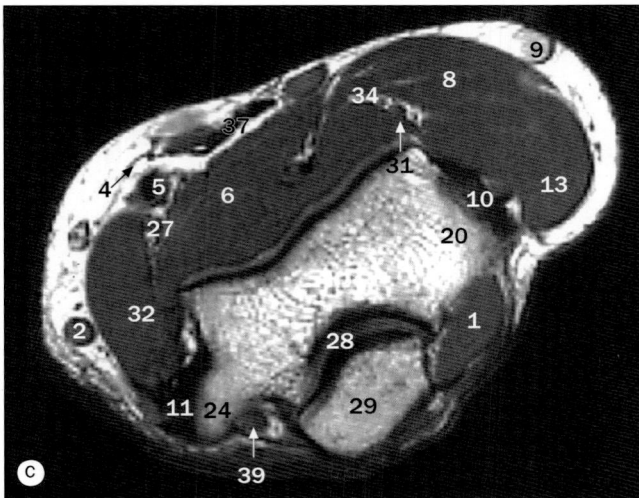

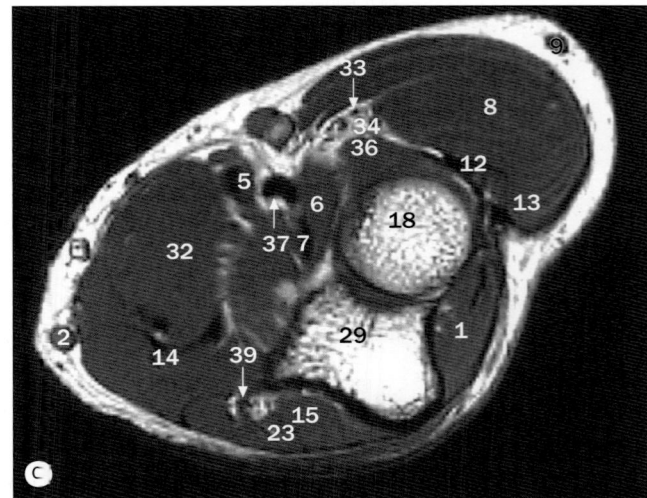

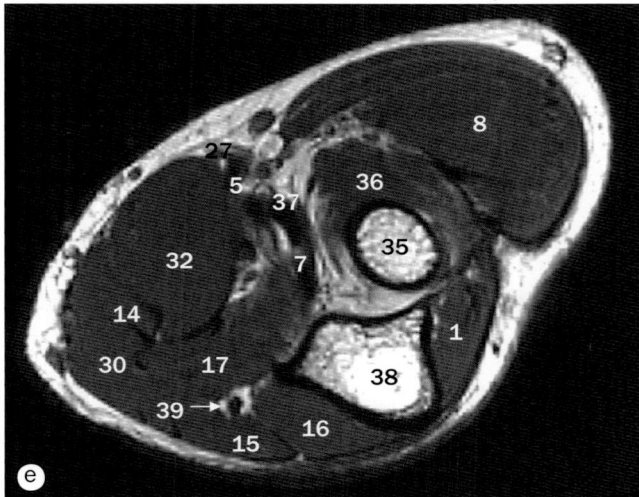

(a)–(e) Elbow, axial MR images.

1 Anconeus muscle	20 Lateral epicondyle
2 Basilic vein	21 Lateral head of triceps
3 Biceps brachii muscle	muscle
4 Bicipital aponeurosis	22 Lateral supracondylar ridge
5 Brachial artery	23 Long head of triceps muscle
6 Brachialis muscle	24 Medial epicondyle
7 Brachialis tendon	25 Medial head of triceps
8 Brachioradialis muscle	muscle
9 Cephalic vein	26 Medial supracondylar ridge
10 Common extensor origin	27 Median nerve
11 Common flexor origin	28 Olecranon fossa of humerus
12 Extensor carpi radialis	29 Olecranon process of ulna
brevis muscle	30 Palmaris longus muscle
13 Extensor carpi radialis	31 Profunda brachii artery
longus muscle	32 Pronator teres muscle
14 Flexor carpi radialis muscle	33 Radial artery
15 Flexor carpi ulnaris muscle	34 Radial nerve
16 Flexor digitorum profundus	35 Radius
muscle	36 Supinator muscle
17 Flexor digitorum	37 Tendon of biceps brachii
superficialis muscle	muscle
18 Head of radius	38 Ulna
19 Humerus	39 Ulnar nerve

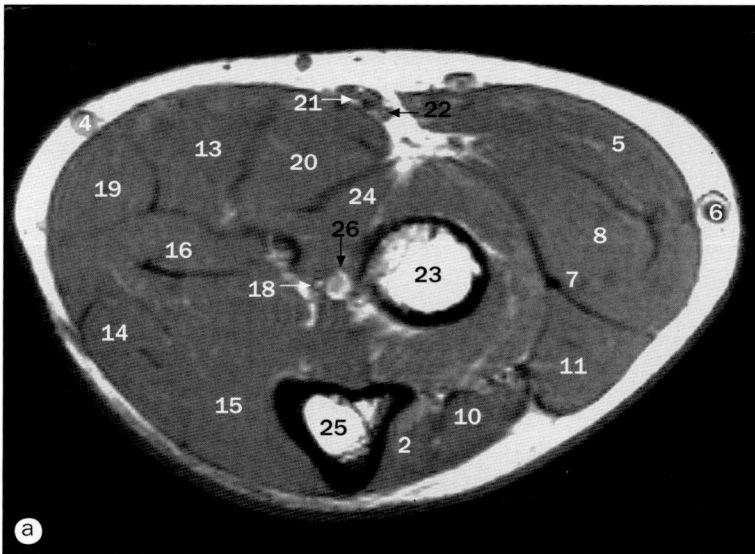

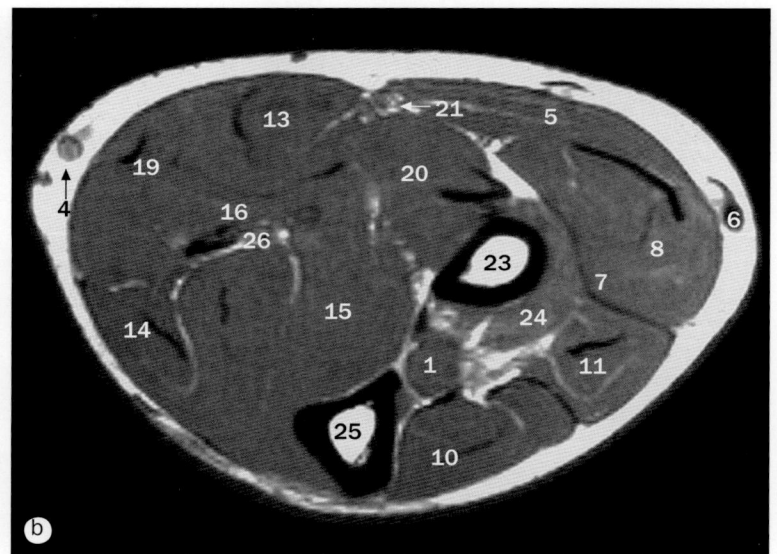

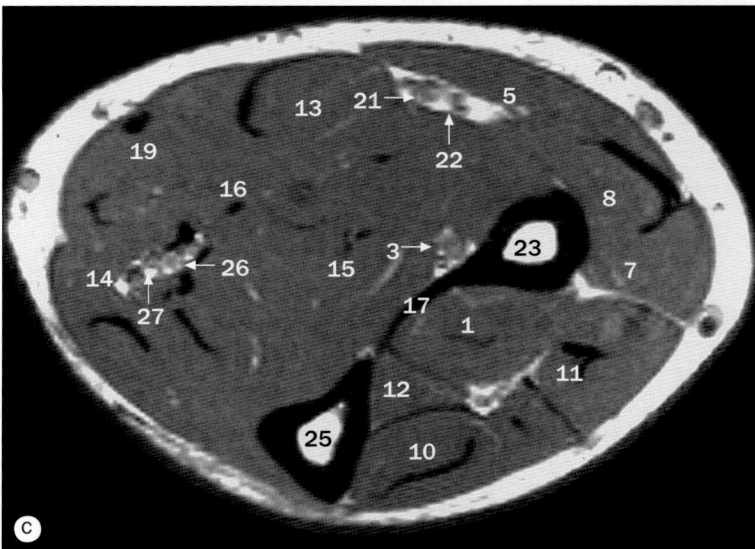

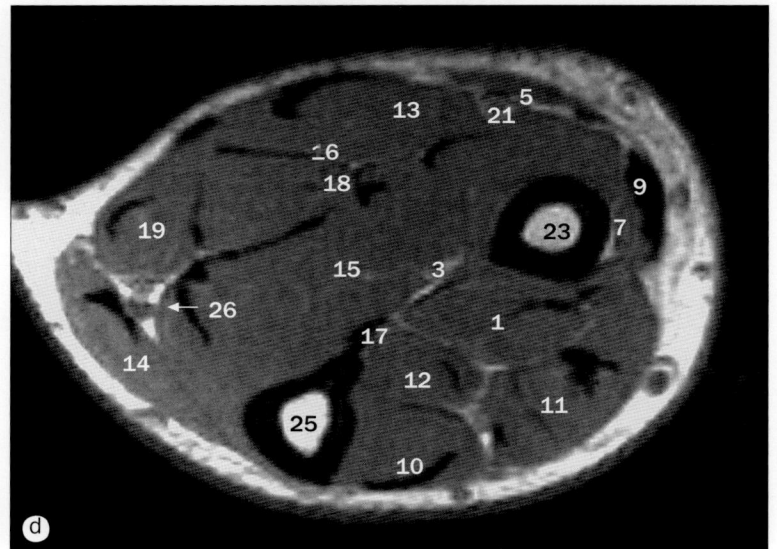

(a)–(d) Forearm, axial MR images.

1 Abductor pollicis longus muscle	10 Extensor carpi ulnaris muscle	19 Palmaris longus muscle
2 Anconeus muscle	11 Extensor digitorum muscle	20 Pronator teres muscle
3 Anterior interosseous artery	12 Extensor pollicis longus muscle	21 Radial artery
4 Basilic vein	13 Flexor carpi radialis muscle	22 Radial nerve
5 Brachioradialis muscle	14 Flexor carpi ulnaris muscle	23 Radius
6 Cephalic vein	15 Flexor digitorum profundus muscle	24 Supinator muscle
7 Extensor carpi radialis brevis muscle	16 Flexor digitorum superficialis muscle	25 Ulna
8 Extensor carpi radialis longus muscle	17 Interosseous membrane	26 Ulnar artery
9 Extensor carpi radialis longus tendon	18 Median nerve	27 Ulnar nerve

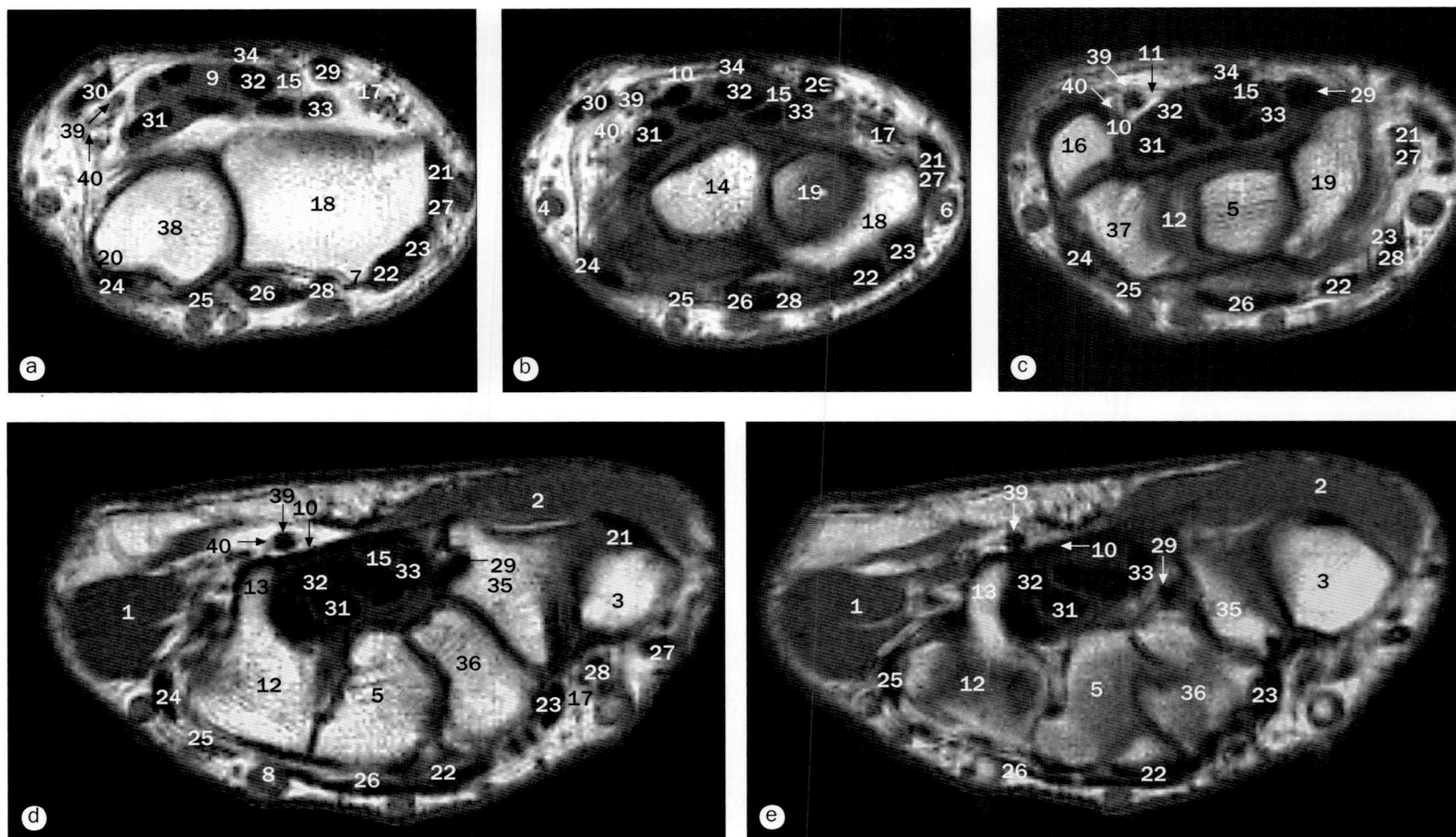

(a)–(e) Wrist, axial MR images.

1 Abductor digiti minimi muscle	16 Pisiform	29 Tendon of flexor carpi radialis muscle
2 Abductor pollicis brevis muscle	17 Radial artery	30 Tendon of flexor carpi ulnaris muscle
3 Base of first metacarpal	18 Radius	31 Tendon of flexor digitorum profundus
4 Basilic vein	19 Scaphoid	muscle
5 Capitate	20 Styloid process of ulna	32 Tendon of flexor digitorum superficialis
6 Cephalic vein	21 Tendon of abductor pollicis longus muscle	muscle
7 Dorsal tubercle of radius	22 Tendon of extensor carpi radialis brevis	33 Tendon of flexor pollicis longus muscle
8 Dorsal venous arch	muscle	34 Tendon of palmaris longus muscle
9 Flexor digitorum superficialis muscle	23 Tendon of extensor carpi radialis longus	35 Trapezium
10 Flexor retinaculum	muscle	36 Trapezoid
11 Guyon's canal	24 Tendon of extensor carpi ulnaris muscle	37 Triquetral
12 Hamate	25 Tendon of extensor digiti minimi muscle	38 Ulna
13 Hook of hamate	26 Tendon of extensor digitorum muscle	39 Ulnar artery
14 Lunate	27 Tendon of extensor pollicis brevis muscle	40 Ulnar nerve
15 Median nerve	28 Tendon of extensor pollicis longus muscle	

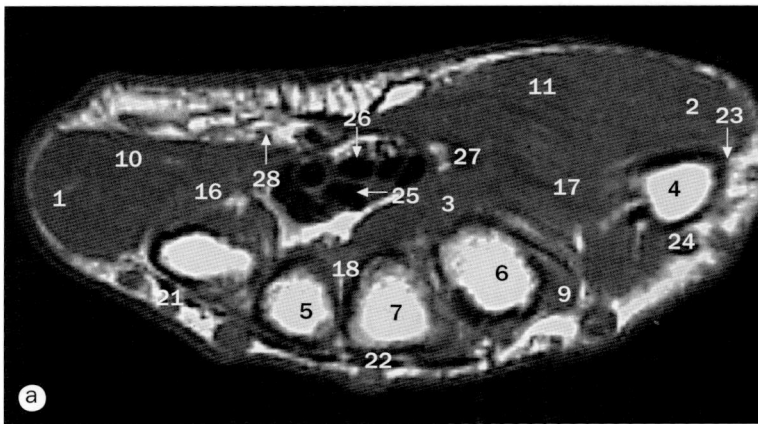

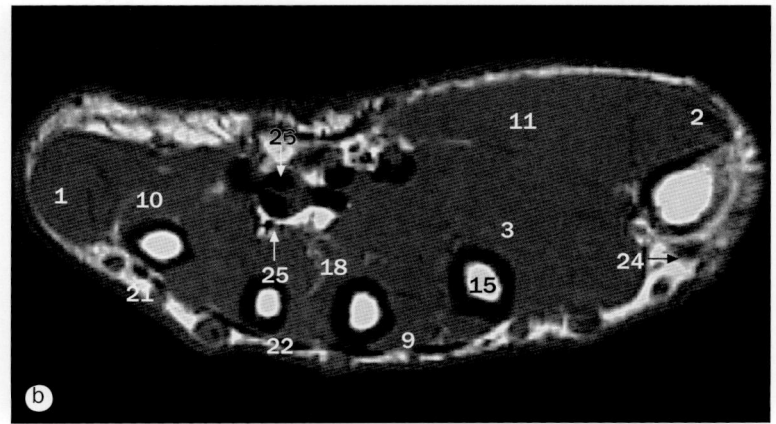

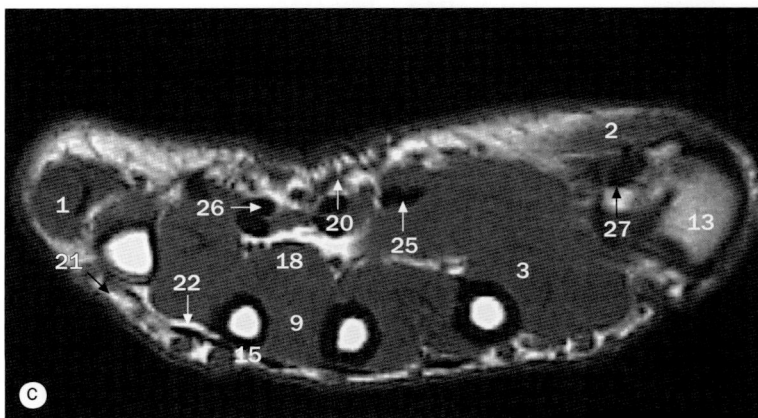

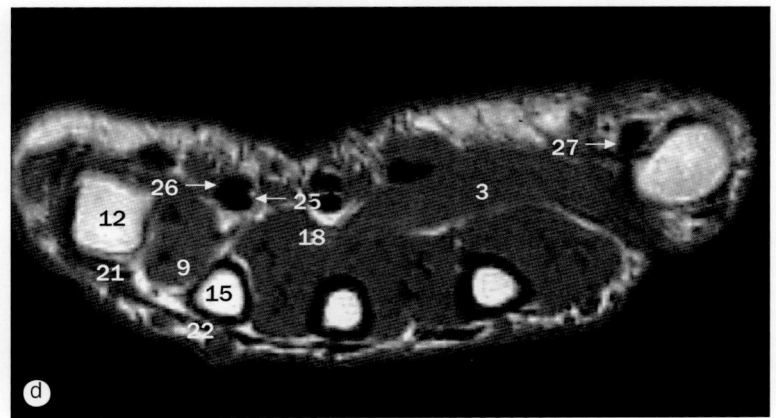

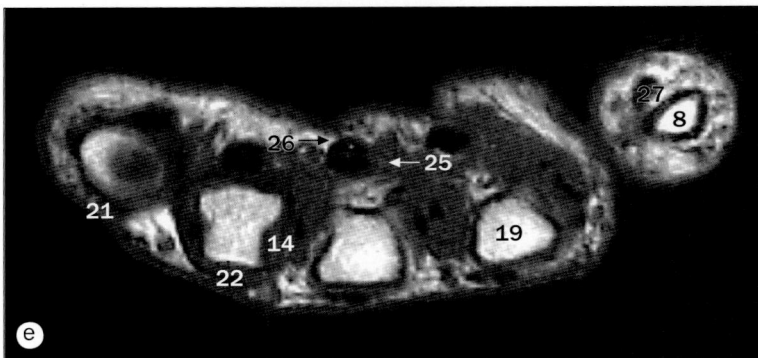

(a)–(e) Hand, axial MR images.

1 Abductor digiti minimi muscle
2 Abductor pollicis brevis muscle
3 Adductor pollicis muscle
4 Base of first metacarpal
5 Base of fourth metacarpal
6 Base of second metacarpal
7 Base of third metacarpal
8 Distal phalanx of thumb
9 Dorsal interossei muscles
10 Flexor digiti minimi muscle
11 Flexor pollicis brevis muscle
12 Head of fifth metacarpal
13 Head of first metacarpal
14 Lumbrical muscle
15 Metacarpal shaft
16 Opponens digiti minimi muscle
17 Opponens pollicis muscle
18 Palmar interossei muscles
19 Proximal phalanx of index finger
20 Superficial palmar arch
21 Tendon of extensor digiti minimi muscle
22 Tendon of extensor digitorum muscle
23 Tendon of extensor pollicis brevis muscle
24 Tendon of extensor pollicis longus muscle
25 Tendon of flexor digitorum profundus muscle
26 Tendon of flexor digitorum superficialis muscle
27 Tendon of flexor pollicis longus muscle
28 Ulnar artery

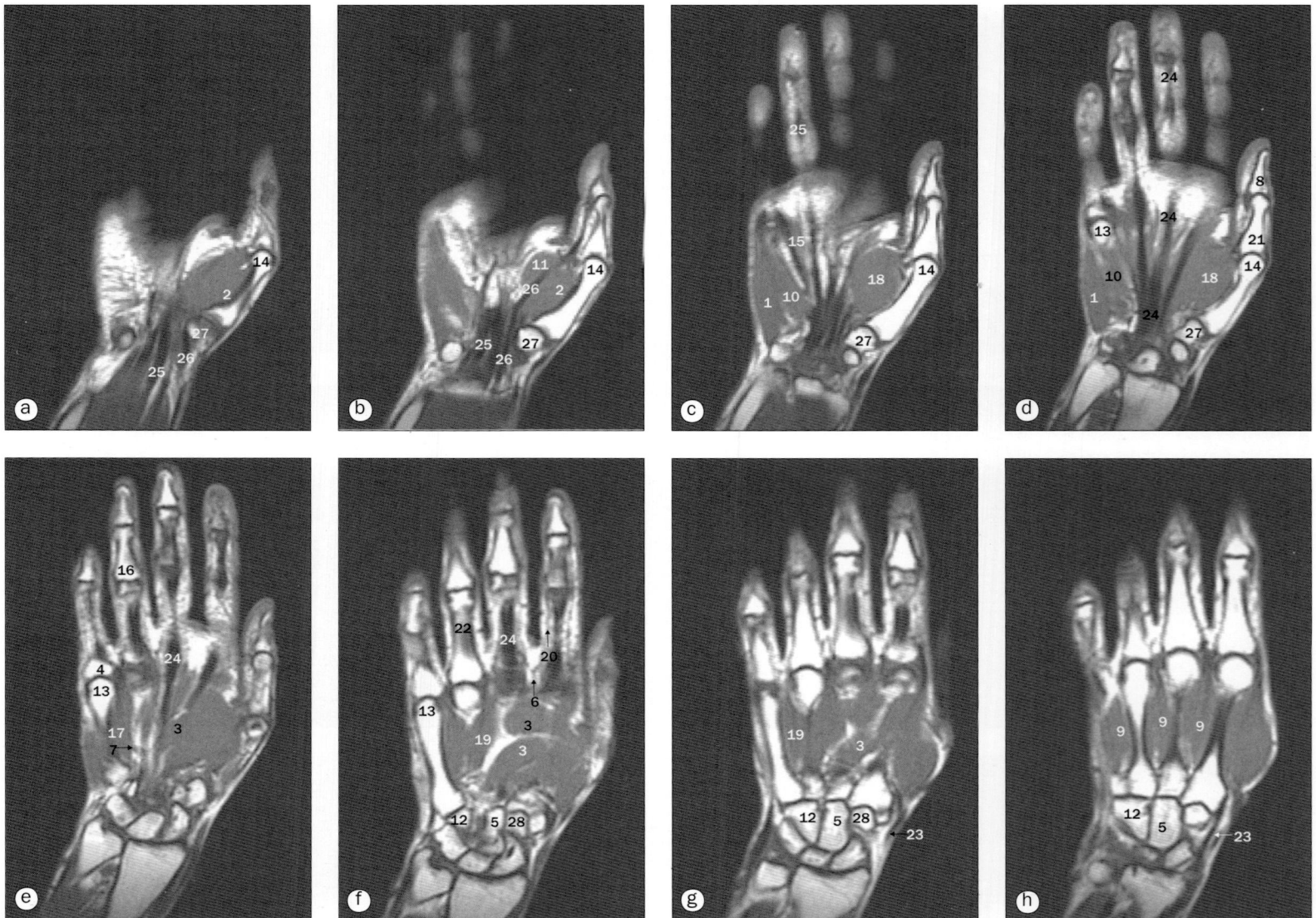

(a)–(h) Hand, coronal MR images.

1 Abductor digiti minimi muscle	**8** Distal phalanx of thumb	**17** Opponens digiti minimi muscle	**24** Tendon of flexor digitorum profundus muscle
2 Abductor pollicis brevis muscle	**9** Dorsal interossei muscles	**18** Opponens pollicis muscle	**25** Tendon of flexor digitorum superficialis muscle
3 Adductor pollicis muscle	**10** Flexor digiti minimi muscle	**19** Palmar interossei muscles	**26** Tendon of flexor pollicis longus muscle
4 Base of proximal phalanx	**11** Flexor pollicis brevis muscle	**20** Proper palmar digital artery	**27** Trapezium
5 Capitate	**12** Hamate	**21** Proximal phalanx of thumb	**28** Trapezoid
6 Common palmar digital artery	**13** Head of fifth metacarpal	**22** Shaft of proximal phalanx	
7 Deep palmar arch	**14** Head of first metacarpal	**23** Tendon of extensor pollicis longus muscle	
	15 Lumbrical muscle		
	16 Middle phalanx		

4 Thorax

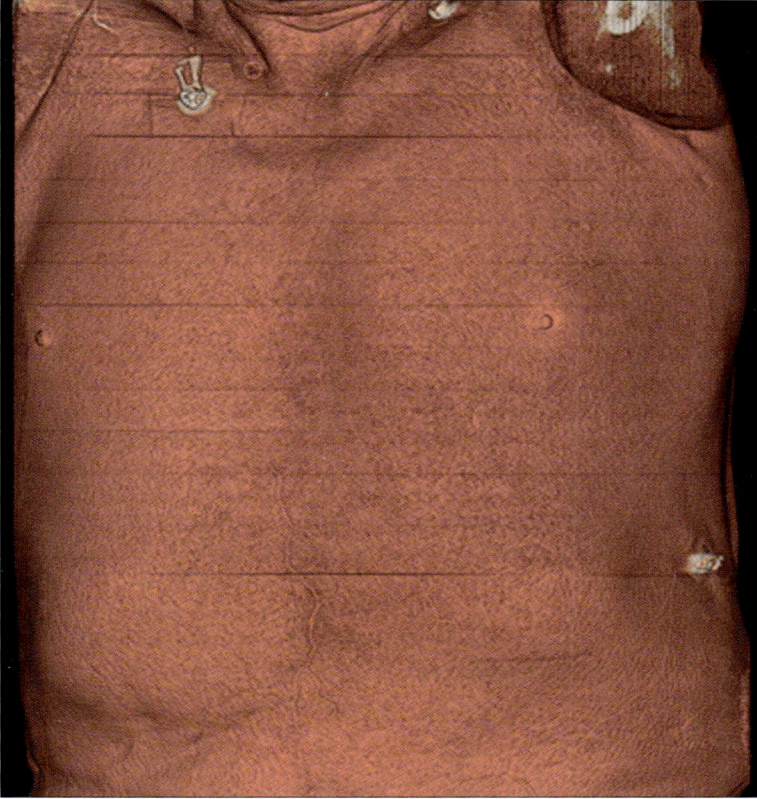
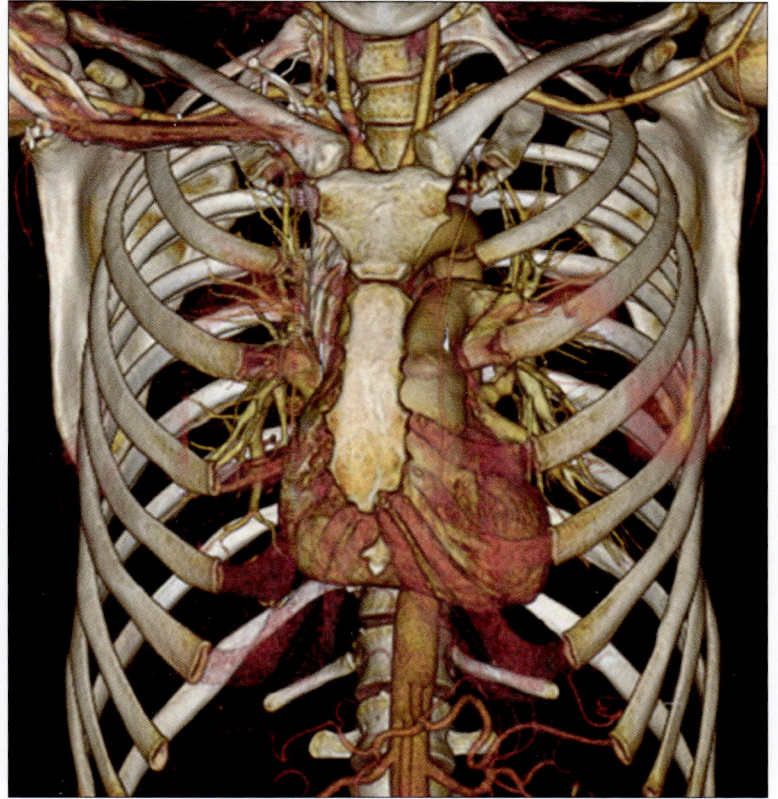
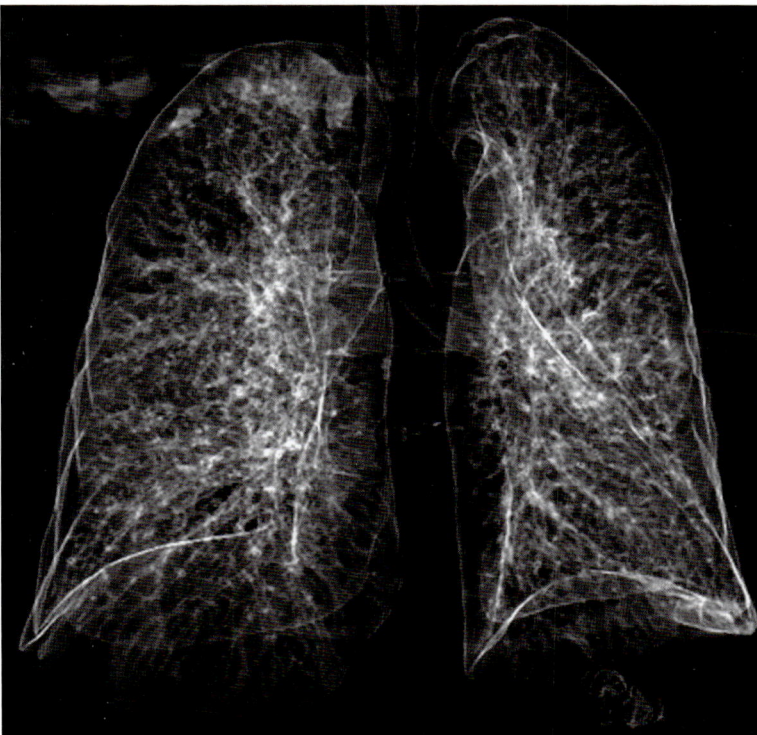
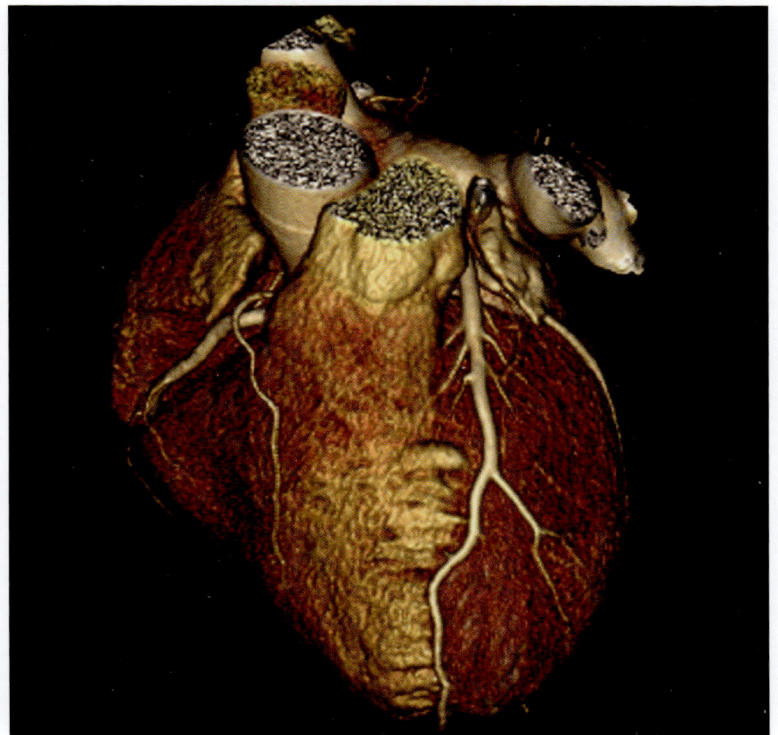

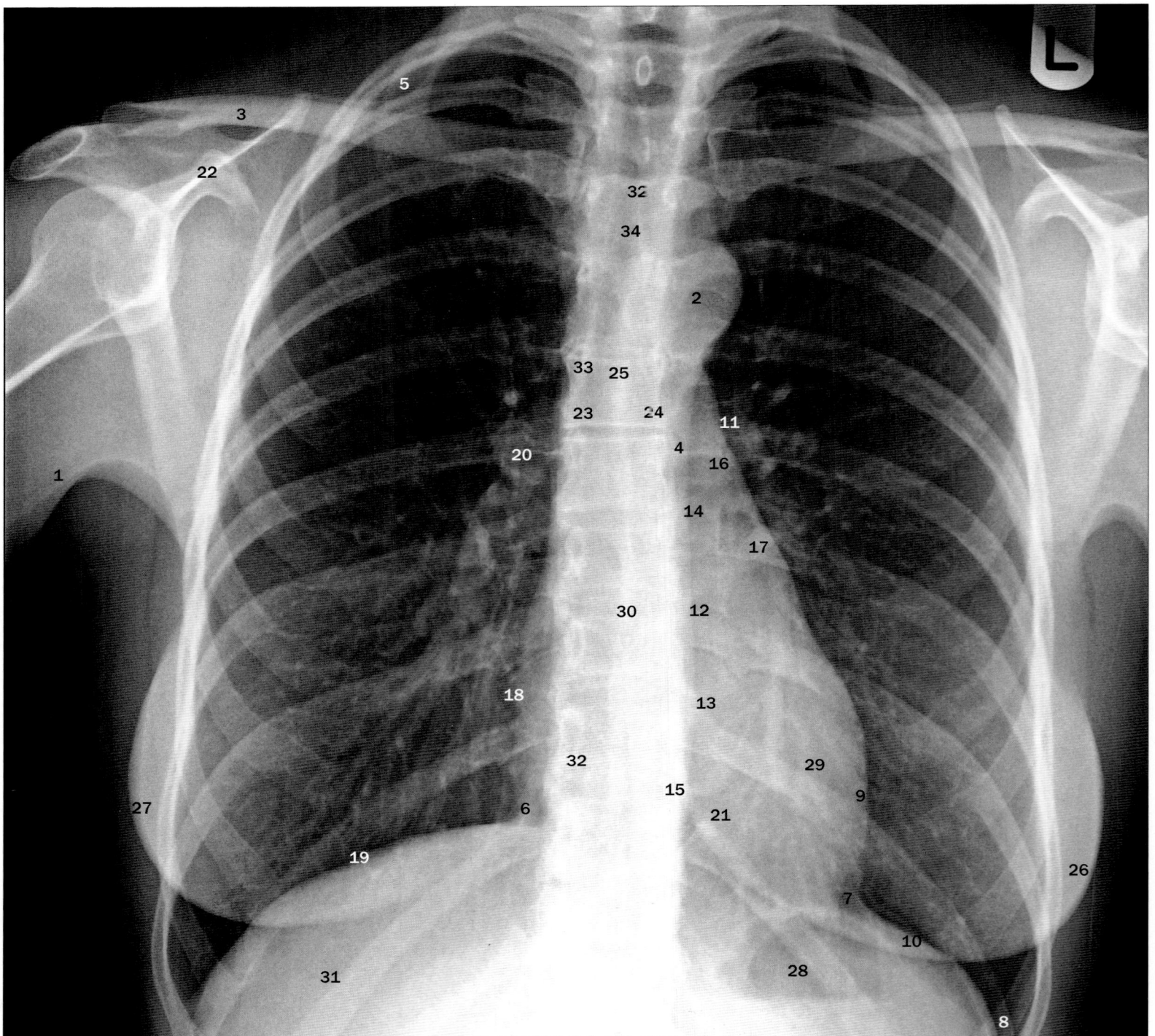

Chest radiograph, postero-anterior projection.

1 Anterior axillary fold
2 Arch of aorta (aortic knuckle or knob)
3 Clavicle
4 Descending aorta
5 First rib
6 Inferior vena cava
7 Left cardiophrenic angle
8 Left costophrenic angle
9 Left ventricular border

10 Left dome of diaphragm
11 Left pulmonary artery
12 Position of aortic valve
13 Position of mitral valve
14 Position of pulmonary valve
15 Position of tricuspid valve
16 Pulmonary trunk
17 Region of tip of auricle of left atrium

18 Right atrial border
19 Right dome of diaphragm
20 Right pulmonary artery
21 Right ventricle
22 Spine of scapula
23 Right main bronchus
24 Left main bronchus
25 Carina
26 Left breast outline

27 Right breast outline
28 Gas in fundus of stomach
29 Position of left ventricle
30 Position of left atrium
31 Position of liver
32 Manubrium
33 Superior vena cava
34 Trachea

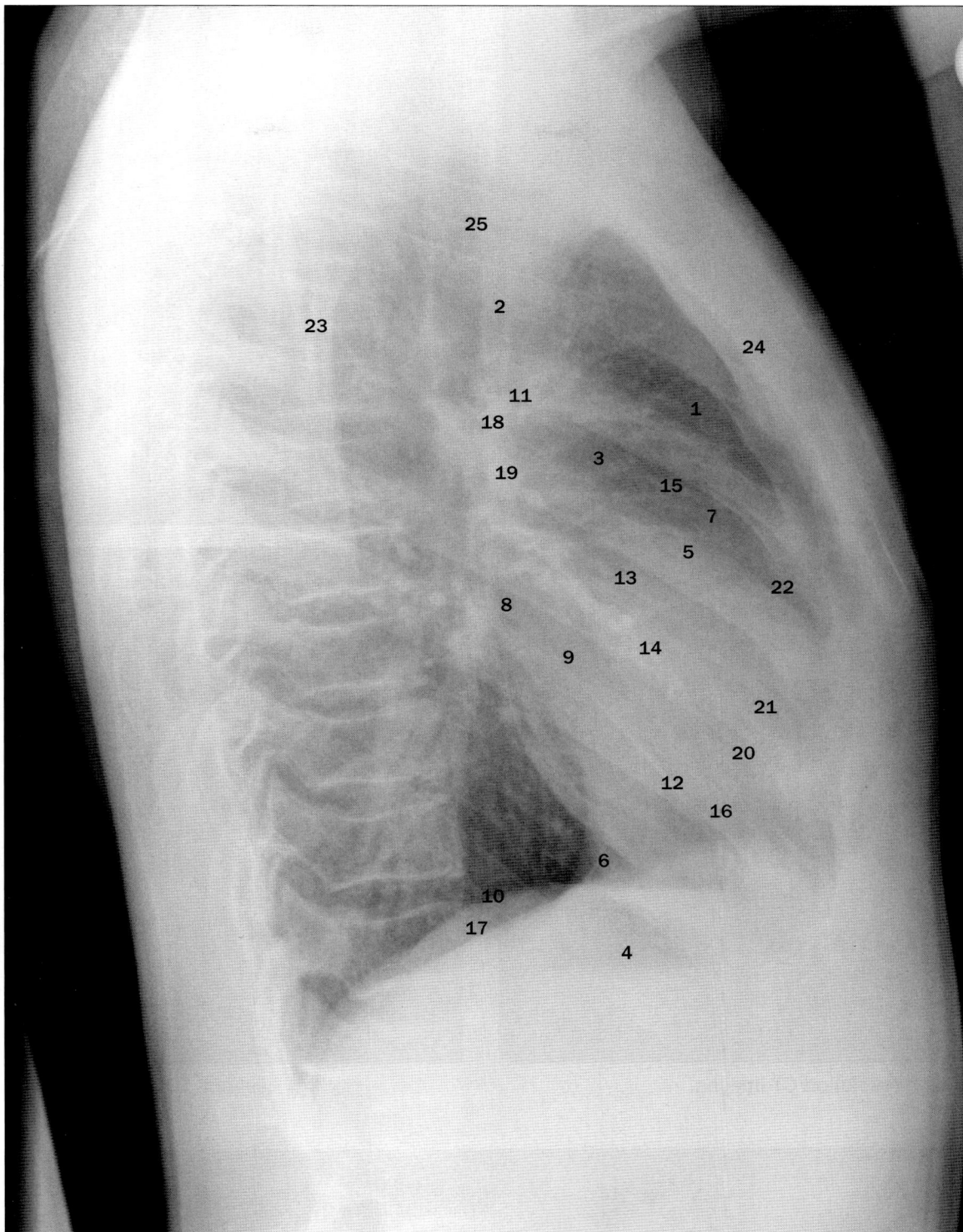

Chest radiograph, lateral projection.

1 Anterior mediastinal space	7 Infundibulum of right ventricle (below) with pulmonary trunk (above)	13 Position of aortic valve	21 Right ventricle
2 Arch of aorta (aortic knuckle or knob		14 Position of mitral valve	22 Right ventricular border of heart
3 Ascending aorta	8 Left atrial border of heart	15 Position of pulmonary valve	23 Scapula
4 Gas in fundus of stomach	9 Left atrium	16 Position of tricuspid valve	24 Sternum
5 Horizontal fissure	10 Left dome of diaphragm	17 Right dome of diaphragm	25 Trachea
6 Inferior vena cava	11 Left main pulmonary artery	18 Right main bronchus	
	12 Left oblique fissure	19 Right main pulmonary artery	
		20 Right oblique fissure	

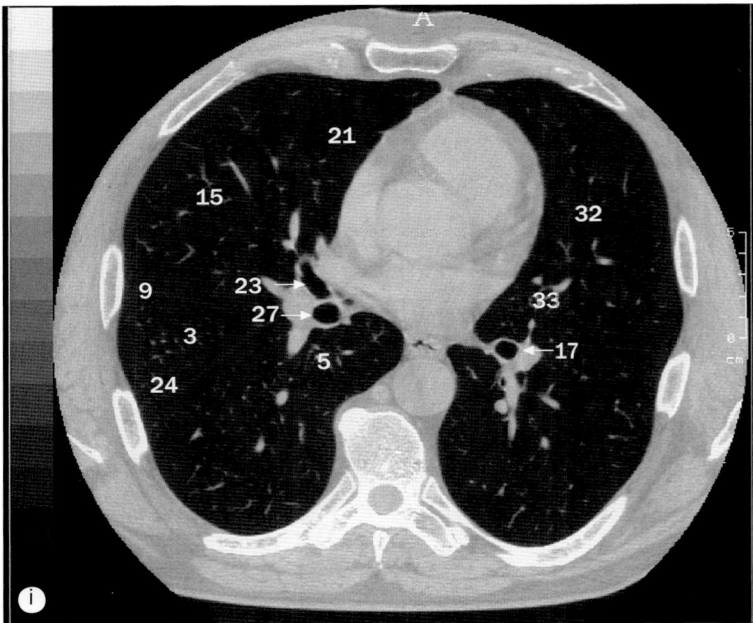

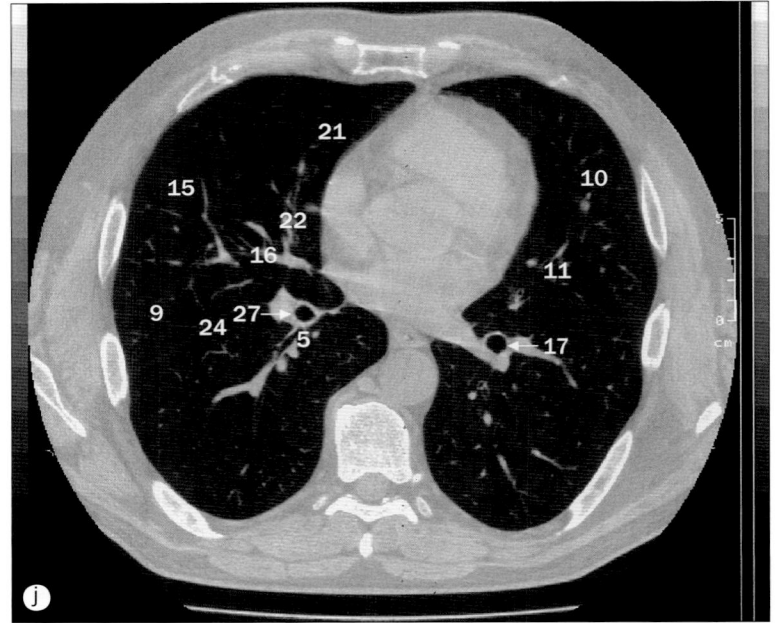

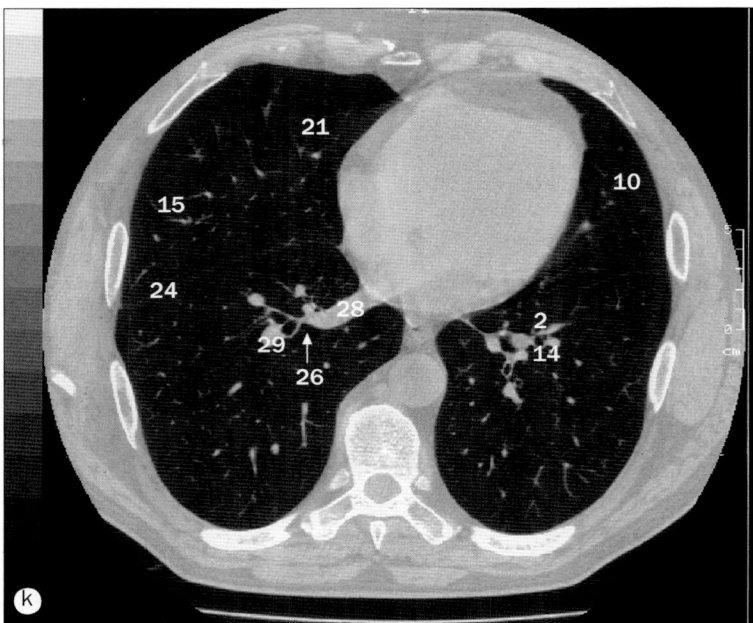

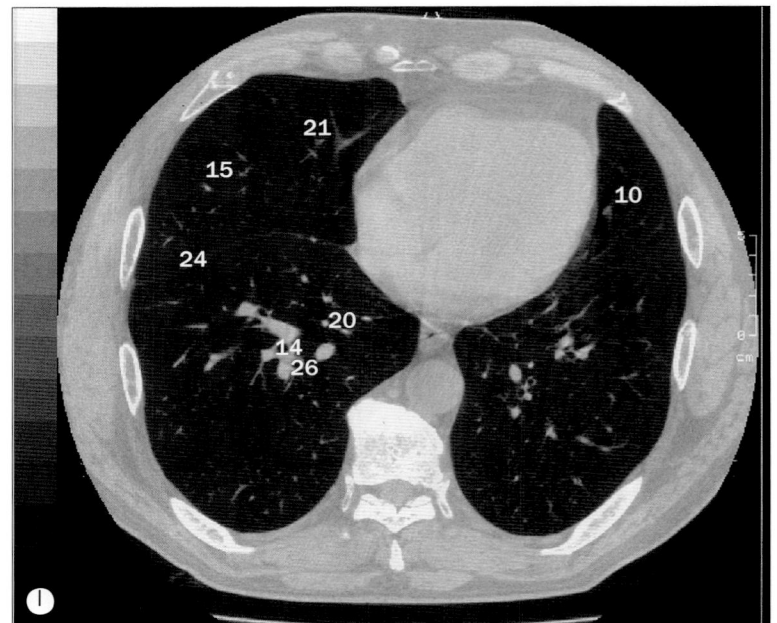

(i)–(p) Lungs, axial high-resolution CT images.

1 Anterior basal segment inferior lobe	**7** Heart	**13** Lateral basal segment inferior lobe
2 Anterior basal segmental bronchus	**8** Hemi-azygos vein	**14** Lateral basal segmental bronchus
3 Anterior segment superior lobe	**9** Horizontal fissure	**15** Lateral segment middle lobe
4 Aorta	**10** Inferior lingular segment	**16** Lateral segmental bronchus of middle
5 Apical segment inferior lobe bronchus	**11** Inferior lingular segmental bronchus	lobe
6 Azygos vein	**12** Inferior vena cava	**17** Left inferior lobe bronchus

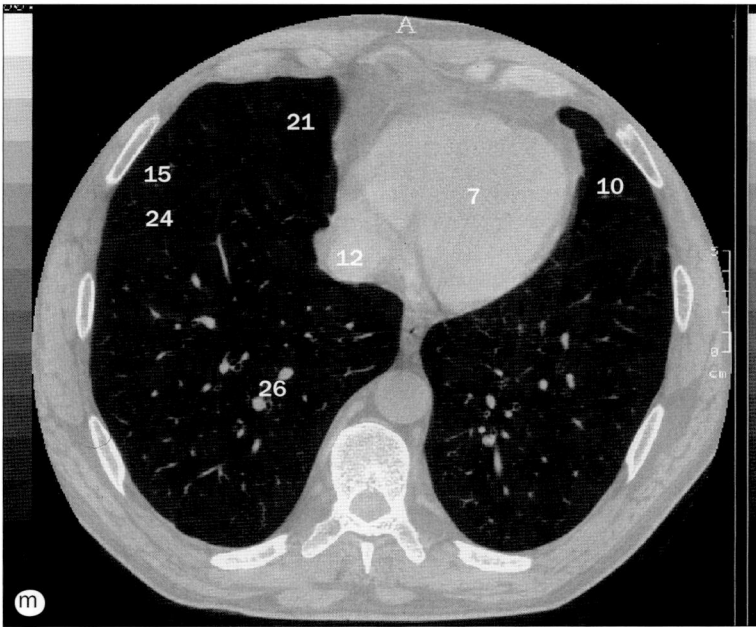

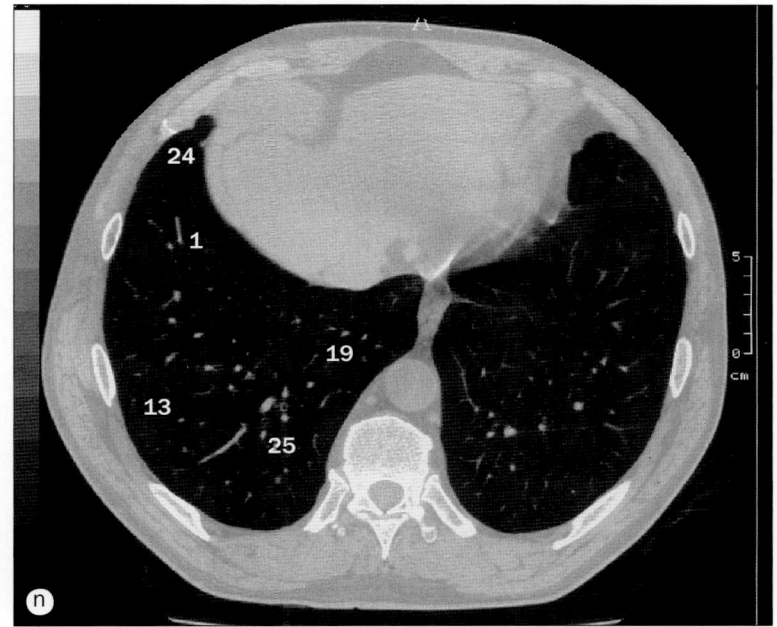

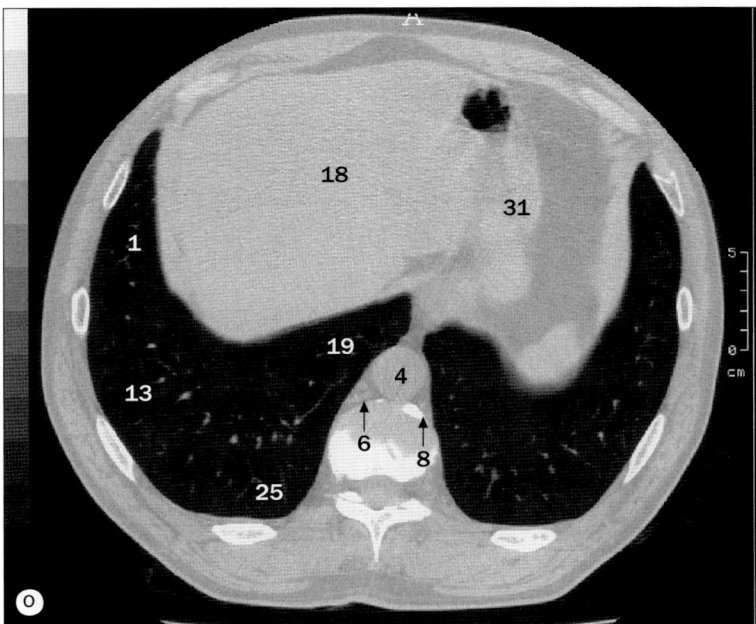

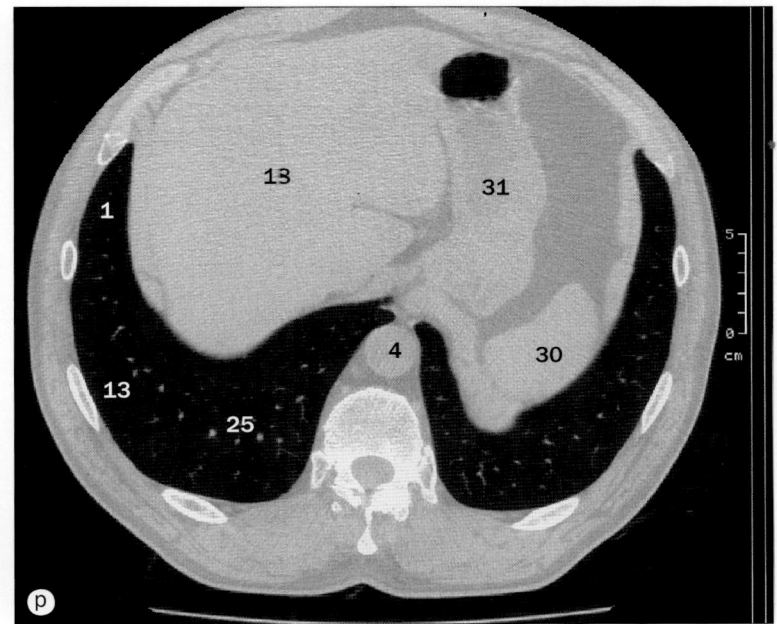

(i)–(p) Lungs, axial high-resolution CT images.

18 Liver	**23** Middle lobe bronchus	**29** Right lower lobe pulmonary artery
19 Medial basal segment inferior lobe	**24** Oblique fissure	**30** Spleen
20 Medial basal segmental bronchus	**25** Posterior basal segment inferior lobe	**31** Stomach
21 Medial segment middle lobe	**26** Posterior basal segmental bronchus	**32** Superior lingular segment
22 Medial segmental bronchus of middle lobe	**27** Right inferior lobe bronchus	**33** Superior lingular segmental bronchus
	28 Right inferior pulmonary vein	

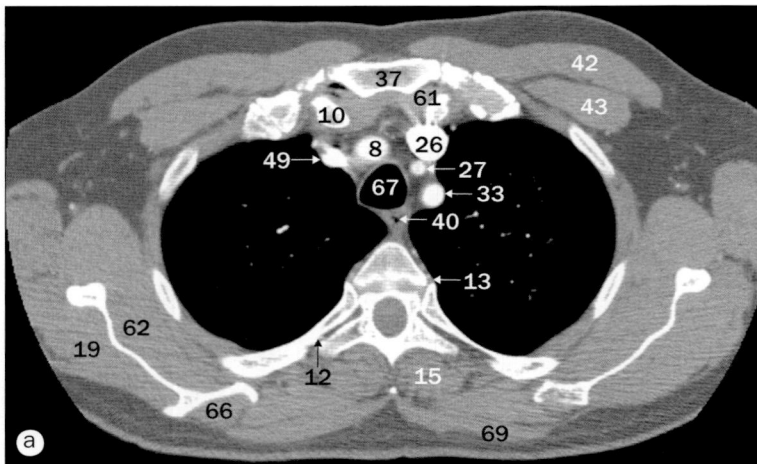

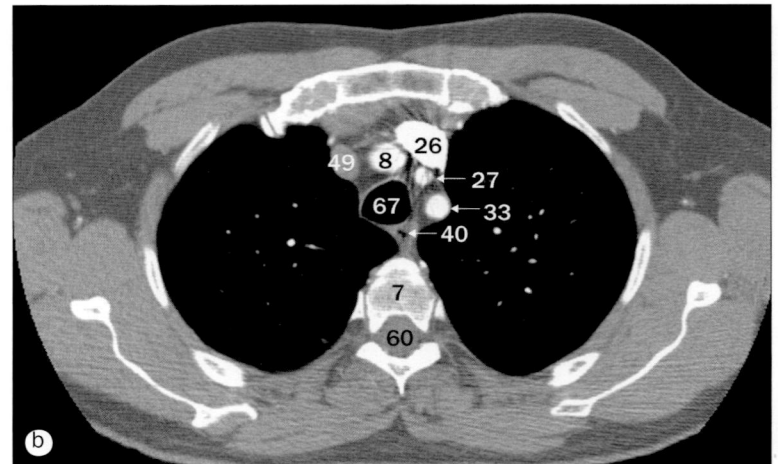

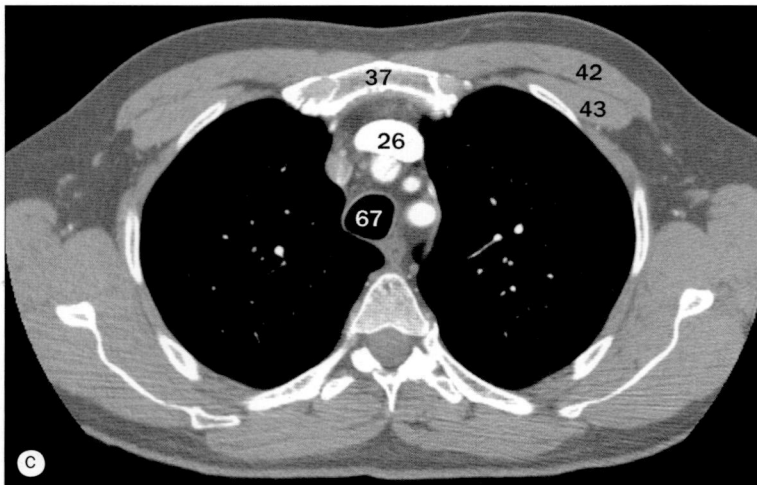

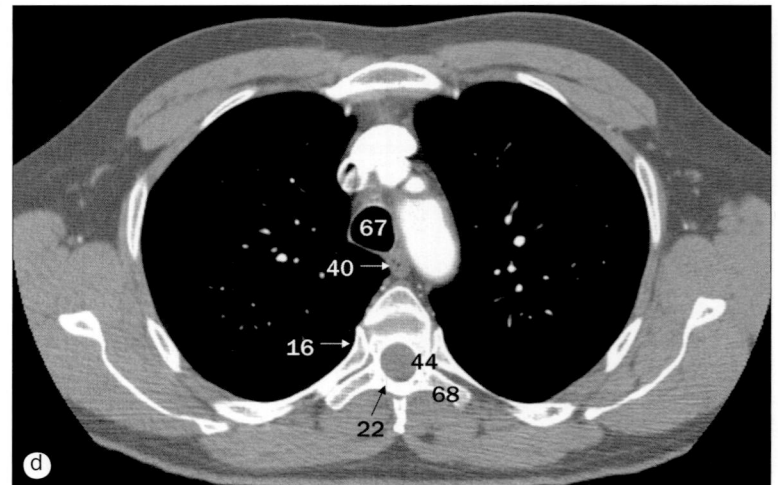

(a)–(t) Chest, axial CT images of mediastinum.

1 Anterior interventricular branch of left coronary artery	12 Costotransverse joint	24 Left atrial appendage (auricle)
2 Aortic valve	13 Costovertebral joint	25 Left atrium
3 Arch of aorta (aortic knuckle or knob)	14 Descending aorta	26 Left brachiocephalic vein
4 Ascending aorta	15 Erector spinae muscle	27 Left common carotid artery
5 Azygos vein	16 Head of rib	28 Left hemidiaphragm
6 Body of sternum	17 Hemi-azygos vein	29 Left inferior lobe bronchus
7 Body of vertebra	18 Inferior vena cava	30 Left inferior pulmonary vein
8 Brachiocephalic trunk	19 Infraspinatus muscle	31 Left main bronchus
9 Carina (bifurcation of trachea)	20 Interatrial septum	32 Left pulmonary artery
10 Clavicle	21 Internal thoracic artery and vein	33 Left subclavian artery
11 Coronary sinus	22 Lamina	34 Left superior lobe bronchus
	23 Latissimus dorsi muscle	35 Left superior pulmonary vein

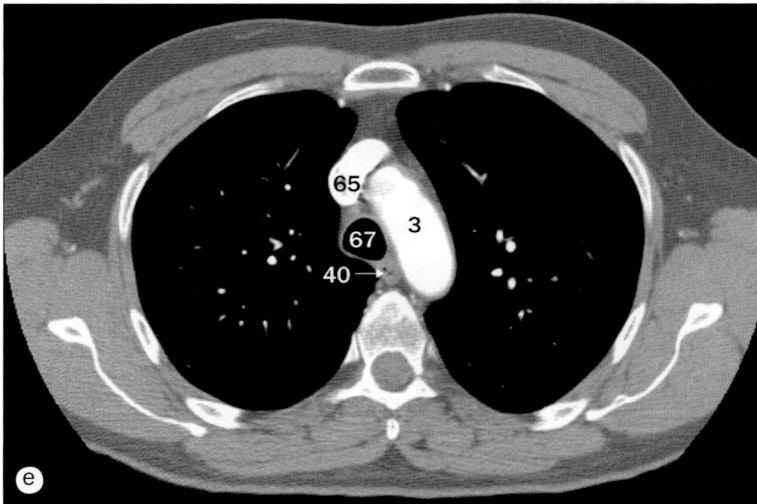

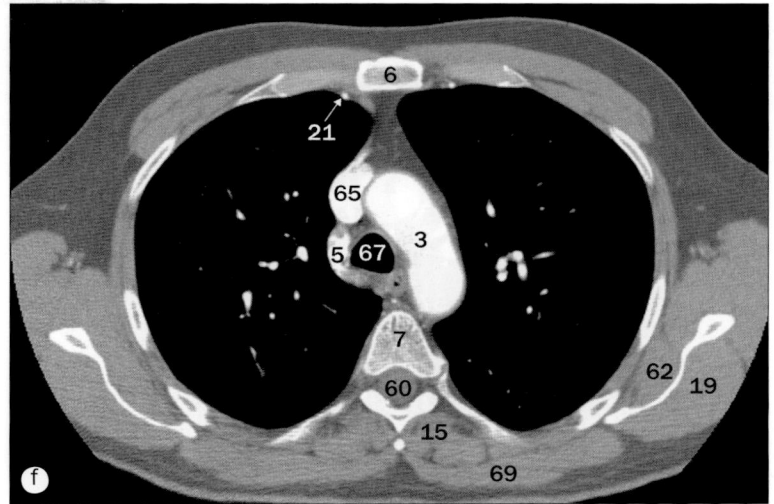

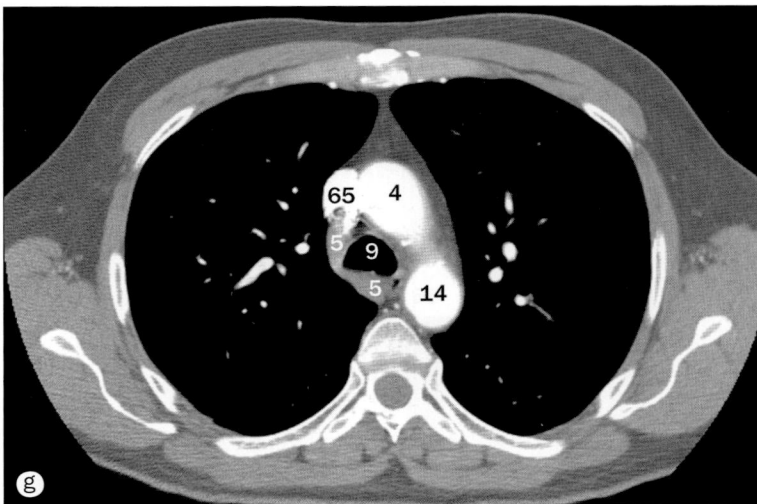

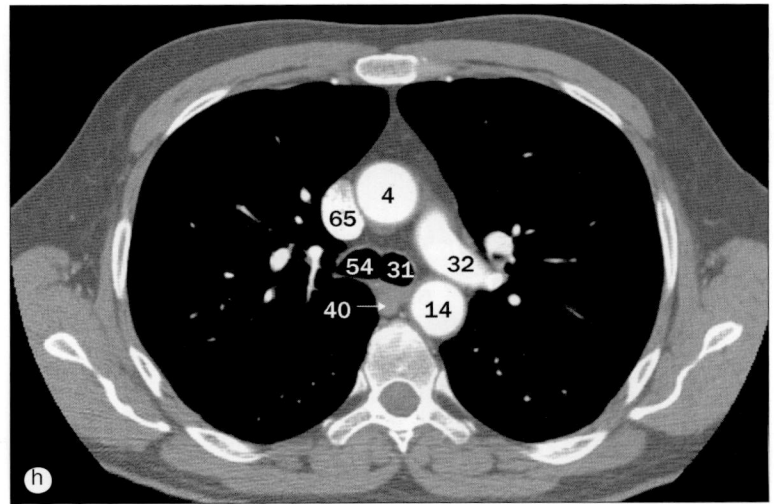

(a)–(t) Chest, axial CT images of mediastinum.

36 Left ventricular cavity
37 Manubrium of sternum
38 Mitral valve
39 Muscular interventricular septum
40 Oesophagus
41 Papillary muscles
42 Pectoralis major muscle
43 Pectoralis minor muscle
44 Pedicle
45 Pericardium
46 Pulmonary trunk
47 Right atrial appendage (auricle)
48 Right atrium

49 Right brachiocephalic vein
50 Right hemidiaphragm
51 Right inferior lobe bronchus
52 Right inferior pulmonary vein
53 Right lobe of liver
54 Right main bronchus
55 Right pulmonary artery
56 Right superior lobe bronchus
57 Right superior pulmonary vein
58 Right ventricular cavity
59 Serratus anterior muscle
60 Spinal canal
61 Sternoclavicular joint

62 Subscapularis muscle
63 Superior lobe branch of right pulmonary artery
64 Superior pericardial recess
65 Superior vena cava
66 Supraspinatus muscle
67 Trachea
68 Transverse process
69 Trapezius muscle
70 Tricuspid valve
71 Xiphisternum

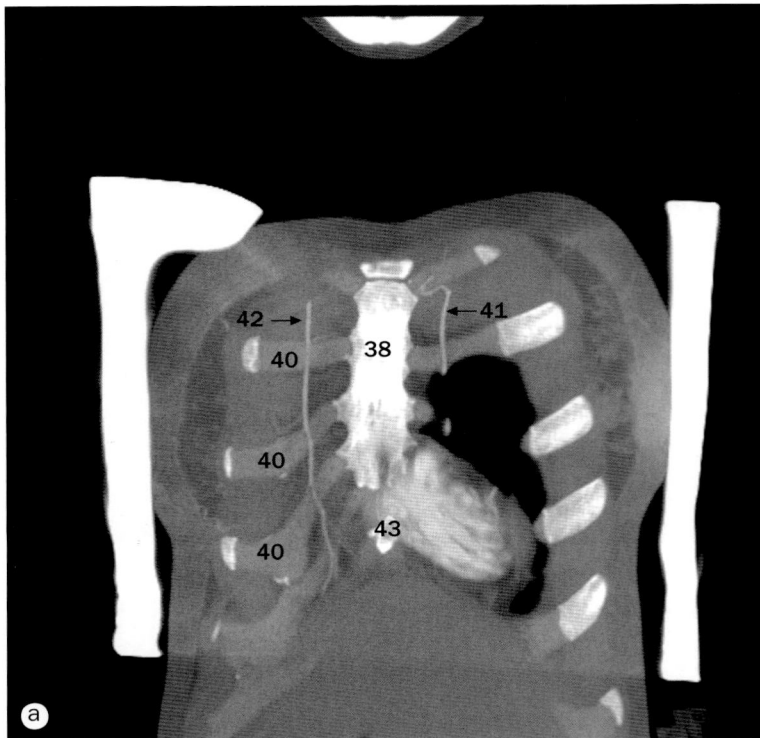

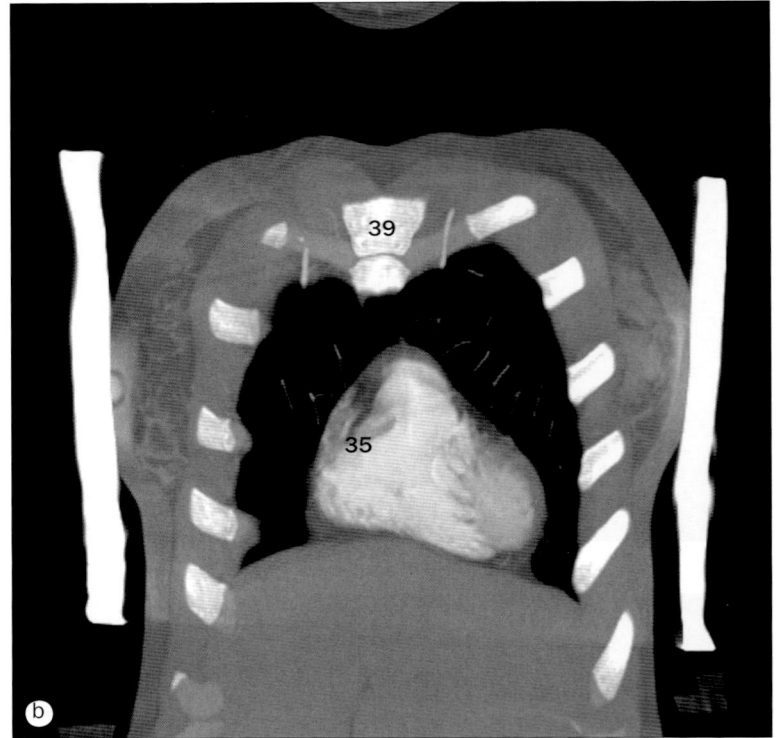

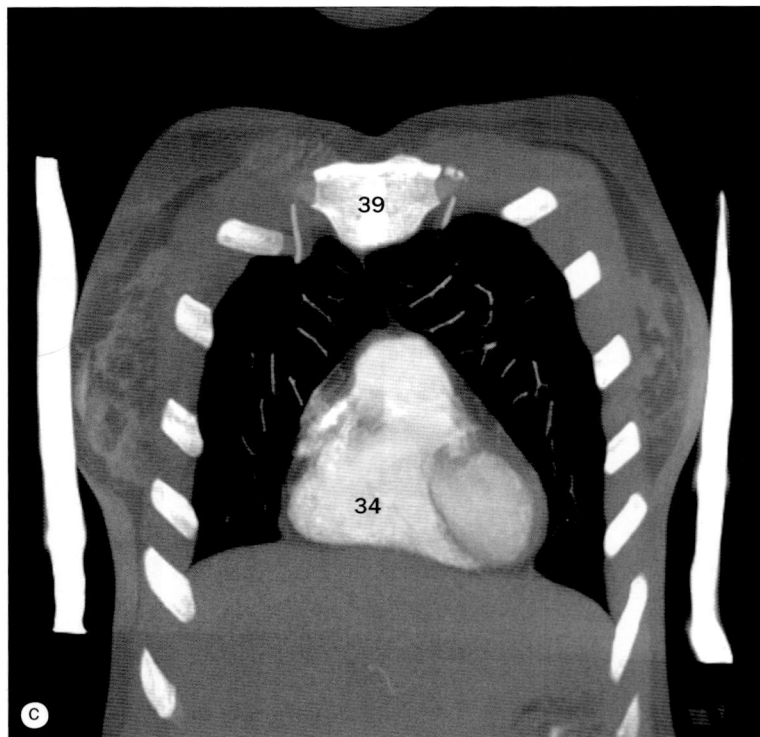

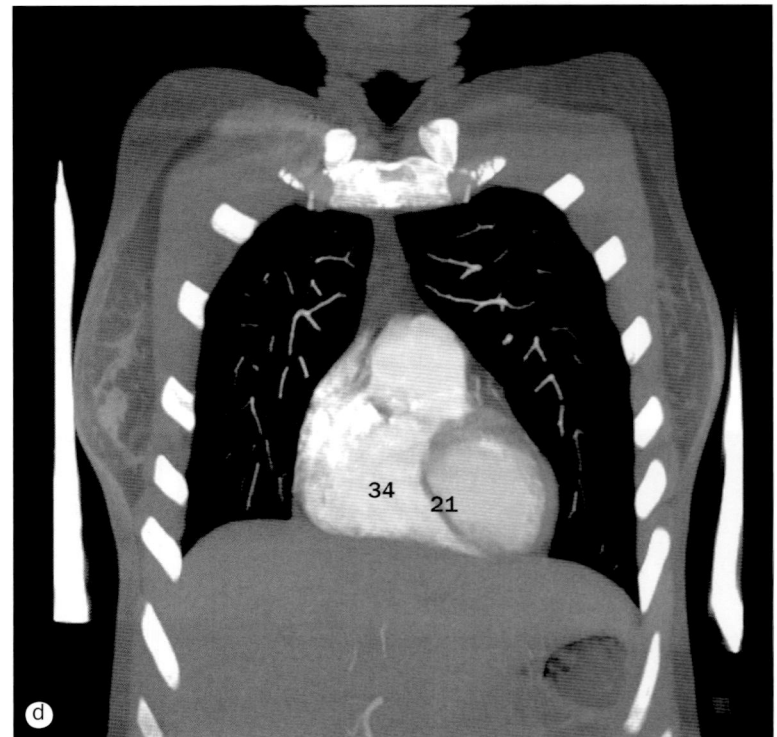

(a)–(p) Chest, coronal CT images, from anterior to posterior.

1 Aortic valve	**9** Interatrial septum	**17** Left superior pulmonary vein
2 Arch of aorta (aortic knuckle or knob)	**10** Left atrial appendage (auricle)	**18** Left ventricular cavity
3 Ascending aorta	**11** Left atrium	**19** Left ventricular wall
4 Brachiocephalic trunk	**12** Left brachiocephalic vein	**20** Membranous interventricular septum
5 Carina (bifurcation of trachea)	**13** Left common carctid artery	**21** Muscular interventricular septum
6 Clavicle	**14** Left main bronchus	**22** Papillary muscles
7 Descending aorta	**15** Left pulmonary artery	**23** Pericardium
8 Inferior vena cava	**16** Left subclavian artery	**24** Pulmonary trunk

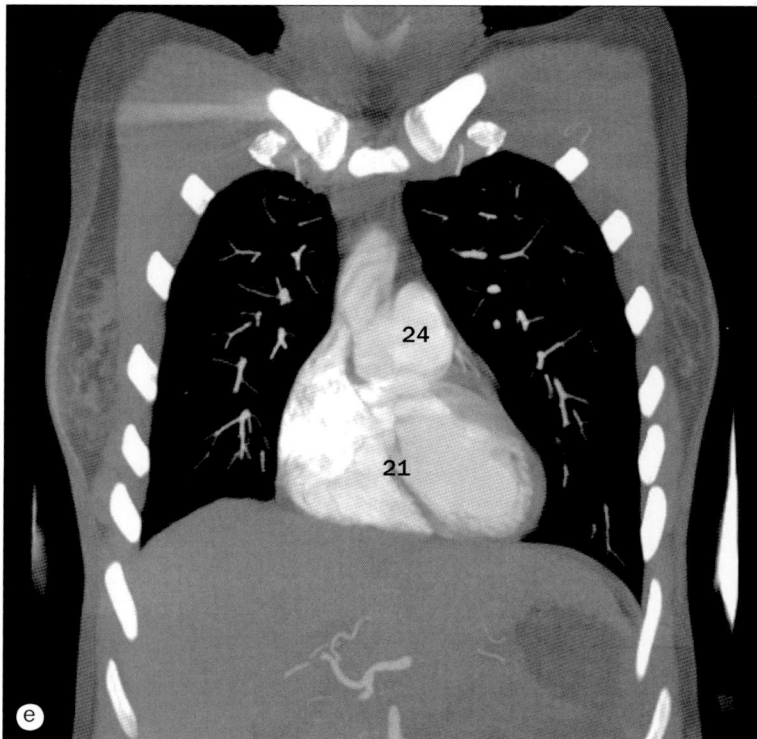

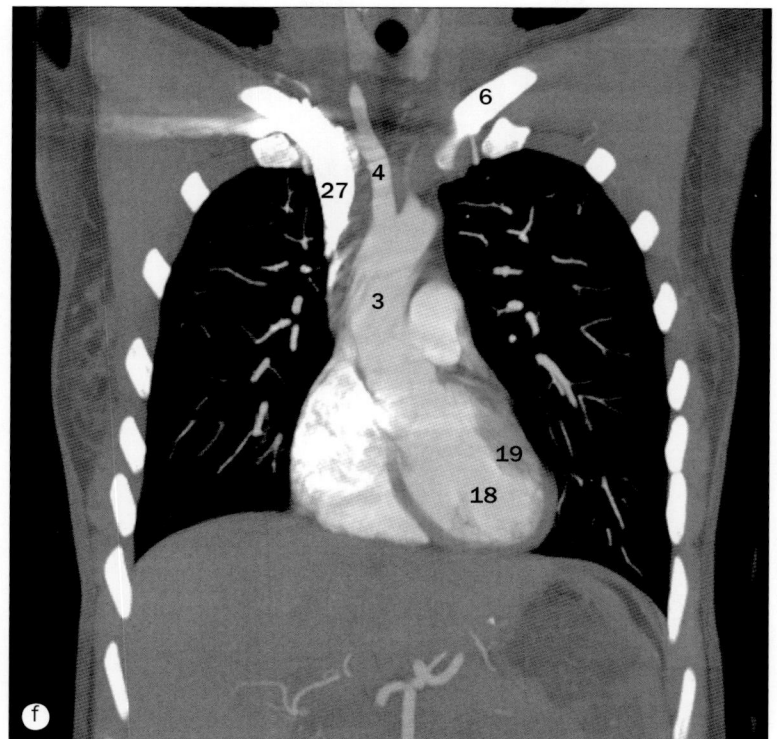

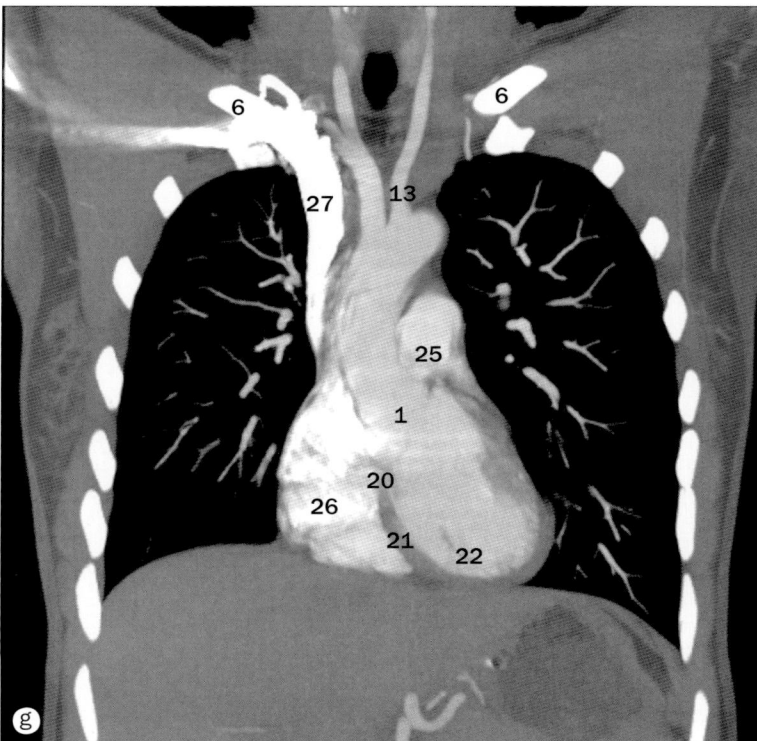

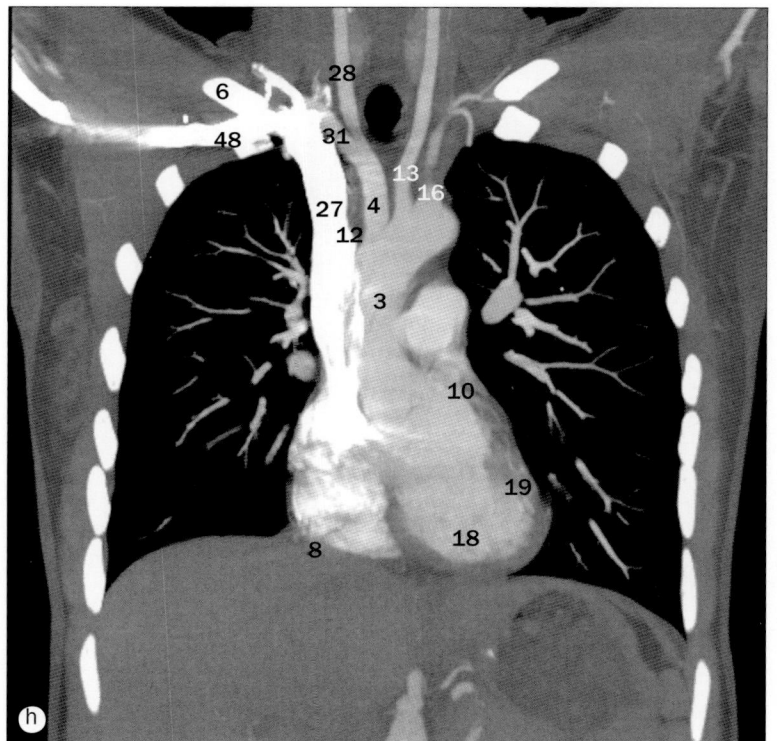

(a)–(p) Chest, coronal CT images, from anterior to posterior.

25 Pulmonary valve	34 Right ventricular cavity	43 Xiphisternum
26 Right atrium	35 Right ventricular wall	44 Tricuspid valve
27 Right brachiocephalic vein	36 Superior vena cava	45 Mitral valve
28 Right common carotid artery	37 Trachea	46 Left axillary artery
29 Right main bronchus	38 Sternum	47 Left subclavian artery
30 Right pulmonary artery	39 Manubrium	48 Right subclavian vein
31 Right subclavian artery	40 Anterior costal cartilage	49 Left inferior pulmonary vein
32 Right superior lobe pulmonary artery	41 Left internal thoracic (mammary) artery	50 Abdominal aorta
33 Right superior pulmonary vein	42 Right internal thoracic (mammary) artery	51 Right inferior pulmonary vein

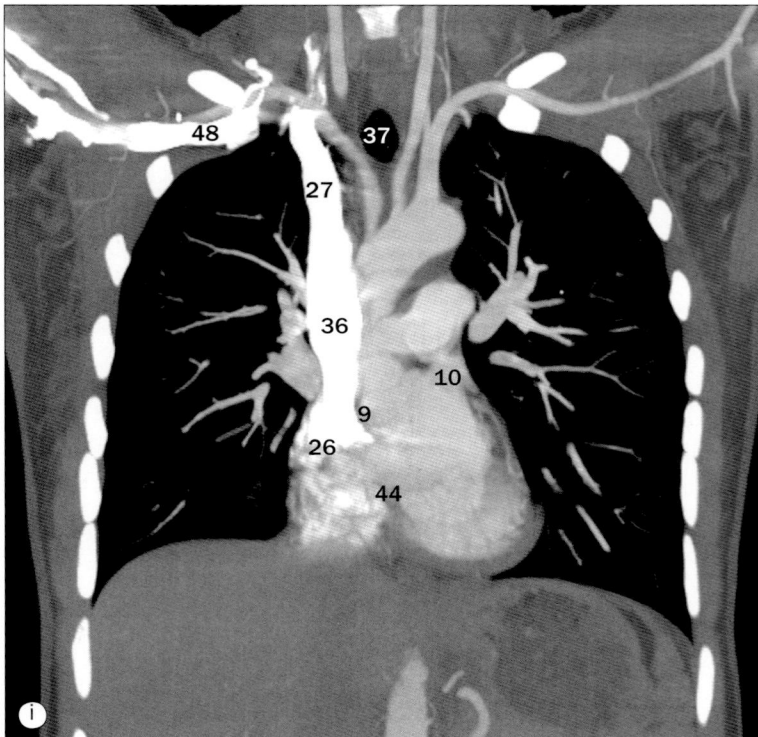

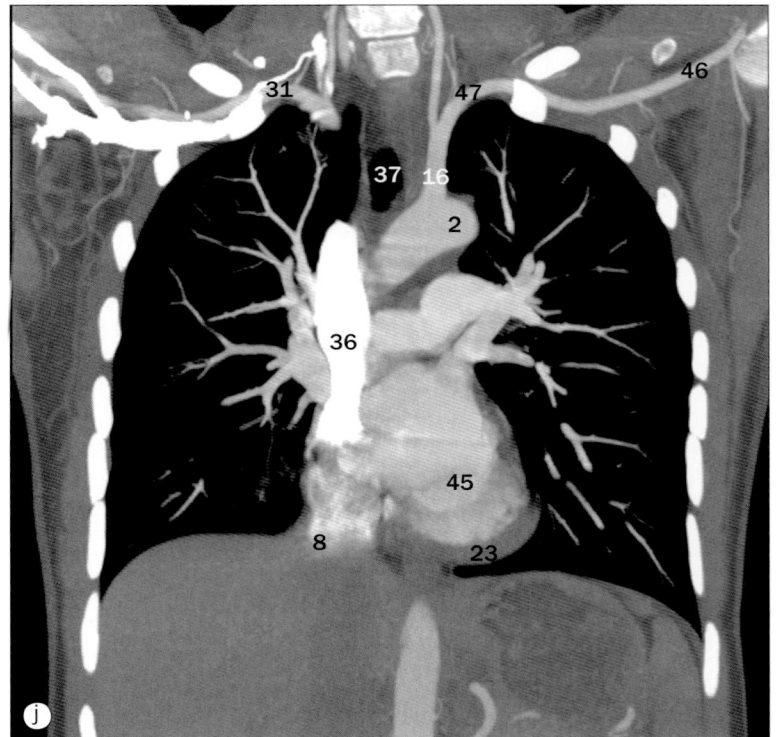

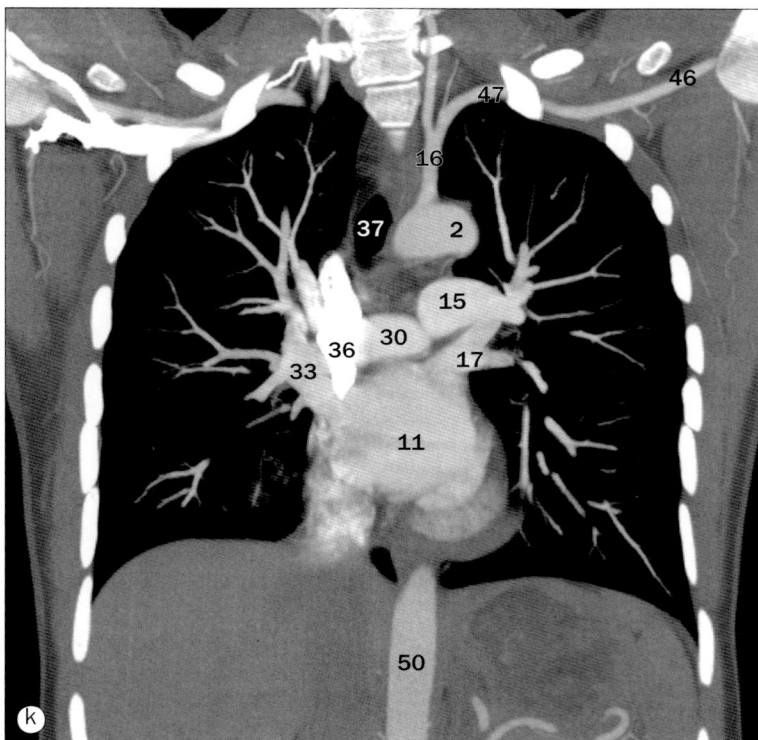

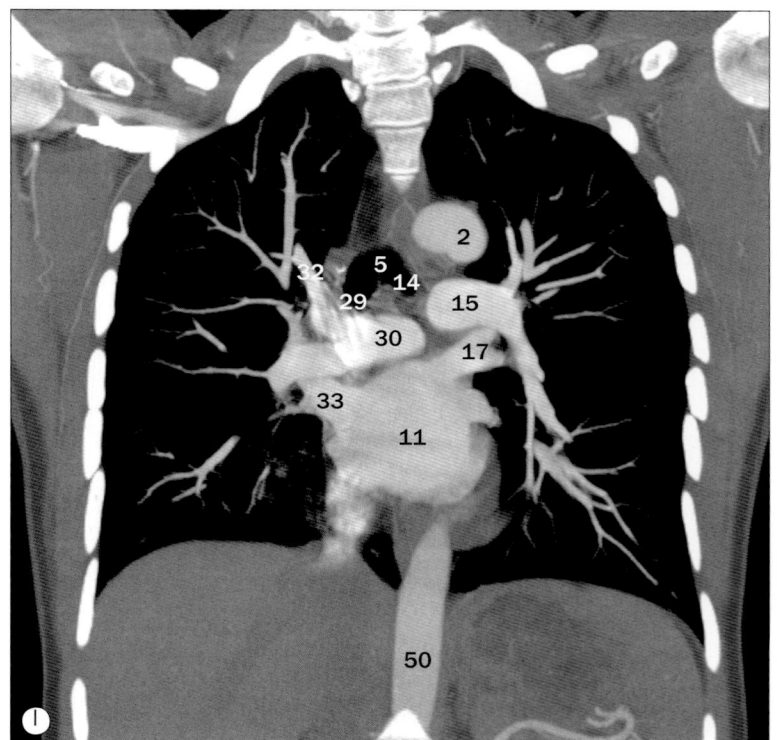

(a)–(p) Chest, coronal CT images, from anterior to posterior.

1 Aortic valve	**9** Interatrial septum	**17** Left superior pulmonary vein
2 Arch of aorta (aortic knuckle or knob)	**10** Left atrial appendage (auricle)	**18** Left ventricular cavity
3 Ascending aorta	**11** Left atrium	**19** Left ventricular wall
4 Brachiocephalic trunk	**12** Left brachiocephalic vein	**20** Membranous interventricular septum
5 Carina (bifurcation of trachea)	**13** Left common carotid artery	**21** Muscular interventricular septum
6 Clavicle	**14** Left main bronchus	**22** Papillary muscles
7 Descending aorta	**15** Left pulmonary artery	**23** Pericardium
8 Inferior vena cava	**16** Left subclavian artery	**24** Pulmonary trunk

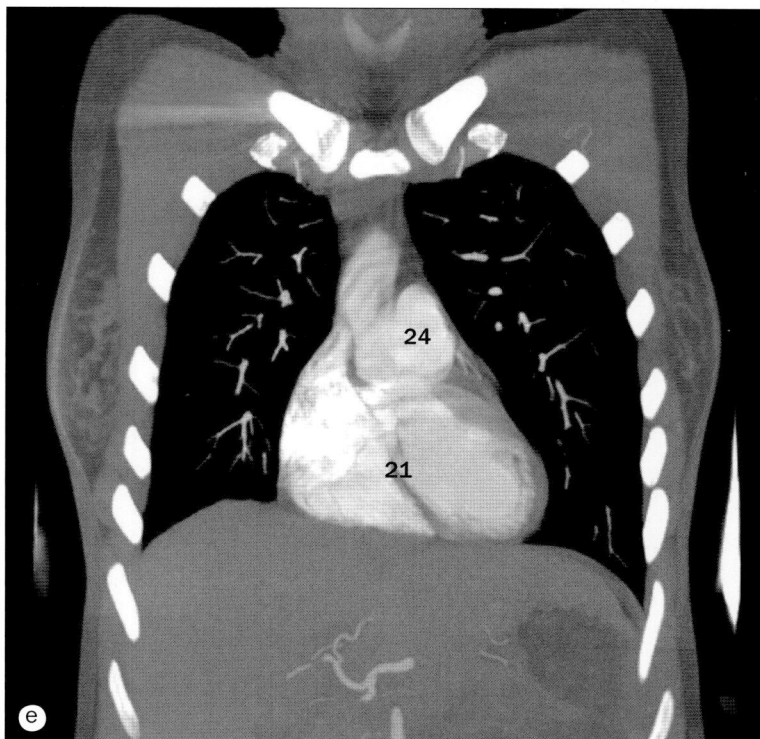

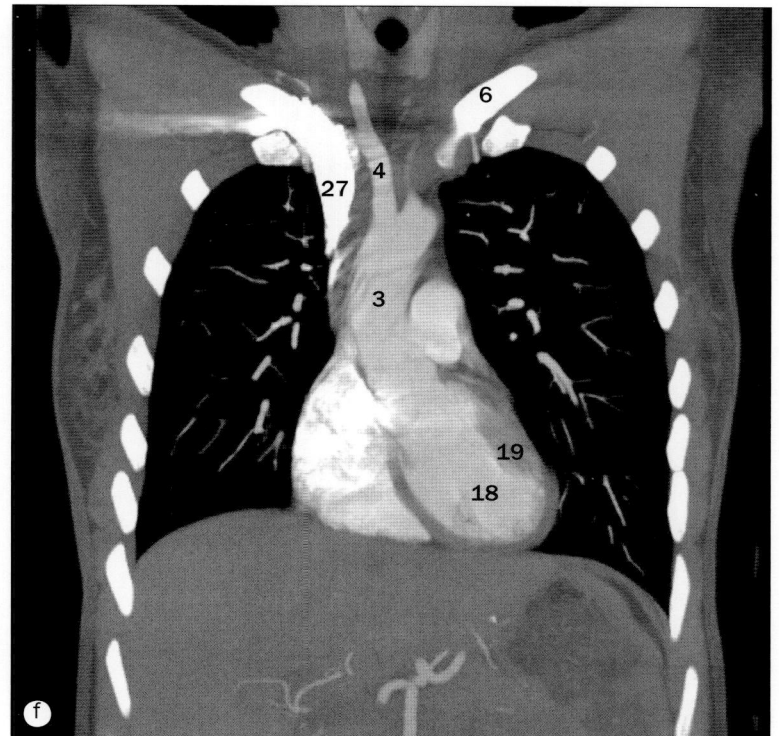

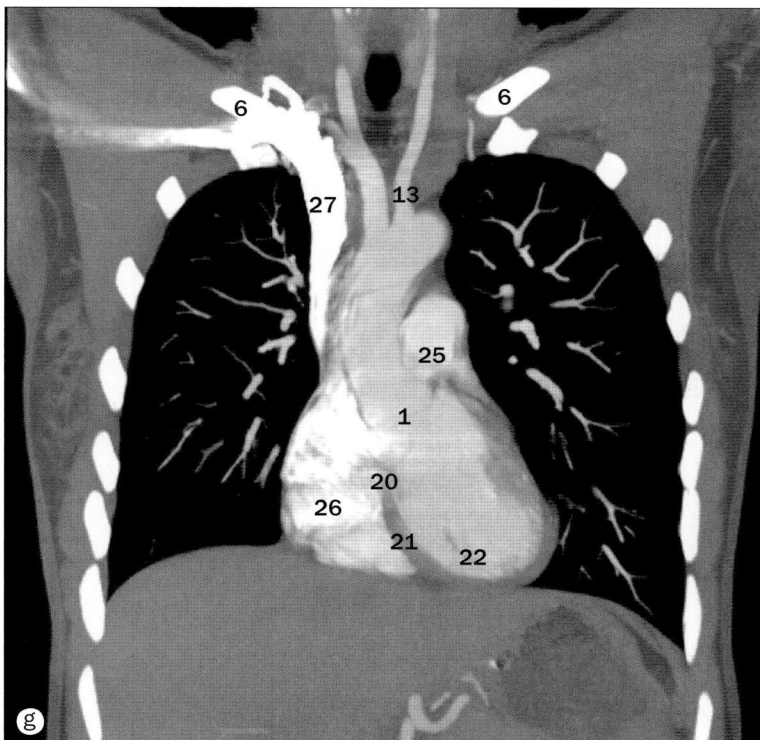

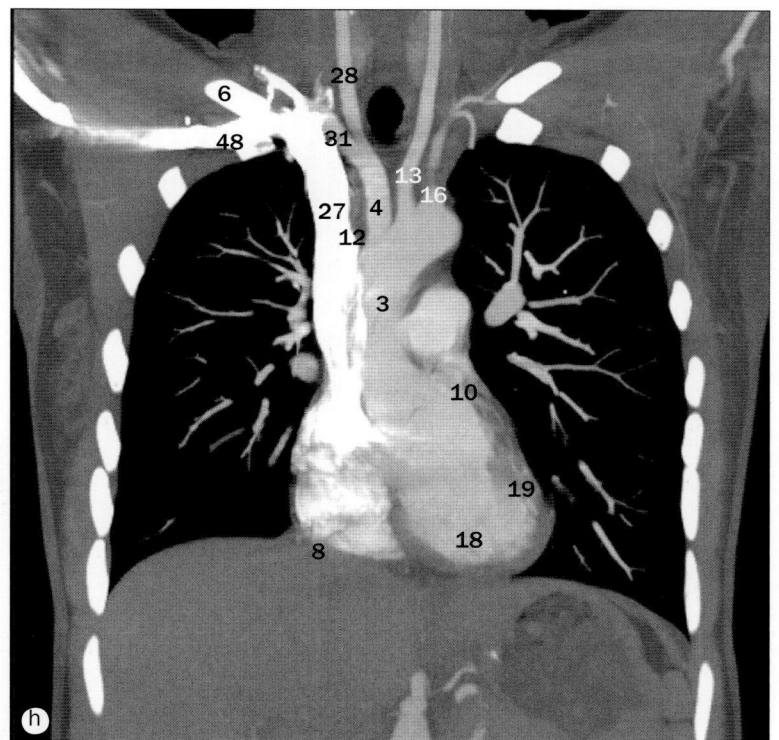

(a)–(p) Chest, coronal CT images, from anterior to posterior.

25 Pulmonary valve	34 Right ventricular cavity	43 Xiphisternum
26 Right atrium	35 Right ventricular wall	44 Tricuspid valve
27 Right brachiocephalic vein	36 Superior vena cava	45 Mitral valve
28 Right common carotid artery	37 Trachea	46 Left axillary artery
29 Right main bronchus	38 Sternum	47 Left subclavian artery
30 Right pulmonary artery	39 Manubrium	48 Right subclavian vein
31 Right subclavian artery	40 Anterior costal cartilage	49 Left inferior pulmonary vein
32 Right superior lobe pulmonary artery	41 Left internal thoracic (mammary) artery	50 Abdominal aorta
33 Right superior pulmonary vein	42 Right internal thoracic (mammary) artery	51 Right inferior pulmonary vein

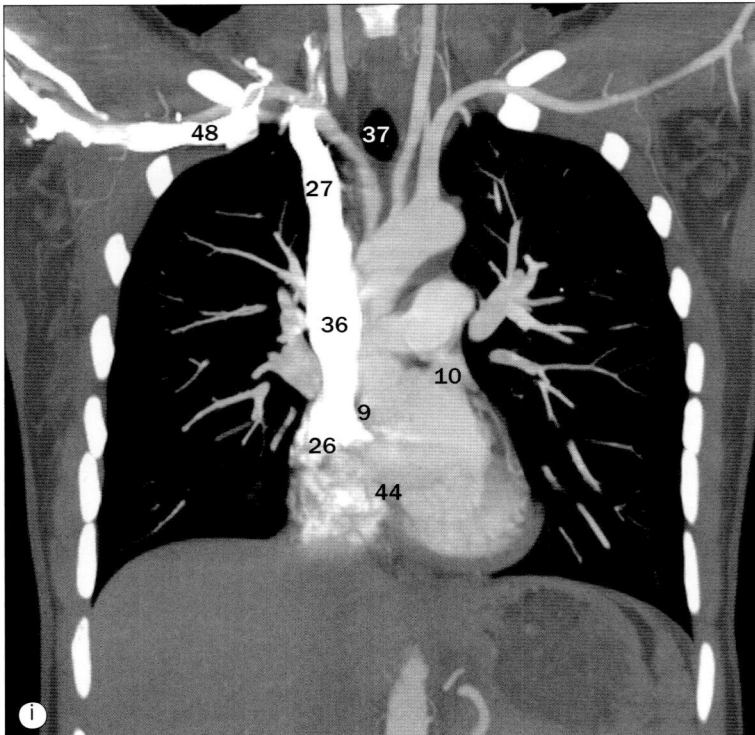

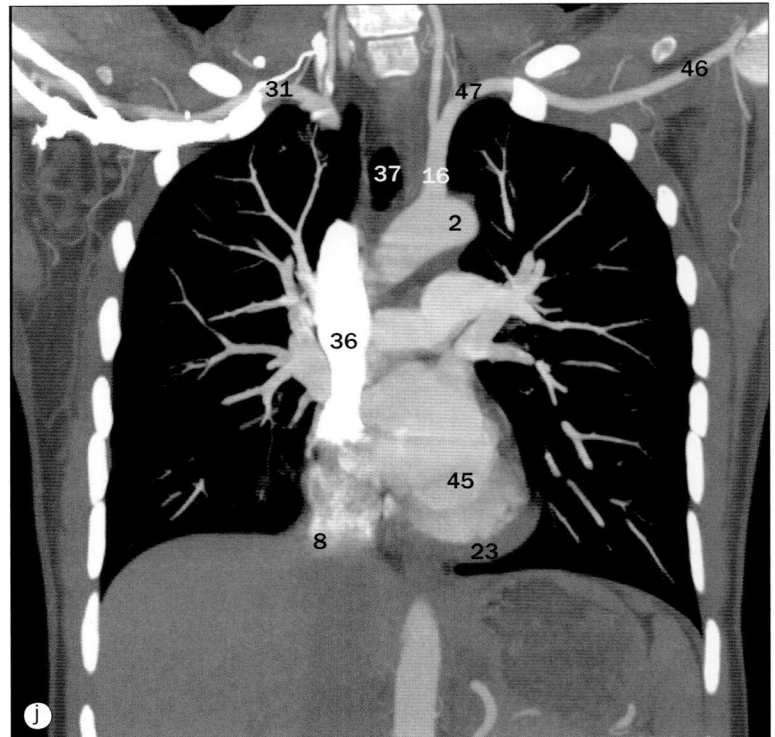

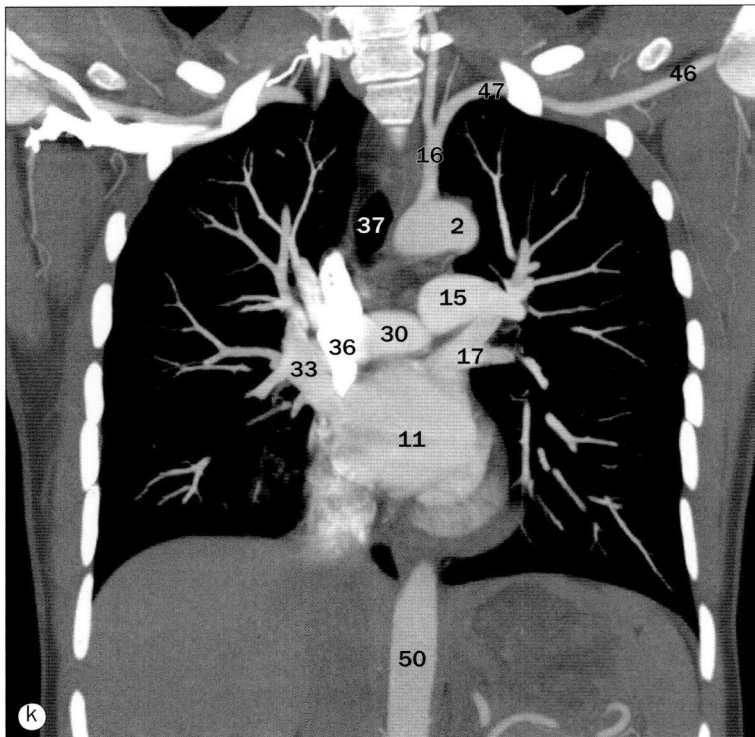

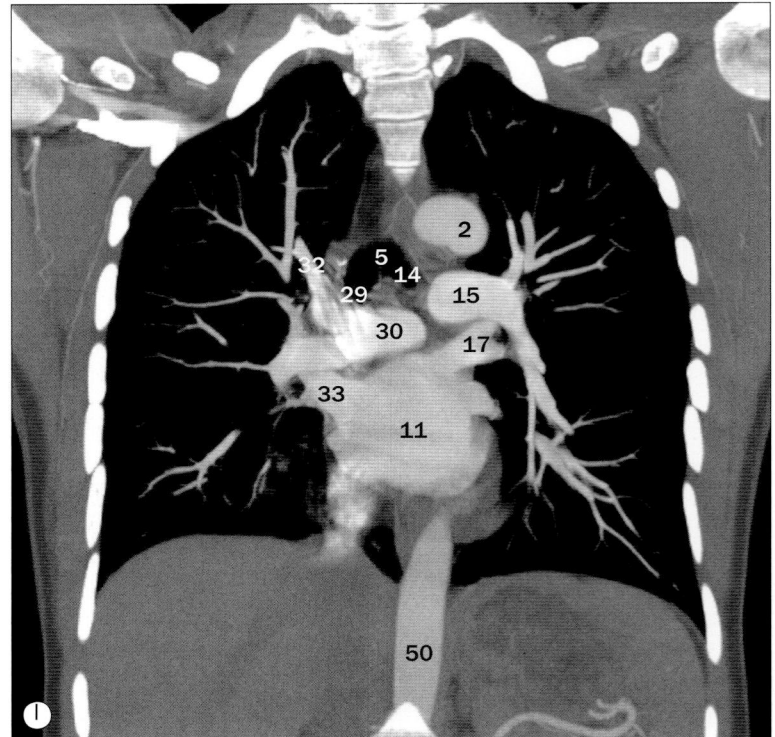

(a)–(p) Chest, coronal CT images, from anterior to posterior.

1 Aortic valve	9 Interatrial septum	17 Left superior pulmonary vein
2 Arch of aorta (aortic knuckle or knob)	10 Left atrial appendage (auricle)	18 Left ventricular cavity
3 Ascending aorta	11 Left atrium	19 Left ventricular wall
4 Brachiocephalic trunk	12 Left brachiocephalic vein	20 Membranous interventricular septum
5 Carina (bifurcation of trachea)	13 Left common carotid artery	21 Muscular interventricular septum
6 Clavicle	14 Left main bronchus	22 Papillary muscles
7 Descending aorta	15 Left pulmonary artery	23 Pericardium
8 Inferior vena cava	16 Left subclavian artery	24 Pulmonary trunk

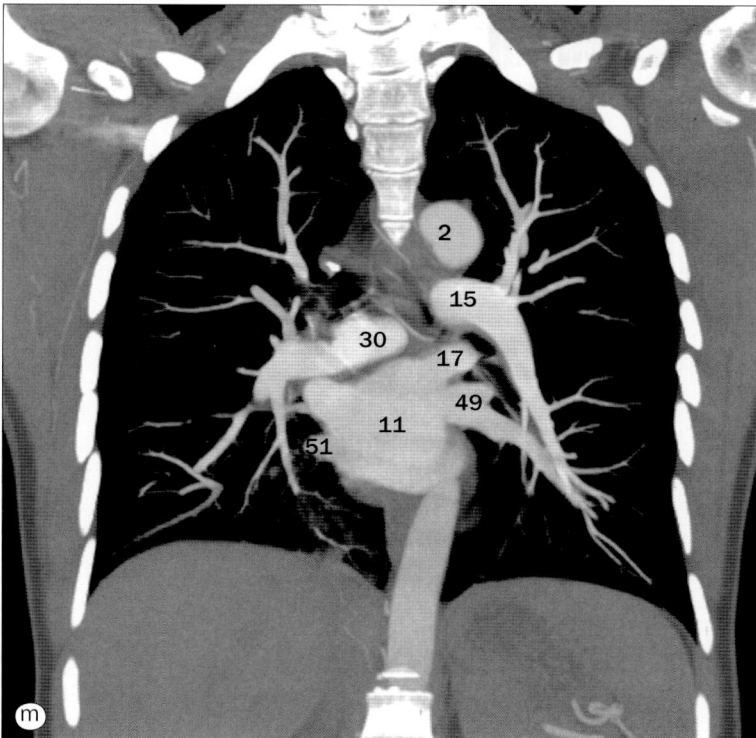

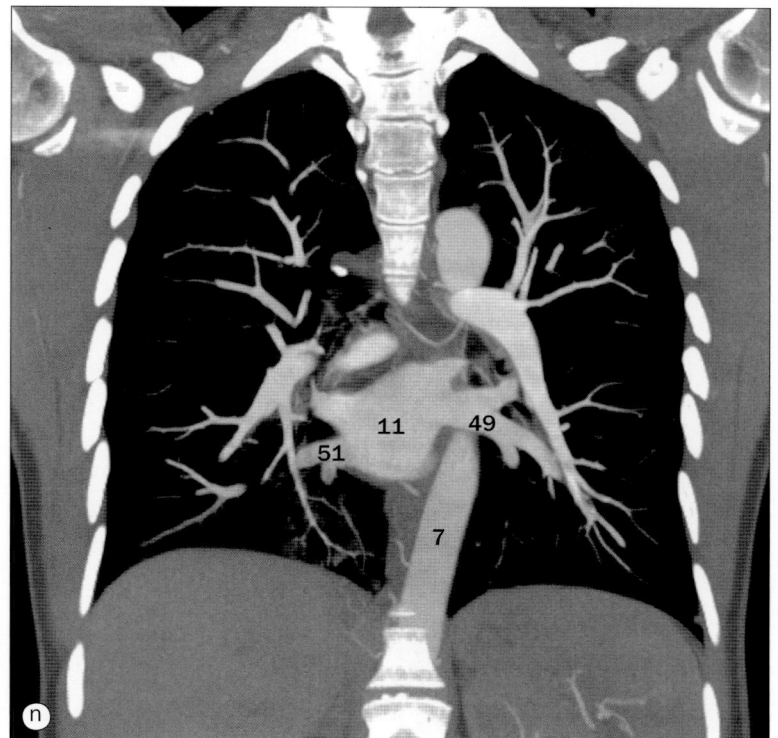

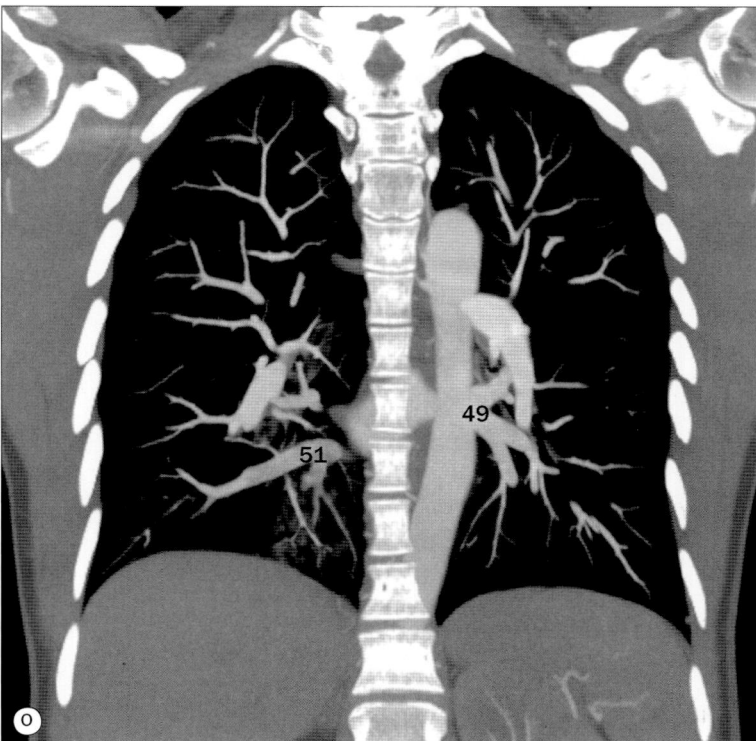

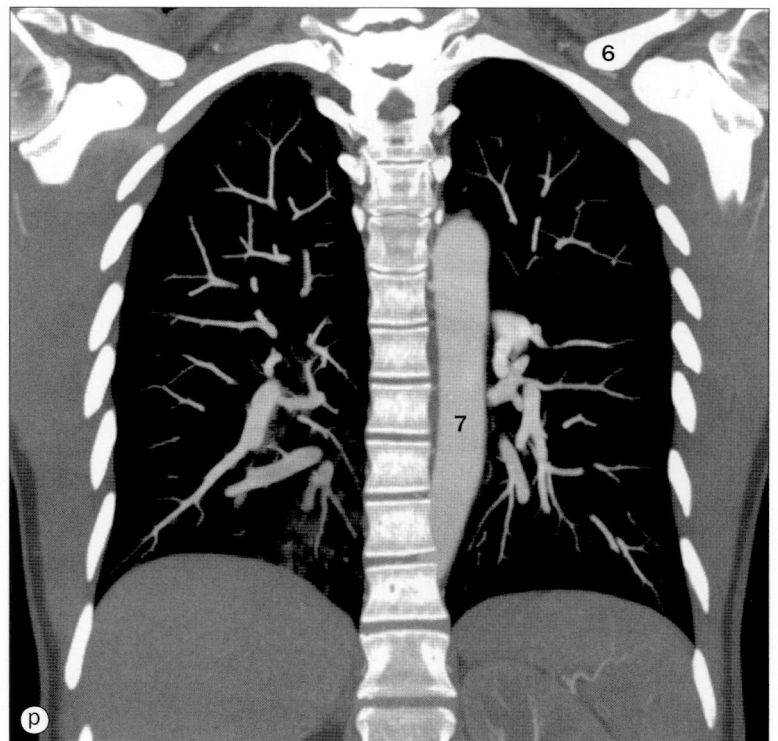

(a)–(p) Chest, coronal CT images, from anterior to posterior.

25 Pulmonary valve
26 Right atrium
27 Right brachiocephalic vein
28 Right common carotid artery
29 Right main bronchus
30 Right pulmonary artery
31 Right subclavian artery
32 Right superior lobe pulmonary artery
33 Right superior pulmonary vein

34 Right ventricular cavity
35 Right ventricular wall
36 Superior vena cava
37 Trachea
38 Sternum
39 Manubrium
40 Anterior costal cartilage
41 Left internal thoracic (mammary) artery
42 Right internal thoracic (mammary) artery

43 Xiphisternum
44 Tricuspid valve
45 Mitral valve
46 Left axillary artery
47 Left subclavian artery
48 Right subclavian vein
49 Left inferior pulmonary vein
50 Abdominal aorta
51 Right inferior pulmonary vein

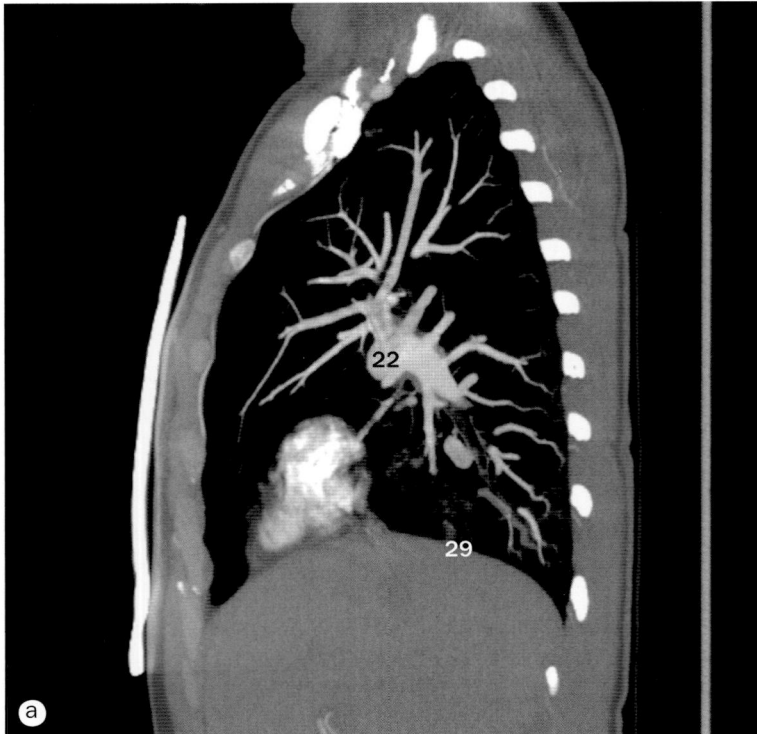

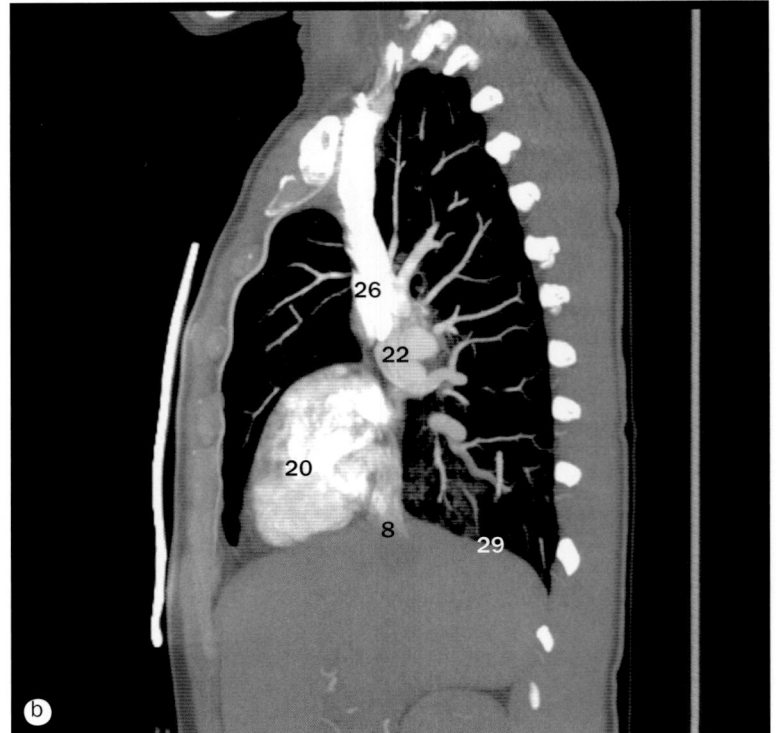

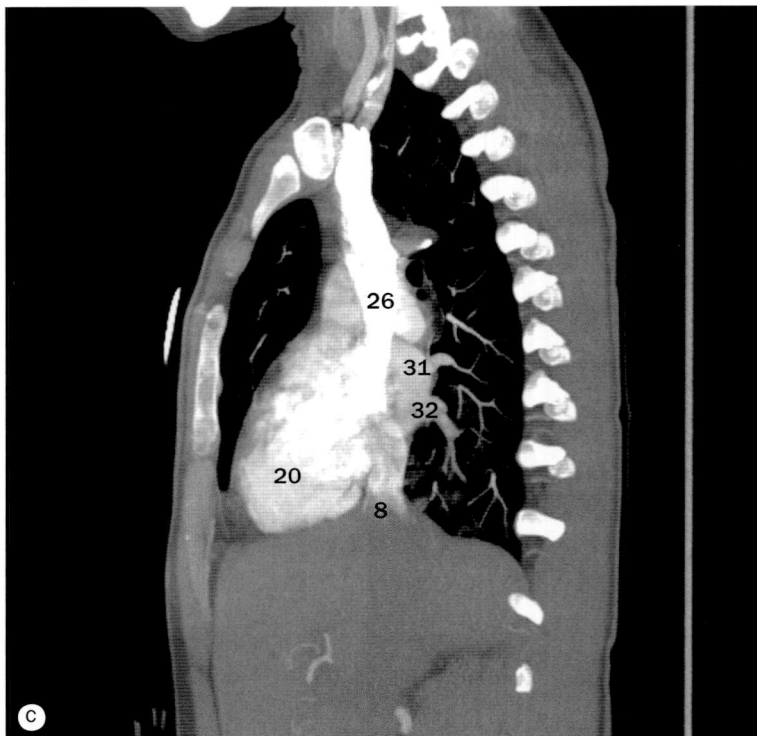

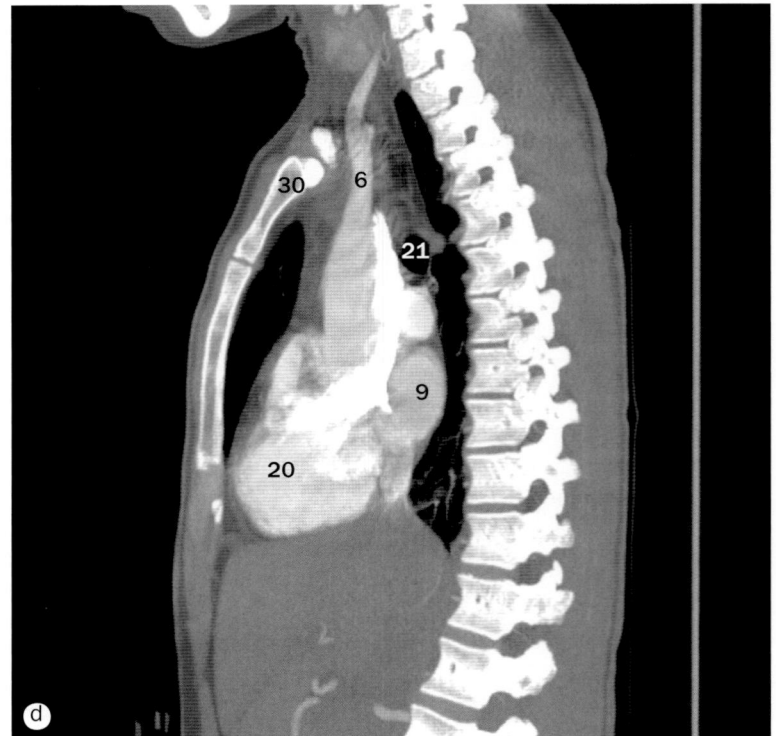

(a)–(p) Chest, sagittal CT images, from right to left.

1 Aortic valve	**8** Inferior vena cava	**15** Mitral valve
2 Arch of aorta (aortic knuckle or knob)	**9** Left atrium	**16** Muscular interventricular septum
3 Ascending aorta	**10** Left common carotid artery	**17** Pericardium
4 Body of sternum	**11** Left main bronchus	**18** Pulmonary trunk
5 Body of vertebra	**12** Left pulmonary artery	**19** Pulmonary valve
6 Brachiocephalic trunk	**13** Left subclavian artery	**20** Right atrium
7 Descending aorta	**14** Left ventricular cavity	**21** Right main bronchus

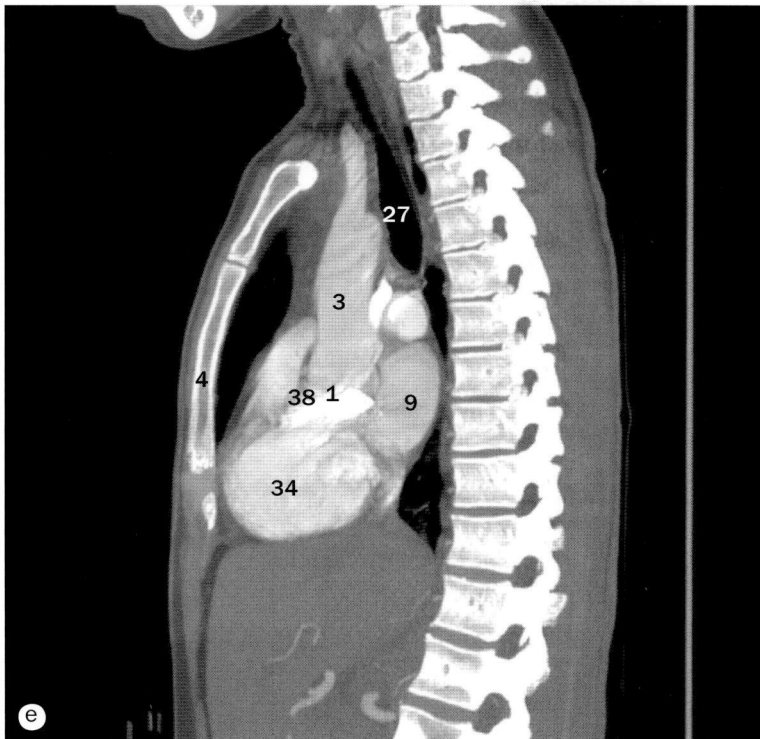

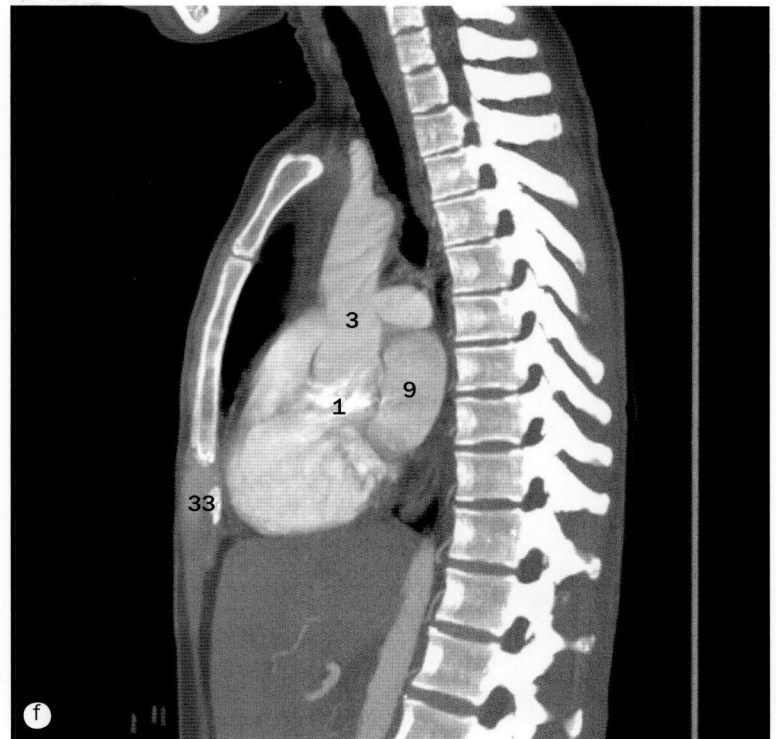

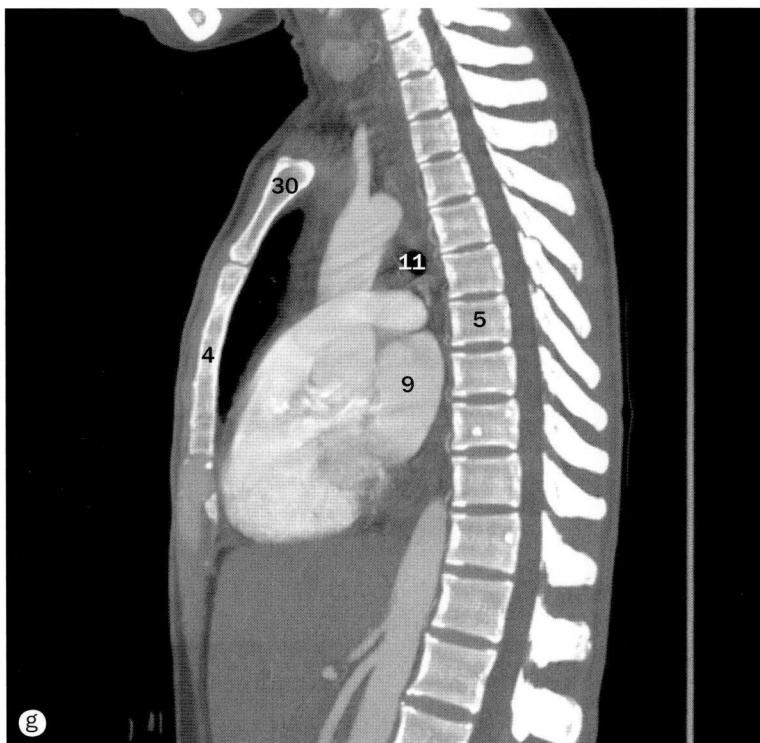

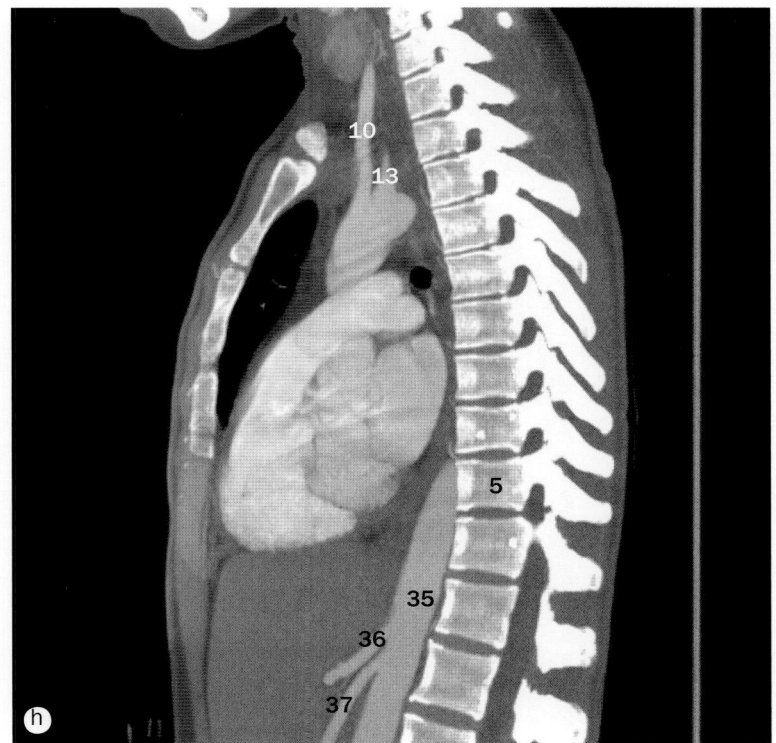

(a)–(p) Chest, sagittal CT images, from right to left.

22 Right pulmonary artery	28 Left dome of diaphragm	34 Tricuspid valve
23 Right ventricular cavity	29 Right dome of diaphragm	35 Abdominal aorta
24 Right ventricular outflow tract	30 Manubrium	36 Coeliac axis
25 Right ventricular wall	31 Right superior pulmonary vein	37 Superior mesenteric artery
26 Superior vena cava	32 Right inferior pulmonary vein	38 Right coronary artery
27 Trachea	33 Xiphisternum	

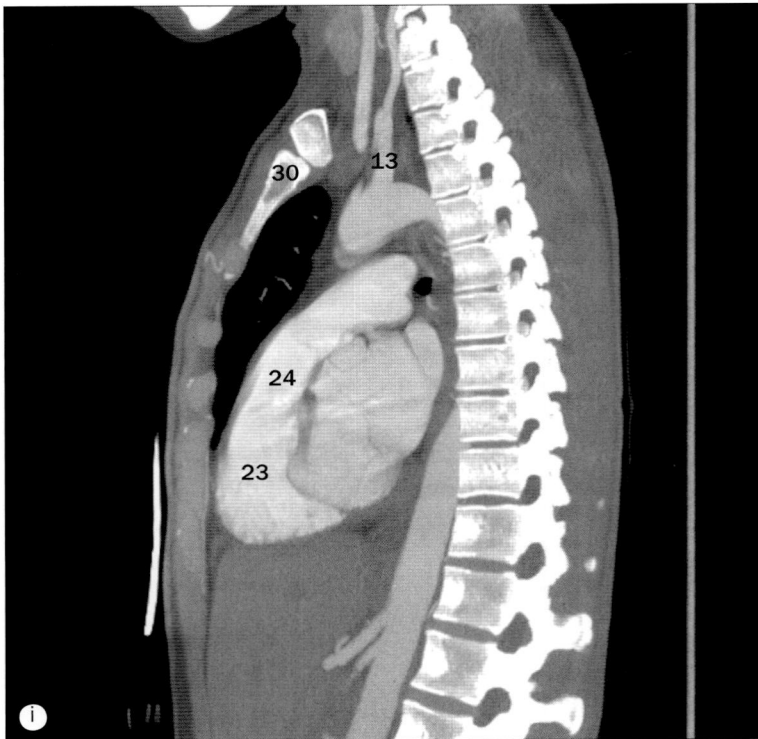

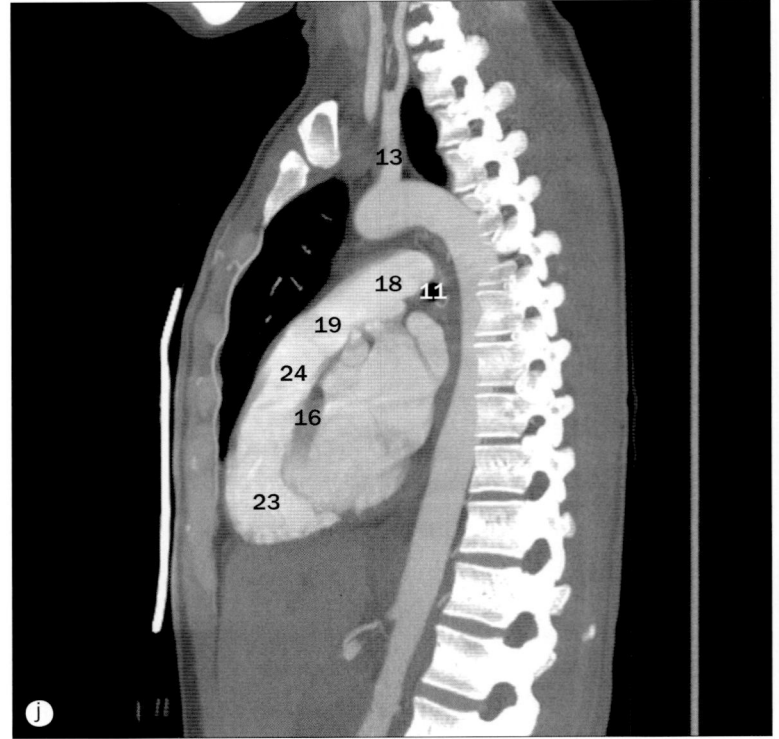

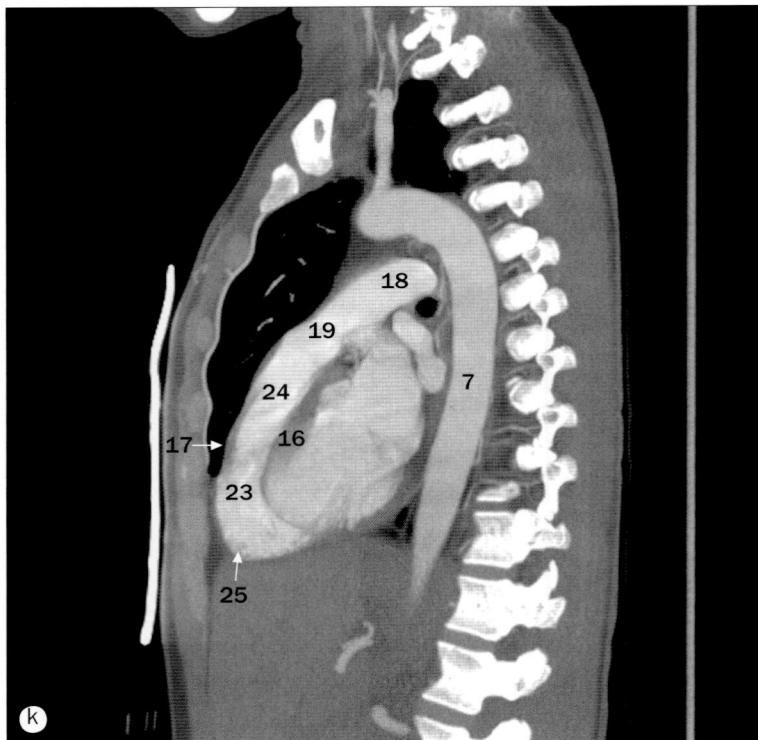

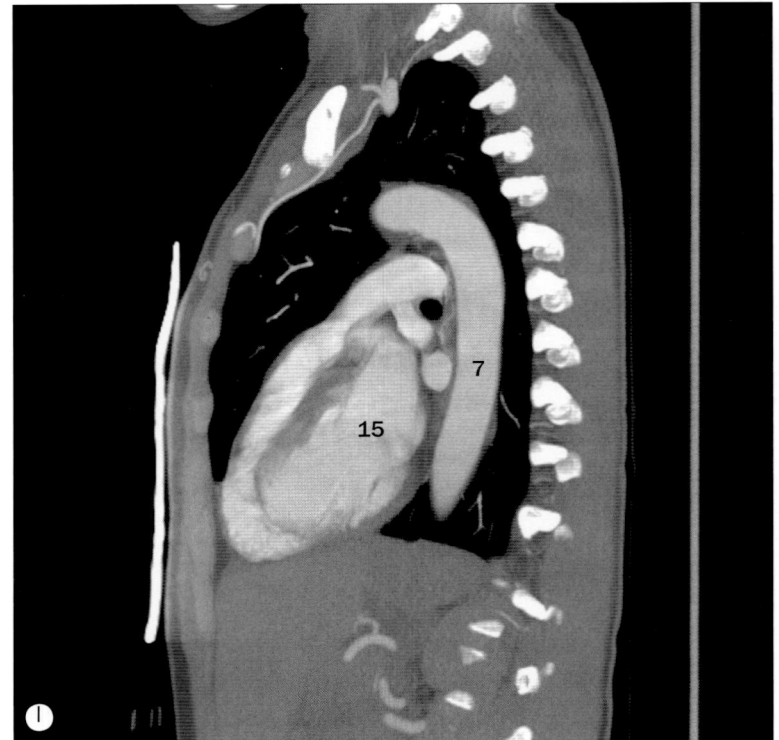

(a)–(p) Chest, sagittal CT images, from right to left.

1 Aortic valve	**8** Inferior vena cava
2 Arch of aorta (aortic knuckle or knob)	**9** Left atrium
3 Ascending aorta	**10** Left common carotid artery
4 Body of sternum	**11** Left main bronchus
5 Body of vertebra	**12** Left pulmonary artery
6 Brachiocephalic trunk	**13** Left subclavian artery
7 Descending aorta	**14** Left ventricular cavity

15 Mitral valve
16 Muscular interventricular septum
17 Pericardium
18 Pulmonary trunk
19 Pulmonary valve
20 Right atrium
21 Right main bronchus

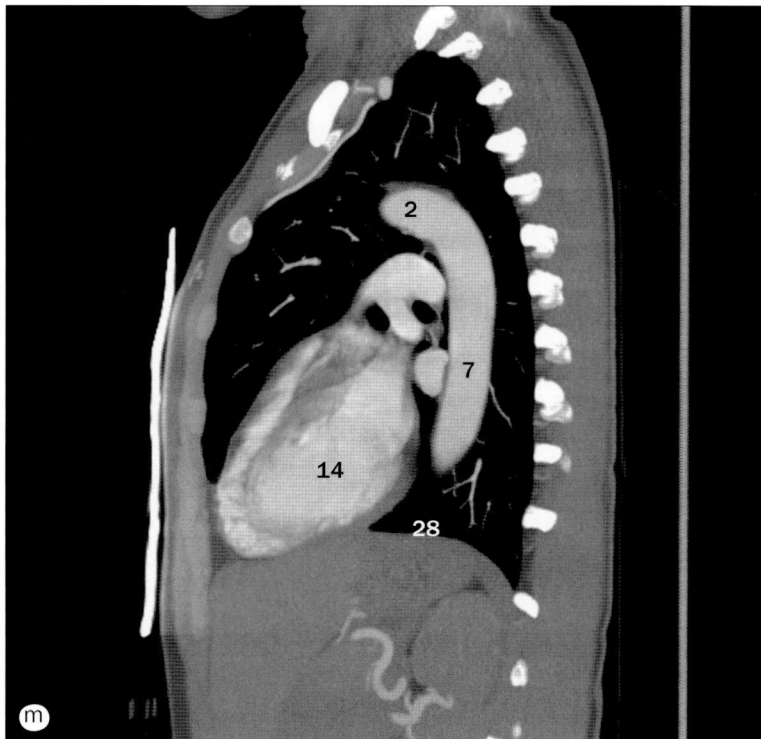

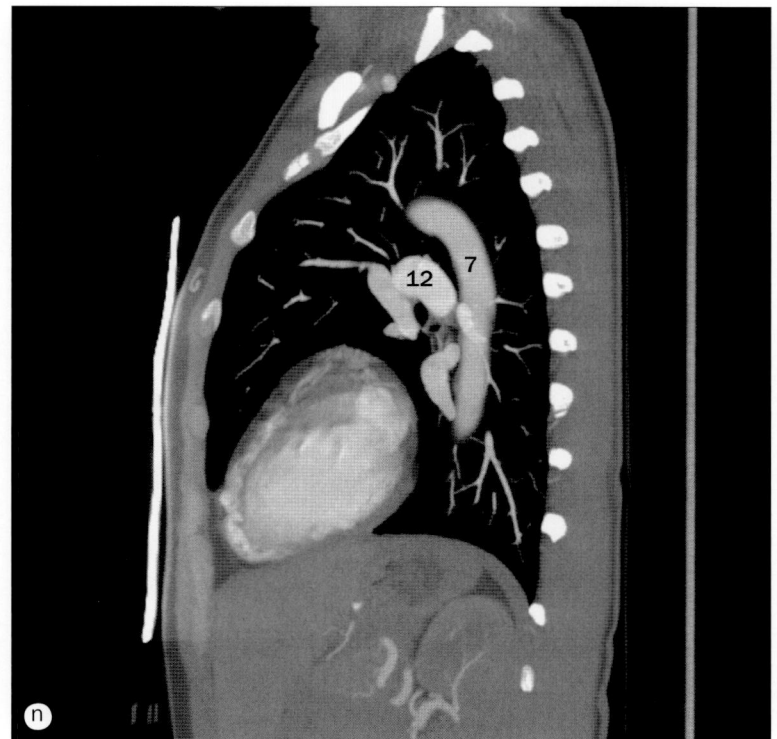

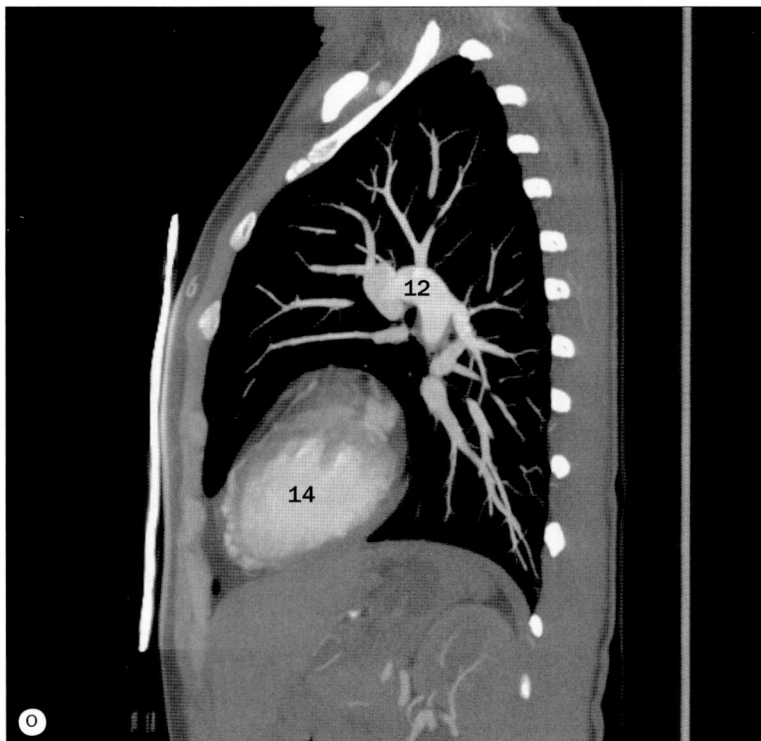

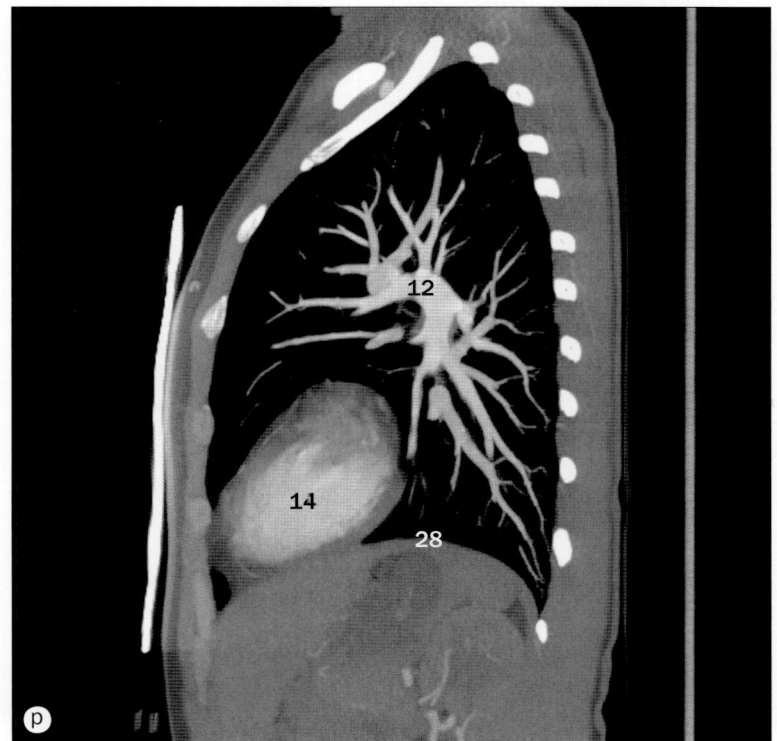

(a)–(p) Chest, sagittal CT images, from right to left.

22 Right pulmonary artery	28 Left dome of diaphragm	34 Tricuspid valve
23 Right ventricular cavity	29 Right dome of diaphragm	35 Abdominal aorta
24 Right ventricular outflow tract	30 Manubrium	36 Coeliac axis
25 Right ventricular wall	31 Right superior pulmonary vein	37 Superior mesenteric artery
26 Superior vena cava	32 Right inferior pulmonary vein	38 Right coronary artery
27 Trachea	33 Xiphisternum	

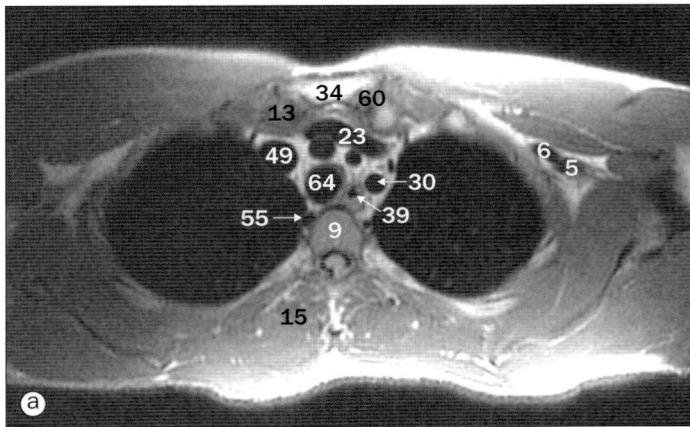

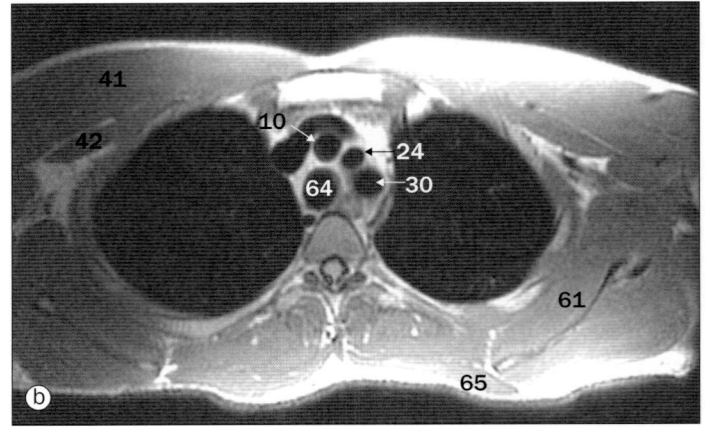

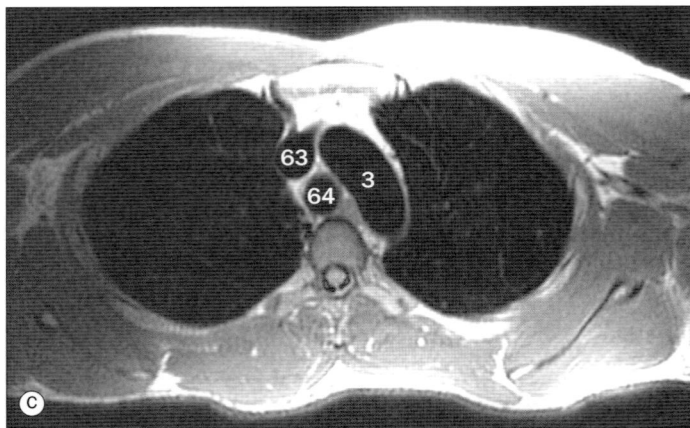

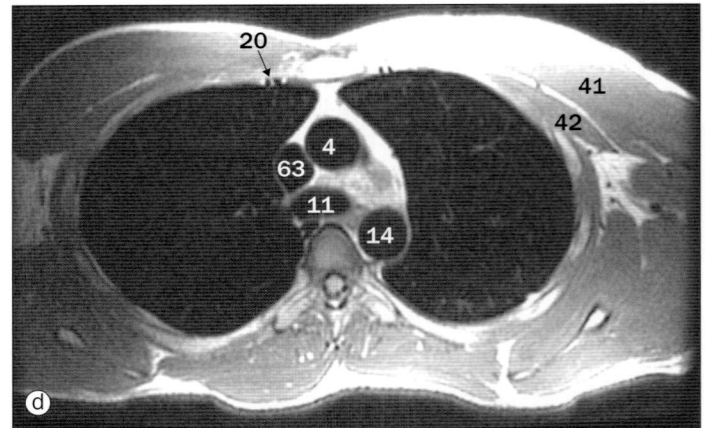

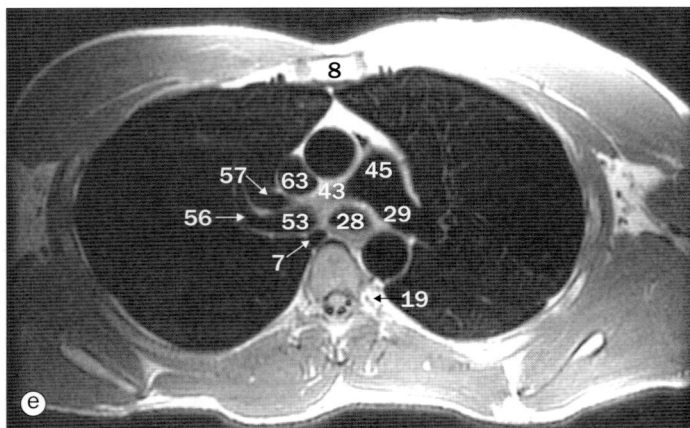

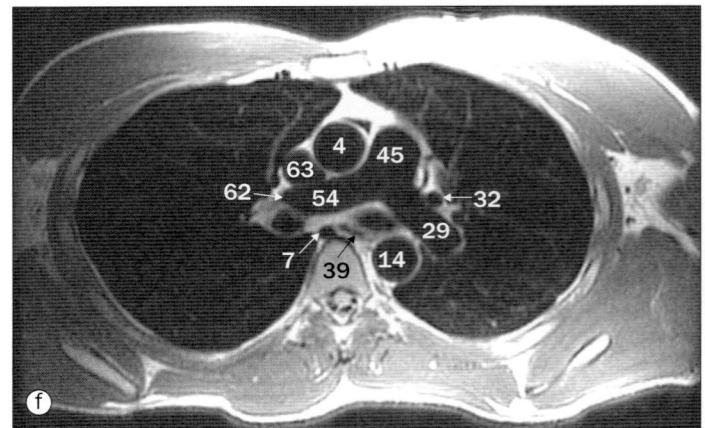

(a)–(l) Chest, axial MR images.

1 Anterior interventricular branch of left coronary artery	12 Circumflex branch of left coronary artery	24 Left common carotid artery
2 Aortic valve	13 Clavicle	25 Left coronary artery
3 Arch of aorta (aortic knuckle or knob)	14 Descending aorta	26 Left inferior lobe bronchus
4 Ascending aorta	15 Erector spinae muscle	27 Left inferior pulmonary vein
5 Axillary artery	16 Hemi-azygos vein	28 Left main bronchus
6 Axillary vein	17 Inferior vena cava	29 Left pulmonary artery
7 Azygos vein	18 Interatrial septum	30 Left subclavian artery
8 Body of sternum	19 Intercostal artery	31 Left superior lobe bronchus
9 Body of vertebra	20 Internal thoracic artery and vein	32 Left superior pulmonary vein
10 Brachiocephalic trunk	21 Left atrial appendage (auricle)	33 Left ventricular cavity
11 Carina (bifurcation of trachea)	22 Left atrium	34 Manubrium of sternum
	23 Left brachiocephalic vein	35 Membranous interventricular septum

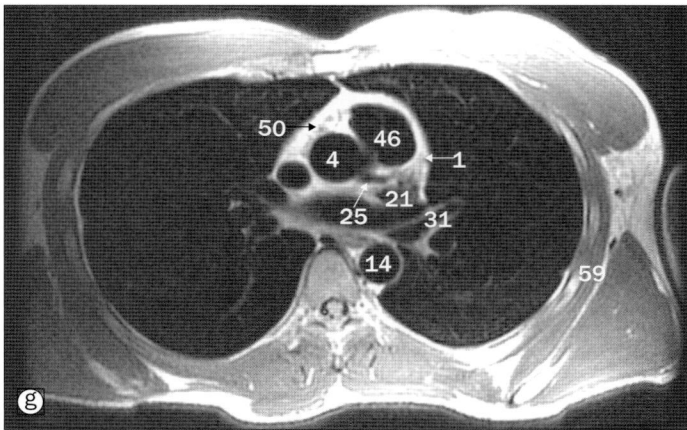

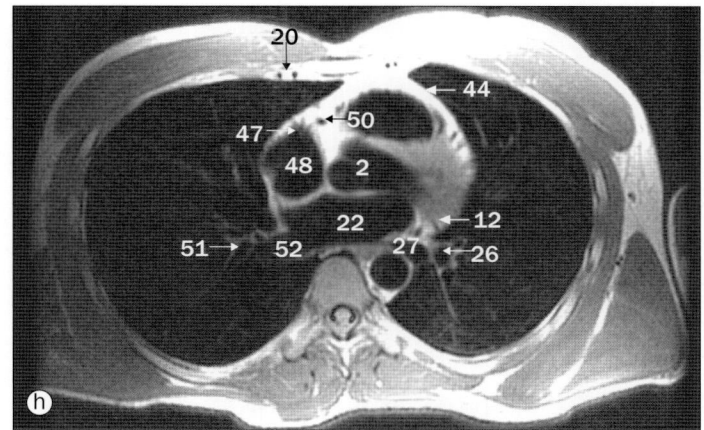

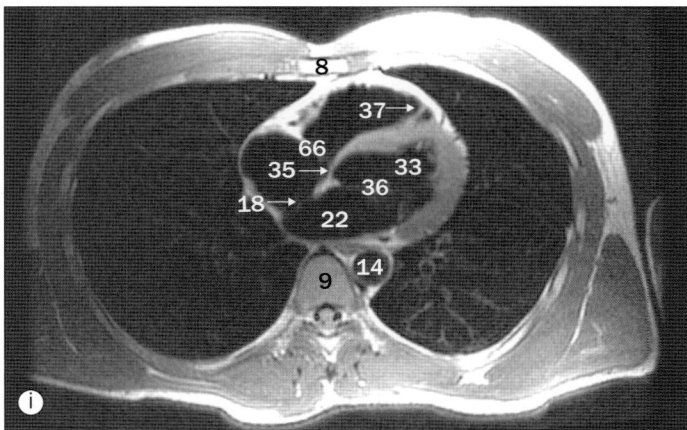

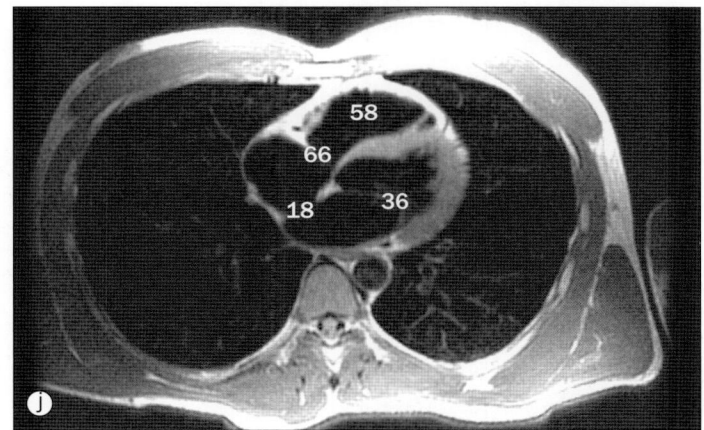

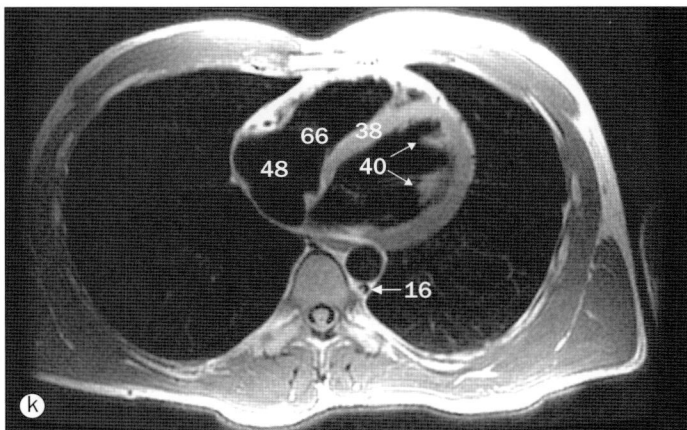

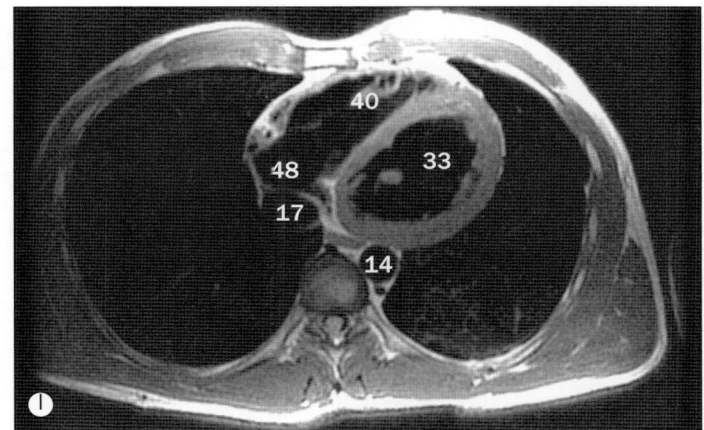

(a)–(l) Chest, axial MR images.

36 Mitral valve	47 Right atrial appendage (auricle)	58 Right ventricular cavity
37 Moderator band	48 Right atrium	59 Serratus anterior muscle
38 Muscular interventricular septum	49 Right brachiocephalic vein	60 Sternoclavicular joint
39 Oesophagus	50 Right coronary artery	61 Subscapularis muscle
40 Papillary muscles	51 Right inferior lobe bronchus	62 Superior lobe branch of
41 Pectoralis major muscle	52 Right inferior pulmonary vein	right pulmonary artery
42 Pectoralis minor muscle	53 Right main bronchus	63 Superior vena cava
43 Pericardial recess	54 Right pulmonary artery	64 Trachea
44 Pericardium	55 Right superior intercostal vein	65 Trapezius muscle
45 Pulmonary trunk	56 Right superior lobe bronchus	66 Tricuspid valve
46 Pulmonary valve	57 Right superior pulmonary vein	

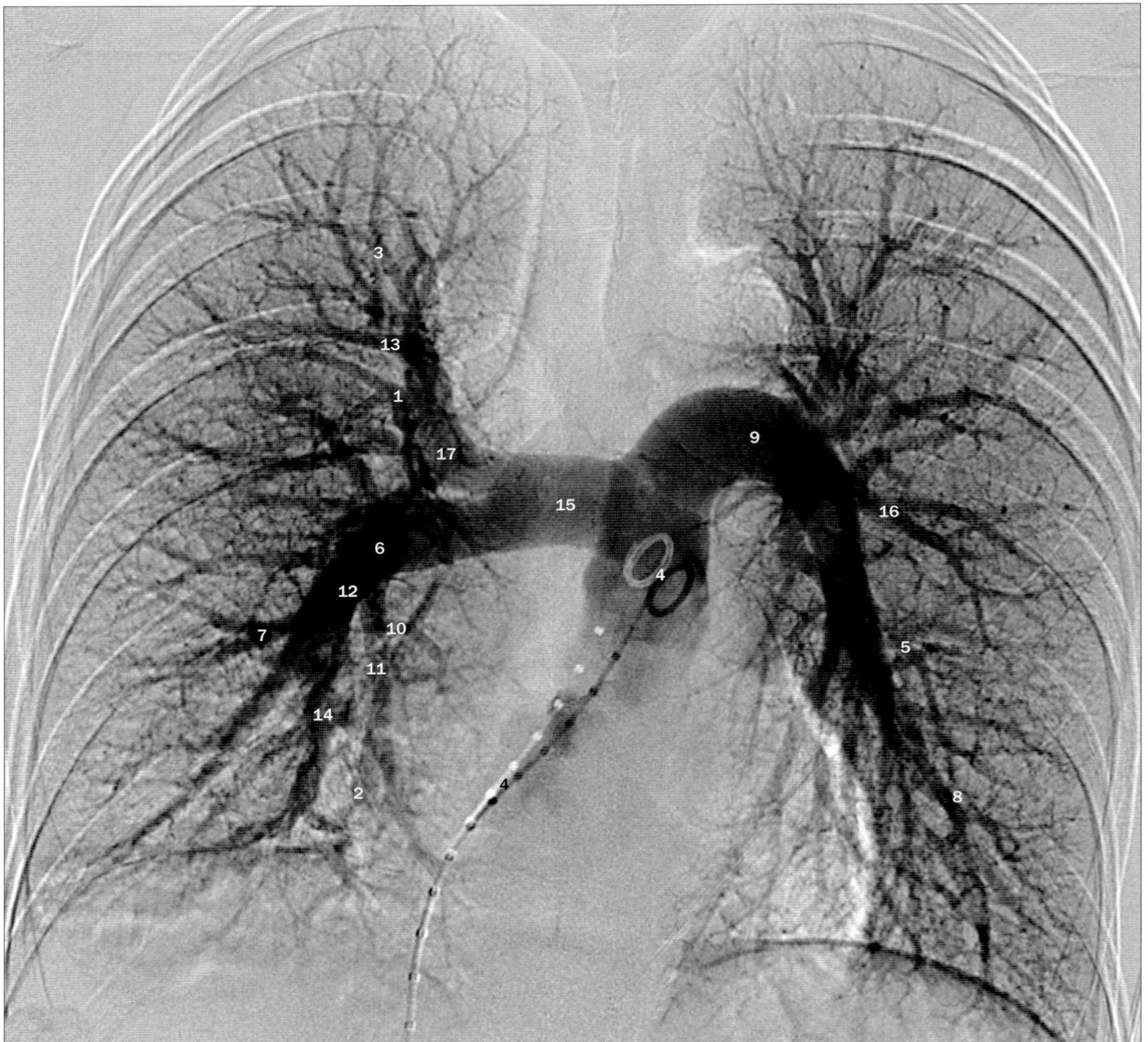

Pulmonary arteriogram, arterial phase.

1 Anterior artery (superior lobe)	**6** Inferior lobe pulmonary artery	**13** Posterior artery (superior lobe)
2 Anterior basal artery	**7** Lateral artery (middle lobe)	**14** Posterior basal artery
3 Apical artery (superior lobe)	**8** Lateral basal artery	**15** Right pulmonary artery
4 Catheter in main pulmonary artery via a femoral vein, inferior vena cava, right atrium and right ventricle	**9** Left pulmonary artery	**16** Superior lingular artery
	10 Medial artery (middle lobe)	**17** Superior lobe pulmonary artery
5 Inferior lingular artery	**11** Medial basal artery	
	12 Middle lobe pulmonary artery	

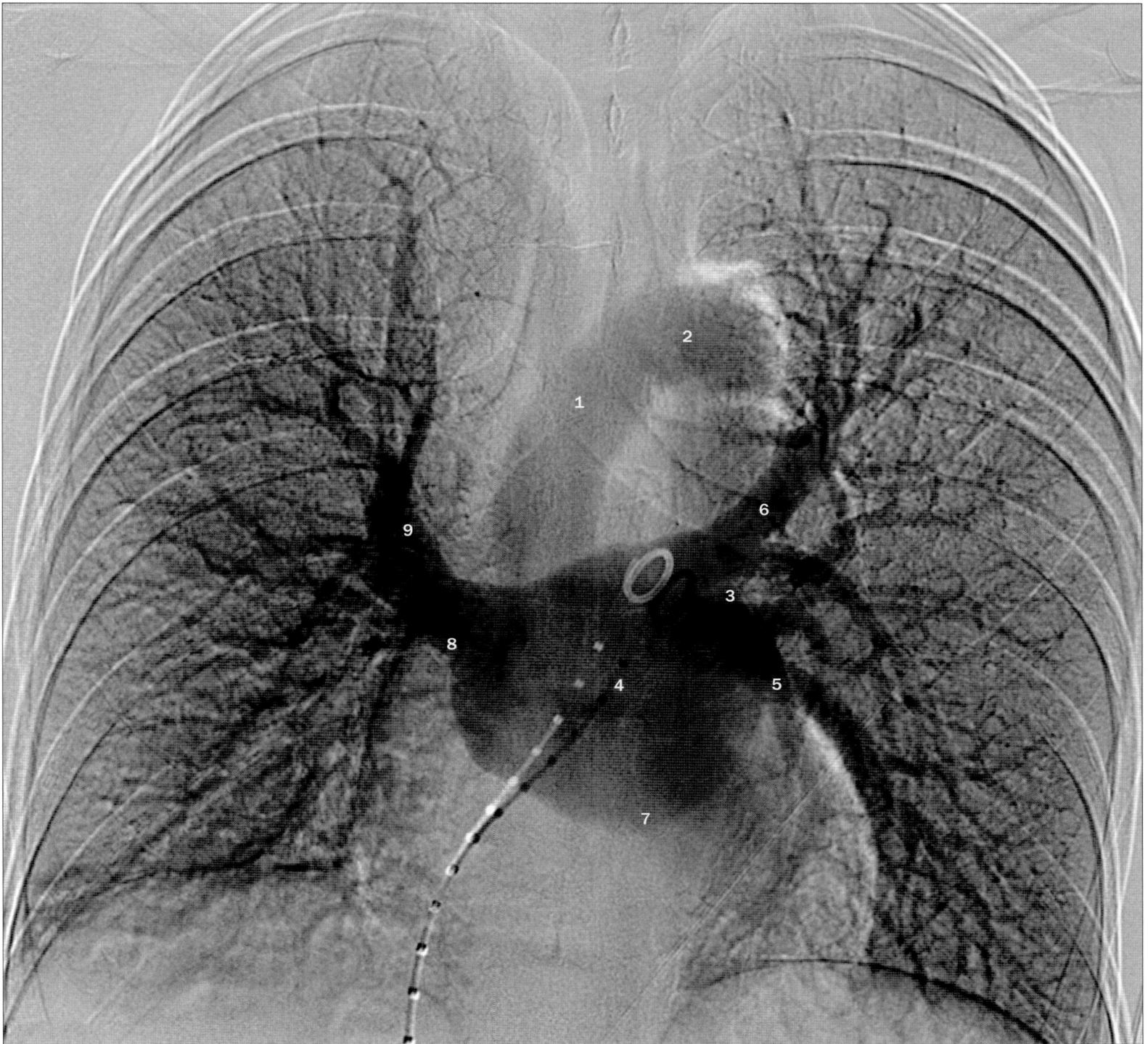

Pulmonary arteriogram, venous phase.

1 Aorta
2 Aortic arch
3 Left atrial appendage (auricle)
4 Left atrium
5 Left inferior pulmonary vein
6 Left superior pulmonary vein
7 Mitral valve
8 Right inferior pulmonary vein
9 Right superior pulmonary vein

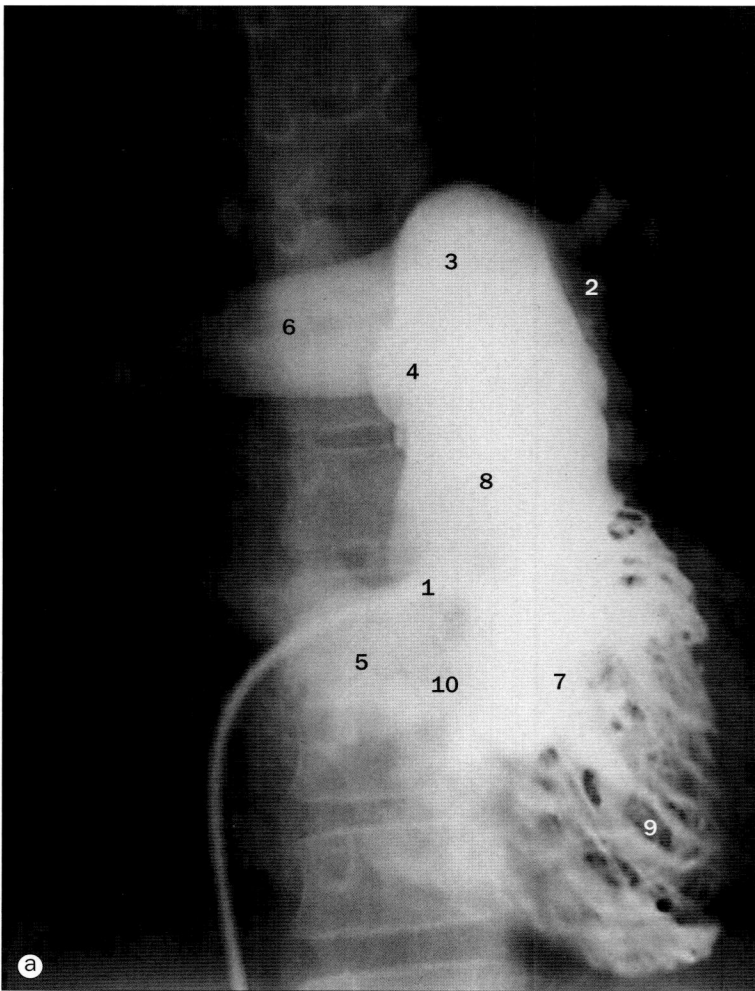

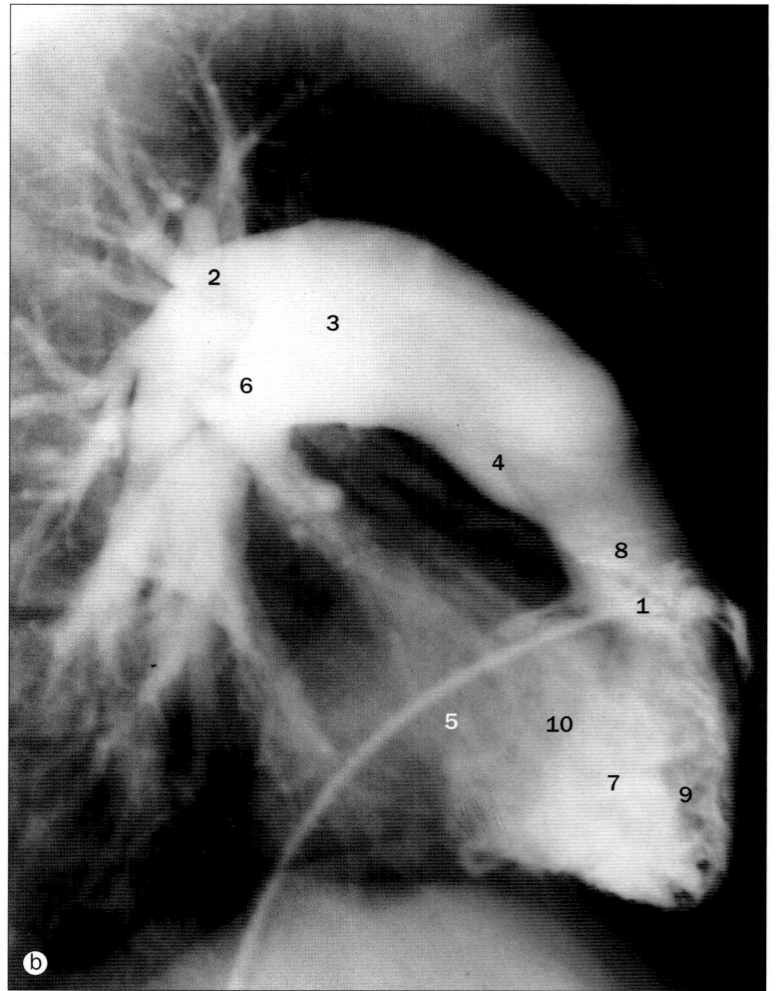

Right ventricular angiograms, (a) anteroposterior projection, (b) lateral projection.

 1 Catheter in right ventricle via inferior vena cava and right atrium
 2 Left main pulmonary artery
 3 Pulmonary artery
 4 Pulmonary valve
 5 Right atrium
 6 Right main pulmonary artery
 7 Right ventricle
 8 Right ventricular outflow tract
 9 Trabeculae of right ventricle
10 Tricuspid valve

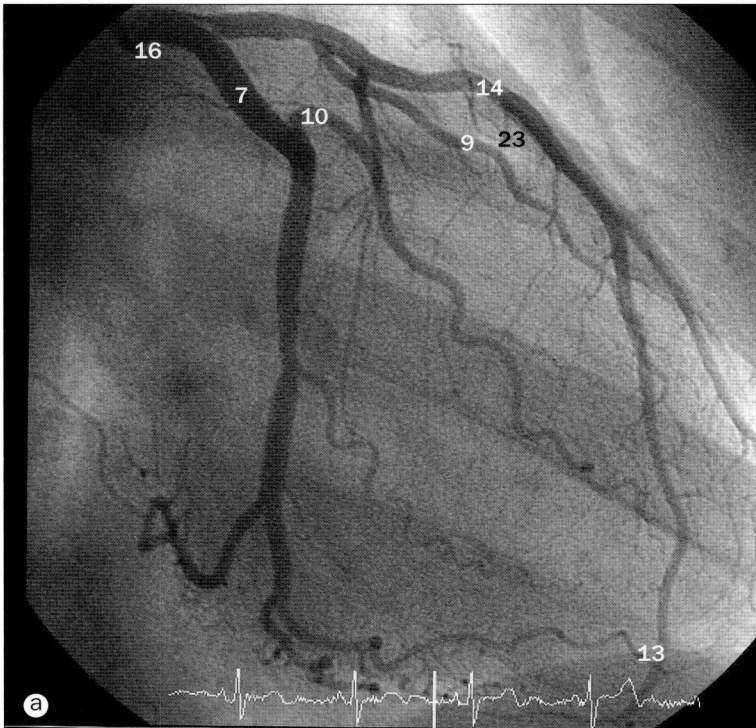

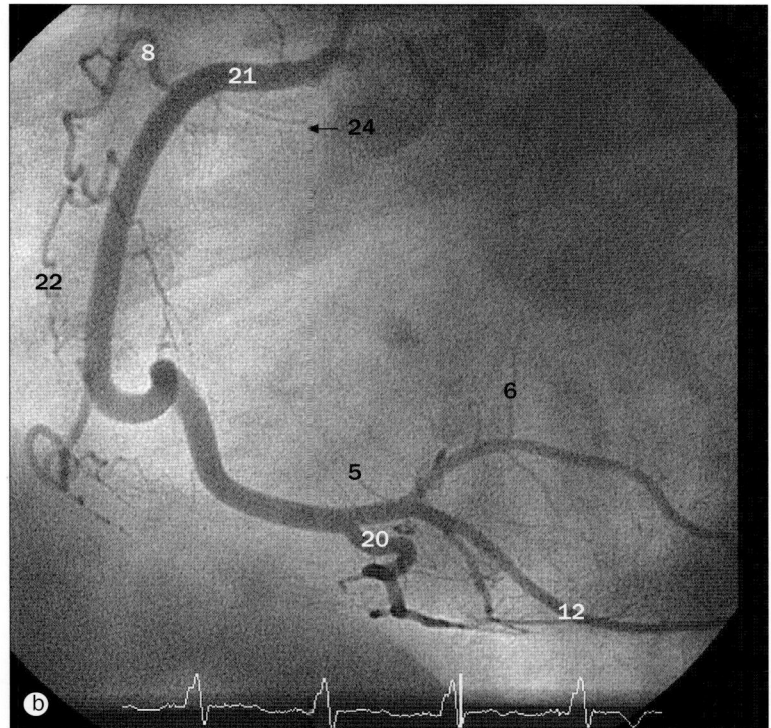

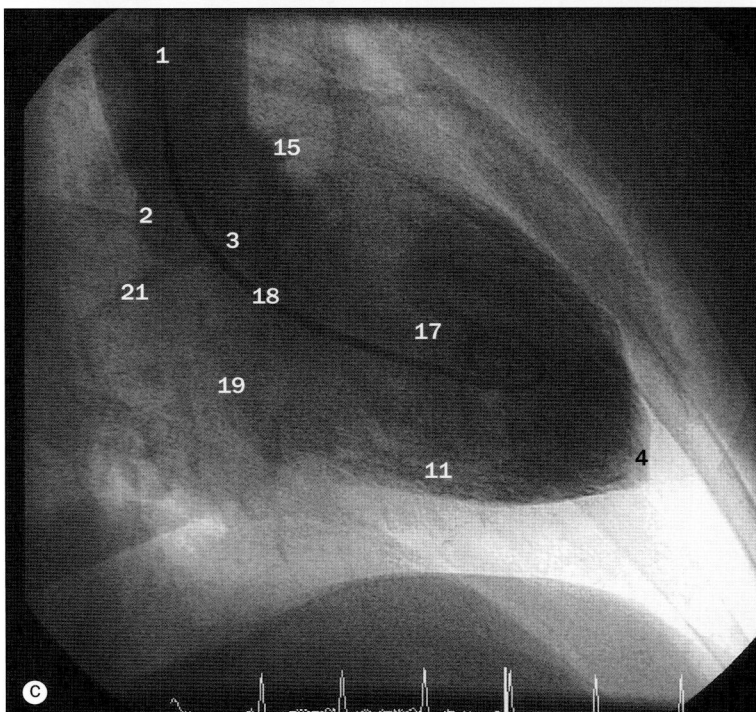

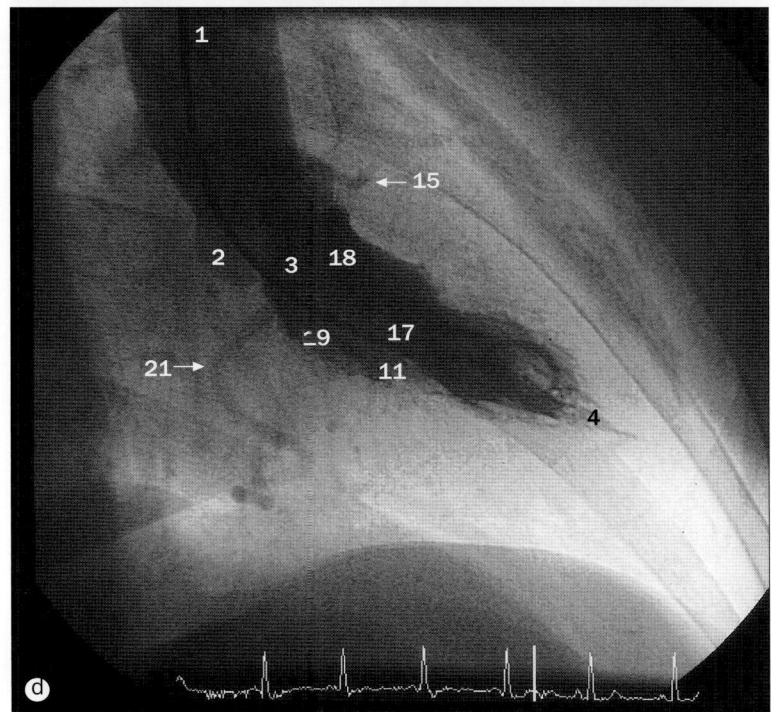

(a) Left coronary arteriogram, (b) right coronary arteriogram, (c) left ventricular angiogram, diastolic phase, (d) left ventricular angiogram, systolic phase.

1 Aorta	**10** First obtuse marginal branch of	**17** Left ventricular cavity
2 Aortic sinus	circumflex artery	**18** Left ventricular outflow tract
3 Aortic valve	**11** Inferior wall of left ventricle	**19** Mitral valve
4 Apex of the left ventricle	**12** Lateral ventricular branch to left ventricle	**20** Posterior interventricular septal artery
5 Atrioventricular nodal artery	**13** Left anterior interventricular artery	(posterior descending artery)
6 Branch to left atrium	curving round apex of heart	**21** Right coronary artery
7 Circumflex artery	**14** Left anterior interventricular branch	**22** Right marginal arteries
8 Conus artery	(left anterior descending)	**23** Septal arteries
9 Diagonal arteries	**15** Left coronary artery	**24** Sinuatrial nodal artery
	16 Left main stem coronary artery	

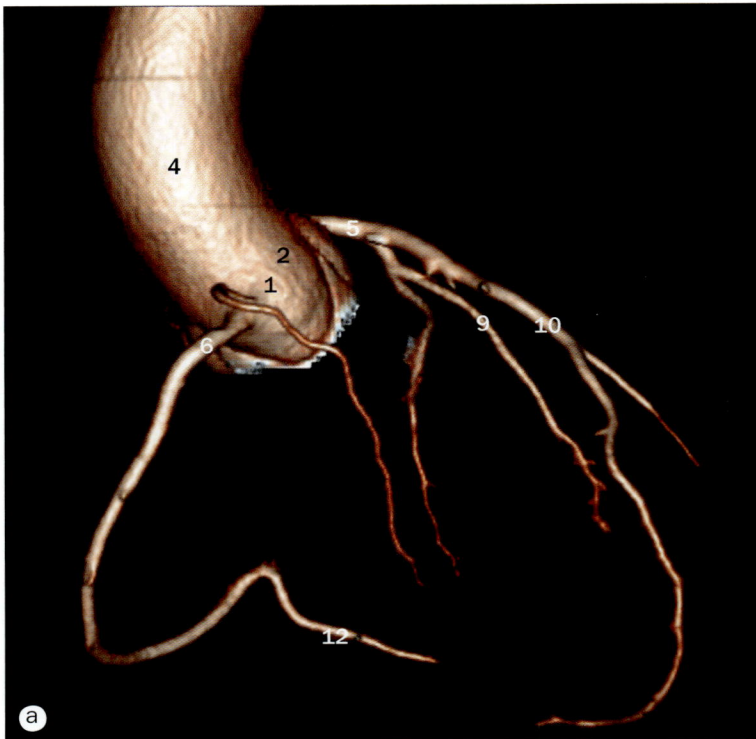

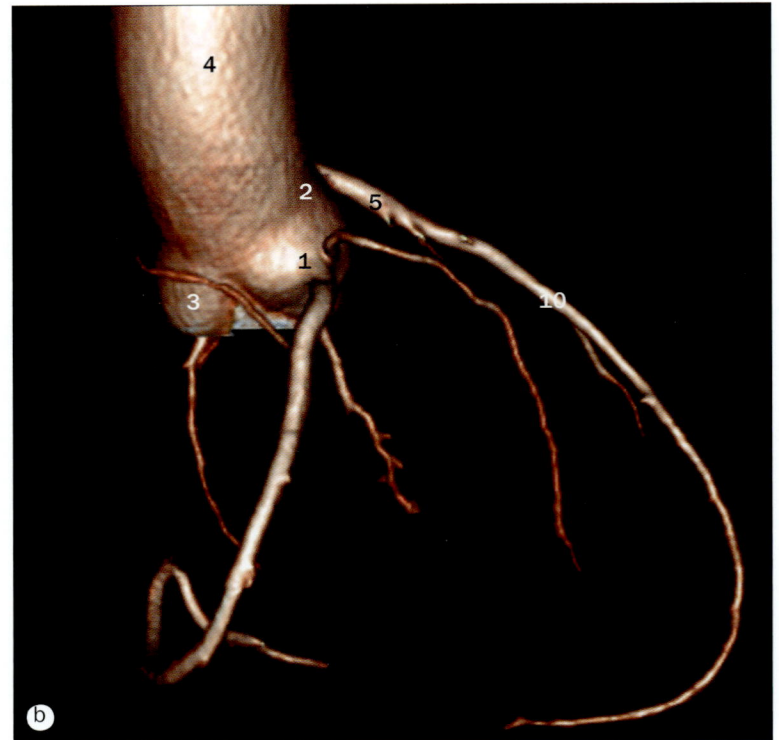

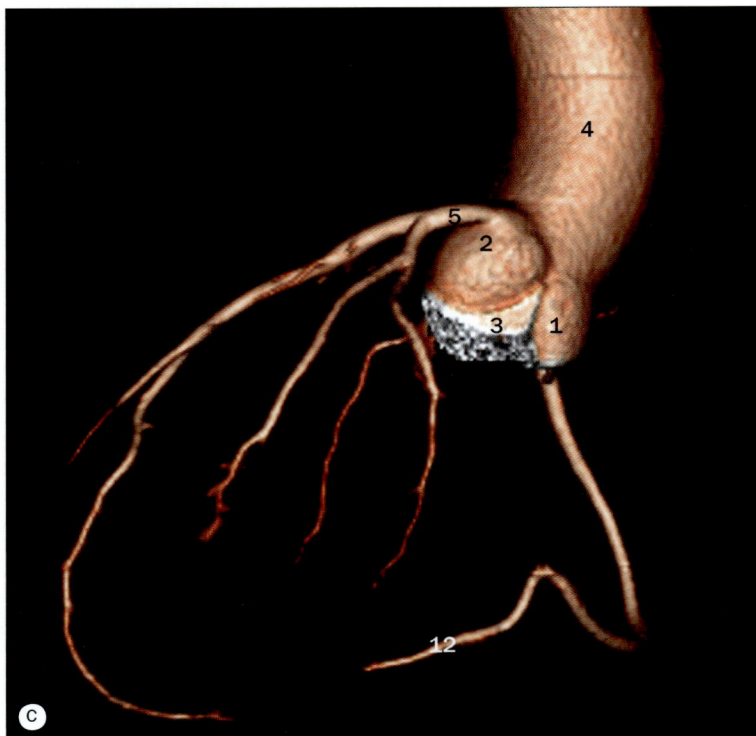

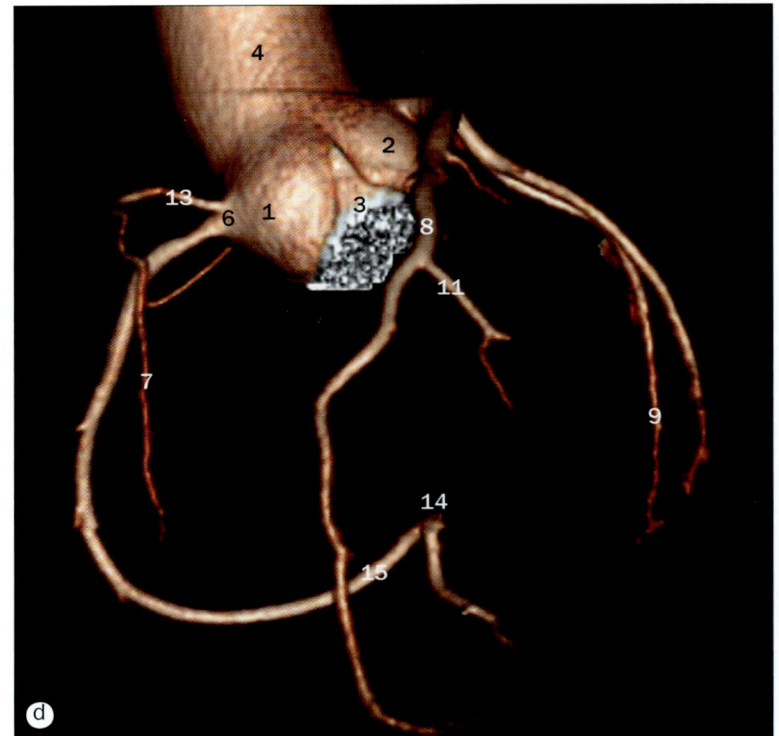

(a)–(d) 3D CT coronary angiograms.

 1 Right coronary sinus
 2 Left coronary sinus
 3 Non coronary sinus
 4 Ascending aorta
 5 Left main coronary artery
 6 Right main coronary artery
 7 Right ventricular branch of right coronary artery
 8 Circumflex artery
 9 Diagonal artery
10 Left anterior descending artery
11 Obtuse marginal artery
12 Marginal artery
13 Right conal artery
14 Atrioventricular nodal artery
15 Posterior interventricular branch, right coronary artery

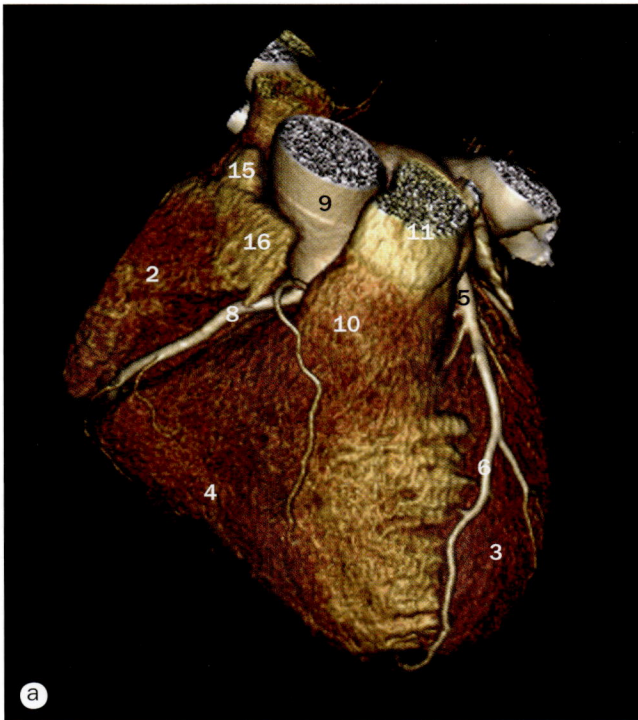

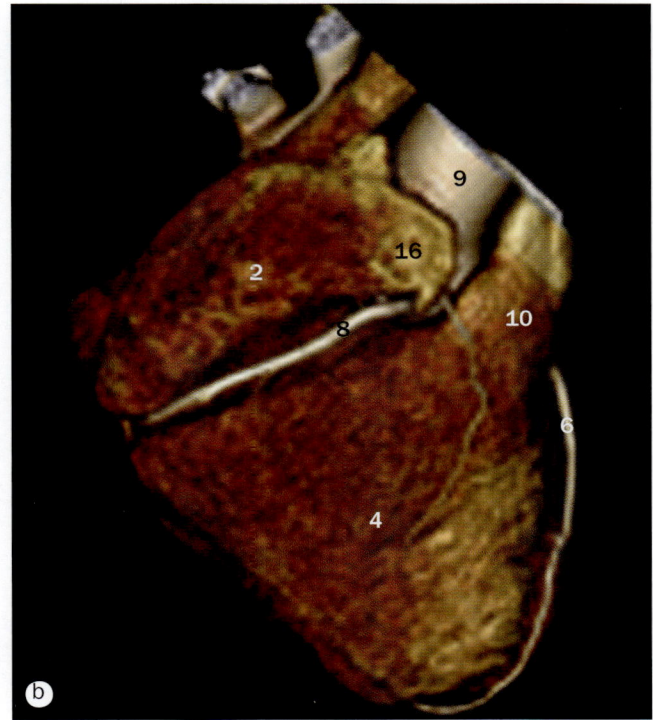

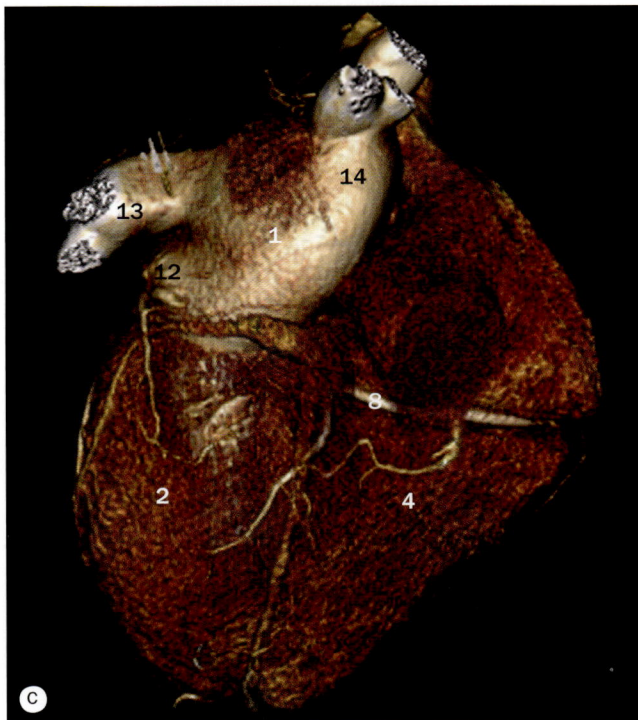

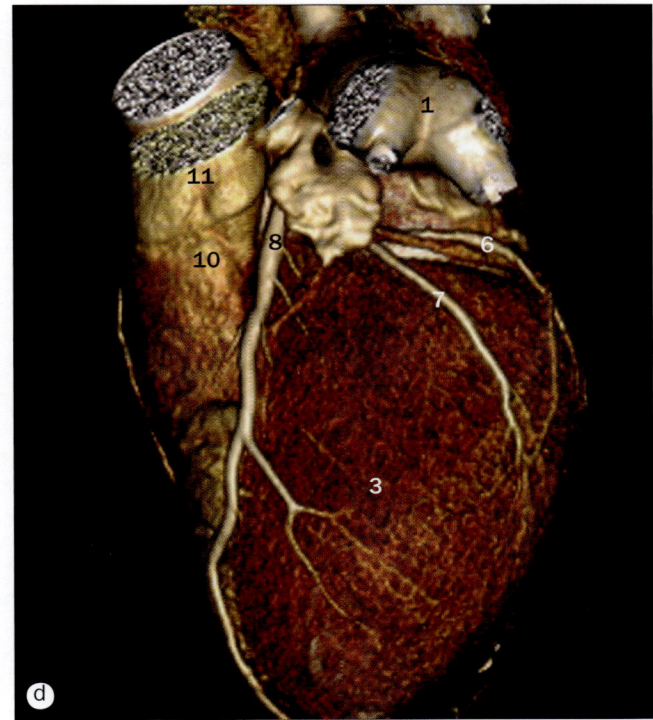

(a)–(d) 3D CT heart reconstructions.

1 Left atrium	7 Circumflex artery	12 Left atrial appendage
2 Right atrium	8 Right coronary artery	13 Right pulmonary veins
3 Left ventricle	9 Aortic root	14 Left pulmonary veins
4 Right ventricle	10 Pulmonary outflow tract	15 Superior vena cava
5 Left main coronary artery	11 Pulmonary artery	16 Right atrial appendage
6 Left anterior descending coronary artery		

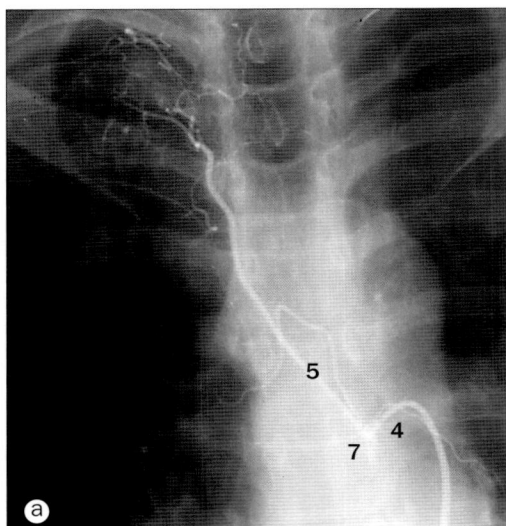

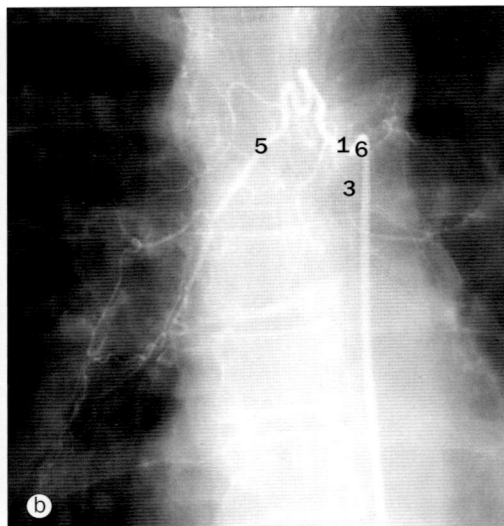

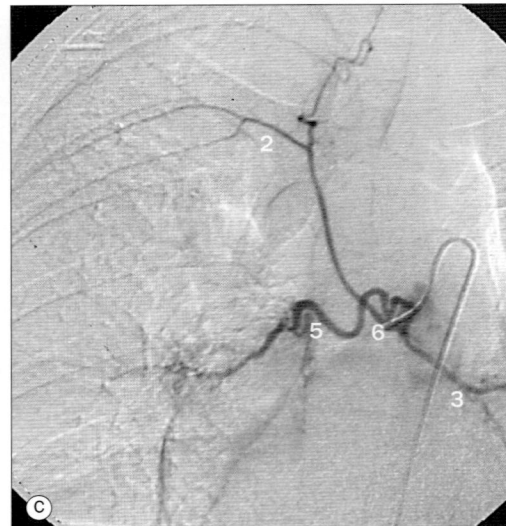

(a)–(c) Right bronchial arteriograms.
There is a great variability in the anatomy of the bronchial arteries, but the majority originate from the descending thoracic aorta, above the level of the left main stem bronchus between the upper border of the fifth thoracic vertebra and the lower border of the sixth thoracic vertebra. The number of bronchial arteries on each side may vary between one and four. Usually, there is one vessel to the right lung and two to the left. Accessory bronchial arteries may arise from the brachiocephalic artery and subclavian arteries, or from other branches such as the internal thoracic, pericardiophrenic and oesophageal arteries. In many cases the right bronchial artery arises from an intercostobronchial trunk, but in this example the trunk is very short and divides almost immediately into a right bronchial artery, which is directed towards the hilum, and the first right aortic intercostal artery. Reflux filling of the left bronchial artery is seen.
A second larger bronchial artery which has been catheterised **(b)** has a common trunk arising from the front of the aorta, giving rise to a right and left bronchial artery.

1 Common bronchial trunk
2 Intercostal artery
3 Left bronchial branches
4 Reflux filling of left bronchial artery
5 Right bronchial artery
6 Tip of catheter in common bronchial arterial trunk
7 Tip of catheter in intercostobronchial trunk

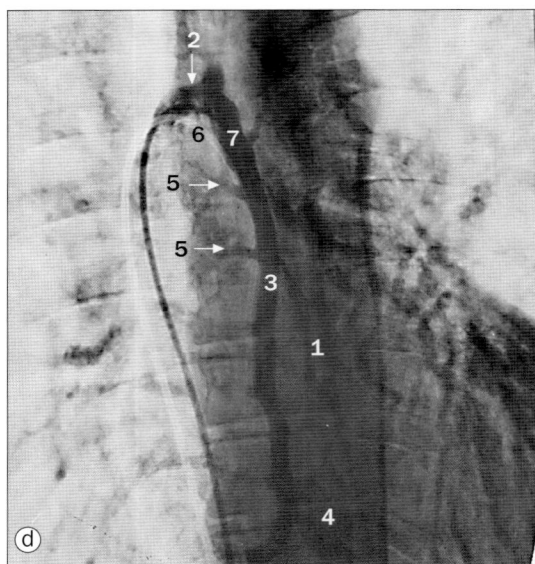

(d) Azygos venogram.
In the thorax the vertebral veins drain into intercostal veins, while in the lumbar region the lumbar veins drain into the ascending lumbar veins. The right ascending lumbar vein becomes the azygos vein on entering the thorax, and the left ascending lumbar vein becomes the hemi-azygos vein. At the level of the fourth thoracic vertebra, the azygos vein turns anteriorly (the arch of the azygos) to enter the superior vena cava. The hemi-azygos vein crosses to join the azygos vein at the level of the eighth or ninth thoracic vertebral body. The accessory hemi-azygos vein is continuous with the hemi-azygos vein inferiorly and the left superior intercostal vein superiorly.

1 Accessory hemi-azygos vein
2 Azygos arch
3 Azygos vein
4 Hemi-azygos vein
5 Intercostal veins
6 Subtraction artefact caused by cardiac and catheter movement
7 Tip of catheter introduced via femoral vein into superior vena cava and azygos vein

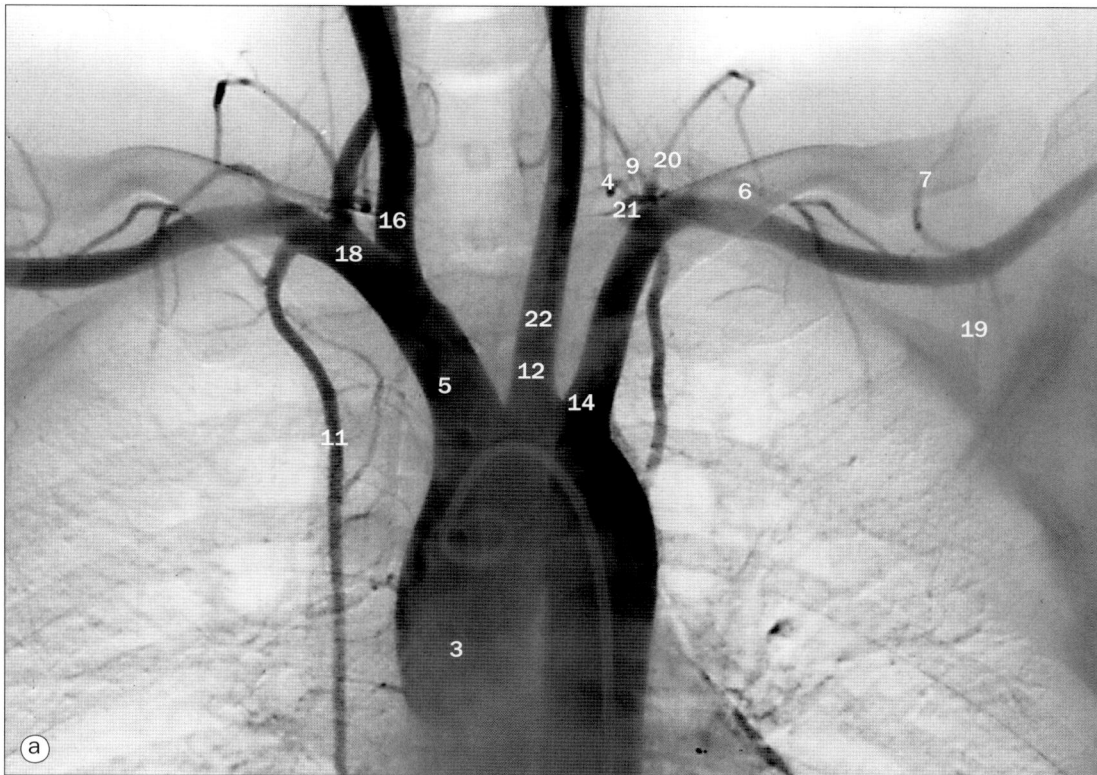

(a) Subtracted arch aortogram, anteroposterior image.
The vertebral artery (22) has a separate origin off the arch, projected over the left common carotid artery in this view. This is a normal variant.

(b) Subtracted arch aortogram, left anterior oblique image.
The origins of the supra-aortic branches are best shown by left anterior oblique projection, so that the origins of the vessels are not superimposed. There are many congenital variations in the way in which the major vessels arise from the aortic arch, but the most common is shown here.

(c) Left ventricular angiogram.

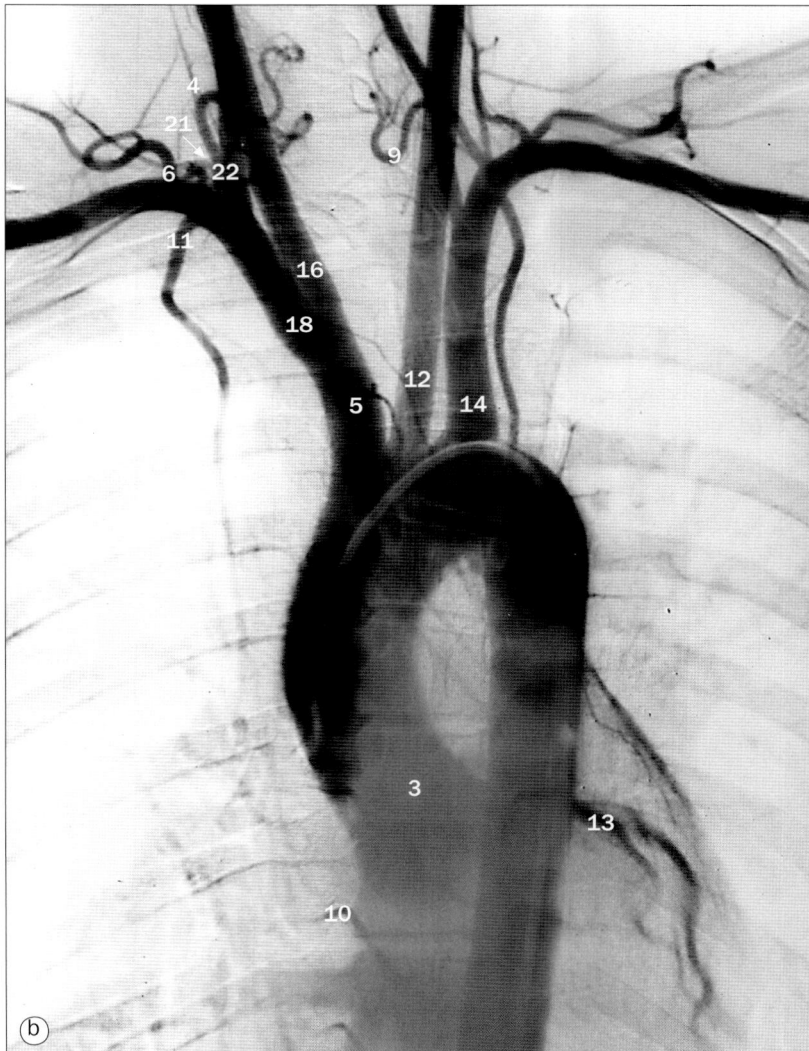

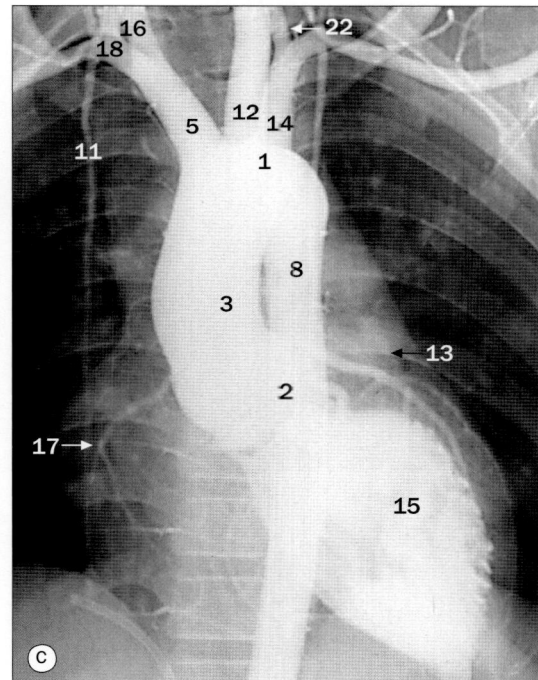

1 Aortic arch	12	Left common carotid artery
2 Aortic valve	13	Left coronary artery
3 Ascending aorta	14	Left subclavian artery
4 Ascending cervical artery	15	Left ventricle
5 Brachiocephalic trunk	16	Right common carotid artery
6 Costocervical trunk	17	Right coronary artery
7 Deltoid branch of thoraco-acromial artery	18	Right subclavian artery
8 Descending aorta	19	Superior thoracic artery
9 Inferior thyroid artery	20	Suprascapular artery
10 Intercostal artery	21	Thyrocervical trunk
11 Internal thoracic artery	22	Vertebral artery

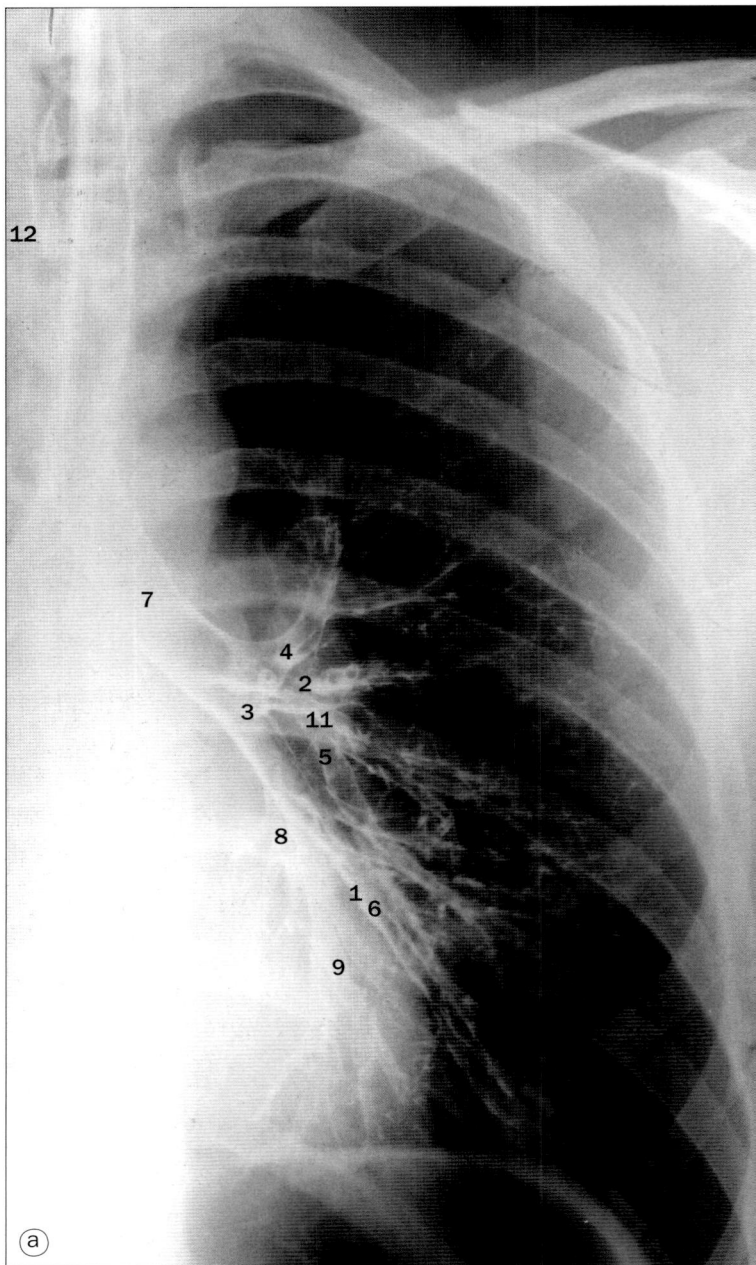

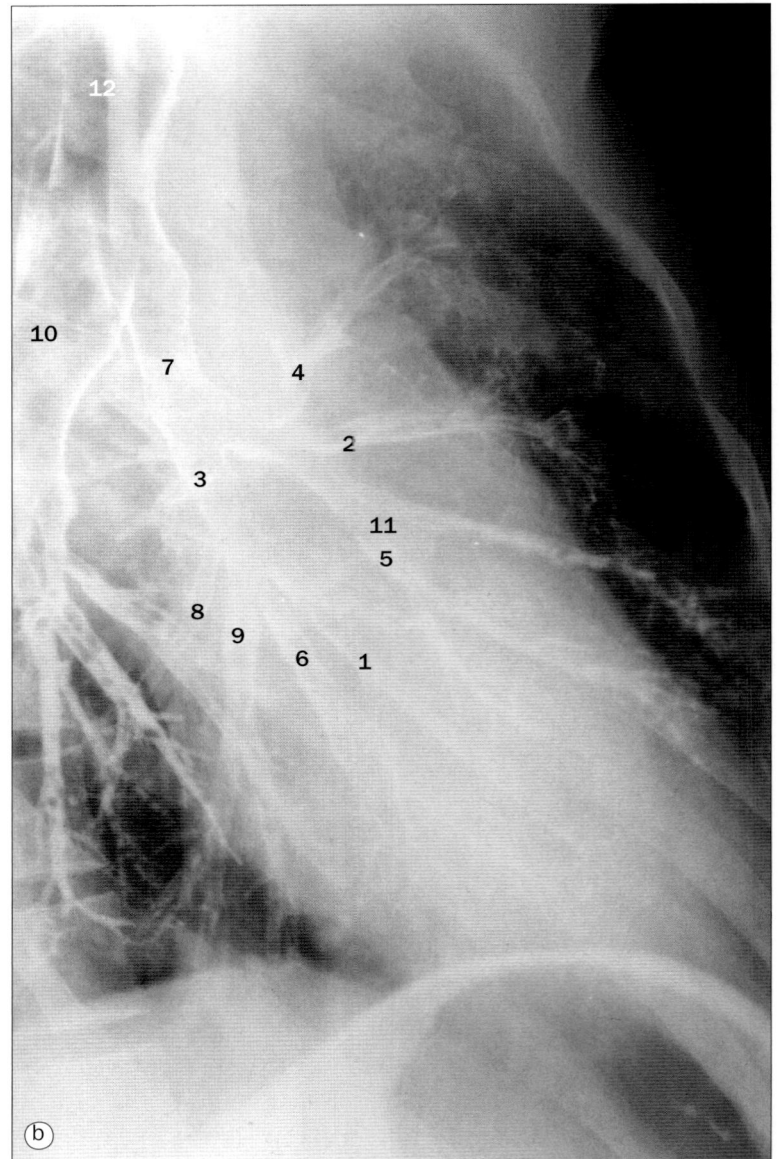

Left lung bronchogram, (a) postero-anterior image, (b) oblique projection.

1 Anterior basal segmental bronchus
2 Anterior segmental bronchus
3 Apical (superior) segmental bronchus
4 Apicoposterior segmental bronchus
5 Inferior lingular segmental bronchus
6 Lateral basal segmental bronchus
7 Left main bronchus
8 Medial basal segmental bronchus
9 Posterior basal segmental bronchus
10 Right main bronchus
11 Superior lingular segmental bronchus
12 Trachea

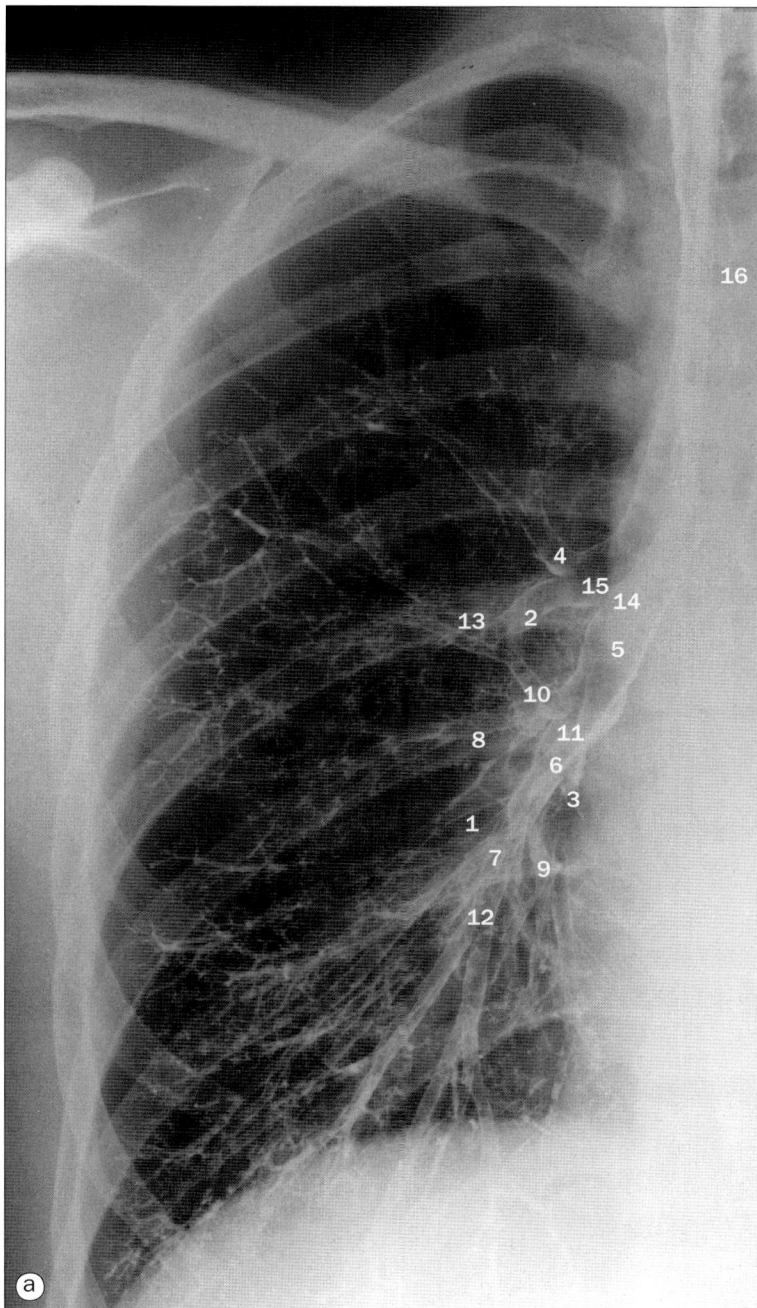

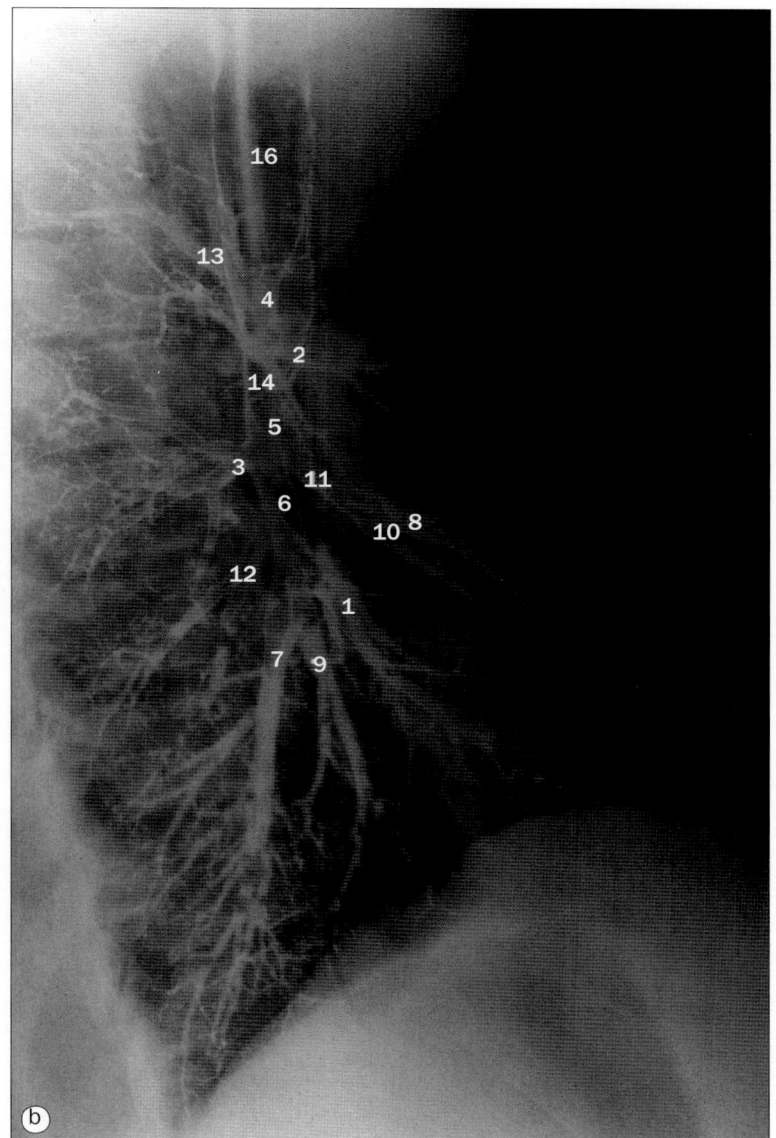

Right lung bronchogram, (a) postero-anterior projection, (b) lateral projection.

1 Anterior basal segmental bronchus	9 Medial basal segmental bronchus
2 Anterior segmental bronchus	10 Medial segmental bronchus of middle lobe
3 Apical (superior) segmental bronchus	11 Middle lobe bronchus
4 Apical segmental bronchus	12 Posterior basal segmental bronchus
5 Bronchus intermedius	13 Posterior segmental bronchus
6 Inferior lobe bronchus	14 Right main bronchus
7 Lateral basal segmental bronchus	15 Right superior lobe bronchus
8 Lateral segmental bronchus of middle lobe	16 Trachea

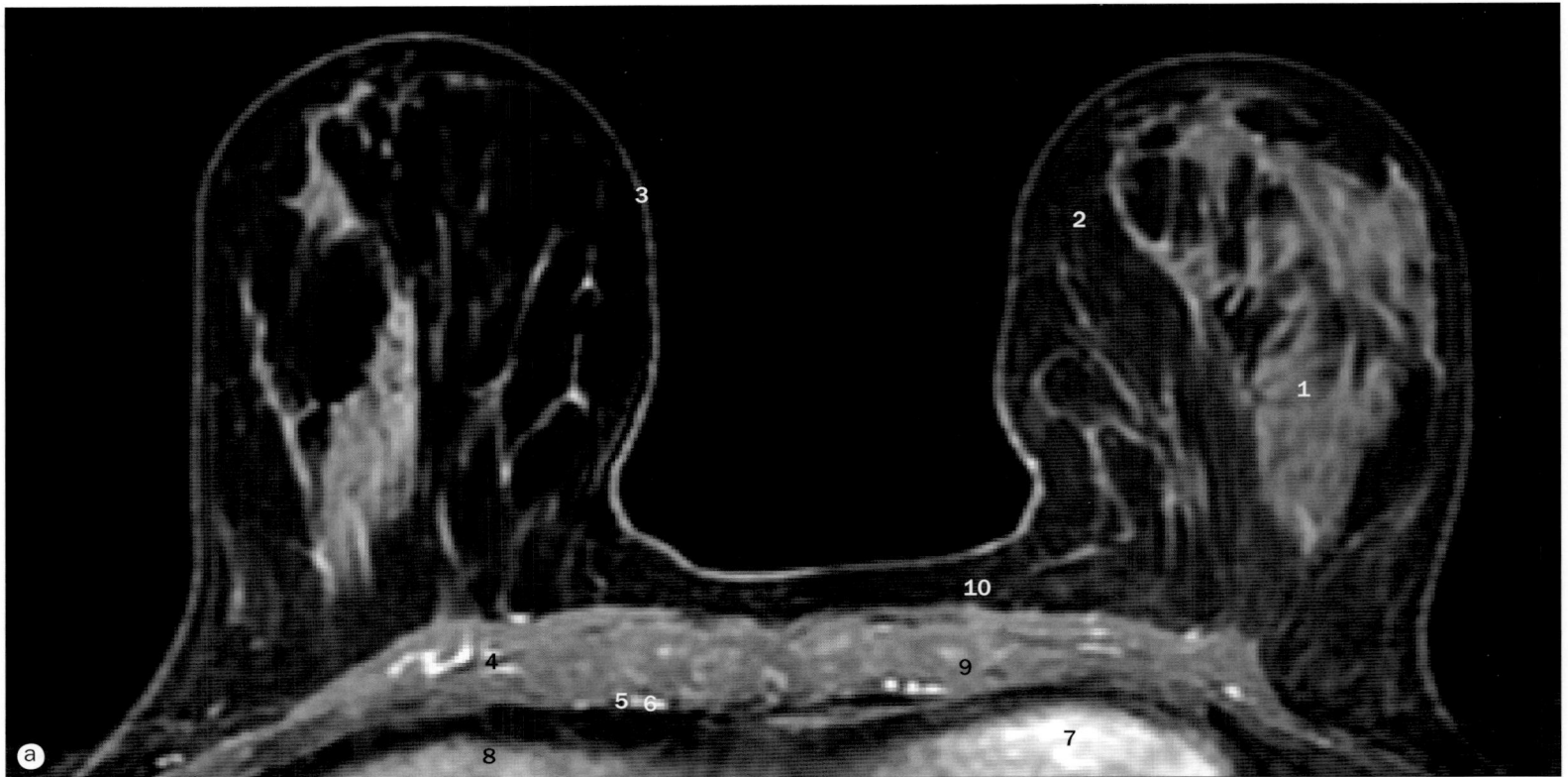

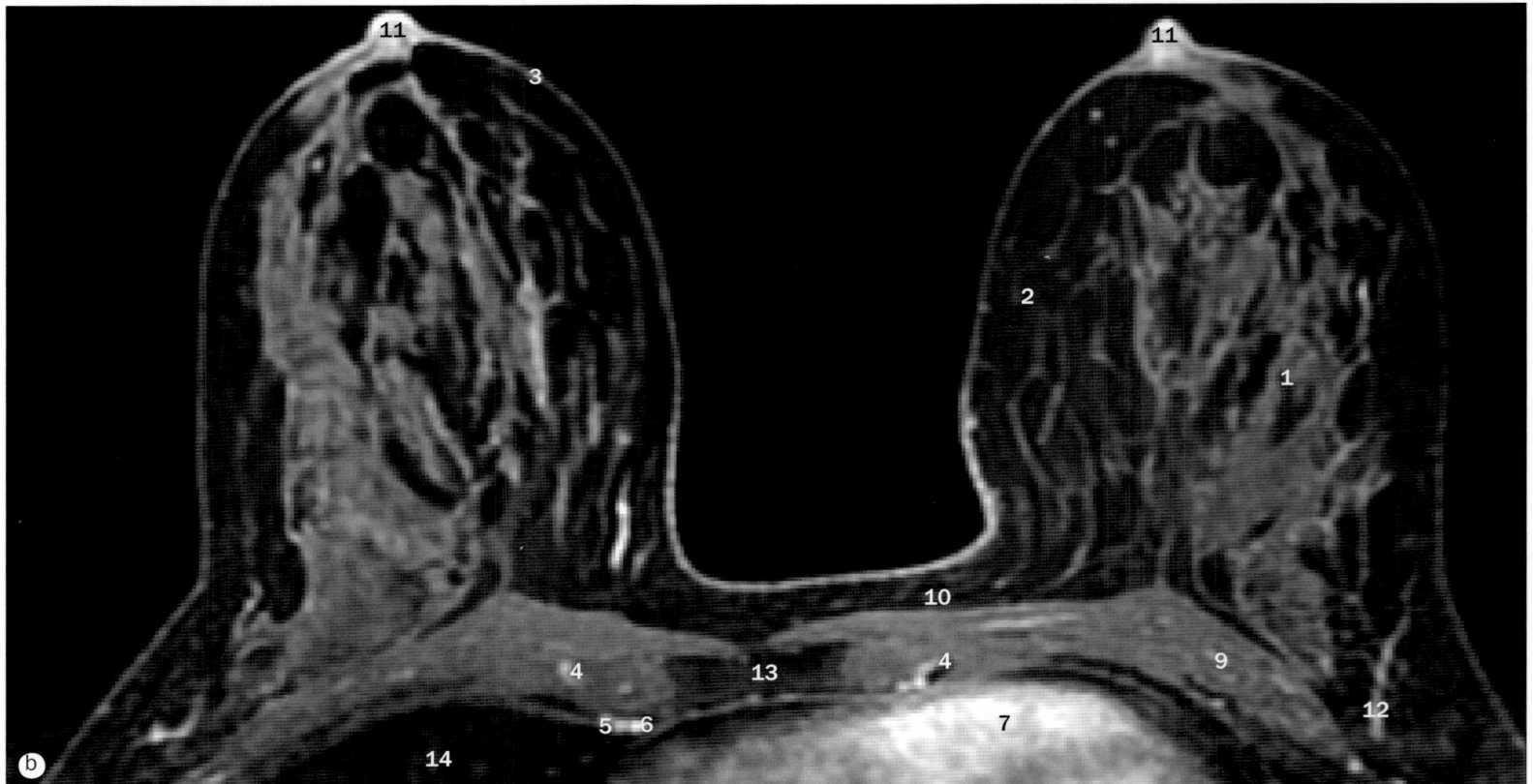

Mammograms, MR images.

1 Fibroglandular tissue (of the right breast)	6 Internal mammary artery	12 Intramammary branches of lateral thoracic artery
2 Adipose tissue of the breast	7 Heart	13 Sternum
3 Skin	8 Liver	14 Middle lobe of the right lung
4 Anterior perforating branch of the internal mammary artery	9 Pectoralis major muscle	
5 Internal mammary vein	10 Anterior pectoralis fascia	
	11 Nipple/areolar complex	

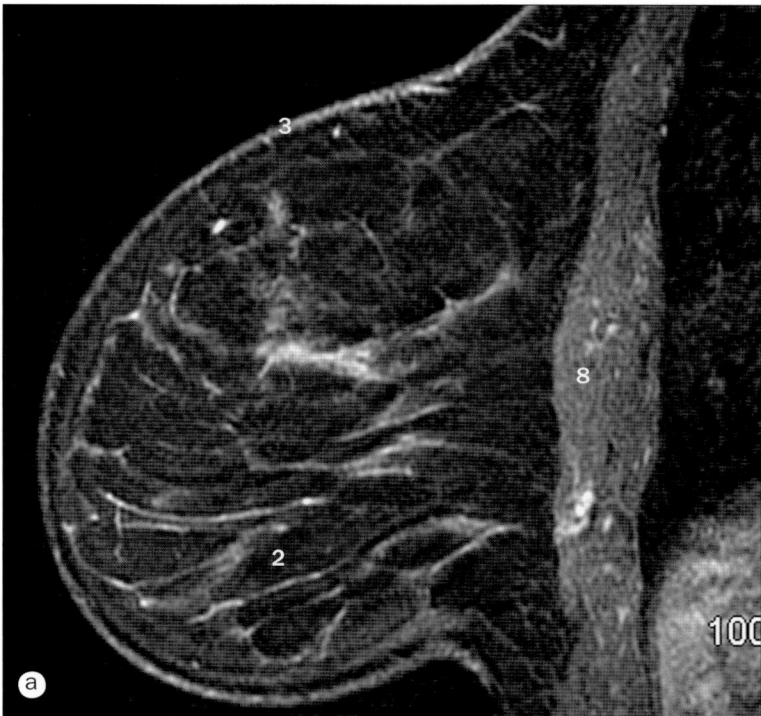

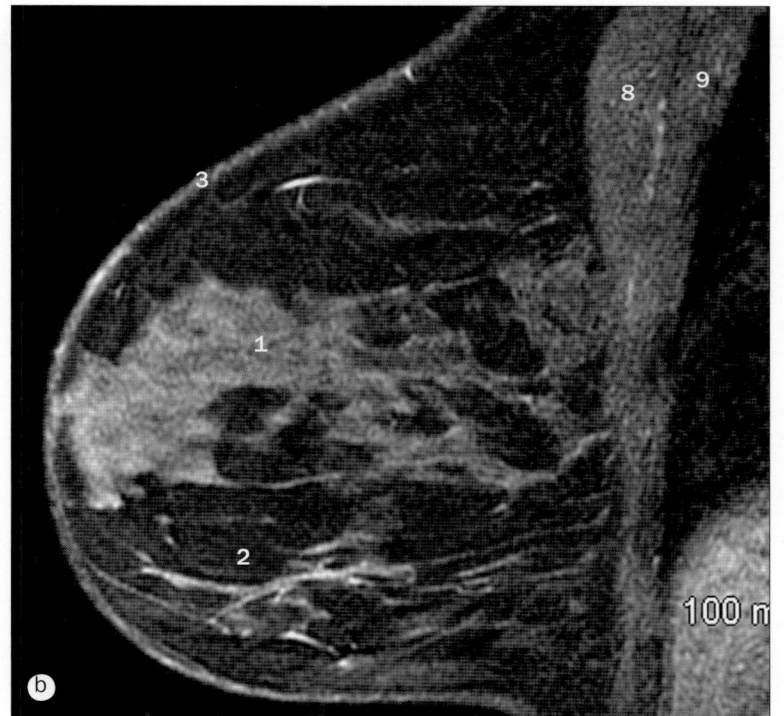

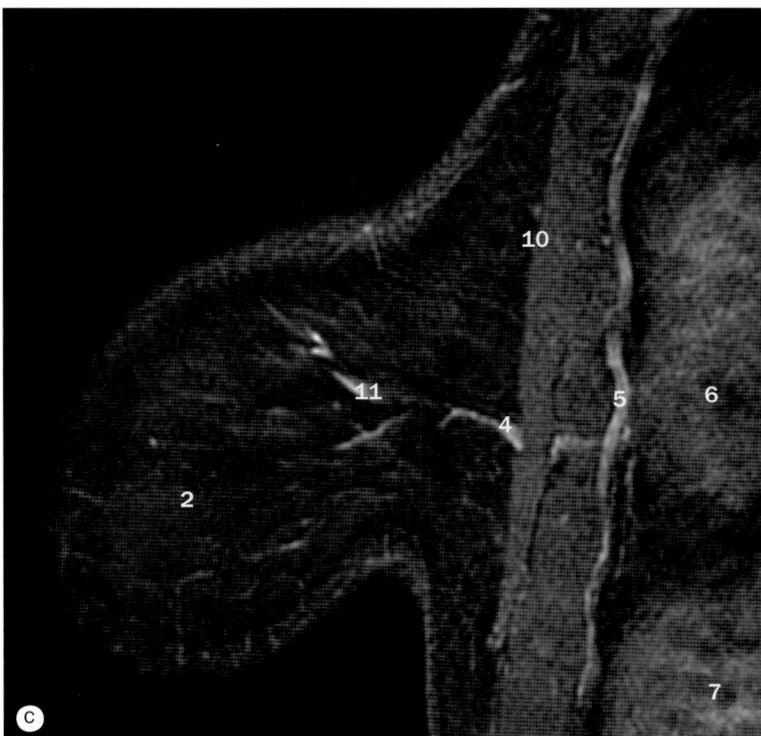

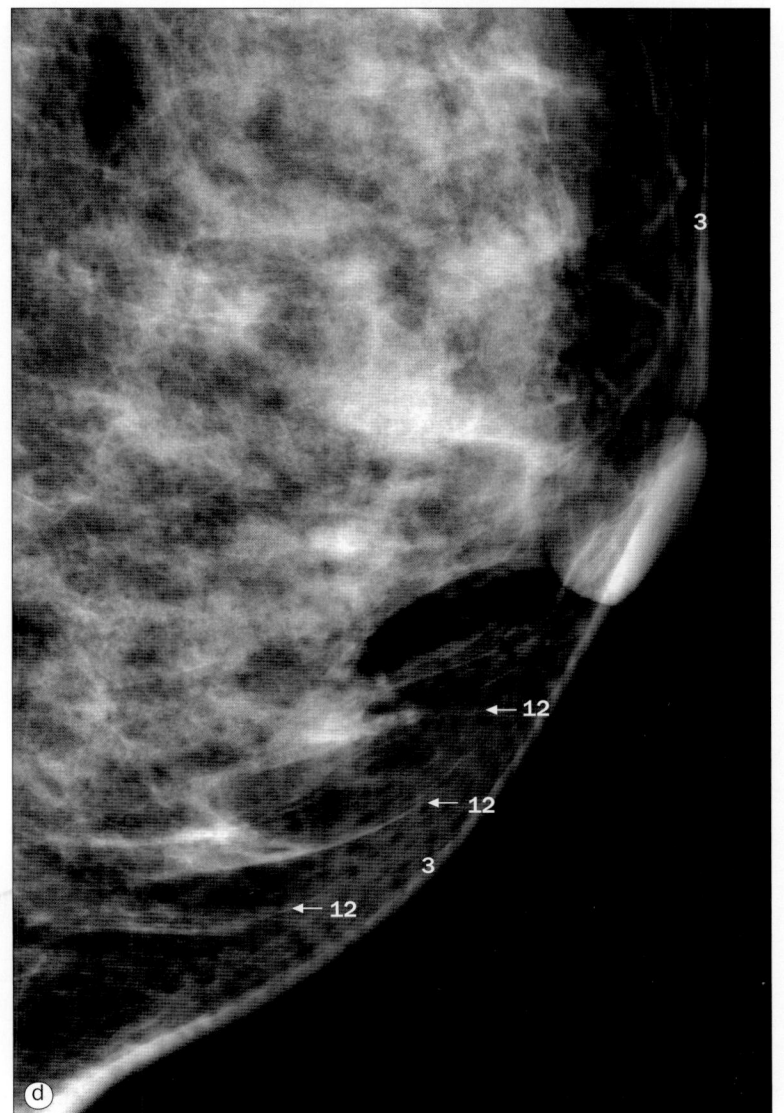

Mammograms, (a)–(c) MR images, (d) mammographic X-ray image.

1 Fibroglandular tissue (of the right breast)
2 Adipose tissue of the breast
3 Skin
4 Anterior perforating branch of the internal mammary artery
5 Internal mammary artery
6 Heart
7 Liver
8 Pectoralis major muscle
9 Pectoralis minor muscle
10 Anterior pectoralis fascia
11 Intramammary vessels
12 Cooper's ligaments

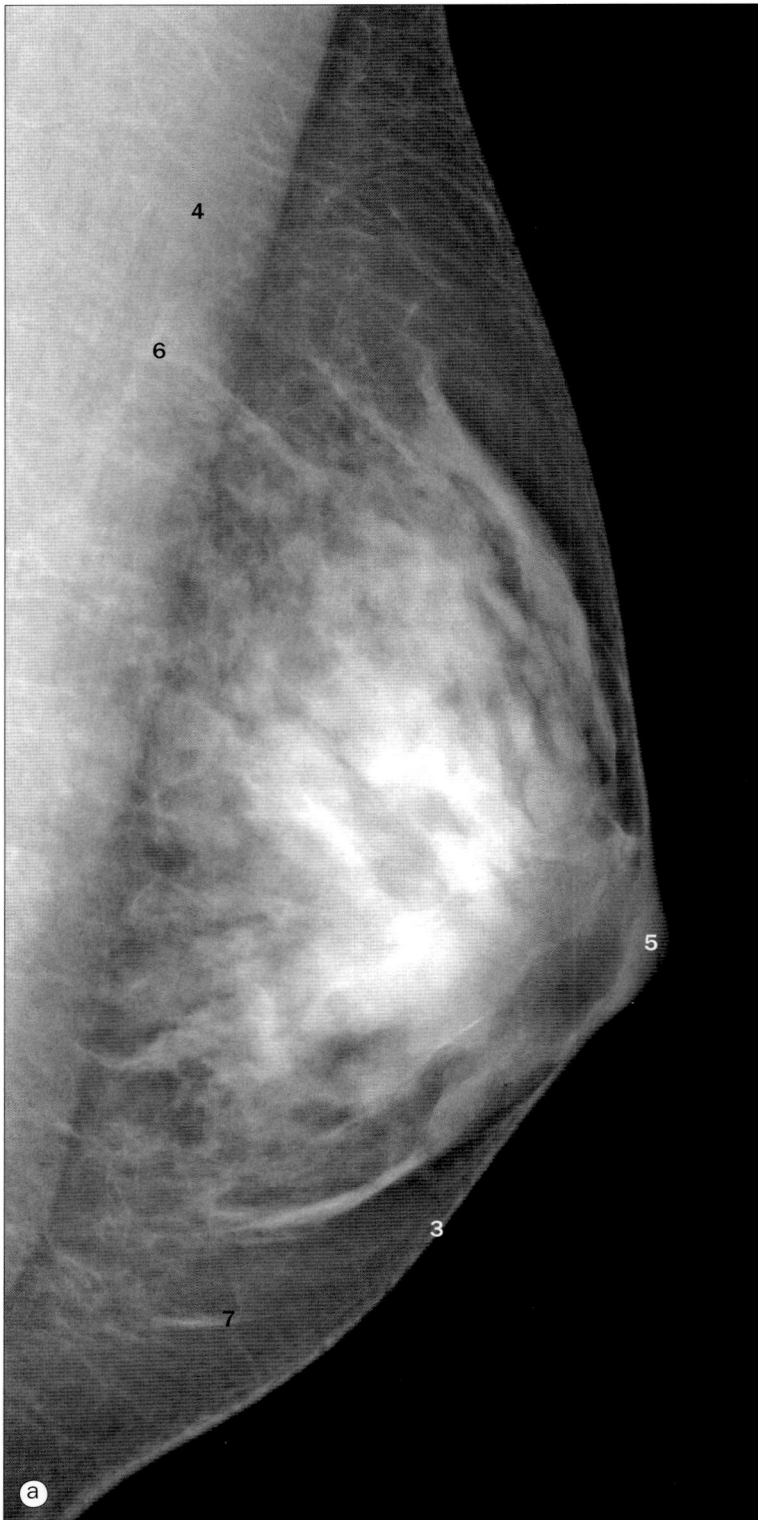

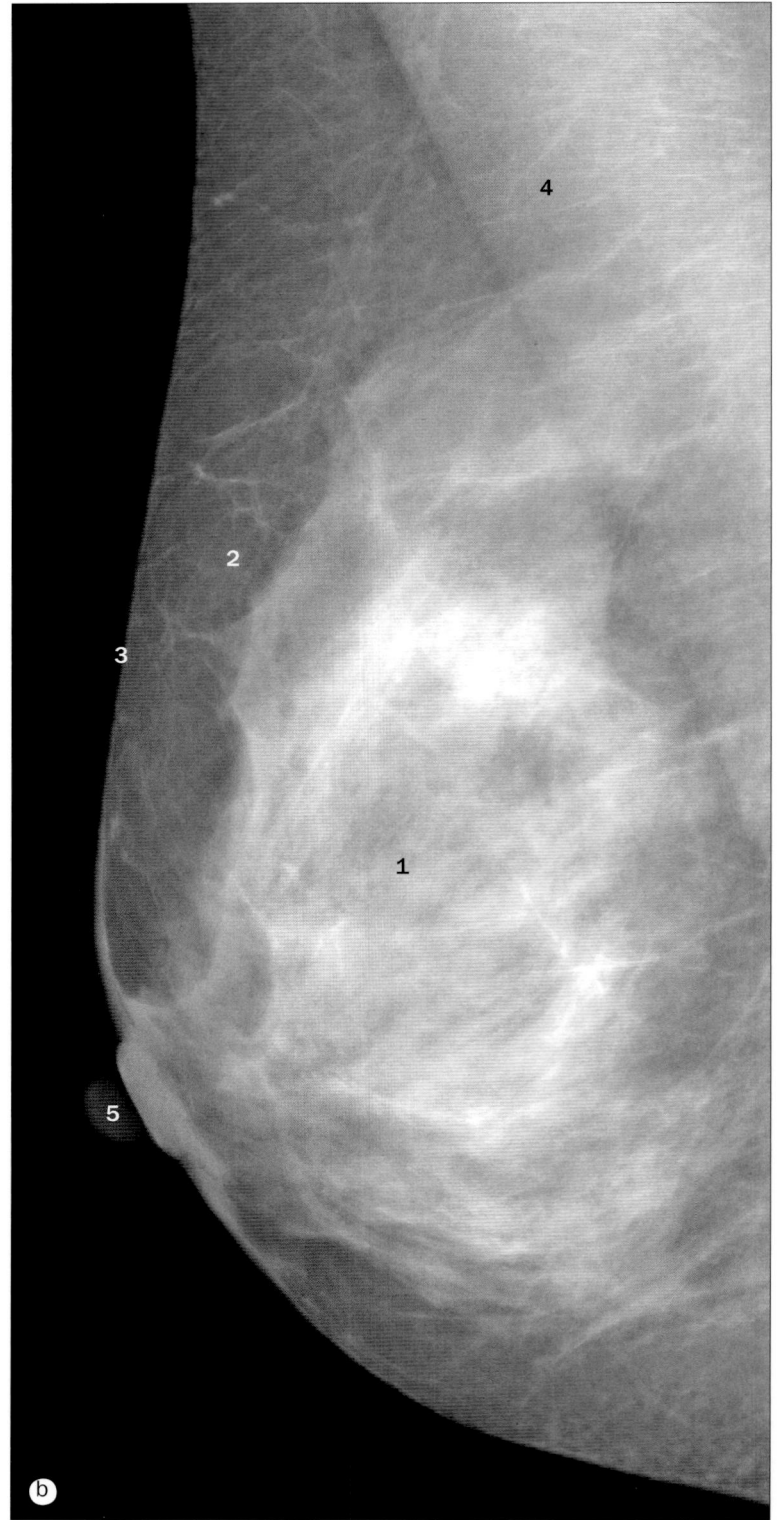

Mammograms.

1 Fibroglandular tissue (of the right breast)
2 Adipose tissue of the breast
3 Skin
4 Pectoralis major muscle
5 Nipple–areolar complex
6 Vessel
7 Cooper's ligament

5 Abdomen and pelvis – Cross-sectional

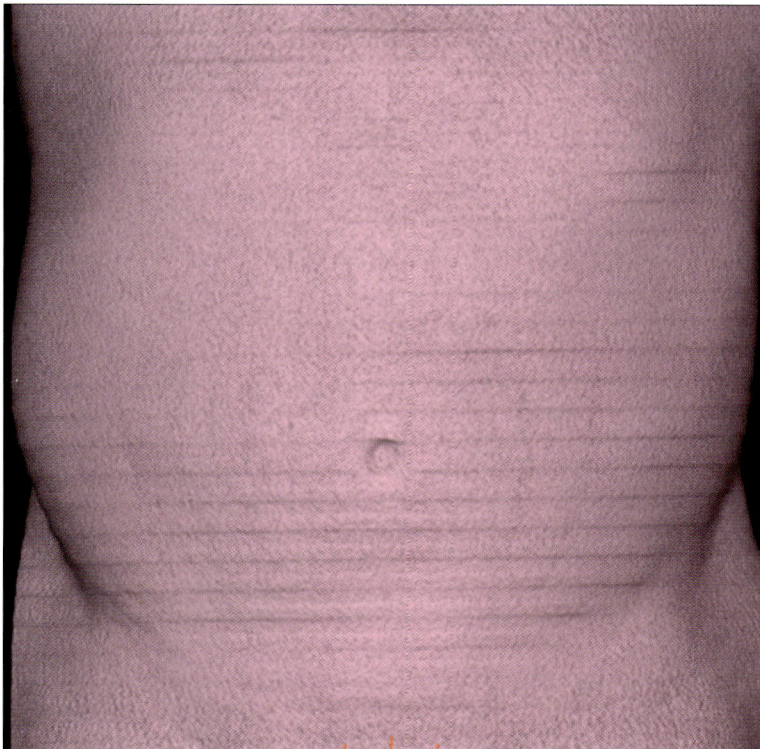

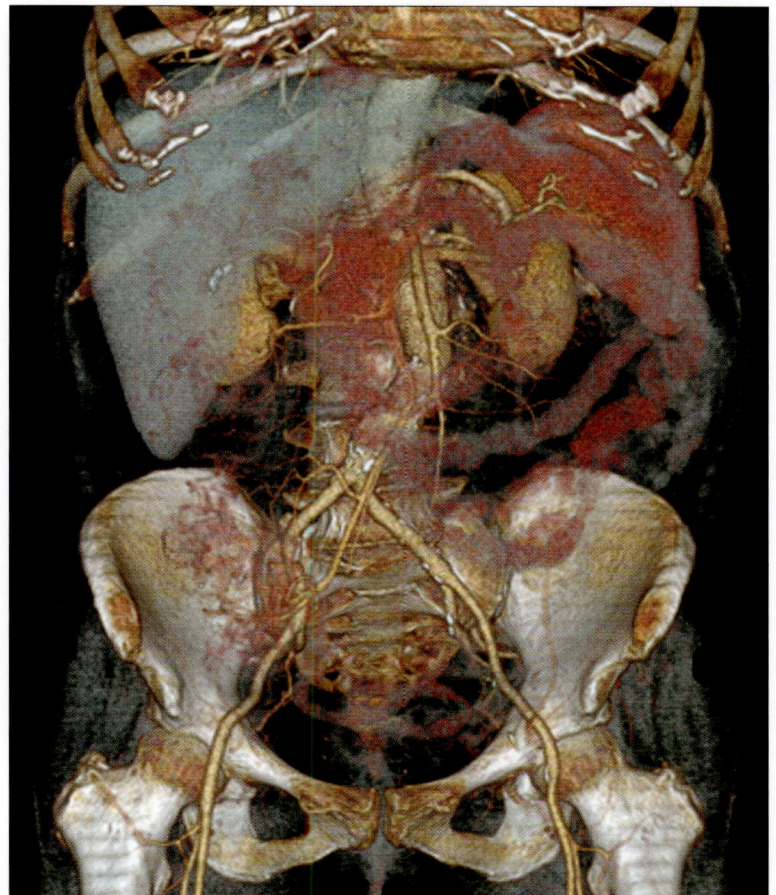

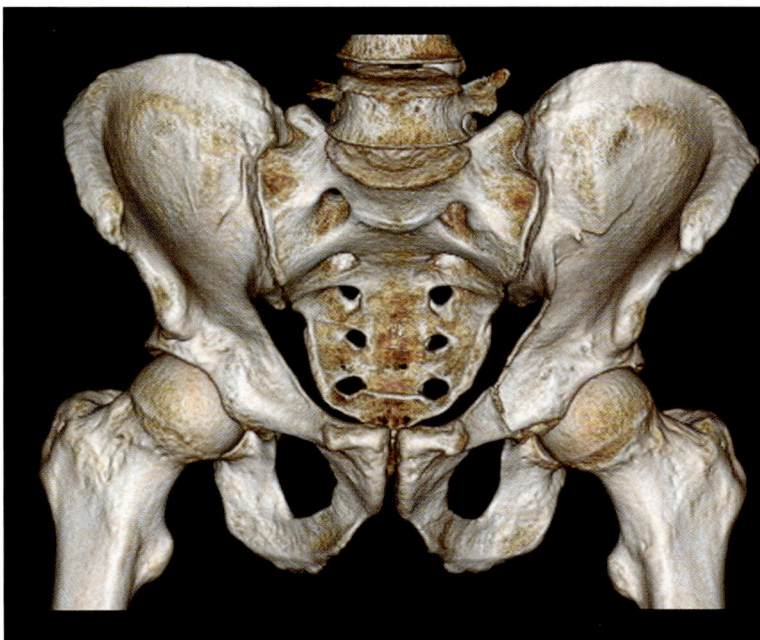

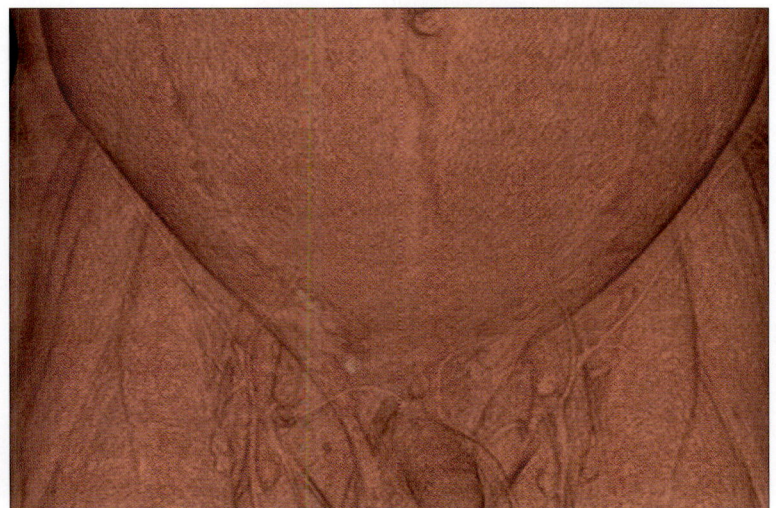

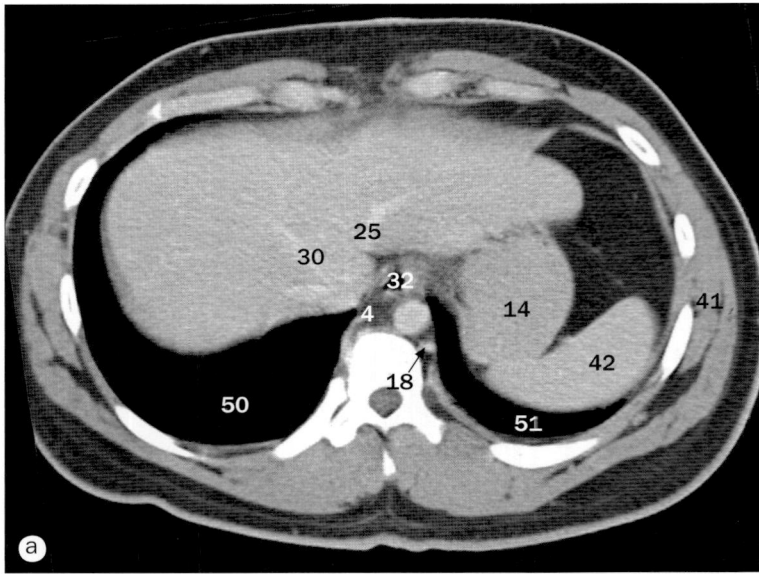

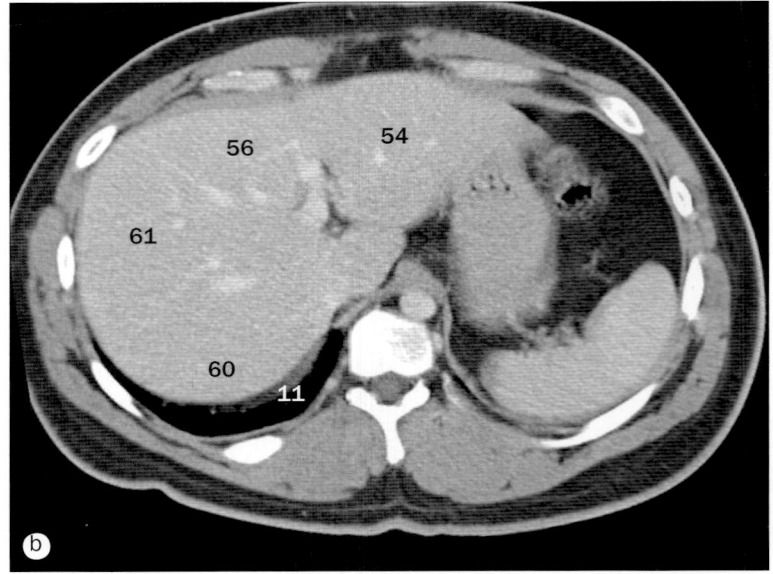

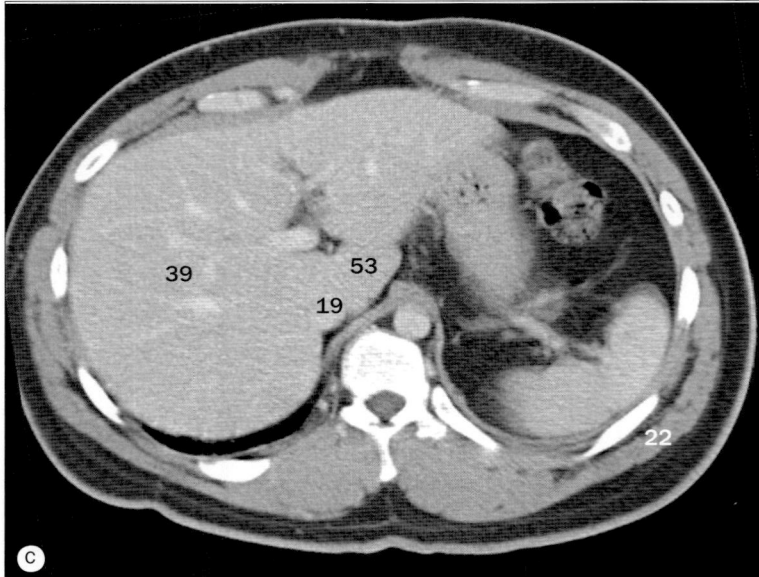

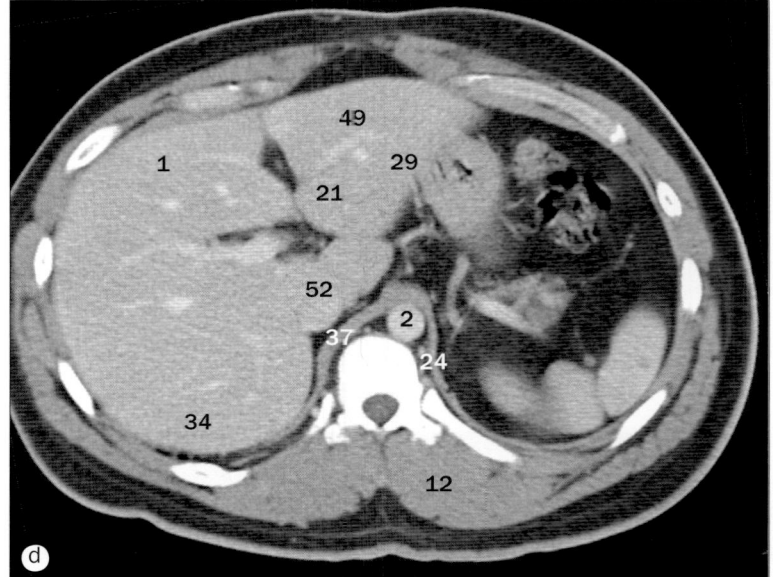

(a)–(h) Sequential axial CT images of abdomen and pelvis in a male, from superior to inferior.
Note: pages 124–135 show sequential images of the abdomen and pelvis of the same male patient.

1 Anterior segment of right lobe of liver	14 Fundus of stomach	27 Left suprarenal gland
2 Aorta	15 Gall bladder	28 Lesser curvature of stomach
3 Decending colon	16 Greater curvature of stomach	29 Medial segment of left lobe of liver
4 Azygos vein	17 Head of pancreas	30 Middle hepatic vein
5 Body of pancreas	18 Hemi-azygos vein	31 Neck of pancreas
6 Body of stomach	19 Inferior vena cava	32 Oesophagus
7 Body of vertebra	20 Jejunum	33 Porta vein
8 Coeliac trunk	21 Lateral segment of left lobe of liver	34 Posterior segment of right lobe of liver
9 Common hepatic artery	22 Latissimus dorsi muscle	35 Renal cortex
10 Descending (second) part of duodenum	23 Left colic (splenic) flexure	36 Renal fascia
11 Diaphragm	24 Left crus of diaphragm	37 Right crus of diaphragm
12 Erector spinae muscle	25 Left hepatic vein	38 Right kidney
13 Fissure for ligamentum venosum	26 Left kidney	39 Right lobe of liver

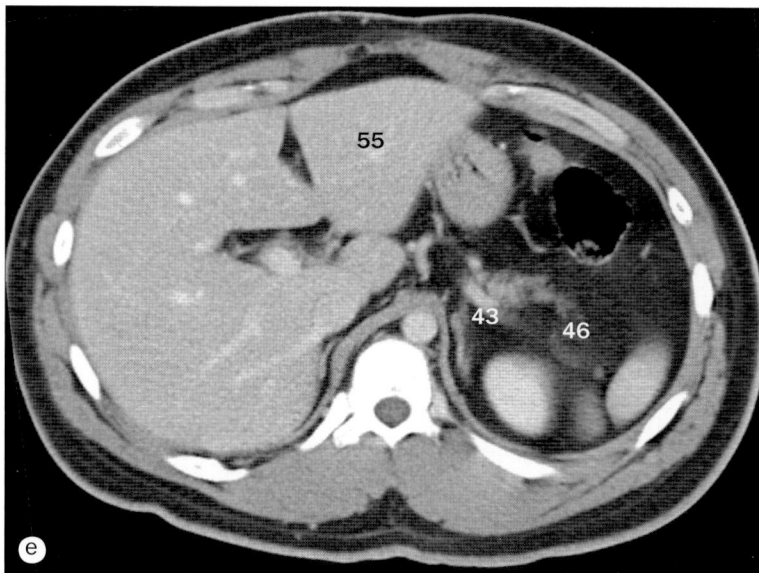

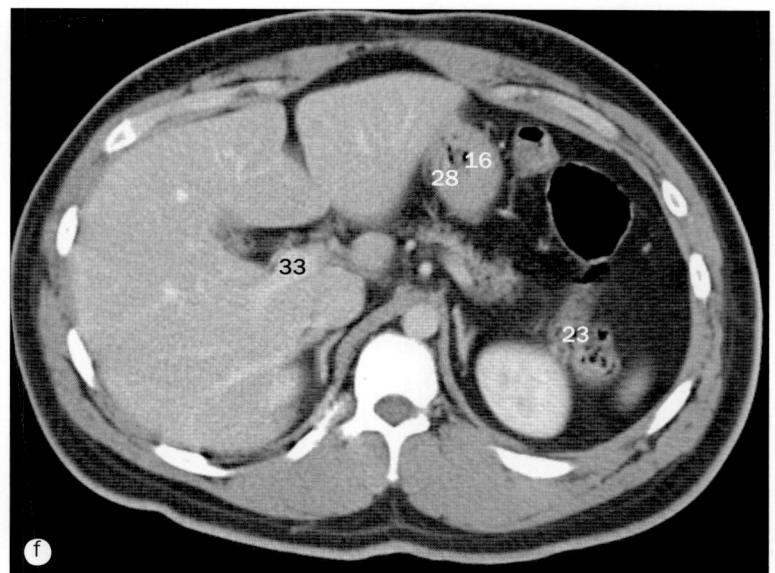

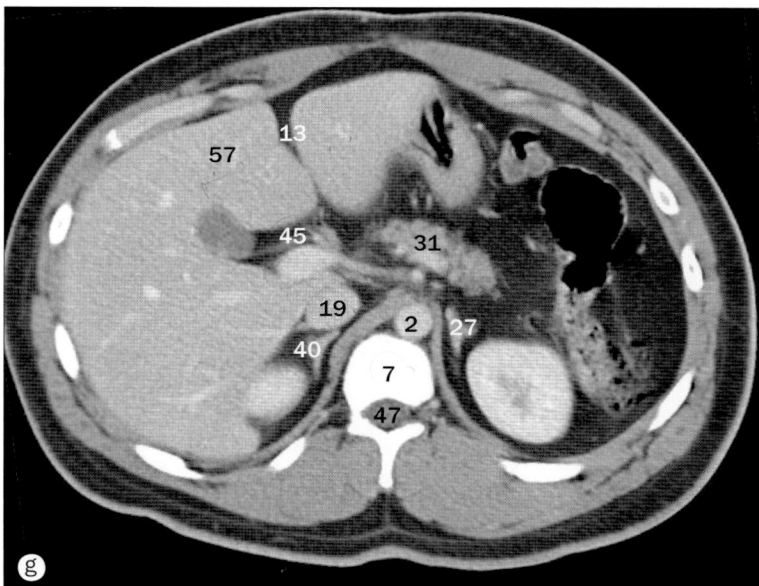

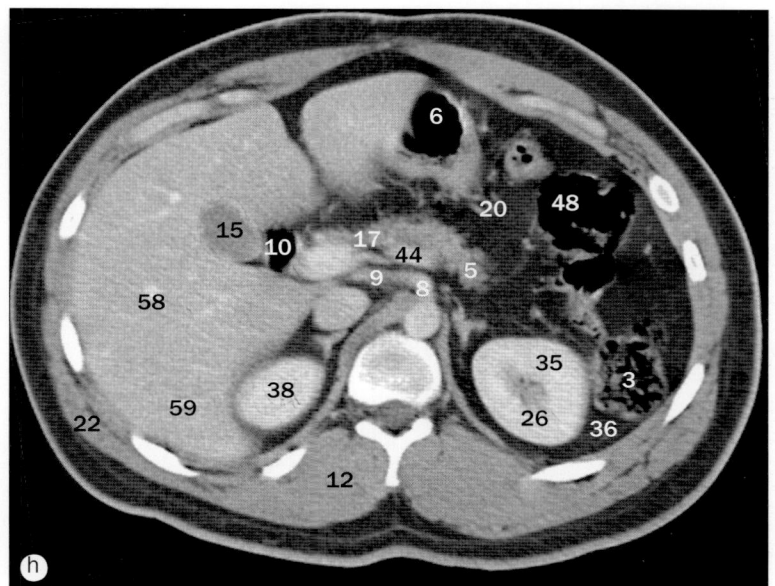

(a)–(h) Sequential axial CT images of abdomen and pelvis in a male, from superior to inferior.

40 Right suprarenal gland
41 Serratus anterior muscle
42 Spleen
43 Splenic artery
44 Splenic vein
45 Superior (first) part of duodenum
46 Tail of pancreas
47 Thecal sac
48 Transverse colon
49 Left lobe of liver

50 Right inferior lobe of lung
51 Left inferior lobe of lung
52 Caudate lobe of liver
53 Segment 1 of liver (caudate)
54 Segment 2 of liver (left lateral superior subsegment)
55 Segment 3 of liver (left lateral inferior subsegment)
56 Segment 4A of liver (left medial superior subsegment)

57 Segment 4B of liver (left medial m inferior subsegment)
58 Segment 5 of liver (right anterior inferior subsegment)
59 Segment 6 of liver (right posterior inferior subsegment)
60 Segment 7 of liver (right posterior superior subsegment)
61 Segment 8 of liver (right anterior superior subsegment)

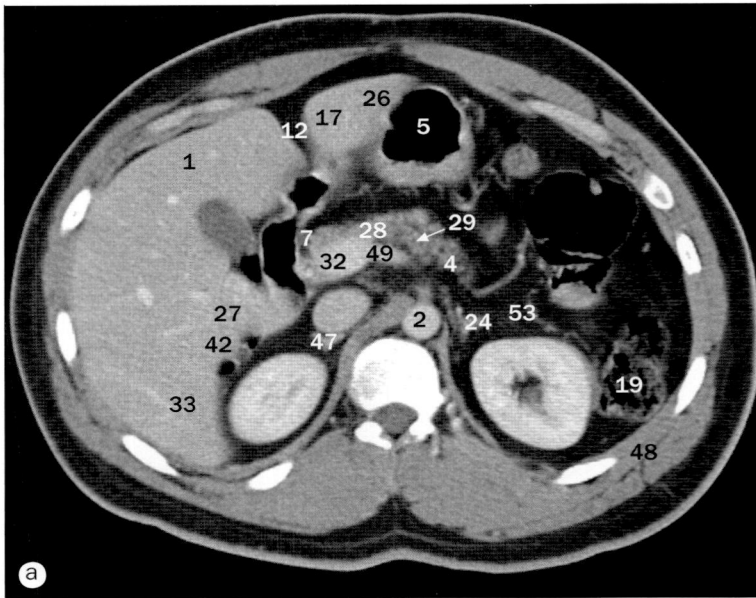

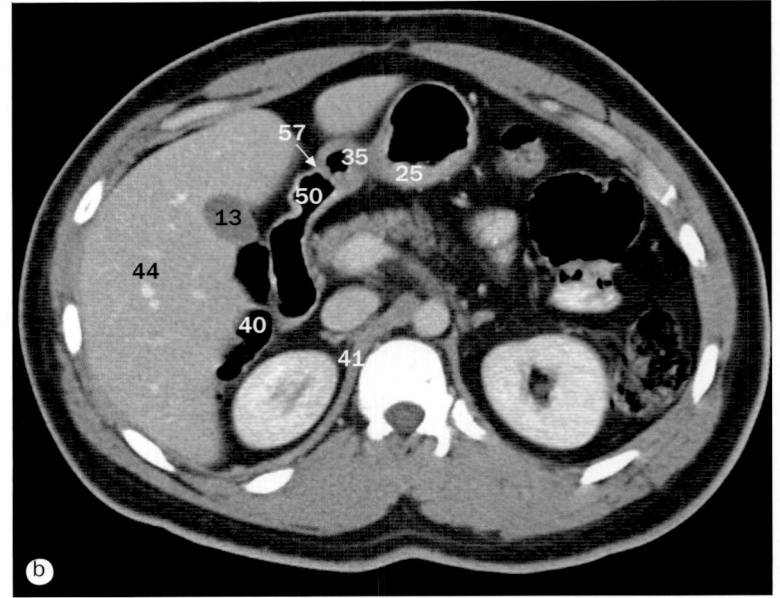

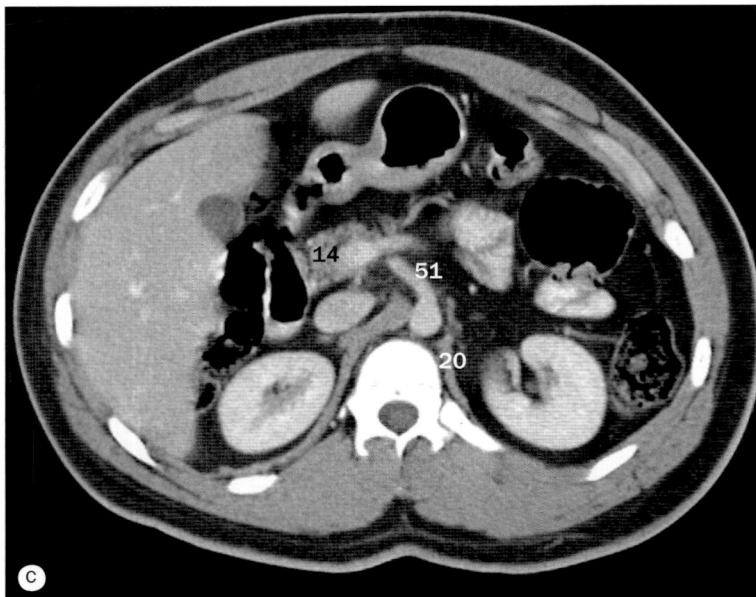

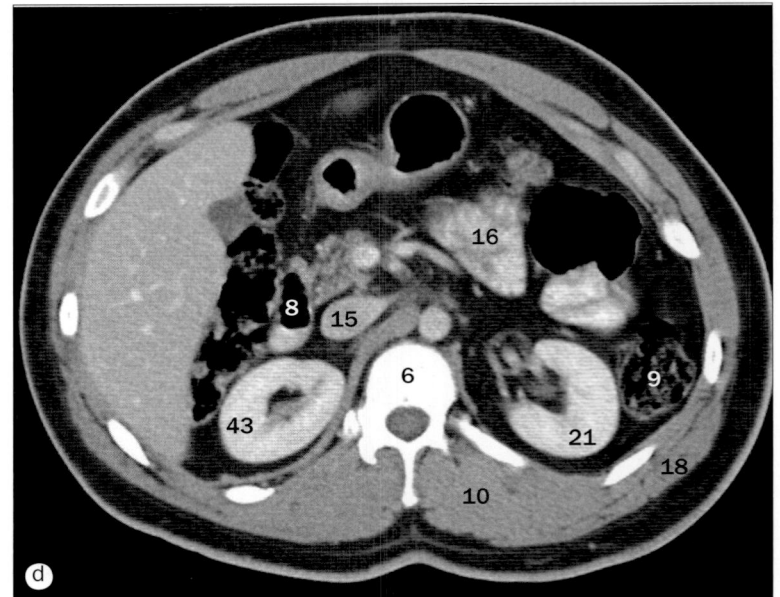

(a)–(h) Sequential axial CT images of abdomen and pelvis in a male, from superior to inferior.

1	Anterior segment of right lobe of liver	11	External oblique muscle	21	Left kidney
2	Aorta	12	Fissure for ligamentum venosum	22	Left renal artery
3	Ascending colon	13	Gall bladder	23	Left renal vein
4	Body of pancreas	14	Head of pancreas	24	Left suprarenal gland
5	Body of stomach	15	Inferior vena cava	25	Lesser curvature of stomach
6	Body of vertebra	16	Jejunum	26	Medial segment of left lobe of liver
7	Common bile duct	17	Lateral segment of left lobe of liver	27	Middle hepatic vein
8	Descending (second) part of duodenum	18	Latissimus dorsi muscle	28	Neck of pancreas
9	Descending colon	19	Left colic (splenic) flexure	29	Pancreatic duct
10	Erector spinae muscle	20	Left crus of diaphragm	30	Pararenal fat

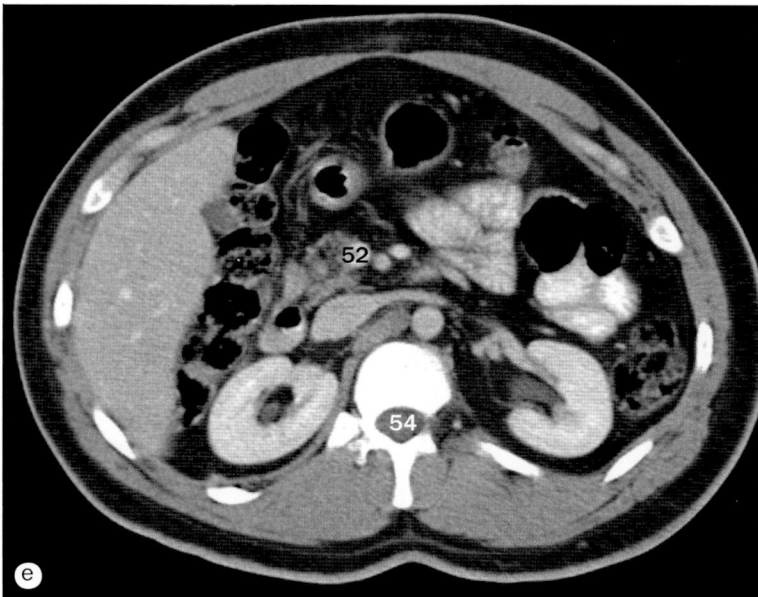

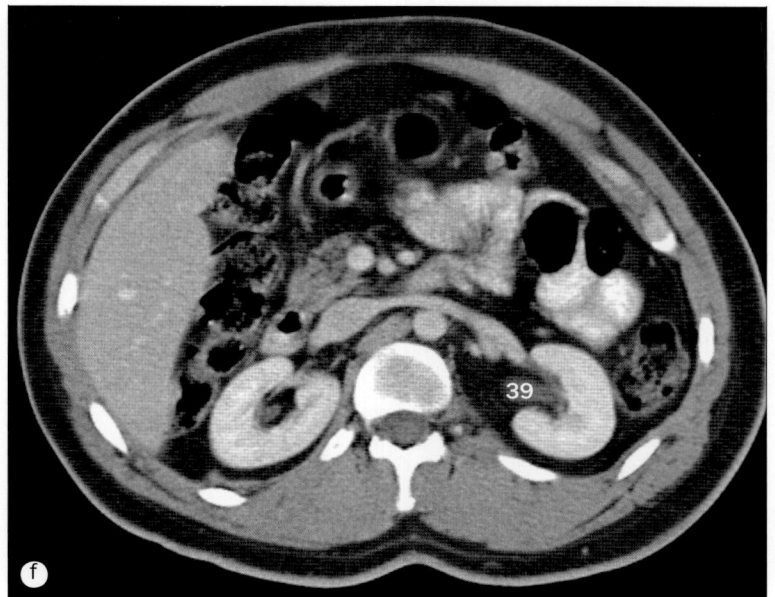

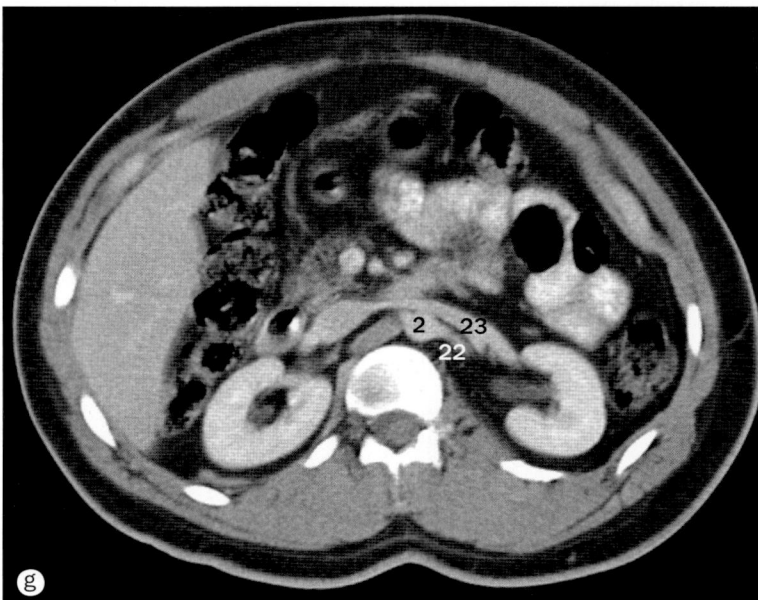

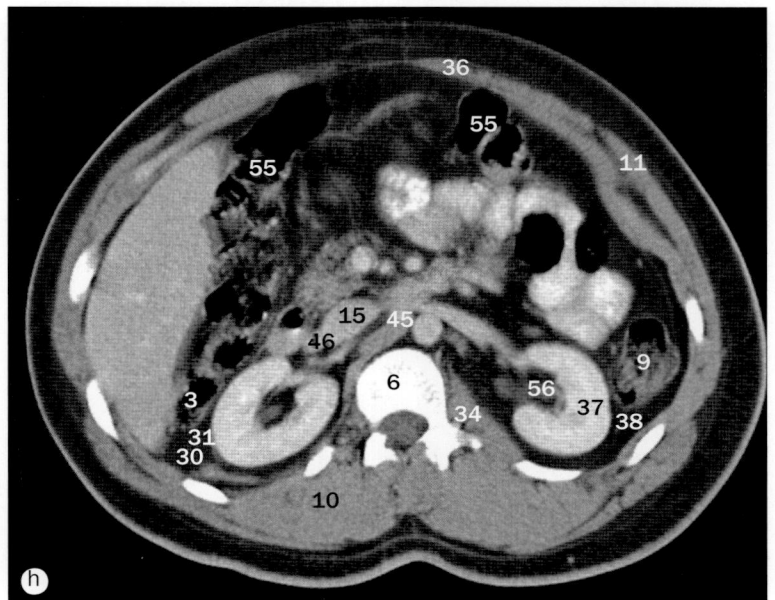

(a)–(h) Sequential axial CT images of abdomen and pelvis in a male, from superior to inferior.

31 Perirenal fat
32 Portal vein
33 Posterior segment of right lobe of liver
34 Psoas major muscle
35 Pyloric part of stomach
36 Rectus abdominis muscle
37 Renal cortex
38 Renal fascia
39 Renal pelvis

40 Right colic (hepatic) flexure
41 Right crus of diaphragm
42 Right hepatic vein
43 Right kidney
44 Right lobe of liver
45 Right renal artery
46 Right renal vein
47 Right suprarenal gland
48 Serratus anterior muscle

49 Splenic vein
50 Superior (first) part of duodenum
51 Superior mesenteric artery
52 Superior mesenteric vein
53 Tail of pancreas
54 Thecal sac
55 Transverse colon
56 Renal sinus fat
57 Pylorus

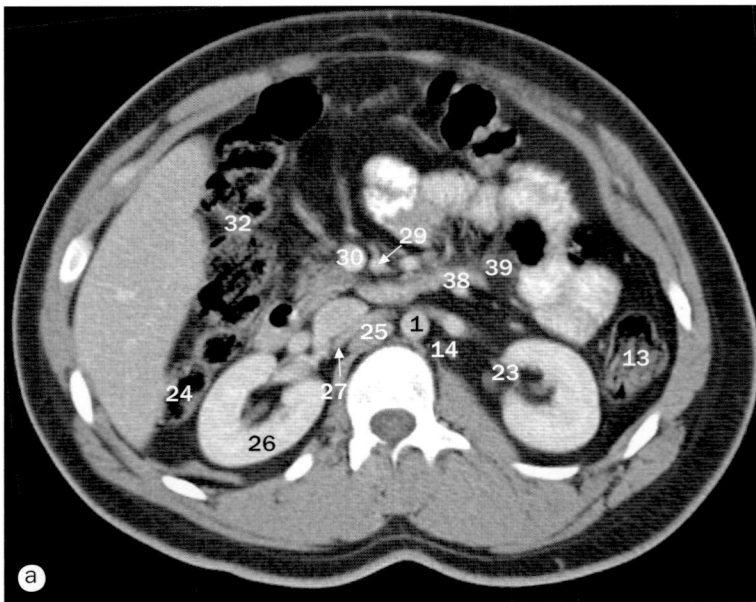

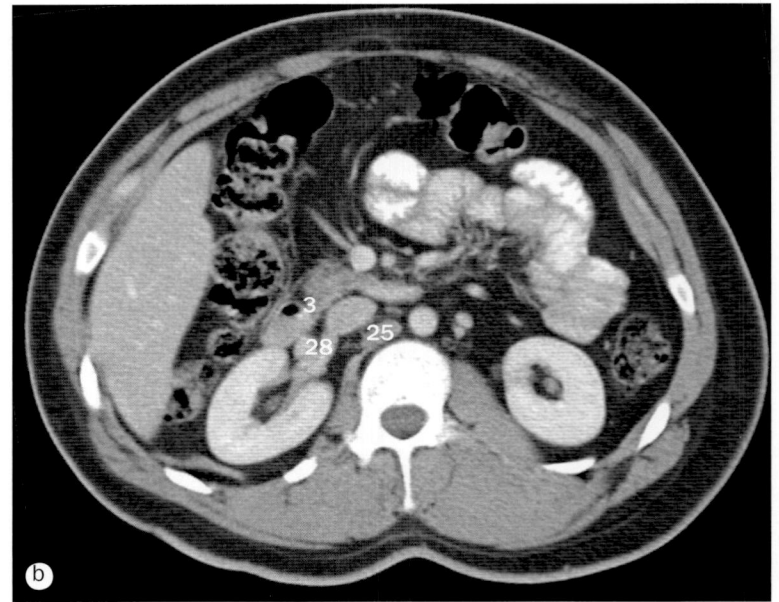

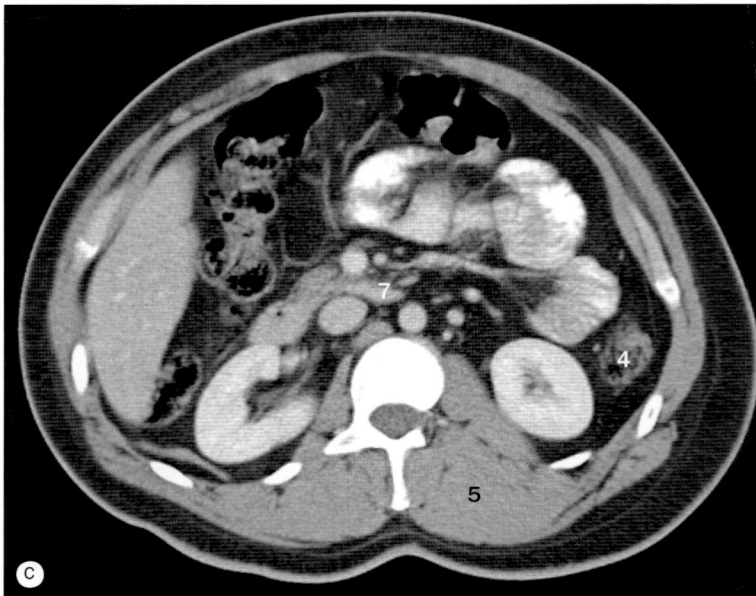

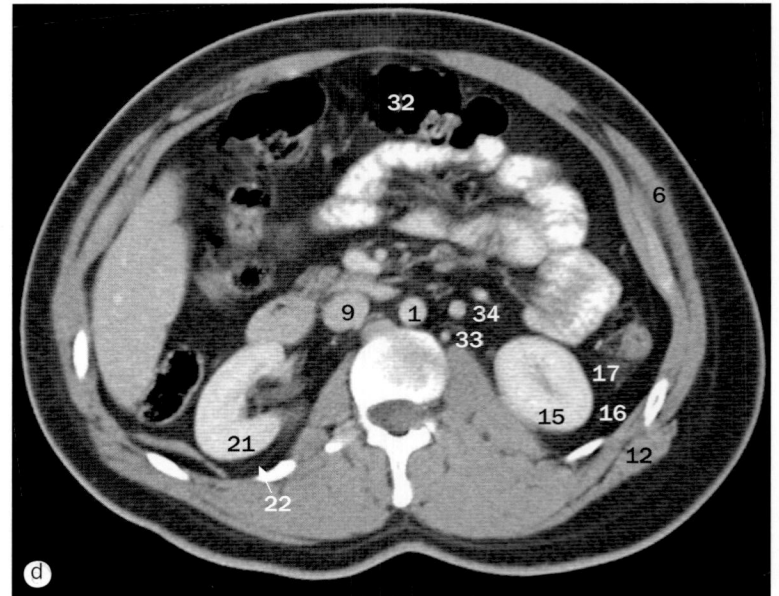

(a)–(h) Sequential axial CT images of abdomen and pelvis in a male, from superior to inferior.

1 Aorta	8 Ileum	15 Left kidney
2 Ascending colon	9 Inferior vena cava	16 Pararenal fat
3 Descending (second) part of duodenum	10 Internal oblique muscle	17 Perirenal fat
4 Descending colon	11 Jejunum	18 Psoas major muscle
5 Erector spinae muscle	12 Latissimus dorsi muscle	19 Quadratus lumborum muscle
6 External oblique muscle	13 Left colic (splenic) flexure	20 Rectus abdominis muscle
7 Horizontal (third) part of duodenum	14 Left crus of diaphragm	21 Renal cortex

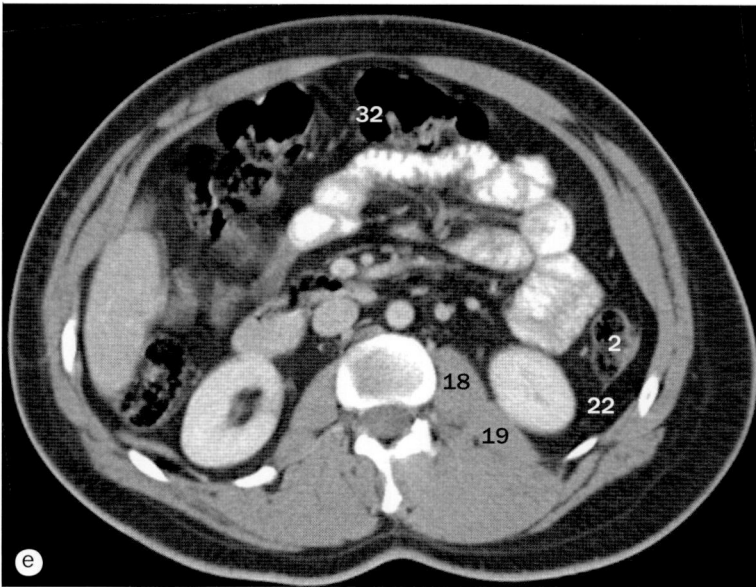

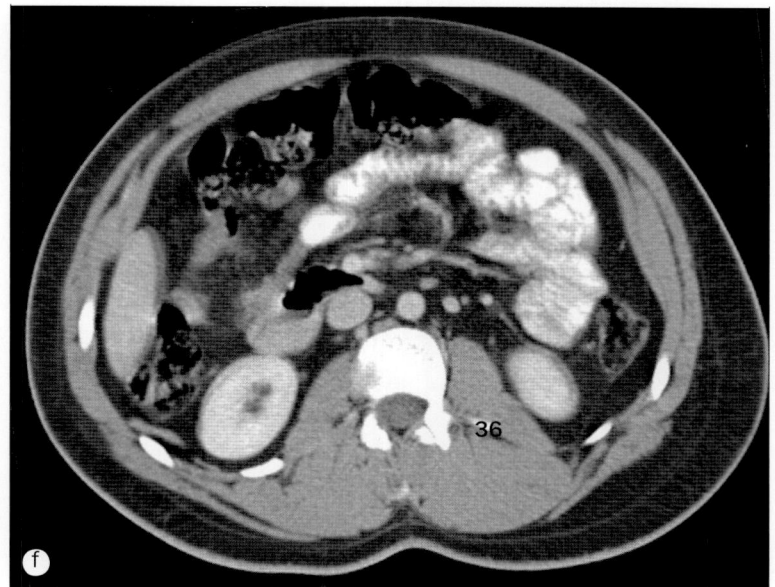

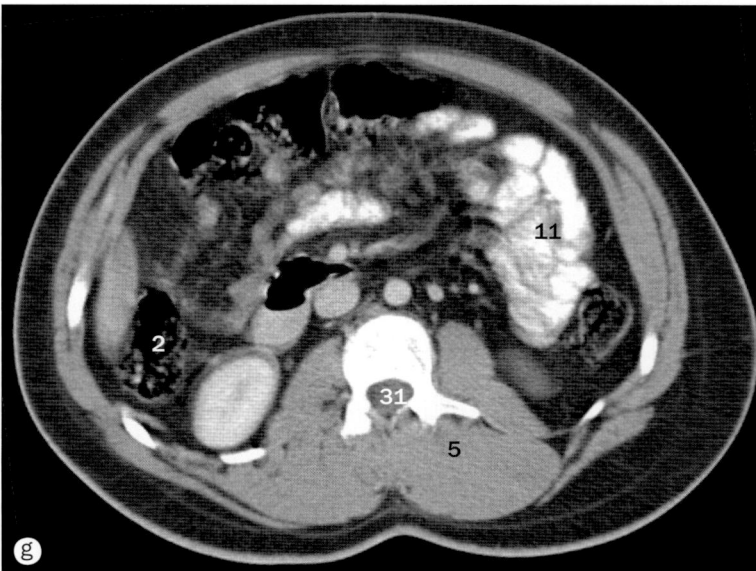

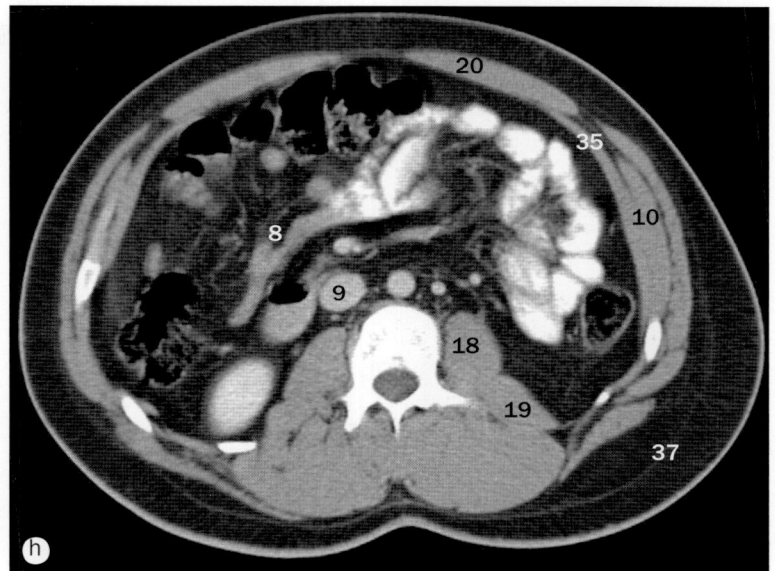

(a)–(h) Sequential axial CT images of abdomen and pelvis in a male, from superior to inferior.

22 Renal fascia	28 Right renal vein	34 Left testicular vein
23 Renal pelvis	29 Superior mesenteric artery	35 Transversus abdominis muscle
24 Right colic (hepatic) flexure	30 Superior mesenteric vein	36 Twelfth rib
25 Right crus of diaphragm	31 Thecal sac	37 Subcutaneous fascia
26 Right kidney	32 Transverse colon	38 Fourth (ascending) part of duodenum
27 Right renal artery	33 Left testicular artery	39 Duodenal–jejunal flexure

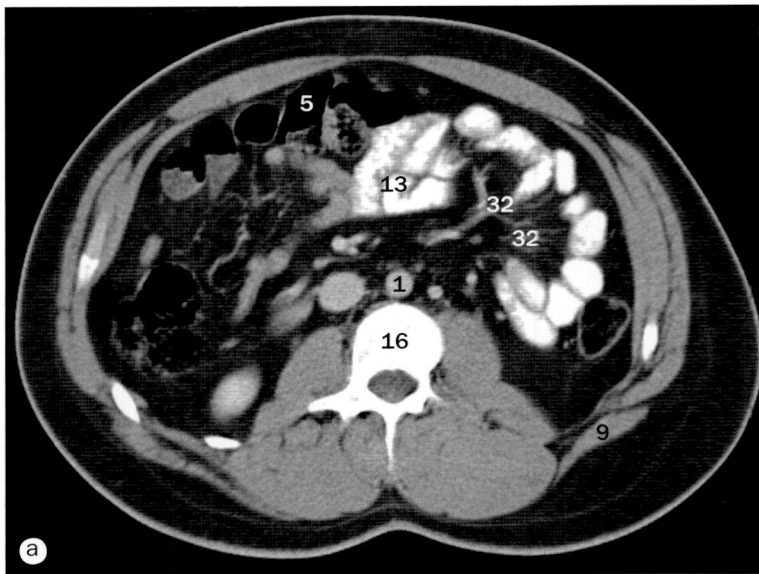

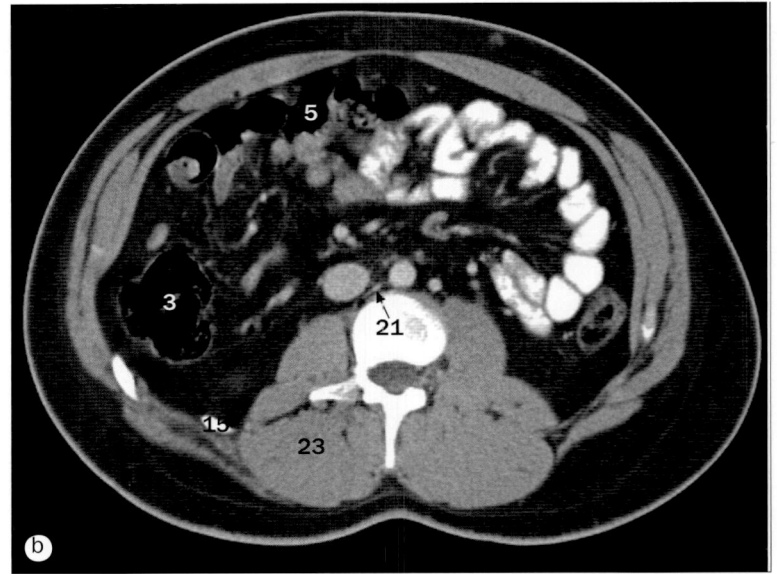

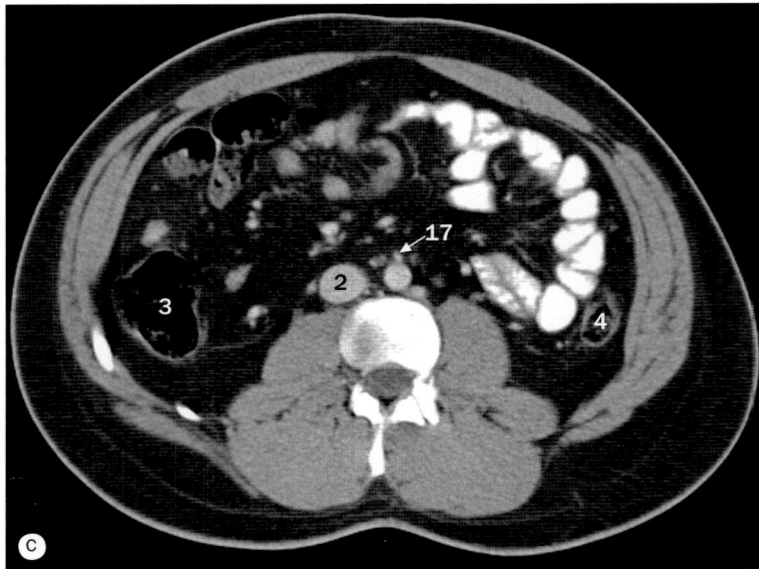

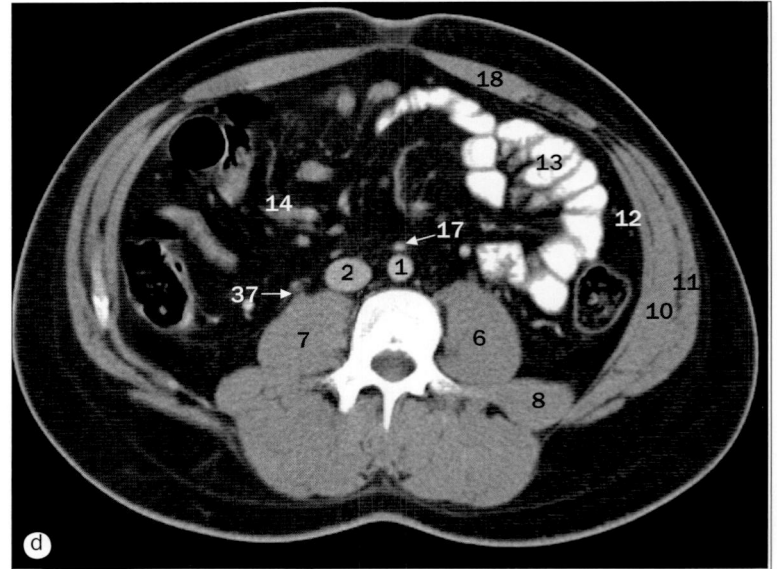

(a)–(h) Sequential axial CT images of abdomen and pelvis in a male, from superior to inferior.

1 Aorta	8 Quadratus lumborum muscle	15 Twelfth rib
2 Inferior vena cava	9 Latissimus dorsi muscle	16 Vertebral body
3 Ascending colon	10 Internal oblique muscle	17 Inferior mesenteric artery
4 Descending colon	11 External oblique muscle	18 Rectus abdominis muscle
5 Transverse colon	12 Transversus abdominis muscle	19 Appendicular artery
6 Left psoas muscle	13 Jejunum	20 Lumbar vein
7 Right psoas muscle	14 Ileum	21 Lumbar artery

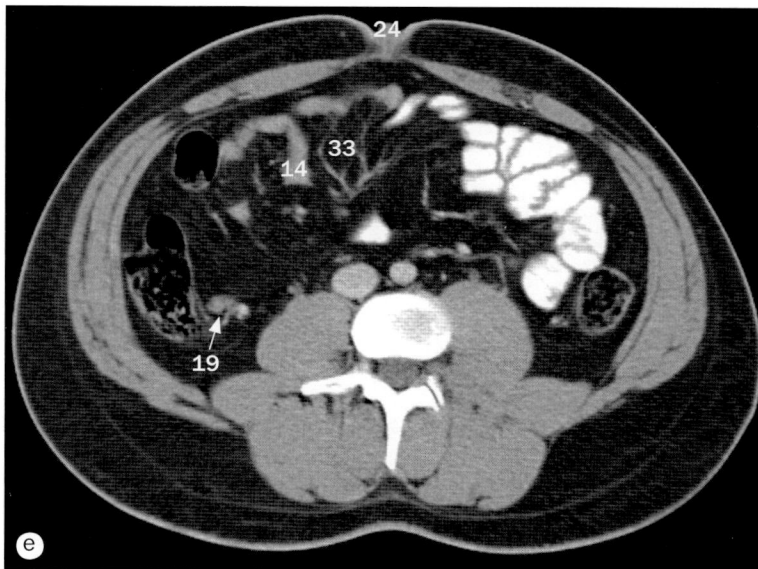

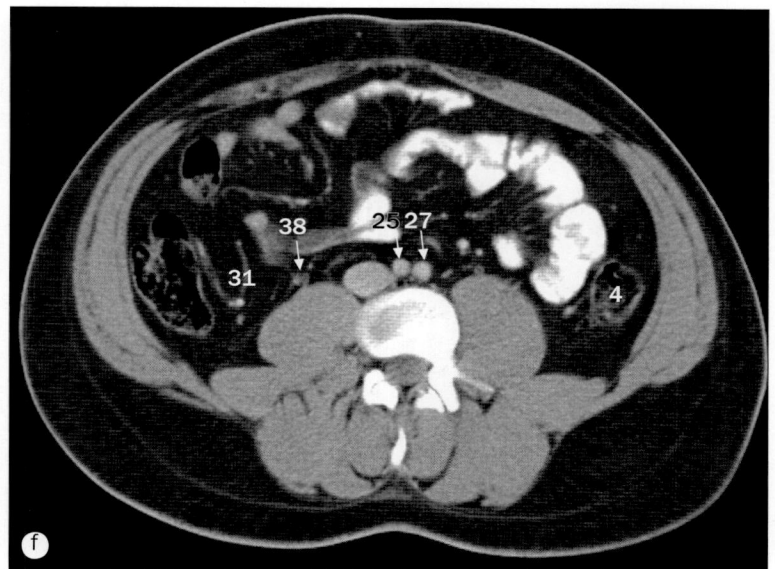

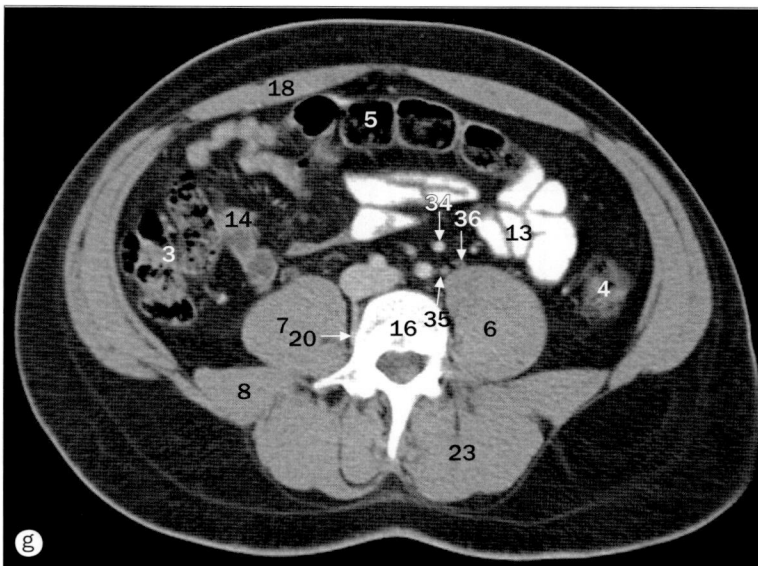

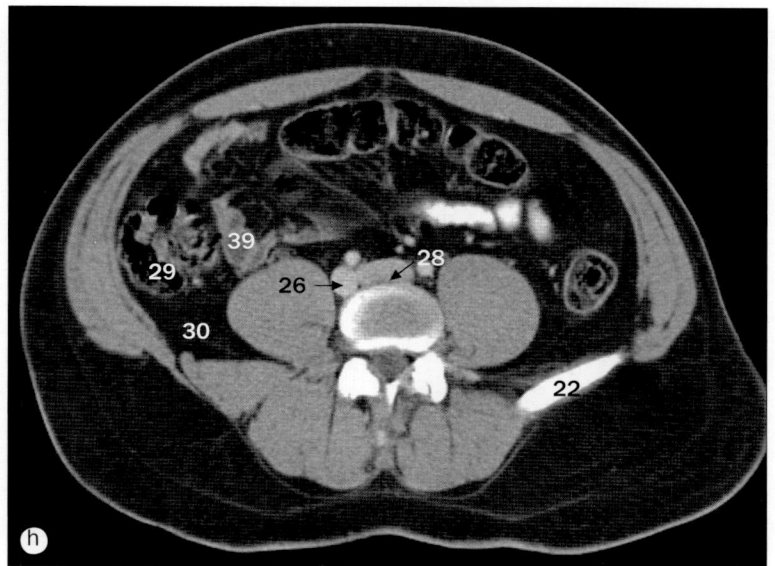

(a)–(h) Sequential axial CT images of abdomen and pelvis in a male, from superior to inferior.

22 Ilium
23 Erector spinae muscles
24 Umbilicus
25 Right common iliac artery
26 Right common iliac vein
27 Left common iliac artery
28 Left common iliac vein

29 Caecum
30 Appendix
31 Ileocolic artery
32 Jejunal branches of superior mesenteric artery
33 Ileal branches of superior mesenteric artery

34 Left testicular artery
35 Left testicular vein
36 Left ureter
37 Right ureter
38 Right testicular vessels
39 Terminal ileum

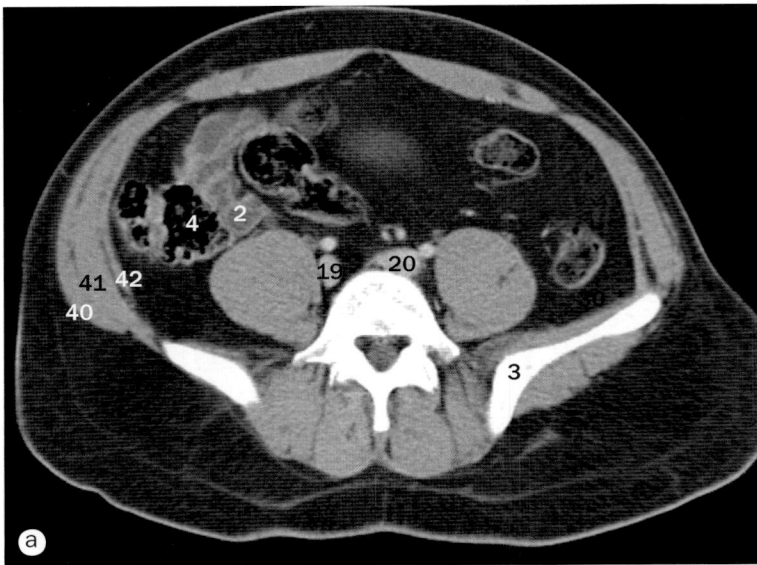

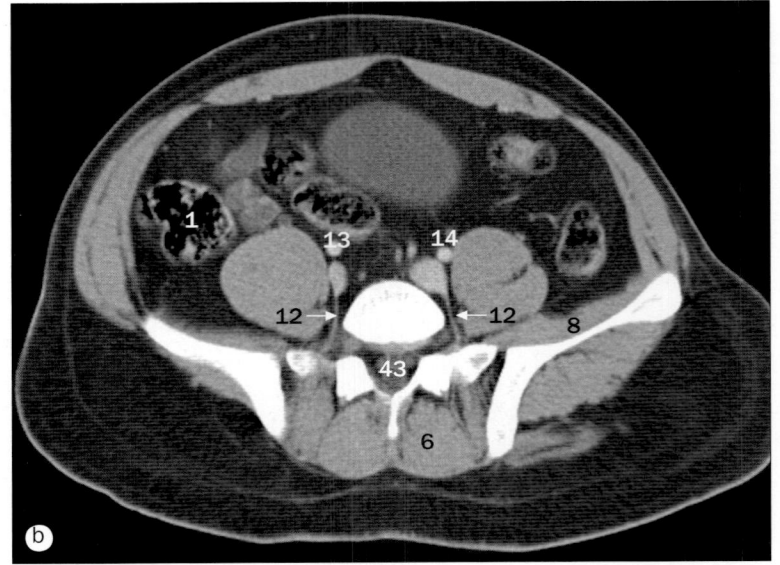

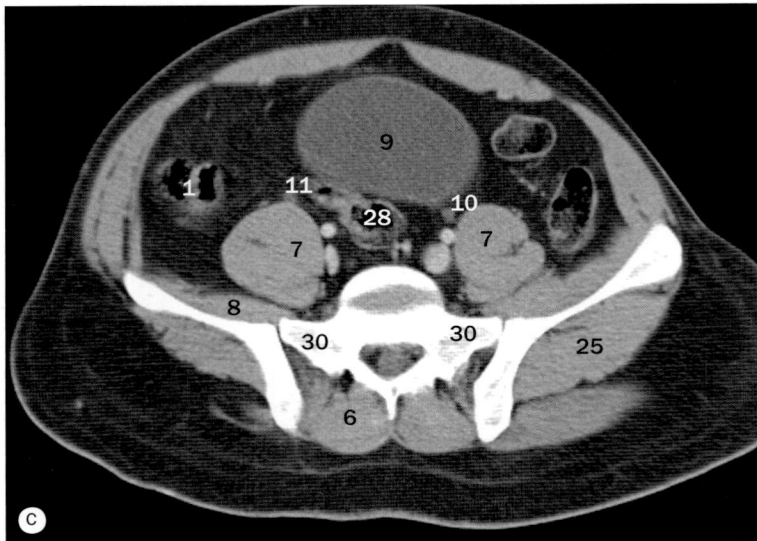

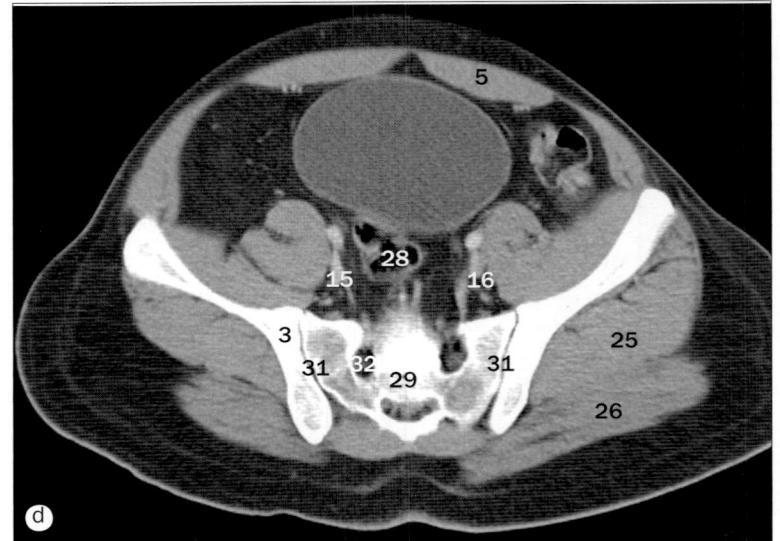

(a)–(h) Sequential axial CT images of abdomen and pelvis in a male, from superior to inferior.

1 Caecum	9 Urinary bladder	17 Right external iliac artery
2 Terminal ileum	10 Left ureter	18 Left external iliac artery
3 Ilium	11 Right ureter	19 Right common iliac vein
4 Ascending colon	12 Lumbar veins	20 Left common iliac vein
5 Rectus abdominis muscle	13 Right common iliac artery	21 Right internal iliac vein
6 Erector spinae muscles	14 Left common iliac artery	22 Left internal iliac vein
7 Psoas major muscle	15 Right internal iliac artery	23 Right external iliac vein
8 Iliacus muscle	16 Left internal iliac artery	24 Left external iliac vein

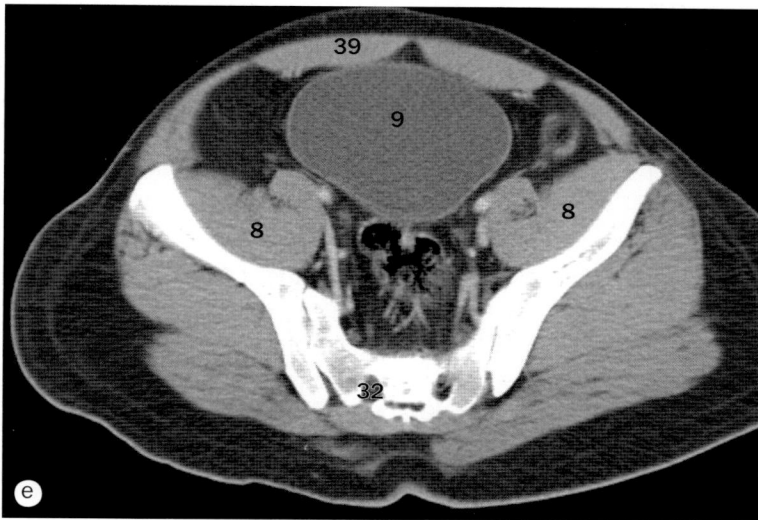

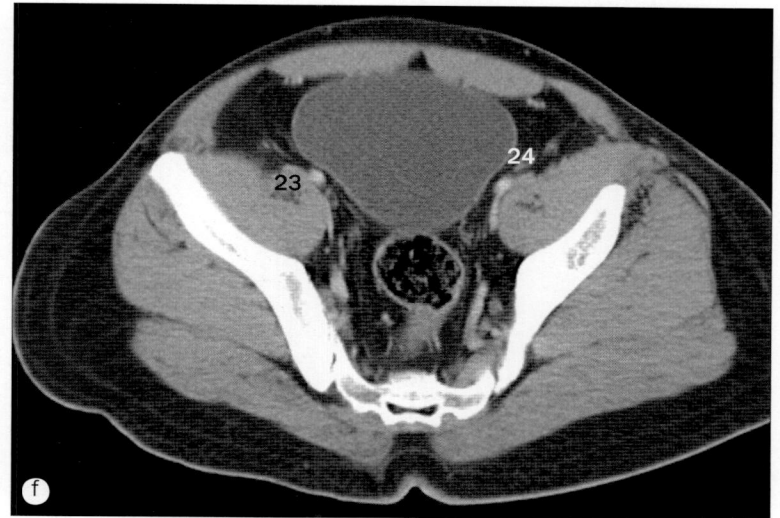

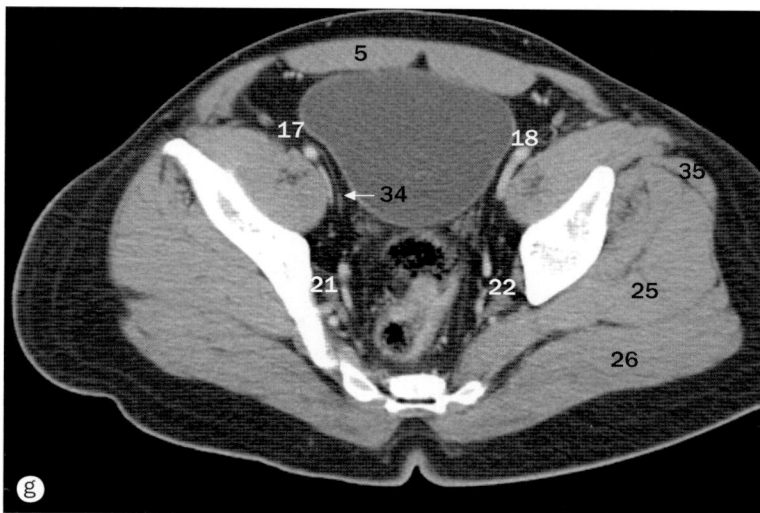

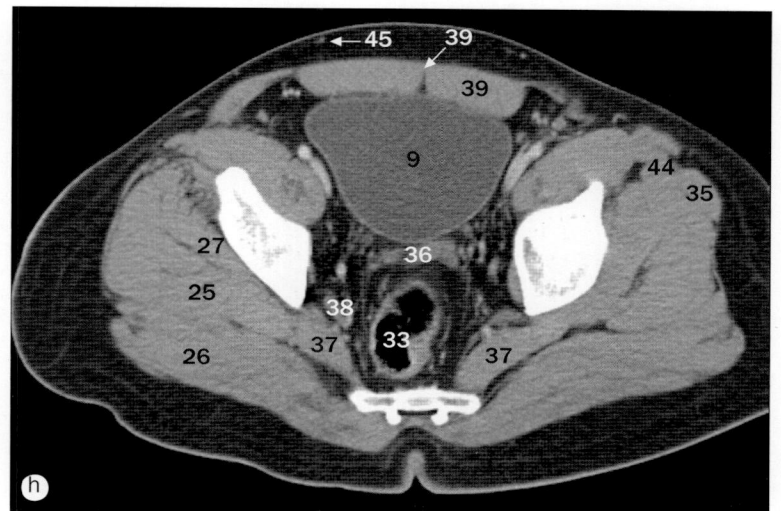

(a)–(h) Sequential axial CT images of abdomen and pelvis in a male, from superior to inferior.

25 Gluteus medius muscle	32 Sacral foramen	39 Linea alba
26 Gluteus maximus muscle	33 Rectum	40 External oblique muscle
27 Gluteus minimus muscle	34 Vas deferens	41 Internal oblique muscle
28 Sigmoid colon	35 Tensor fasciae latae muscle	42 Transversus abdominis muscle
29 Sacrum	36 Seminal vesicle	43 Thecal sac
30 Sacral alum	37 Piriformis muscle	44 Sartorius muscle
31 Sacroiliac joint	38 Superior gluteal artery and vein	45 Superficial inferior epigastric artery

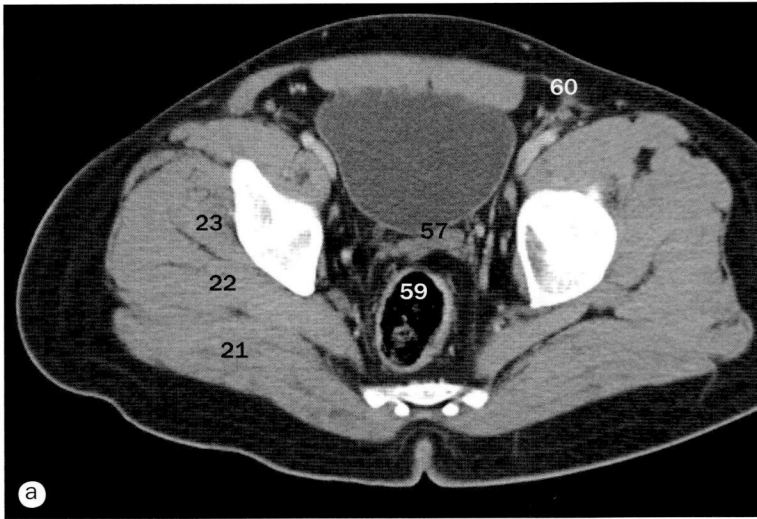

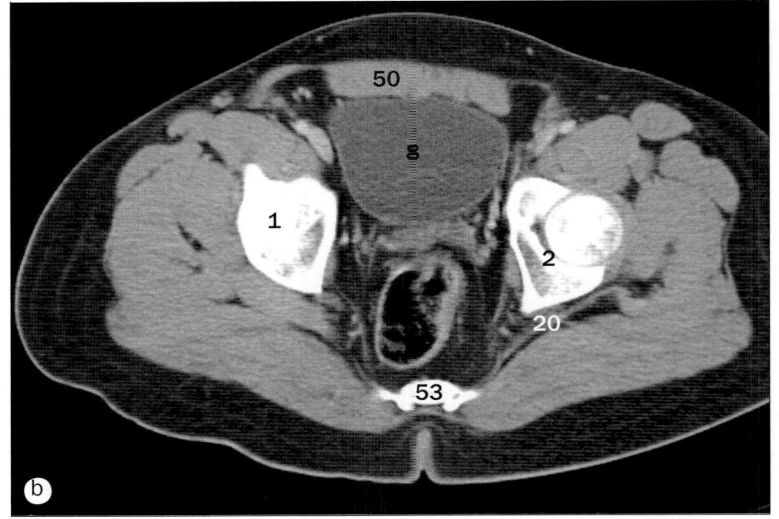

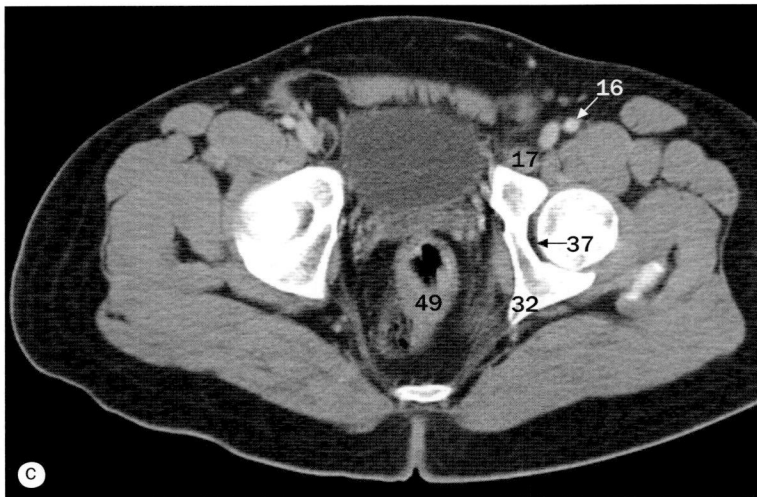

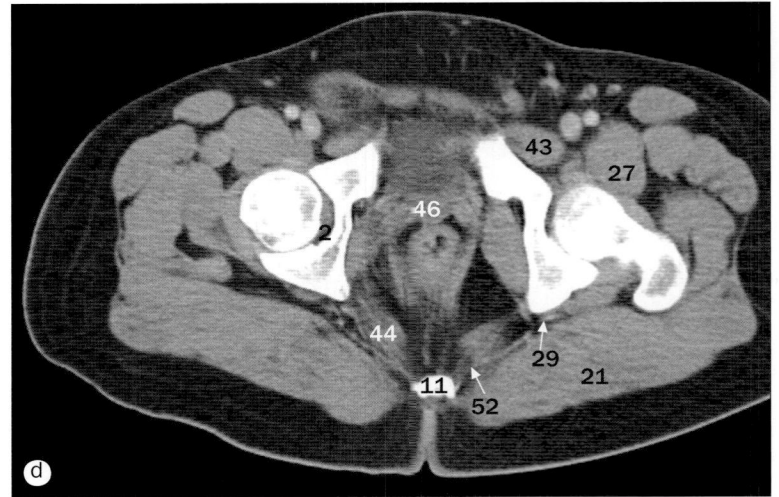

(a)–(h) Sequential axial CT images of abdomen and pelvis in a male, from superior to inferior.

1 Acetabular roof	**12** Corpus cavernosum	**23** Gluteus minimus muscle
2 Acetabulum	**13** Crus of corpus cavernosum	**24** Gracilis muscle
3 Adductor brevis muscle	**14** Epididymis	**25** Greater trochanter of femur
4 Adductor longus muscle	**15** External anal sphincter	**26** Head of femur
5 Adductor magnus muscle	**16** External iliac artery	**27** Iliopsoas muscle
6 Anal canal	**17** External iliac vein	**28** Iliotibial tract
7 Biceps femoris muscle	**18** Femoral artery	**29** Inferior gluteal artery and vein
8 Bladder	**19** Femoral vein	**30** Inferior ramus of pubis
9 Body of pubis	**20** Gemellus muscle	**31** Internal pudendal artery and vein
10 Bulb of penis	**21** Gluteus maximus muscle	**32** Ischial spine
11 Coccyx	**22** Gluteus medius muscle	**33** Ischio-anal fossa

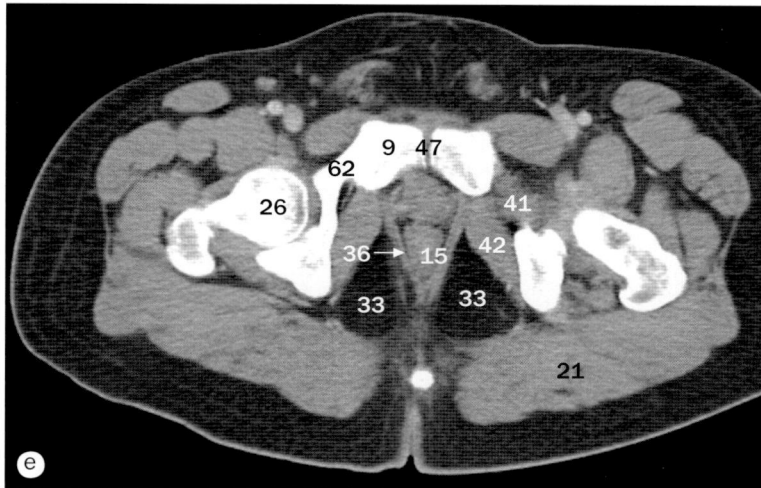

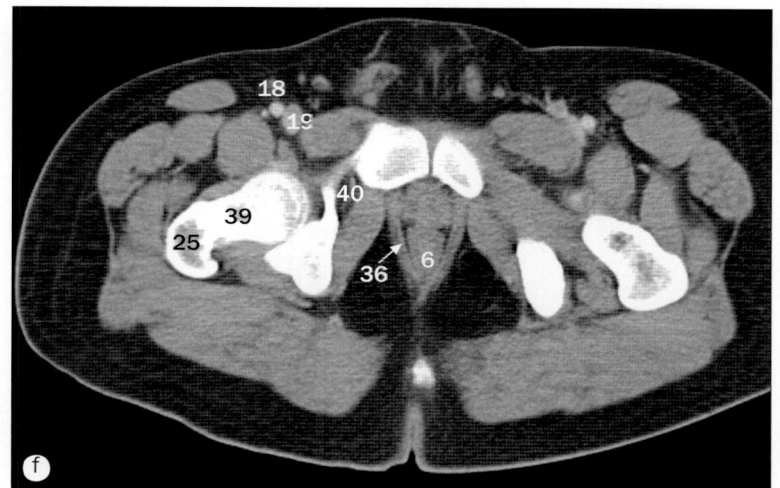

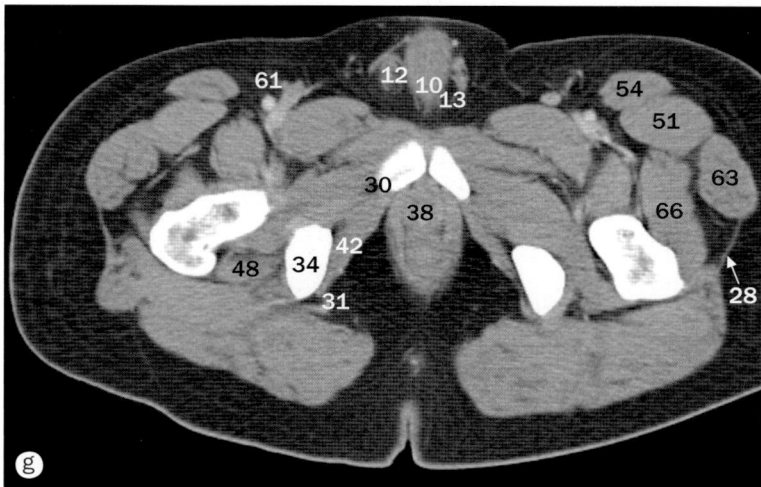

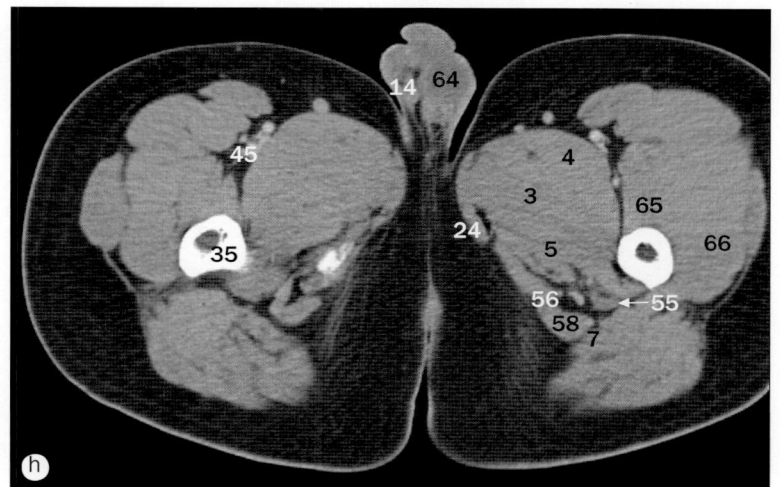

(a)–(h) Sequential axial CT images of abdomen and pelvis in a male, from superior to inferior.

34 Ischium	45 Profunda femoris artery	56 Semimembranosus muscle
35 Lesser trochanter of femur	46 Prostate	57 Seminal vesicle
36 Levator ani muscle	47 Pubic symphysis	58 Semitendinosus muscle
37 Ligament of head of femur	48 Quadratus femoris muscle	59 Sigmoid colon
38 Membranous urethra	49 Rectum	60 Spermatic cord
39 Neck of femur	50 Rectus abdominis muscle	61 Superficial femoral artery
40 Obturator artery and vein	51 Rectus femoris muscle	62 Superior ramus of pubis
41 Obturator externus muscle	52 Sacrospinous ligament	63 Tensor fasciae latae muscle
42 Obturator internus muscle	53 Sacrum	64 Testis
43 Pectineus muscle	54 Sartorius muscle	65 Vastus intermedius muscle
44 Piriformis muscle	55 Sciatic nerve	66 Vastus lateralis muscle

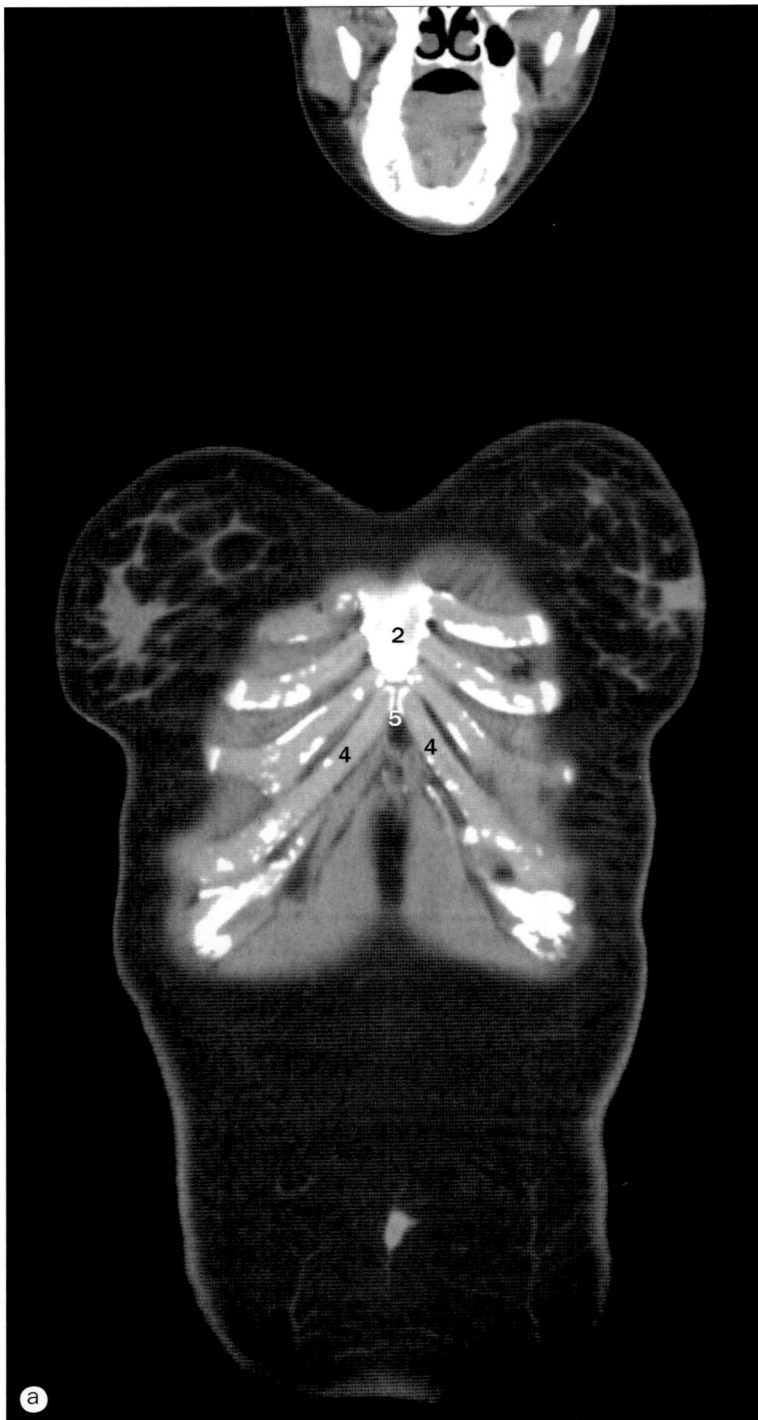

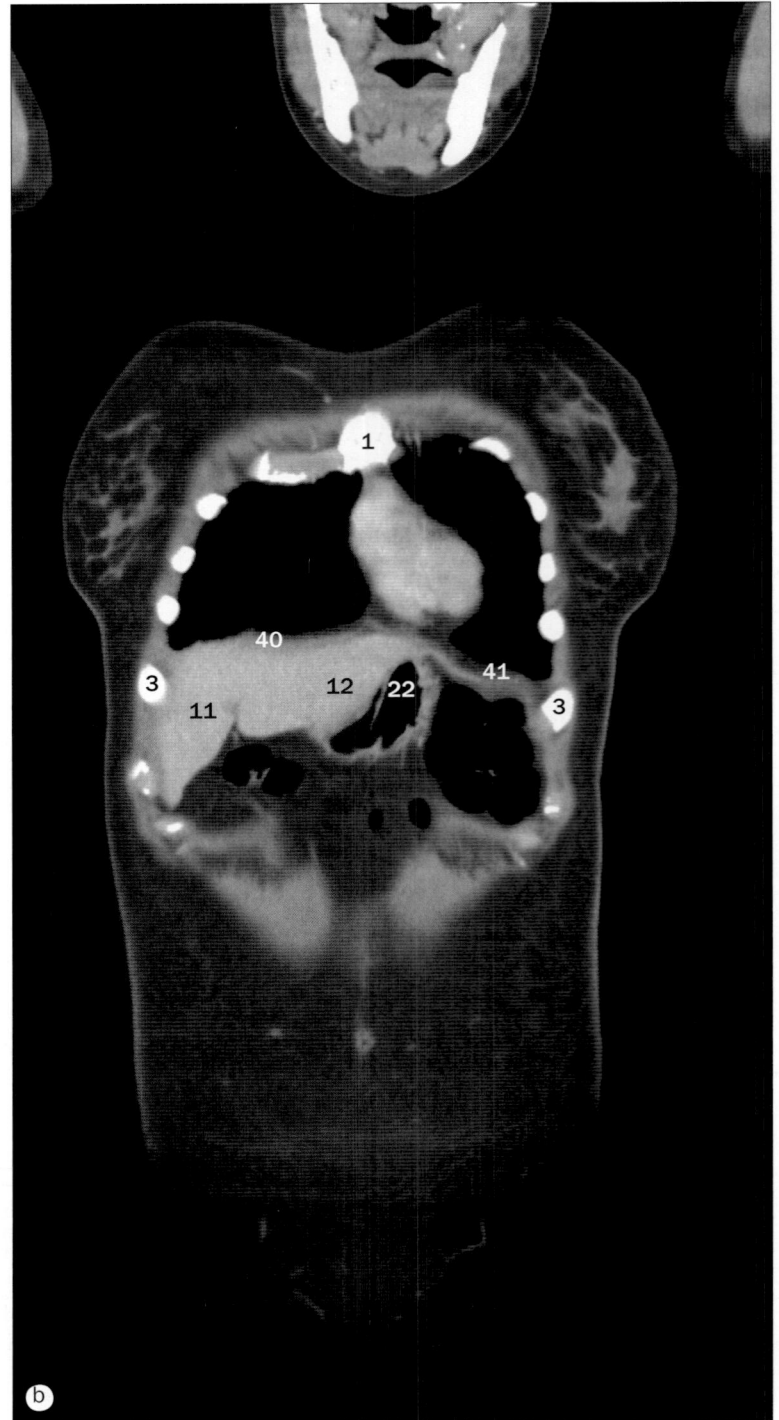

(a)–(d) Sequential coronal CT images of the chest, abdomen and pelvis in a female, from anterior to posterior.
Note: pages 136–145 show sequential images of the same female patient.

1 Manubrium	8 Right ventricle	15 Rectus abdominis muscle
2 Body of sternum	9 Left ventricle	16 Internal oblique muscle
3 Rib	10 Pulmonary conus	17 External oblique muscle
4 Costal cartilage	11 Right lobe of liver	18 Tranversus abdominis muscle
5 Xiphisternum	12 Left lobe of liver	19 Transverse colon
6 Breast	13 Gall bladder	20 Left colic flexure
7 Clavicle	14 Fissure for ligamentum venosum	21 Right colic flexure

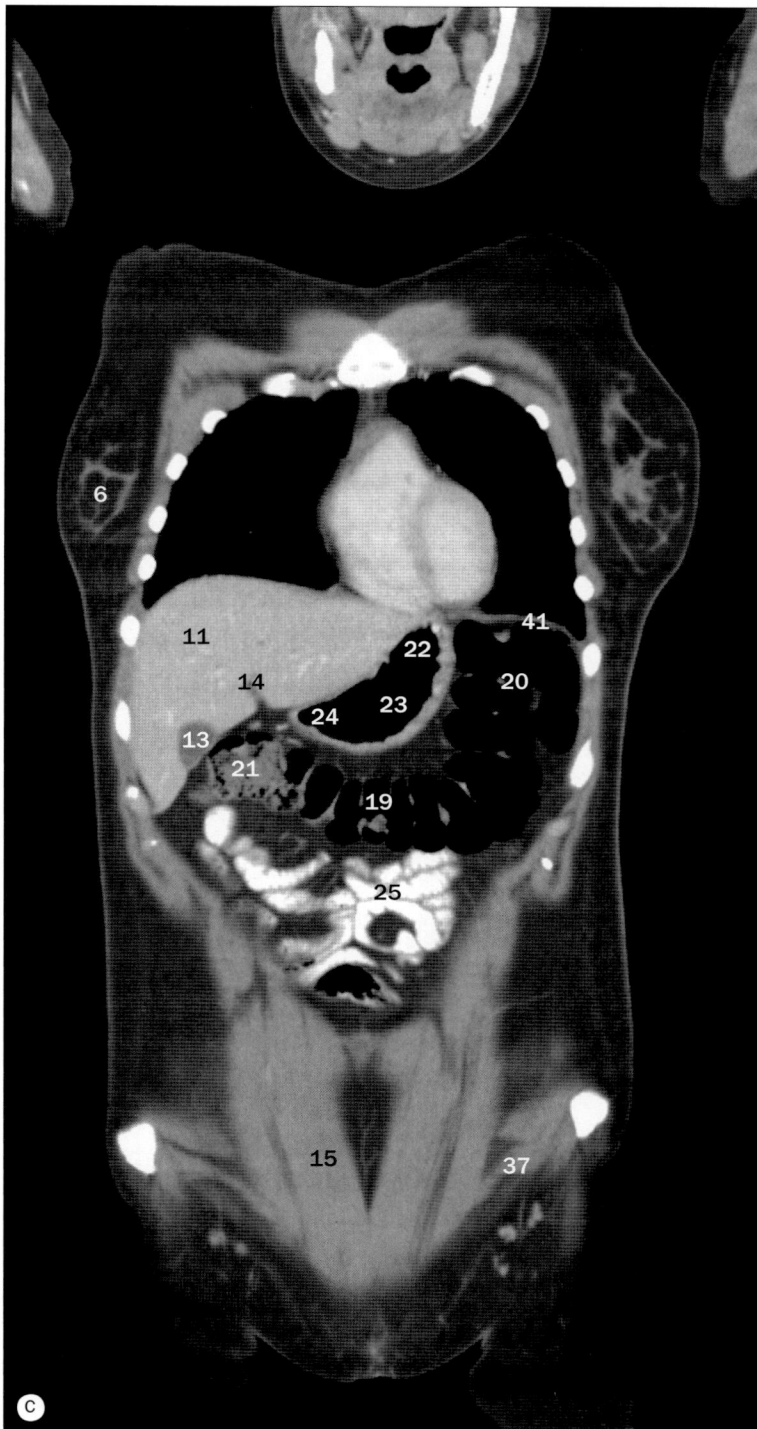

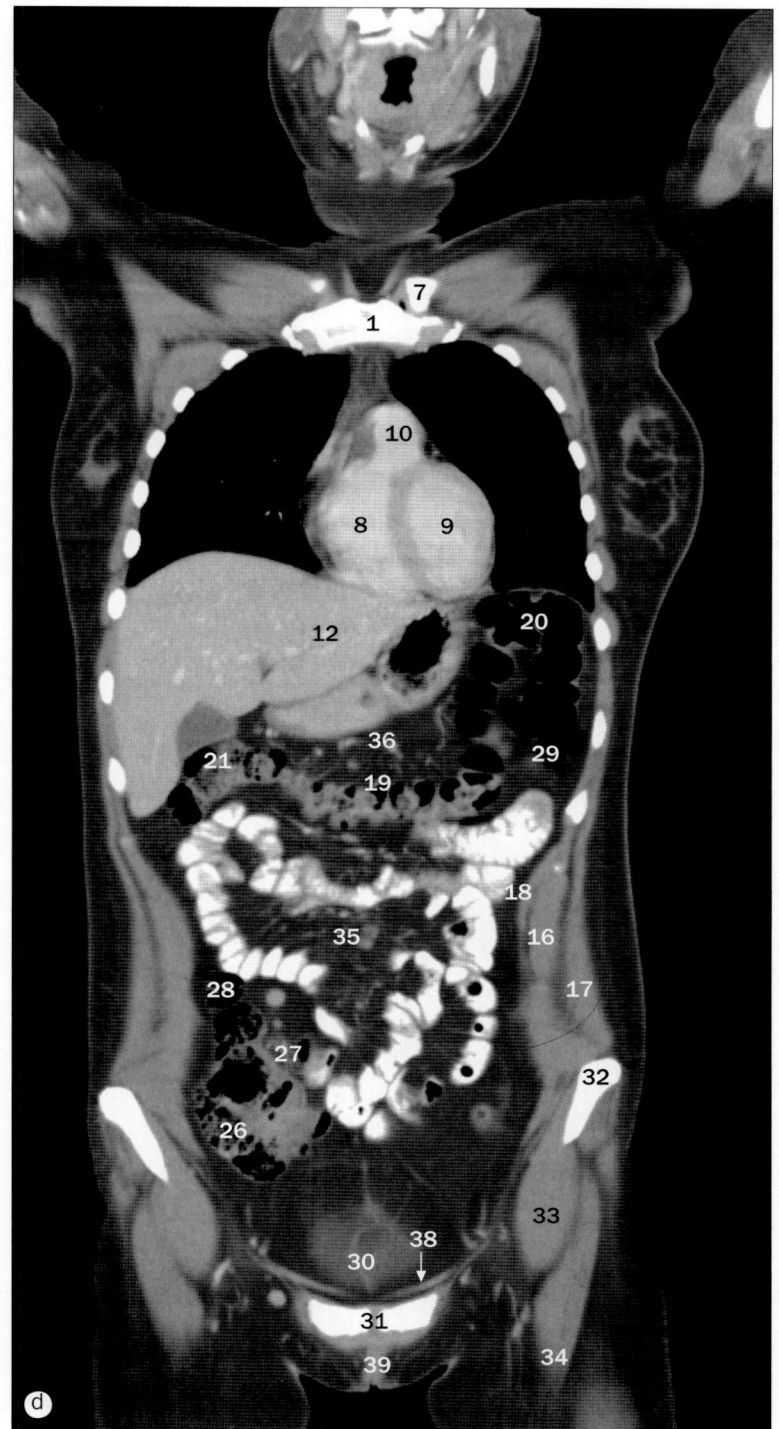

(a)–(d) Sequential coronal CT images of the chest, abdomen and pelvis in a female, from anterior to posterior.

22 Fundus of stomach	29 Descending colon	36 Transverse mesocolon
23 Body of stomach	30 Urinary bladder	37 Pectineus muscle
24 Antrum of stomach	31 Pubic symphysis	38 Levator ani muscle
25 Jejunum	32 Iliac crest	39 Labium majus
26 Caecum	33 Iliopsoas muscle	40 Right hemidiaphragm
27 Ileum	34 Sartorius muscle	41 Left hemidiaphragm
28 Ascending colon	35 Small bowel mesentery	

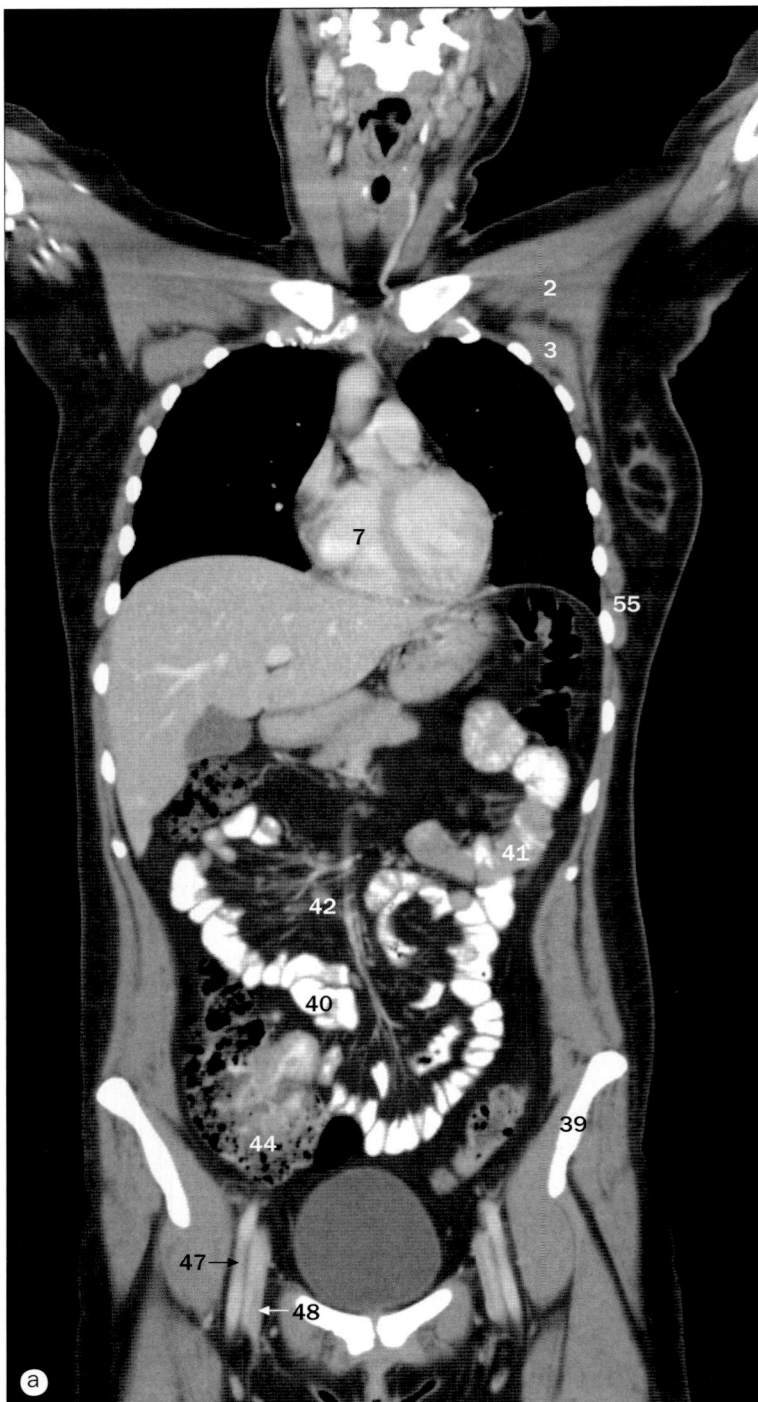

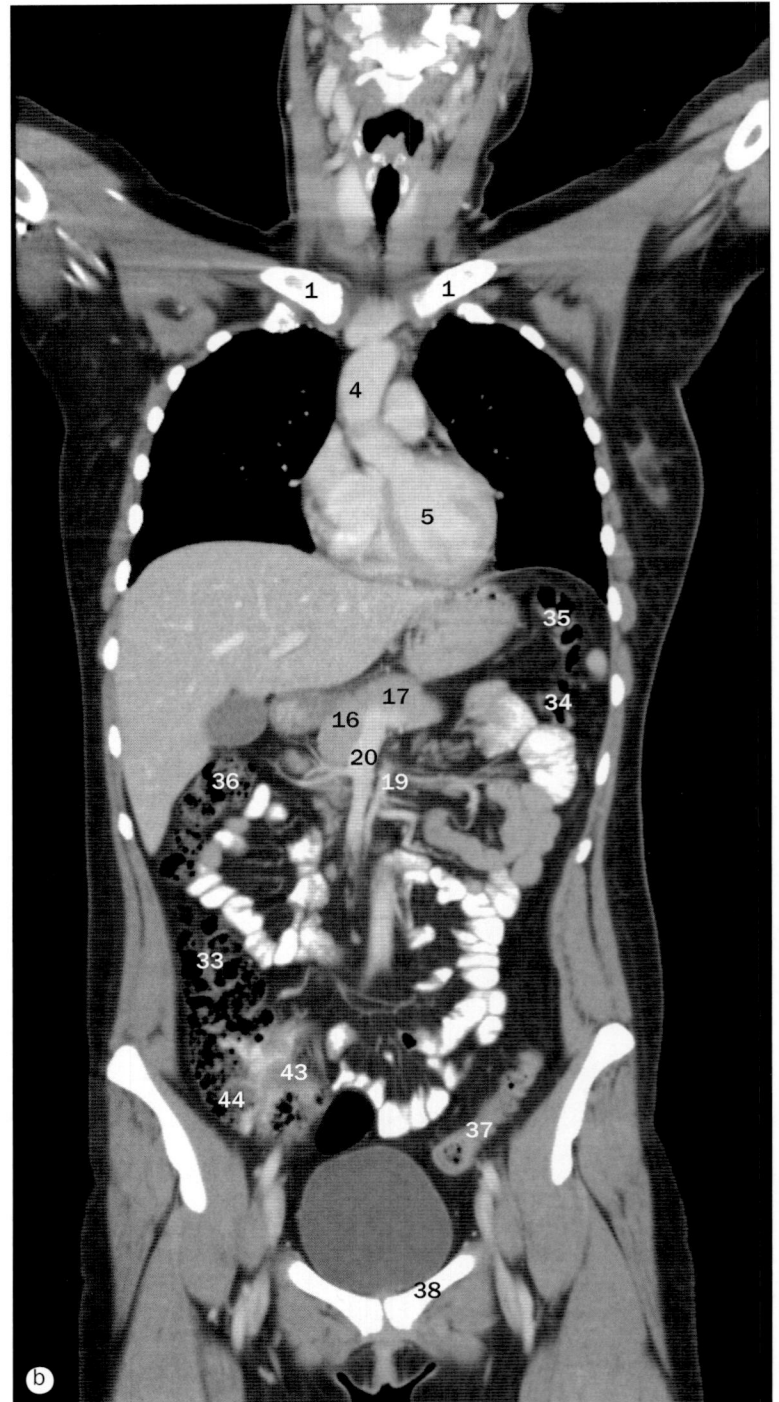

(a)–(d) Sequential coronal CT images of the chest, abdomen and pelvis in a female, from anterior to posterior.

1 Clavicle	11 Brachiocephalic trunk	21 Splenic vein
2 Pectoralis major muscle	12 Right lung	22 Portal vein
3 Pectoralis minor muscle	13 Left lung	23 Gall bladder
4 Ascending aorta	14 Right lobe of liver	24 Inferior vena cava
5 Left ventricle	15 Left lobe of liver	25 Aorta
6 Pulmonary artery	16 Head of pancreas	26 Right common iliac artery
7 Right ventricle	17 Neck of pancreas	27 Left common iliac artery
8 Right atrium	18 Body of pancreas	28 Psoas muscle
9 Superior vena cava	19 Superior mesenteric artery (SMA)	29 Iliacus muscle
10 Left brachiocephalic vein	20 Superior mesenteric vein (SMV)	30 Iliopsoas muscle

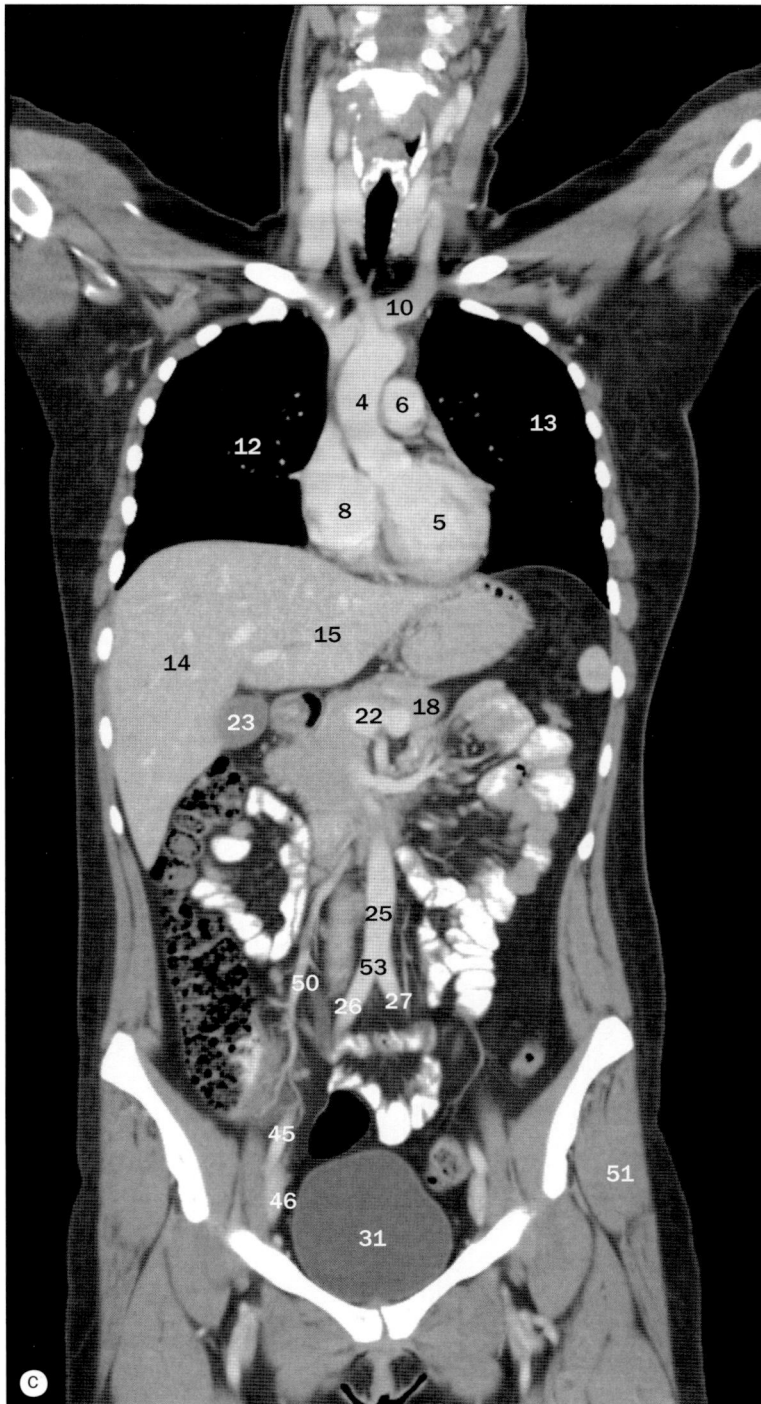

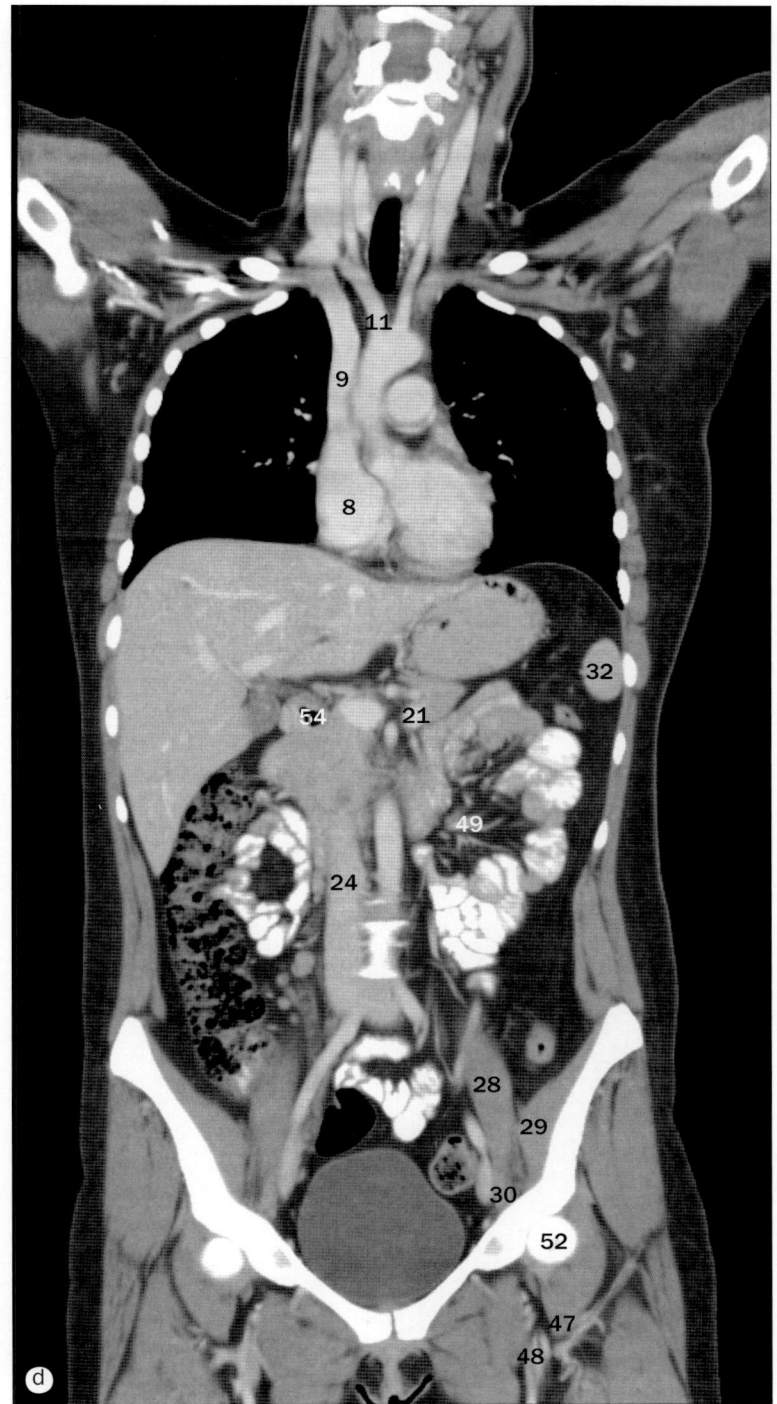

(a)–(d) Sequential coronal CT images of the chest, abdomen and pelvis in a female, from anterior to posterior.

31 Urinary bladder	**40** Ileum	**49** Jejunal branches of SMA
32 Spleen	**41** Jejunum	**50** Ileal branches of SMA
33 Ascending colon	**42** Small bowel mesentery	**51** Gluteus medius muscle
34 Descending colon	**43** Terminal ileum	**52** Head of femur
35 Left colic flexure	**44** Caecum	**53** Aortic bifurcation
36 Right colic flexure	**45** External iliac artery	**54** First part of duodenum
37 Sigmoid colon	**46** External iliac vein	**55** Serratus anterior muscle
38 Superior pubic ramus	**47** Femoral artery	
39 Ilium	**48** Femoral vein	

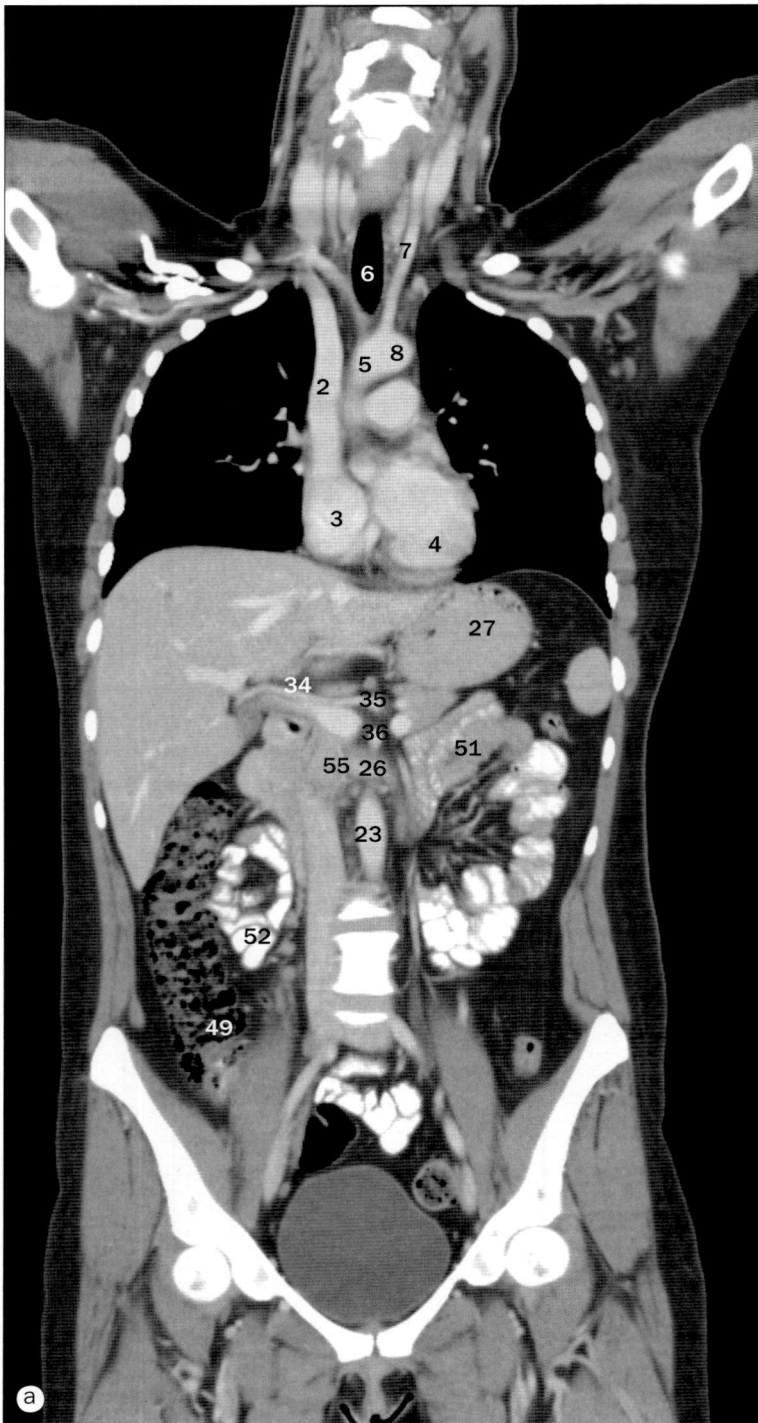

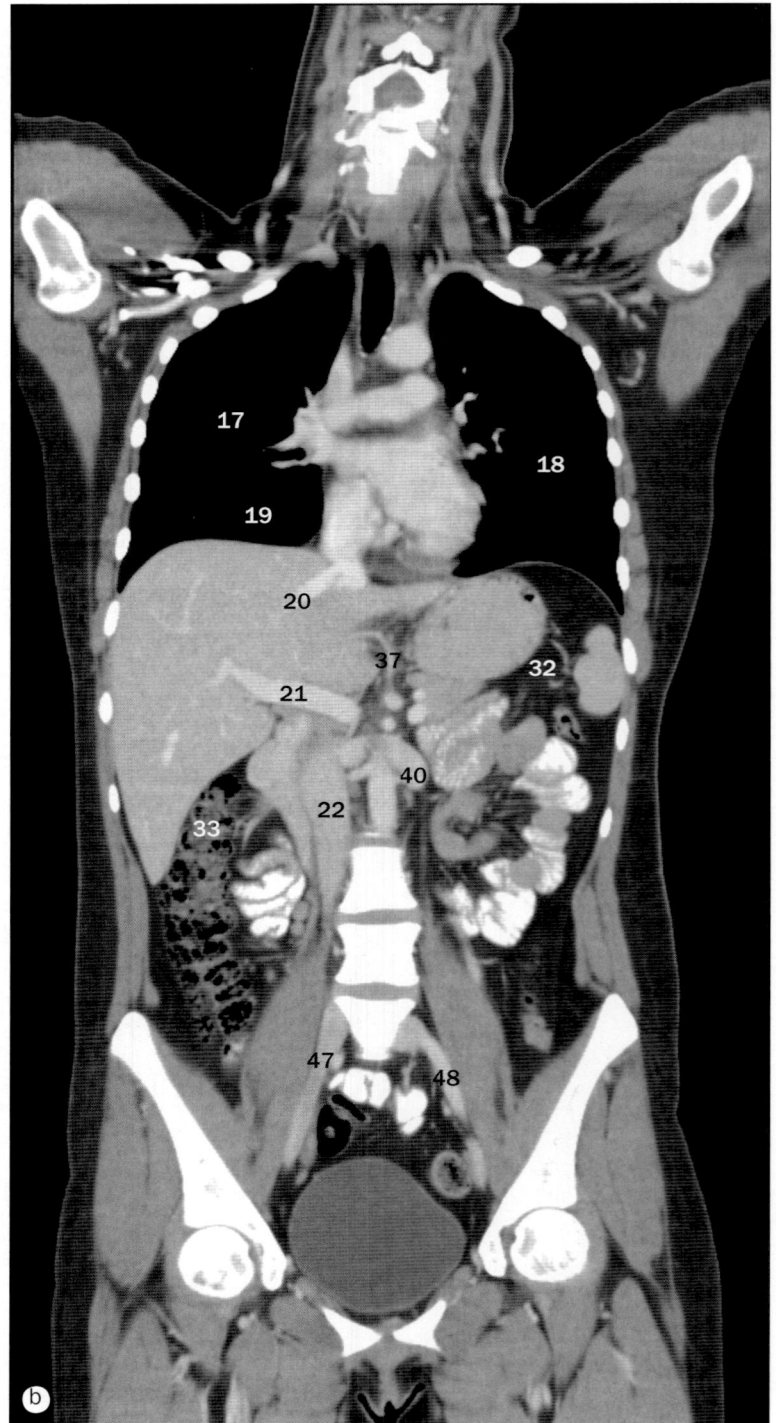

(a)–(d) Sequential coronal CT images of the chest, abdomen and pelvis in a female, from anterior to posterior.

1 Oesophagus	12 Right upper lobe bronchus	23 Aorta
2 Superior vena cava	13 Bronchus intermedius	24 Right kidney
3 Right atrium	14 Left main bronchus	25 Right renal artery
4 Left ventricle	15 Left upper lobe bronchus	26 Left renal vein
5 Ascending aorta	16 Left atrium	27 Fundus of stomach
6 Trachea	17 Right lung	28 Spleen
7 Left common carotid artery	18 Left lung	29 Ascending colon
8 Aortic arch	19 Right lower lobe	30 Descending colon
9 Right pulmonary artery	20 Hepatic vein	31 Sigmoid colon
10 Left pulmonary artery	21 Portal vein	32 Left colic flexure
11 Right main bronchus	22 Inferior vena cava	33 Right colic flexure

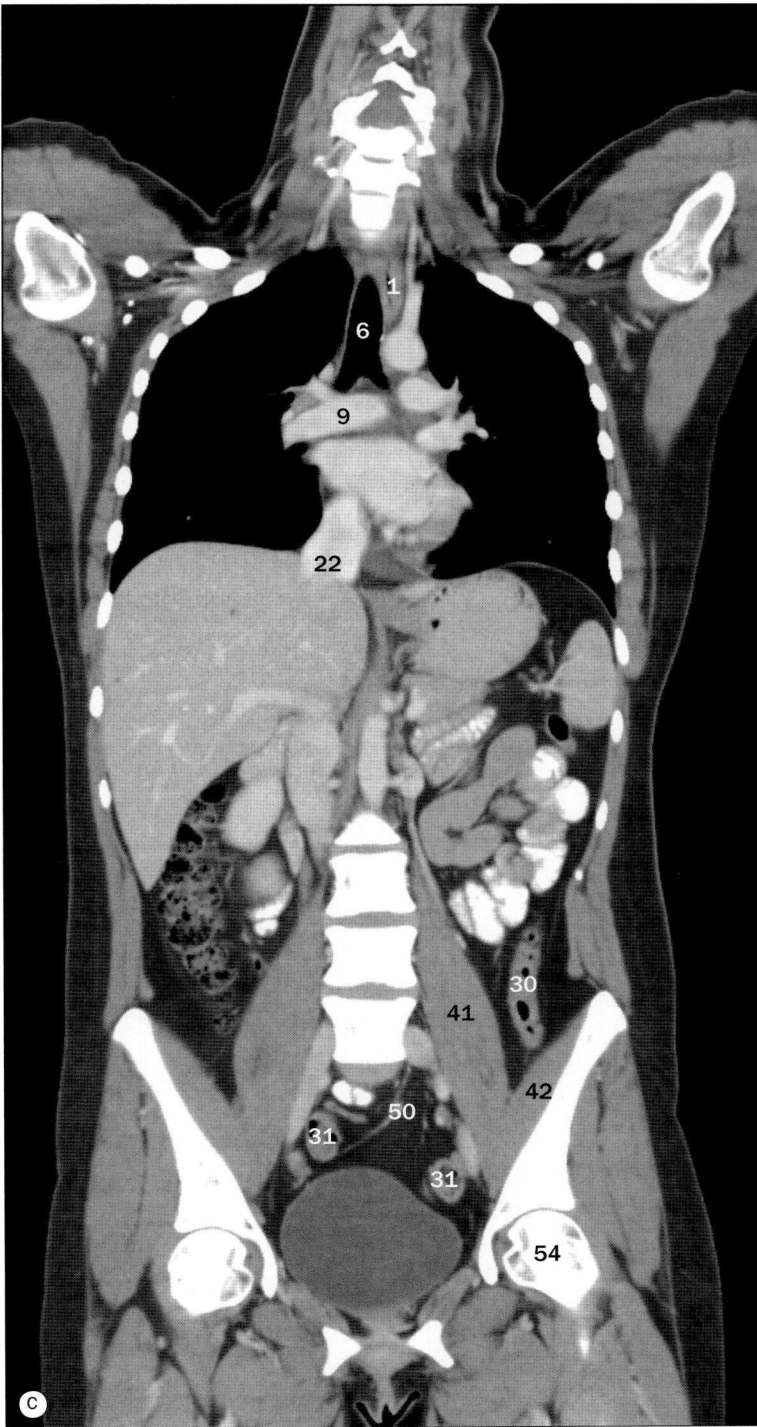

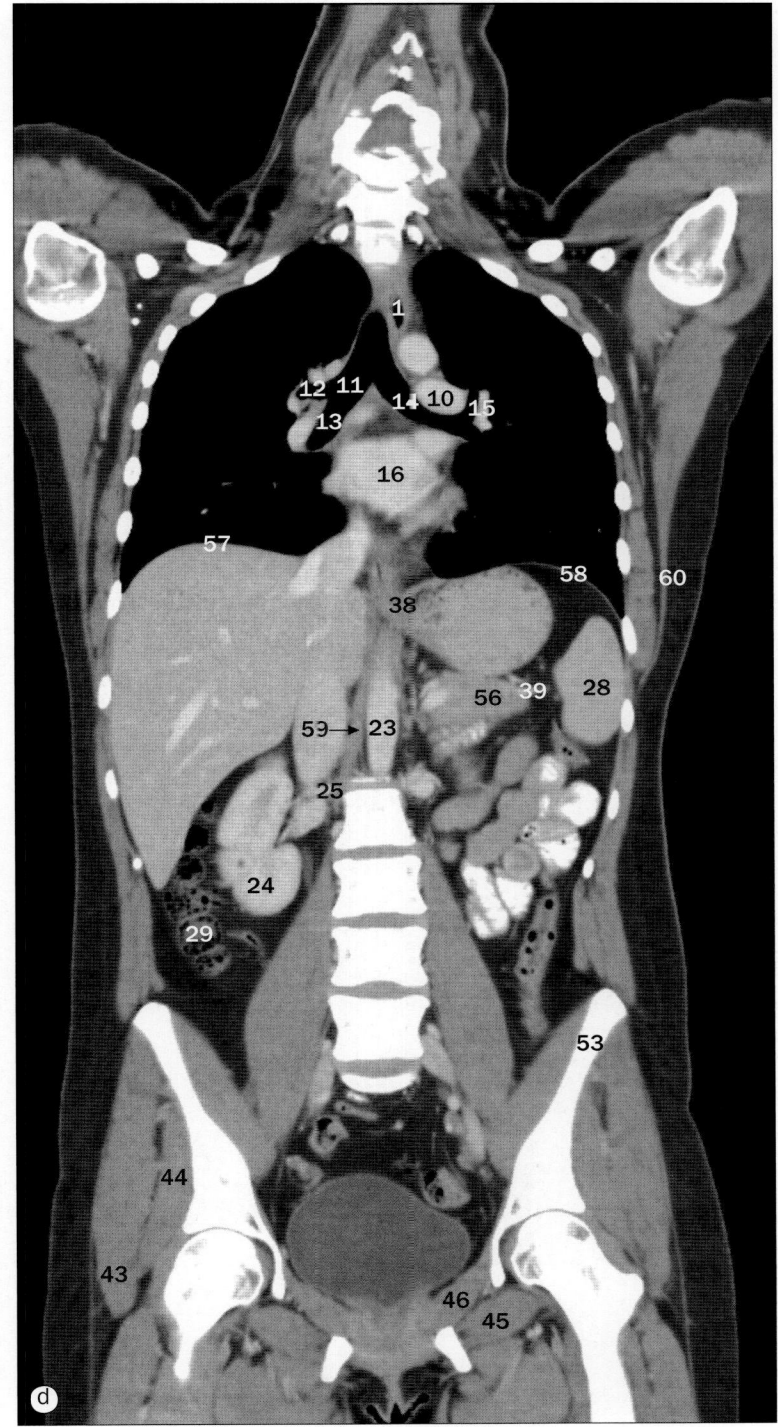

(a)–(d) Sequential coronal CT images of the chest, abdomen and pelvis in a female, from anterior to posterior.

34 Common hepatic artery
35 Coeliac axis
36 Superior mesenteric artery
37 Left gastric artery
38 Oesophagogastric junction
39 Splenic artery
40 Left renal artery
41 Psoas muscle
42 Iliacus muscle
43 Gluteus maximus muscle

44 Gluteus medius muscle
45 Obturator externus muscle
46 Obturator internus muscle
47 Right common iliac vein
48 Left common iliac vein
49 Caecum
50 Sigmoid arteries (from inferior mesenteric artery)
51 Jejunum
52 Ileum

53 Iliac bone
54 Head of femur
55 Body of pancreas
56 Tail of pancreas
57 Right hemidiaphragm
58 Left hemidiaphragm
59 Right crus of diaphragm
60 Latissimus dorsi muscle

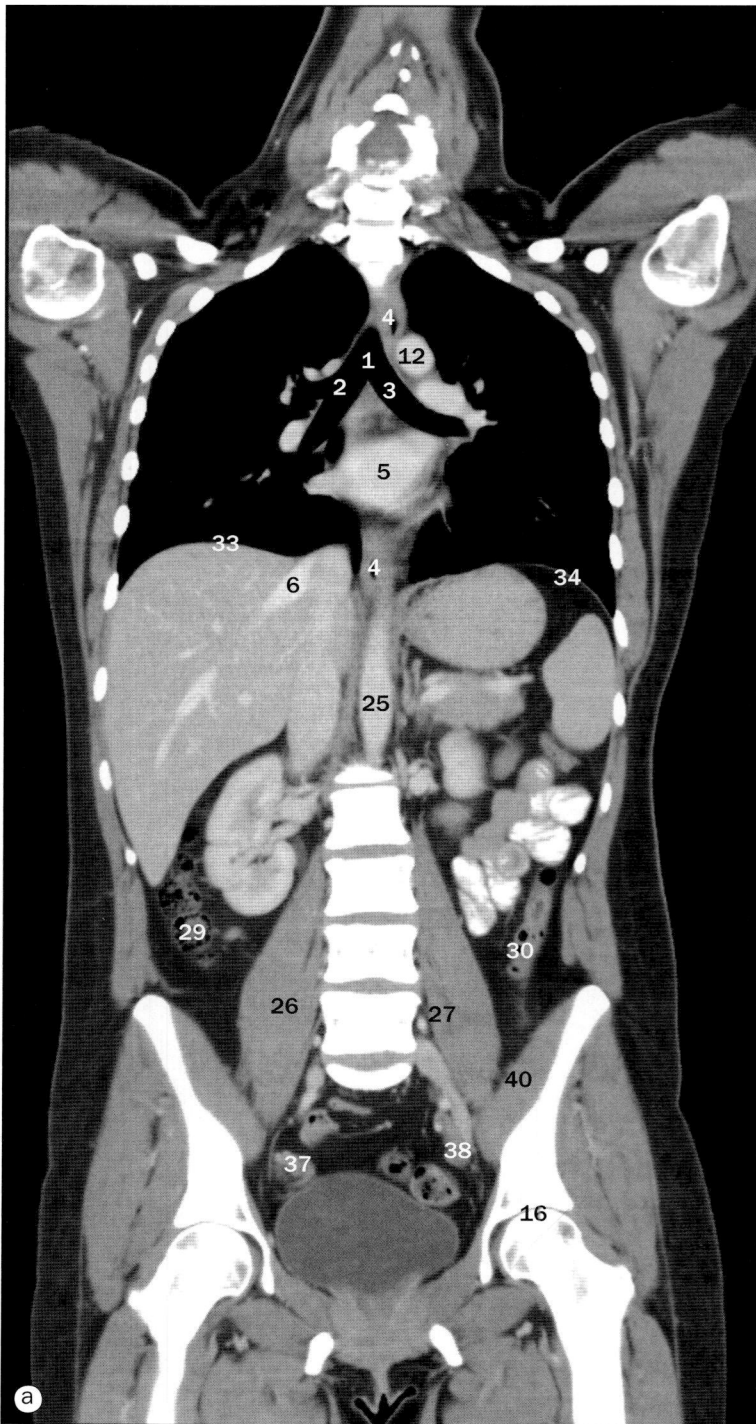

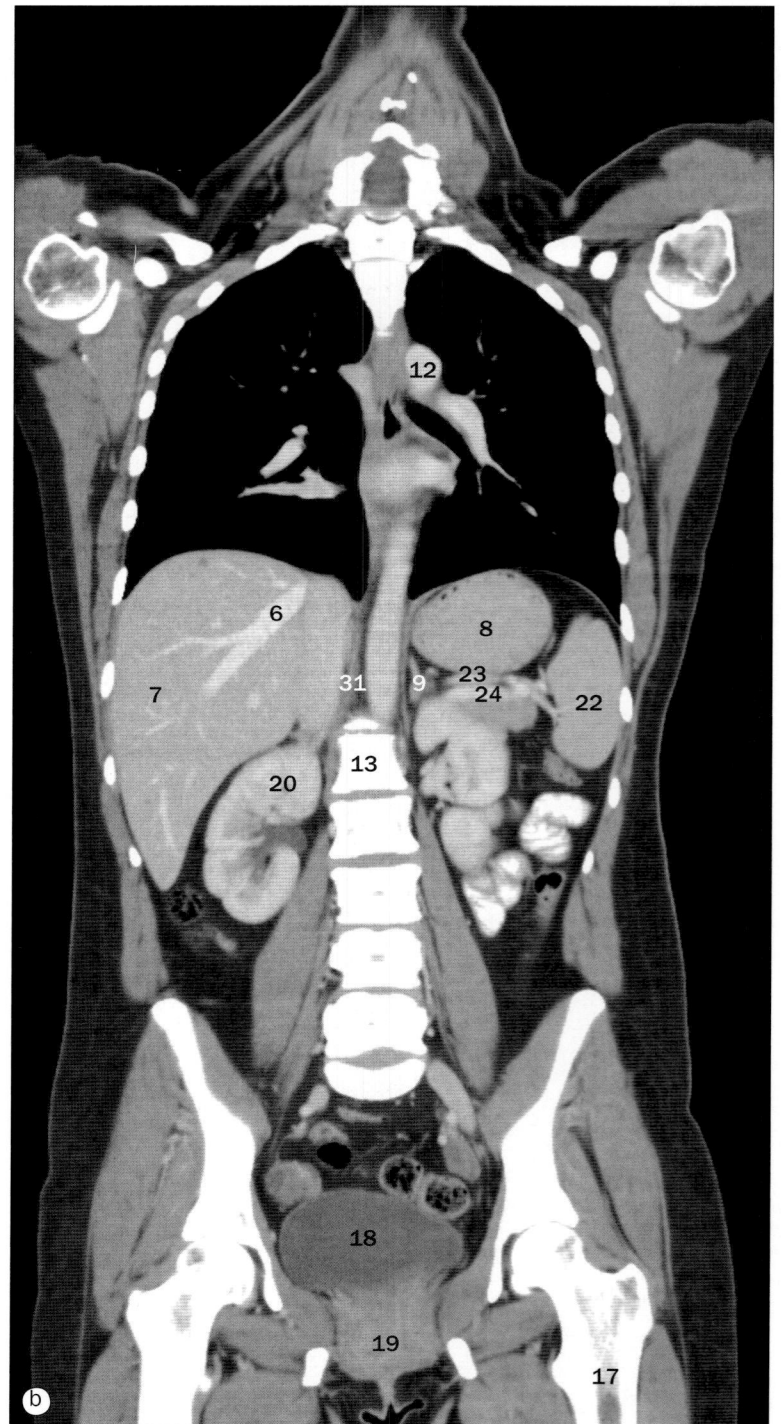

(a)–(d) Sequential coronal CT images of the chest, abdomen and pelvis in a female, from anterior to posterior.

1 Carina	9 Left suprarenal gland	17 Femur
2 Right main bronchus	10 Right suprarenal gland	18 Urinary bladder
3 Left main bronchus	11 Descending thoracic aorta	19 Vagina
4 Oesophagus	12 Aortic arch (knuckle)	20 Right kidney
5 Left atrium	13 Vertebral body of L1	21 Left kidney
6 Hepatic vein	14 Sacrum	22 Spleen
7 Right lobe of liver	15 Sacroiliac joint	23 Splenic artery
8 Fundus of stomach	16 Acetabulum	24 Splenic vein

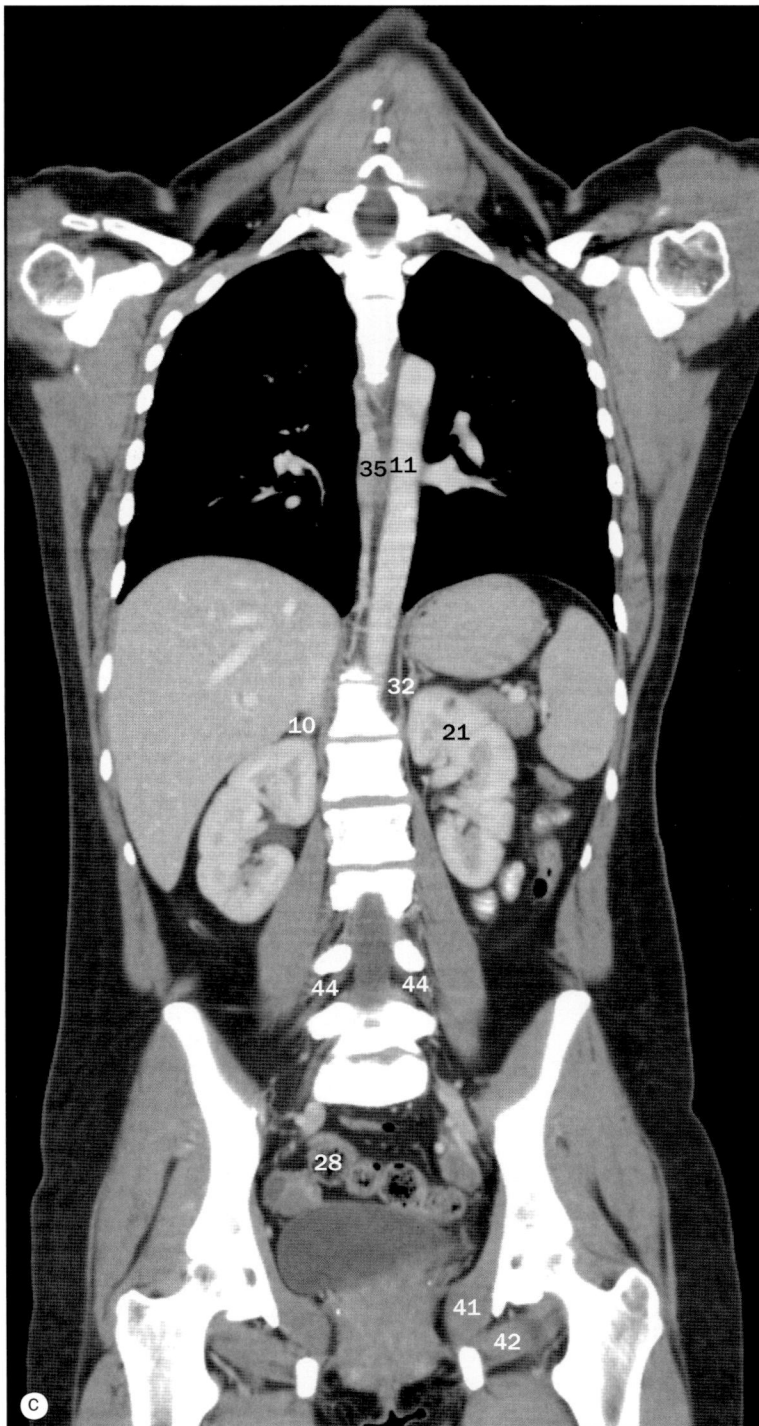

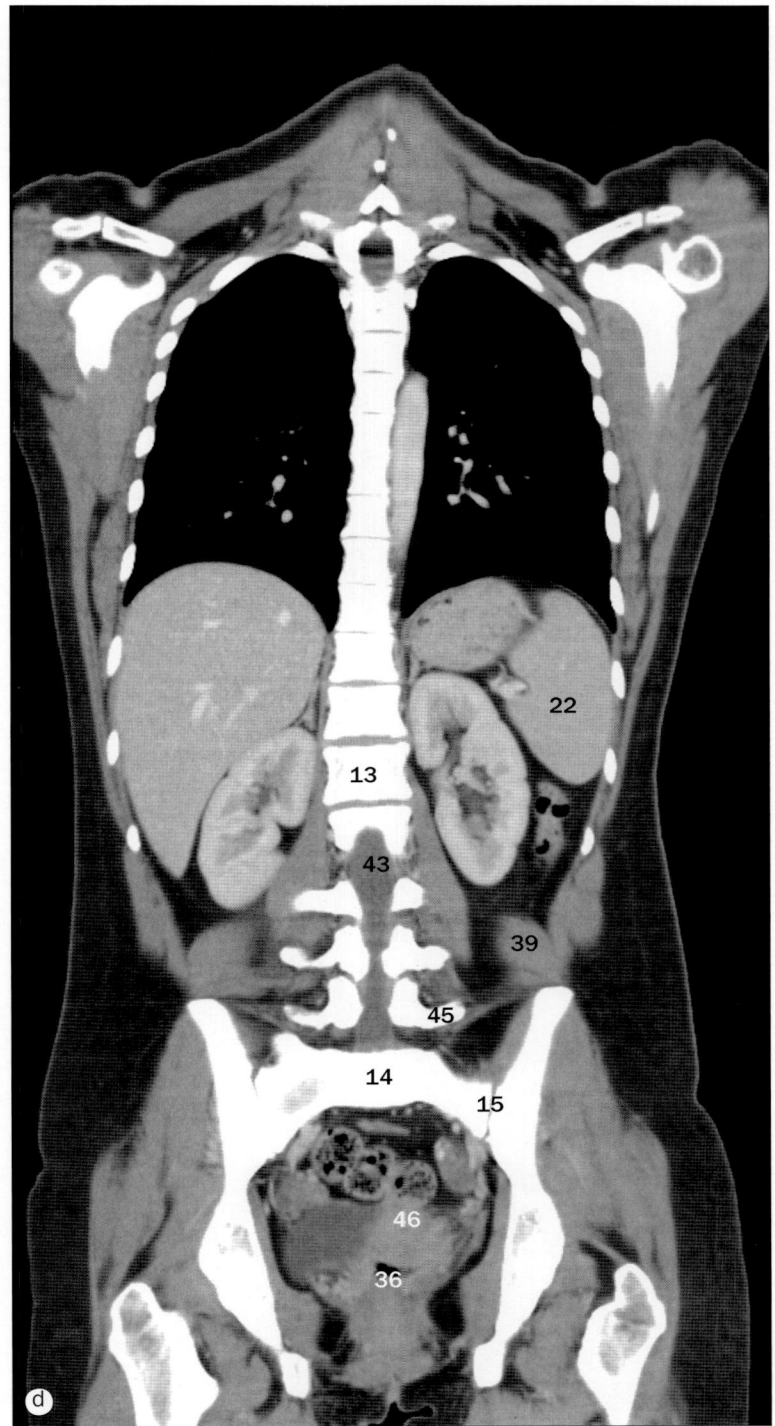

(a)–(d) Sequential coronal CT images of the chest, abdomen and pelvis in a female, from anterior to posterior.

25 Abdominal aorta
26 Psoas major muscle
27 Psoas minor muscle
28 Sigmoid colon
29 Ascending colon
30 Descending colon
31 Right crus of diaphragm
32 Left crus of diaphragm

33 Right hemidiaphragm
34 Left hemidiaphragm
35 Azygos vein
36 Rectum
37 Right internal iliac vessels
38 Left internal iliac vessels
39 Quadratus lumborum muscle
40 Iliacus muscle

41 Obturator internus muscle
42 Obturator externus muscle
43 Spinal canal
44 Lumbar nerve roots
45 Transverse process of L5
46 Uterus

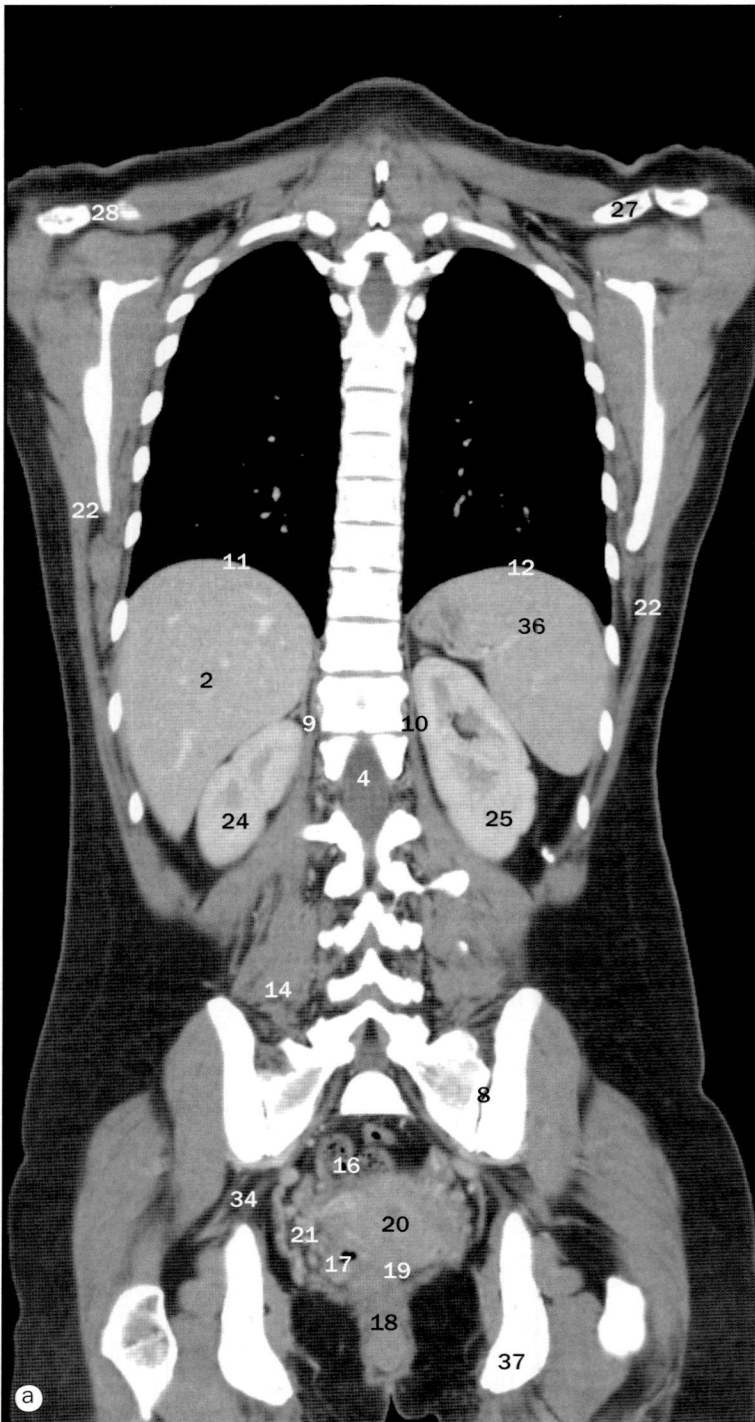

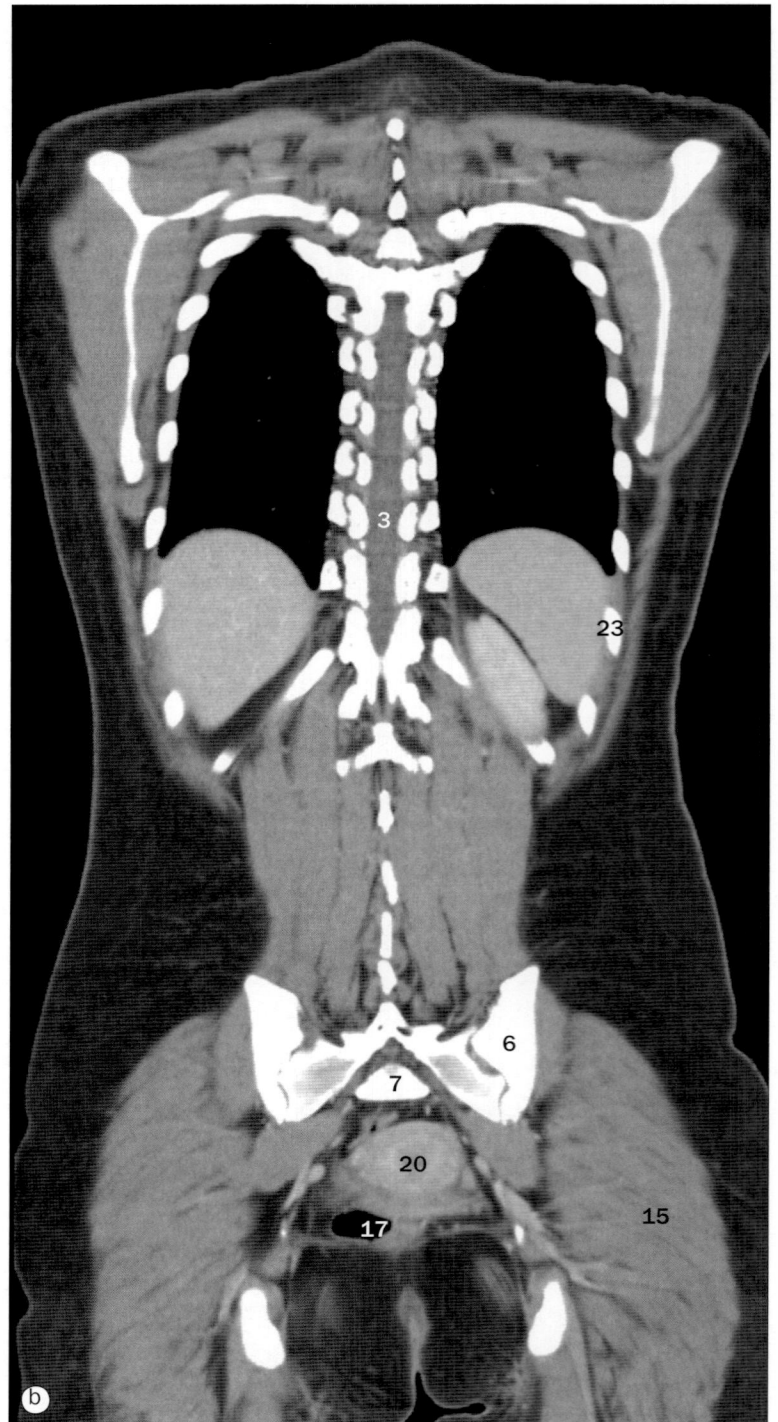

(a)–(d) Sequential coronal CT images of the chest, abdomen and pelvis in a female, from anterior to posterior.

1 Twelfth rib	**8** Sacroiliac joint	**15** Gluteus maximus muscle
2 Liver	**9** Right crus of diaphragm	**16** Sigmoid colon
3 Spinal cord	**10** Left crus of diaphragm	**17** Rectum
4 Spinal canal	**11** Right hemidiaphragm	**18** Vagina
5 Spinous process	**12** Left hemidiaphragm	**19** Cervix
6 Ilium	**13** Erector spinae muscles	**20** Uterus
7 Sacrum	**14** Quadratus lumborum muscle	**21** Uterine veins

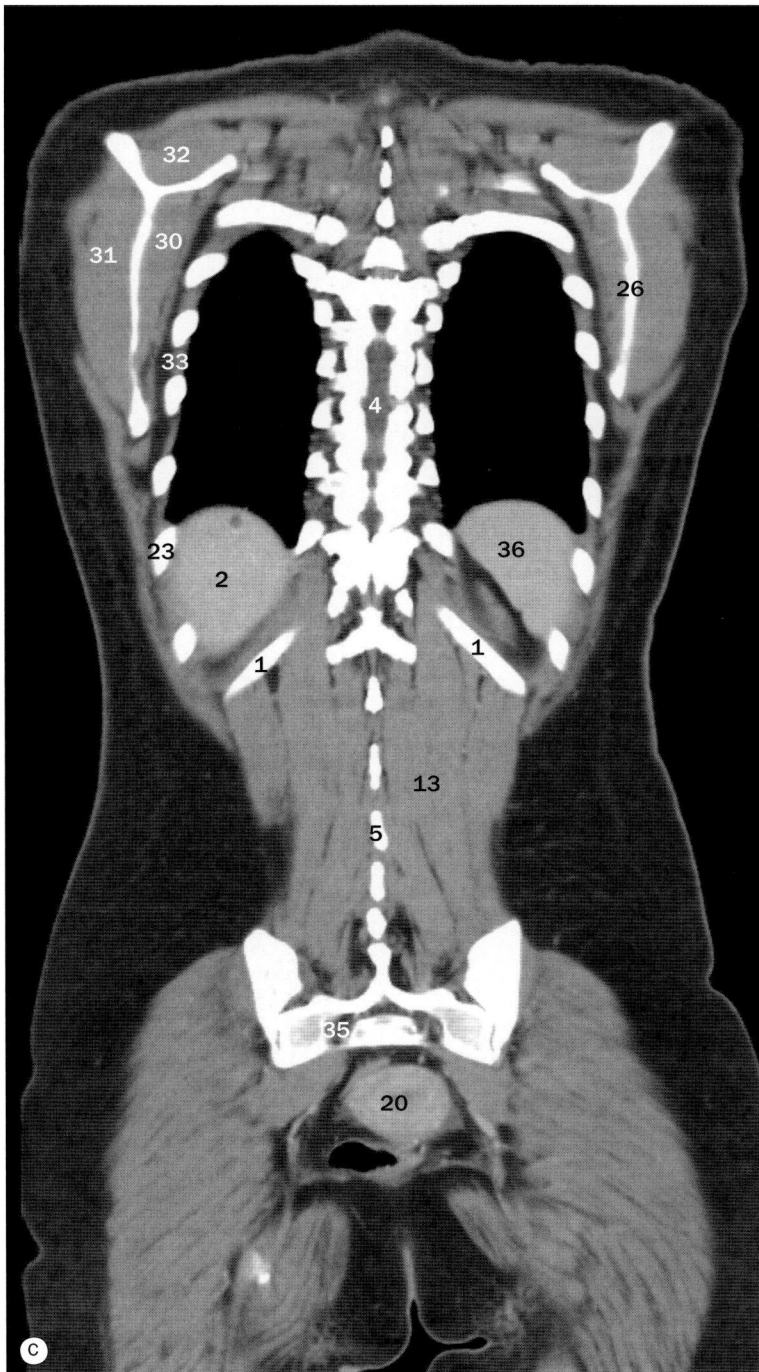

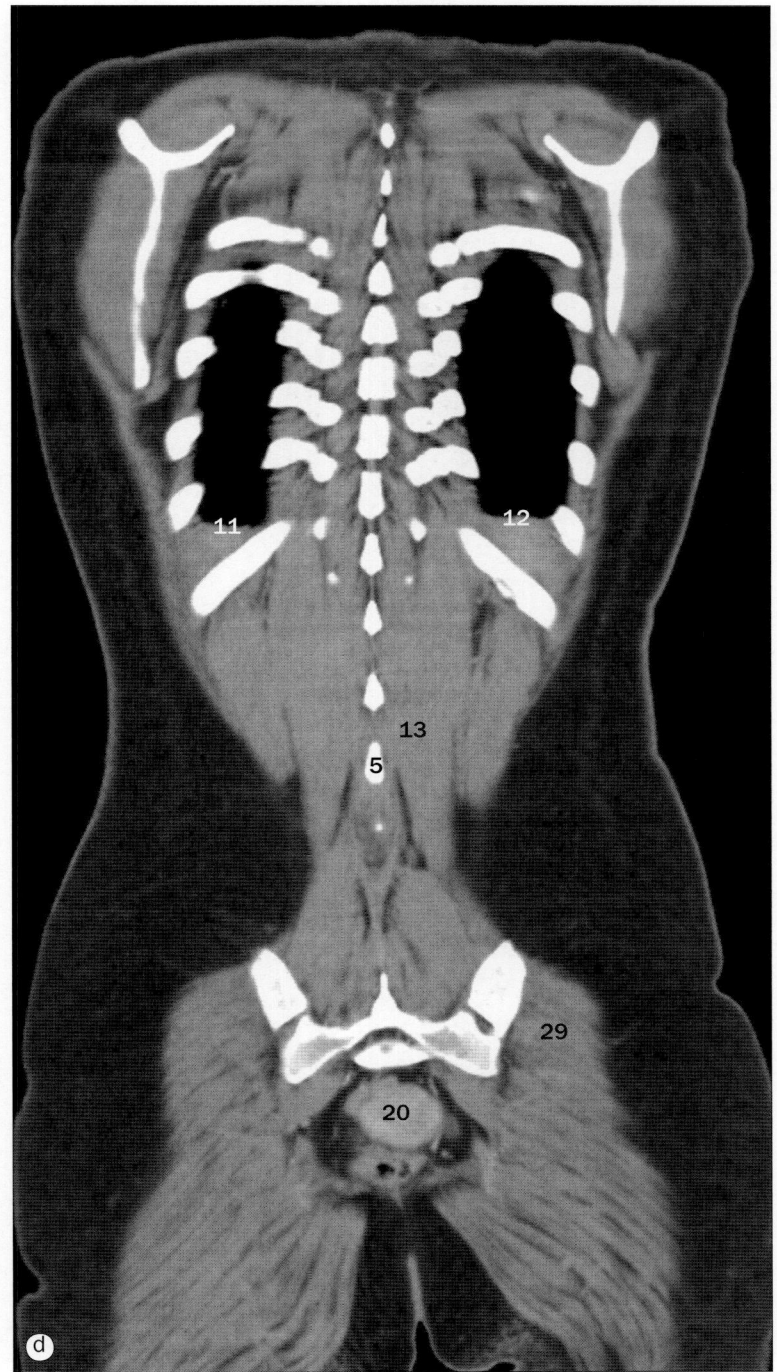

(a)–(d) Sequential coronal CT images of the chest, abdomen and pelvis in a female, from anterior to posterior.

22 Latissimus dorsi muscle	**28** Acromioclavicular joint	**34** Sciatic nerve
23 Tenth rib	**29** Gluteus medius muscle	**35** Sacral nerve foramen
24 Right kidney	**30** Subscapularis muscle	**36** Spleen
25 Left kidney	**31** Infraspinatus muscle	**37** Ischium
26 Scapula	**32** Supraspinatus muscle	
27 Clavicle	**33** Intercostal muscle	

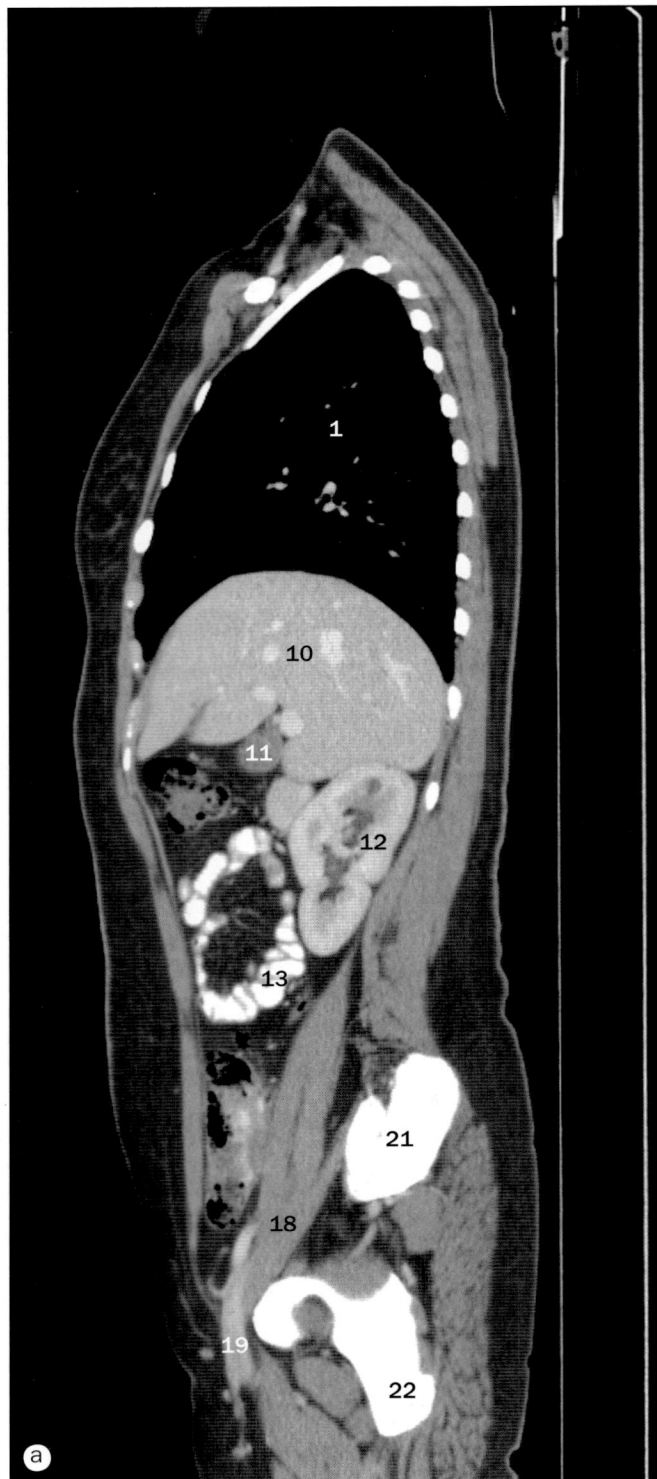

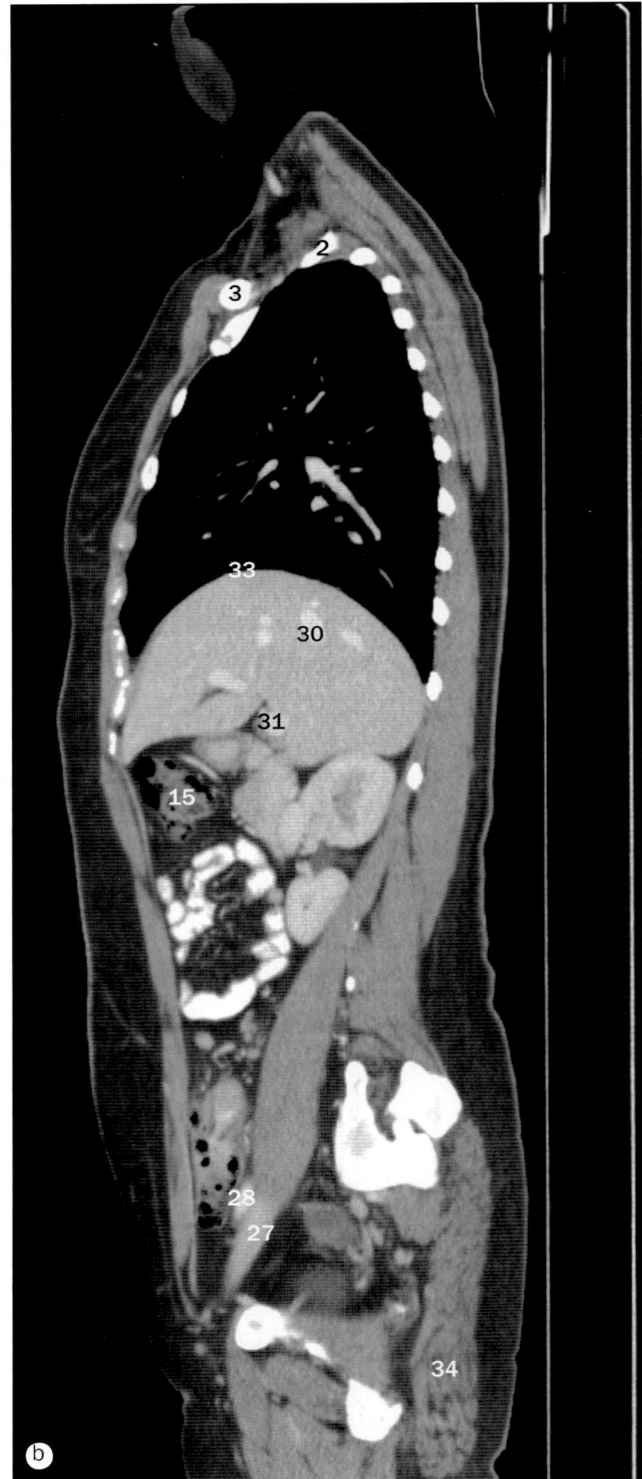

(a)–(d) Sequential sagittal CT images of the chest, abdomen and pelvis in a female, from right to left.
Note: pages 146–149 show sequential images of the same female patient.

1 Right lung	7 Inferior vena cava	13 Jejunum
2 Right first rib	8 Superior vena cava	14 Ileum
3 Right clavicle	9 Right atrium	15 Right colic flexure
4 Manubrium	10 Right lobe of liver	16 Pancreas
5 Right internal jugular vein	11 Gall bladder	17 Psoas major muscle
6 Aorta	12 Right kidney	18 Iliopsoas muscle

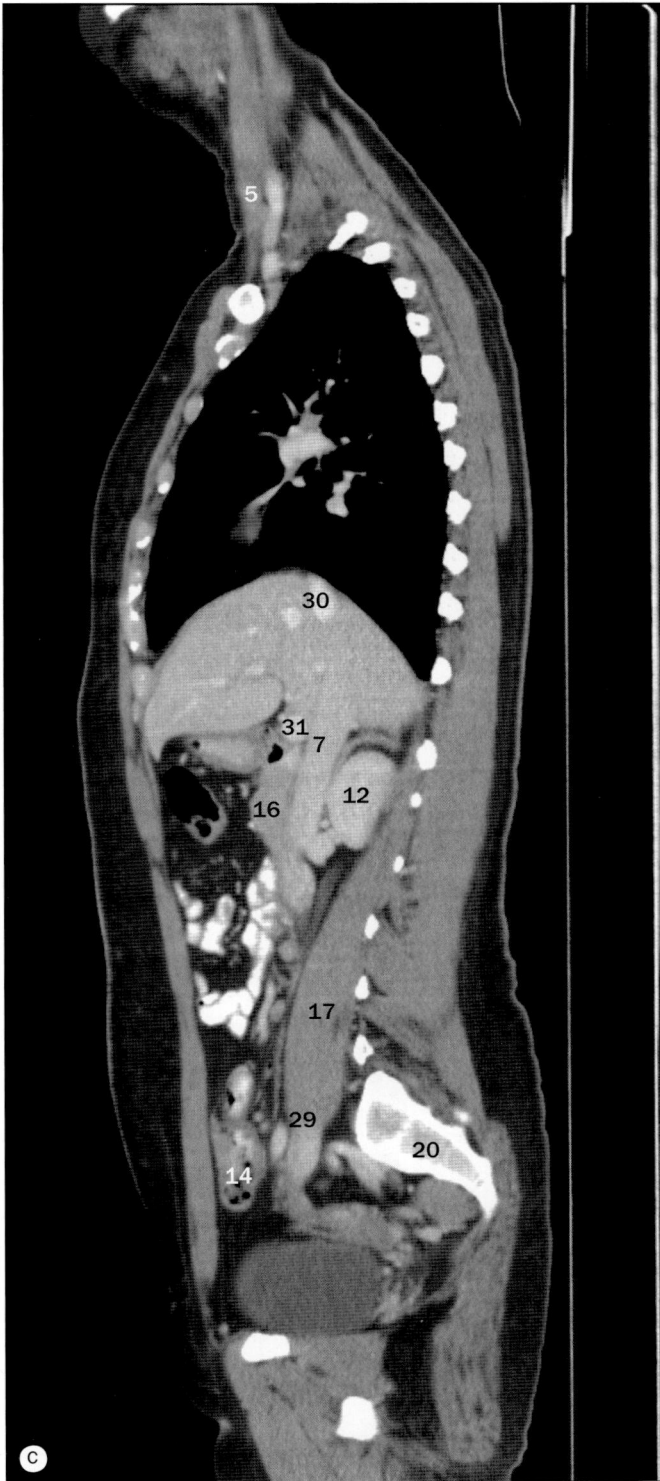

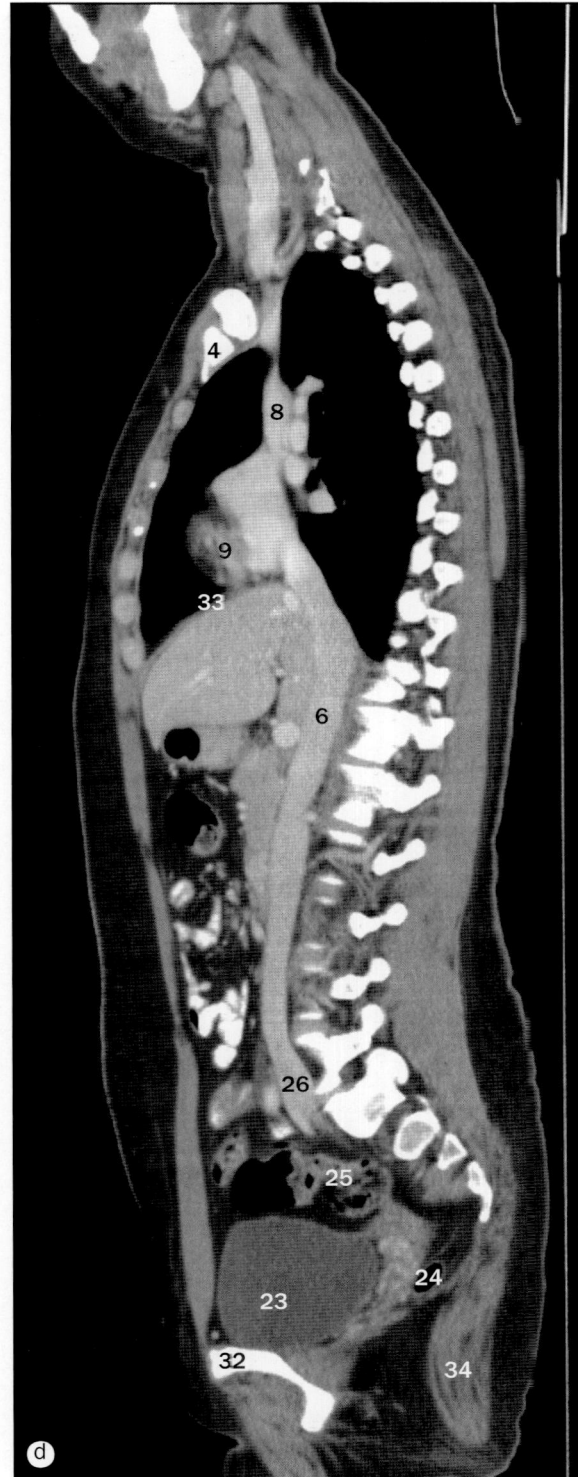

(a)–(d) Sequential sagittal CT images of the chest, abdomen and pelvis in a female, from right to left.

19 Common femoral vessels	25 Sigmoid colon	31 Portal vein
20 Sacrum	26 Right common iliac artery	32 Pubic bone
21 Ilium	27 Right external iliac vein	33 Right hemidiaphragm
22 Ischium	28 Right external iliac artery	34 Gluteus maximus muscle
23 Urinary bladder	29 Right common iliac vein	
24 Rectum	30 Hepatic vein	

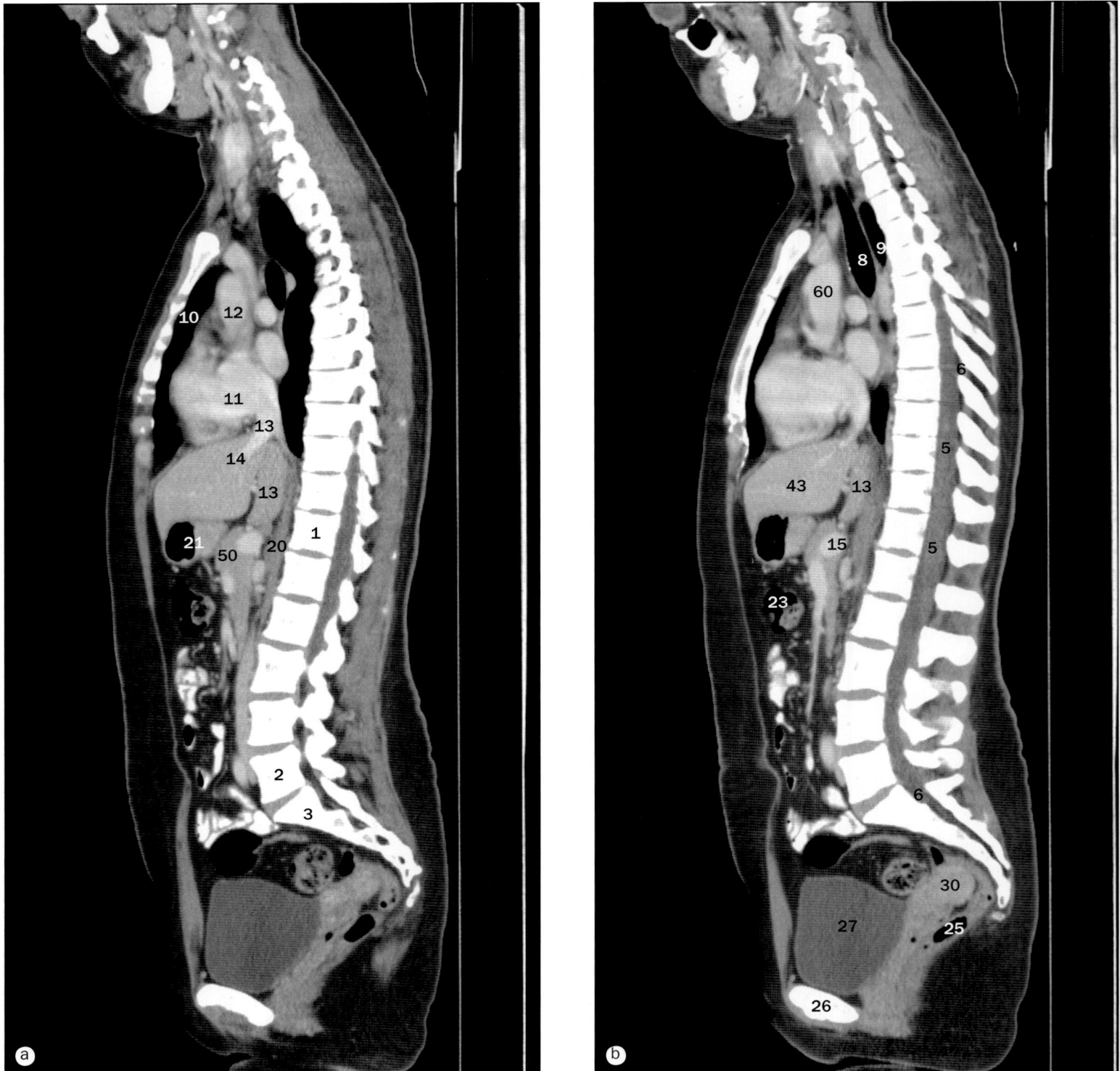

(a)–(d) Sequential sagittal CT images of the chest, abdomen and pelvis in a female, from right to left.

1 Body of T12 vertebra	11 Right atrium	21 Stomach
2 Body of L5 vertebra	12 Superior vena cava	22 Descending colon
3 Sacrum	13 Inferior vena cava	23 Transverse colon
4 Coccyx	14 Hepatic vein	24 Sigmoid colon
5 Spinal cord	15 Splenic vein	25 Rectum
6 Spinal canal	16 Superior mesenteric vein	26 Pubic bone
7 Filum terminale	17 Superior mesenteric artery	27 Urinary bladder
8 Trachea	18 Coeliac axis	28 Cervix
9 Oesophagus	19 Aorta	29 Vagina
10 Right lung	20 Right crus of diaphragm	30 Uterus

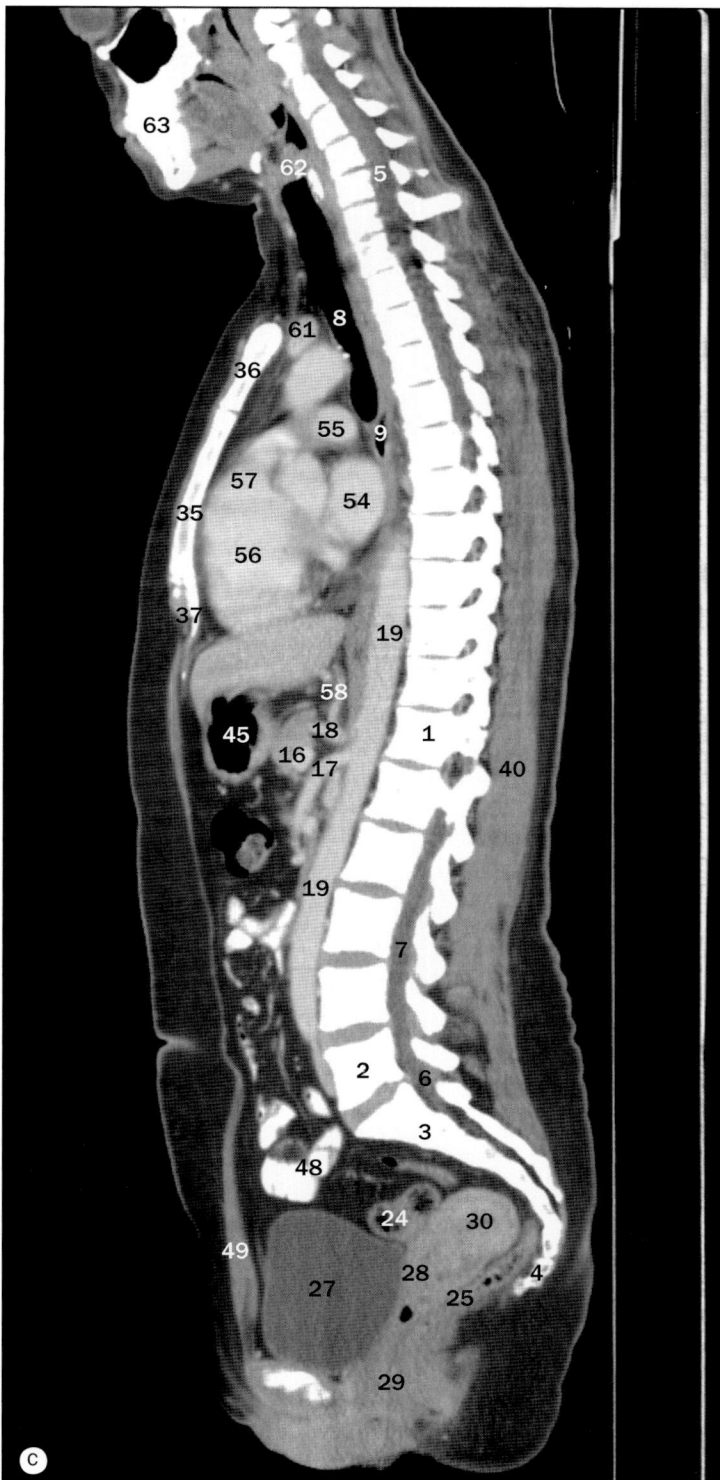

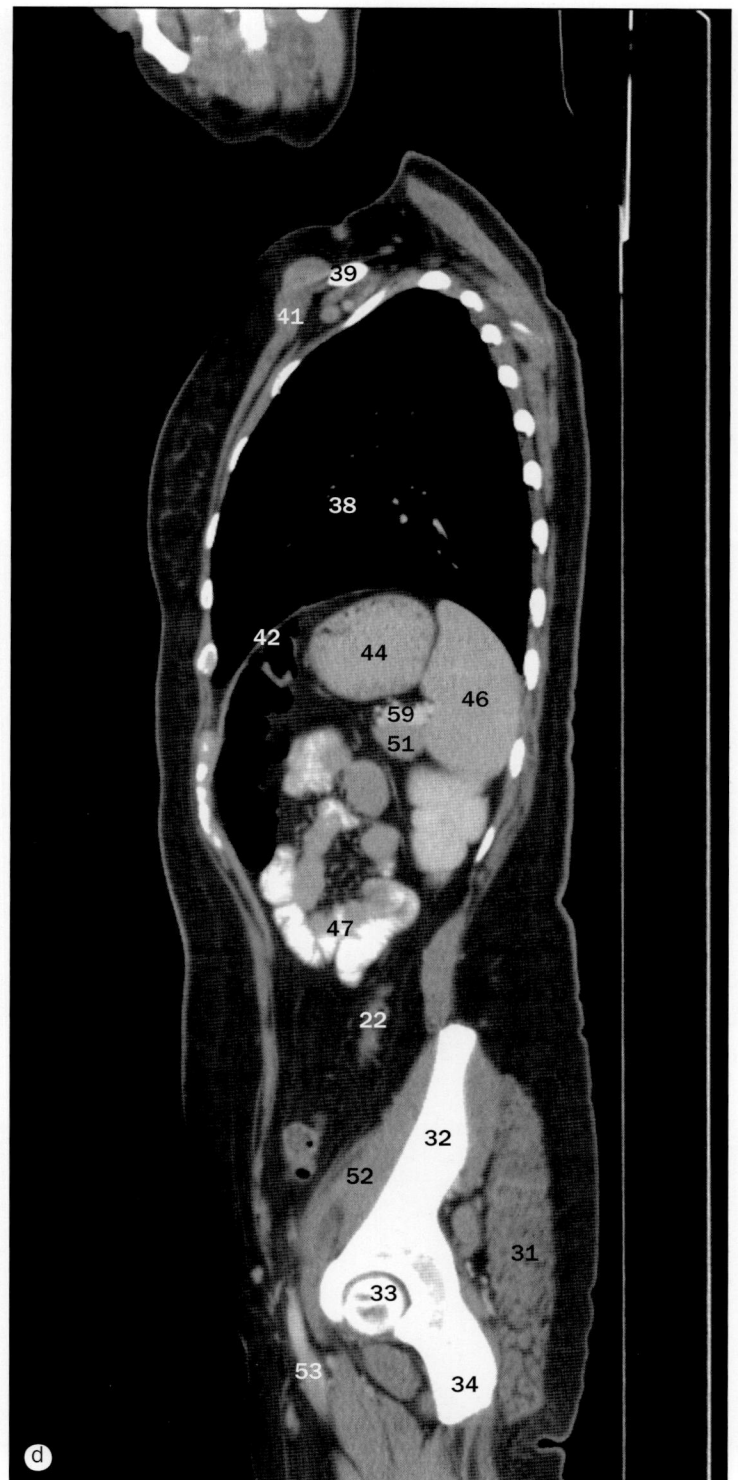

(a)–(d) Sequential sagittal CT images of the chest, abdomen and pelvis in a female, from right to left.

31 Gluteus maximus muscle	42 Left hemidiaphragm	53 Left femoral vessels
32 Ilium	43 Liver	54 Left atrium
33 Head of femur	44 Fundus of stomach	55 R ght pulmonary artery
34 Ischium	45 Body of stomach	56 R ght ventricle
35 Sternum	46 Spleen	57 Pulmonary outflow tract
36 Manubrium	47 Jejunum	58 Common hepatic artery
37 Xiphisternum	48 Ileum	59 Splenic artery
38 Left lung	49 Rectus abdominis muscle	60 Ascending thoracic aorta
39 Left clavicle	50 Body of pancreas	61 Left brachiocephalic vein
40 Erector spinae muscles	51 Tail of pancreas	62 Larynx
41 Left pectoralis major muscle	52 Iliacus muscle	63 Mandible

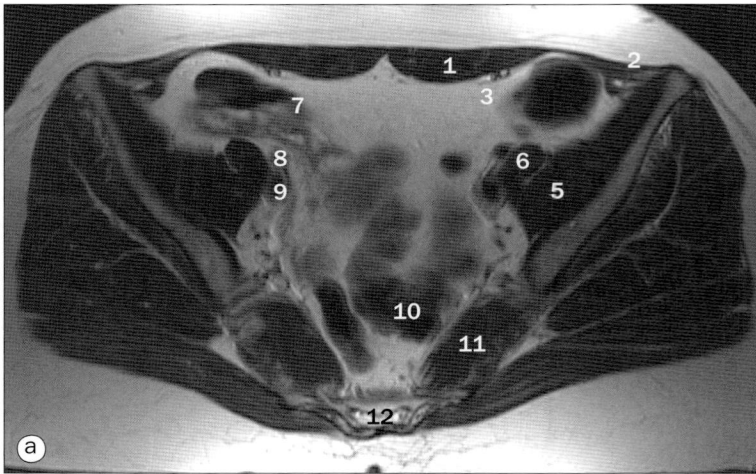

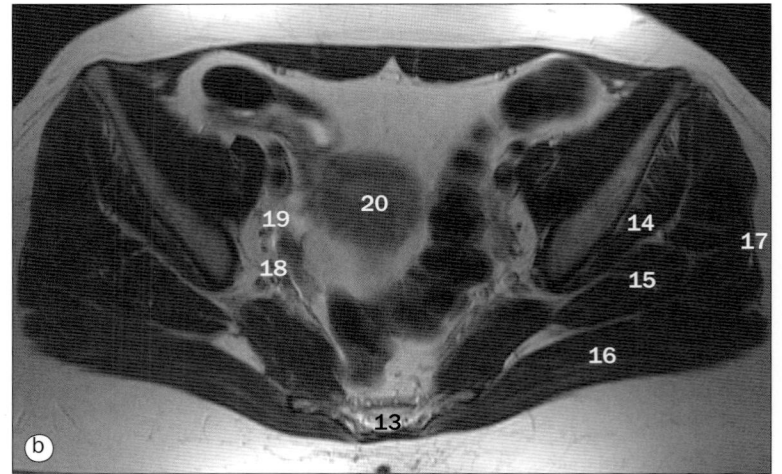

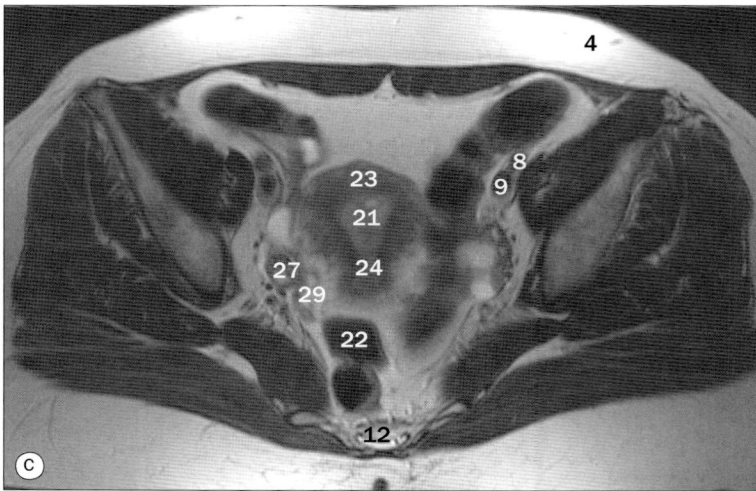

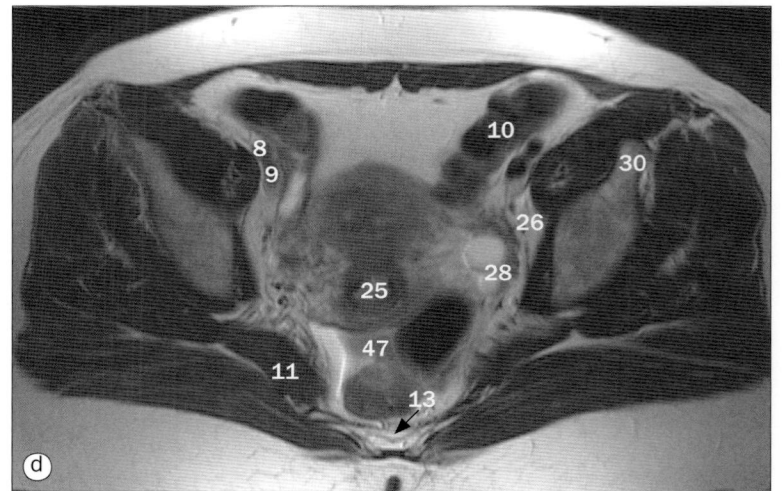

(a)–(p) Sequential axial T2w MR images of the female pelvis, from superior to inferior.

1 Rectus abdominis muscle	11 Piriformis muscle	21 Uterine cavity
2 External oblique aponeurosis	12 Sacrum	22 Rectosigmoid junction
3 Inferior epigastric vessels	13 Central sacral canal	23 Myometrium of uterus
4 Superficial epigastric vessels	14 Gluteus minimis muscle	24 Internal cervical os
5 Iliacus muscle	15 Gluteus medius muscle	25 External cervical os
6 Psoas muscle	16 Gluteus maximus muscle	26 Obturator vessels
7 Ileum	17 Fascia lata	27 Right ovary
8 External iliac artery	18 Superior gluteal vessels	28 Left ovary
9 External iliac vein	19 Ovarian vessels	29 Right uterine tube
10 Sigmoid colon	20 Uterine fundus	30 Antero-inferior iliac spine

(a)–(p) Sequential axial T2w MR images of the female pelvis, from superior to inferior.

31 Round ligament of uterus	41 Obturator internus muscle	51 Ischio-anal fossa
32 Acetabular roof	42 Bladder	52 Greater trochanter of femur
33 Rectus femoris muscle	43 Rectum	53 Natal cleft
34 Ischial spine	44 Mesorectum	54 Common femoral artery
35 Ligamentum teres	45 Waldeyer's fascia	55 Common femoral vein
36 Sacrospinous ligament	46 Ischium	56 Femoral nerve branches
37 Iliopsoas muscle	47 Recto-uterine pouch (of Douglas)	57 Transverse cervical ligament
38 Cervical wall	48 Posterior vaginal fornix	58 Uterosacral ligament
39 Coccyx	49 Cervical os	59 Broad ligament
40 Sciatic nerve	50 Levator ani muscle (puborectalis)	

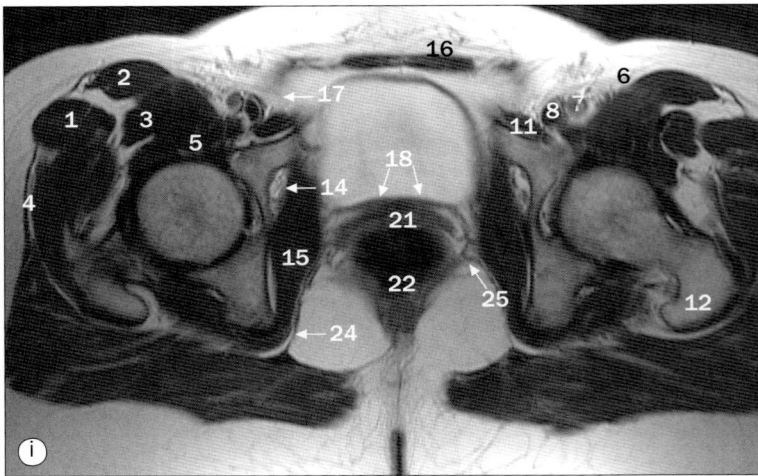

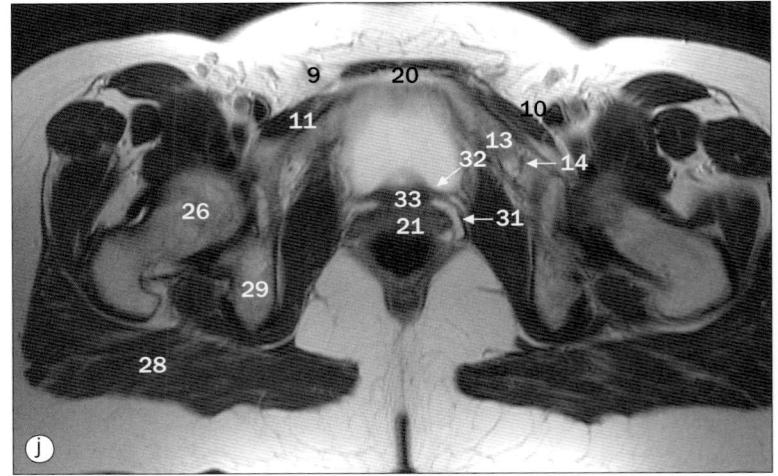

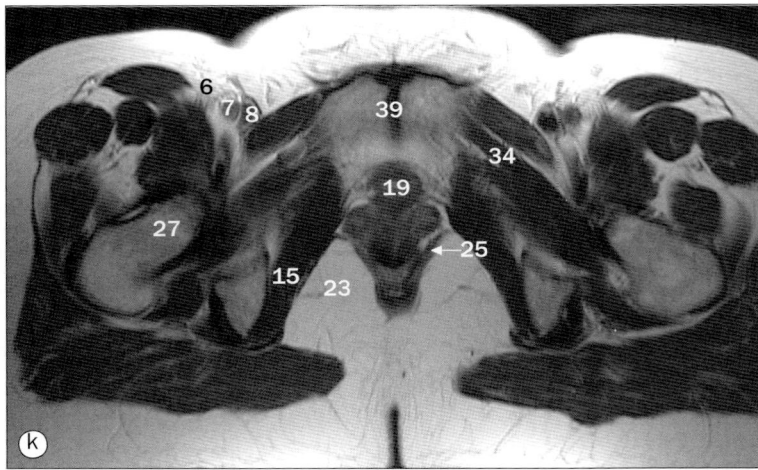

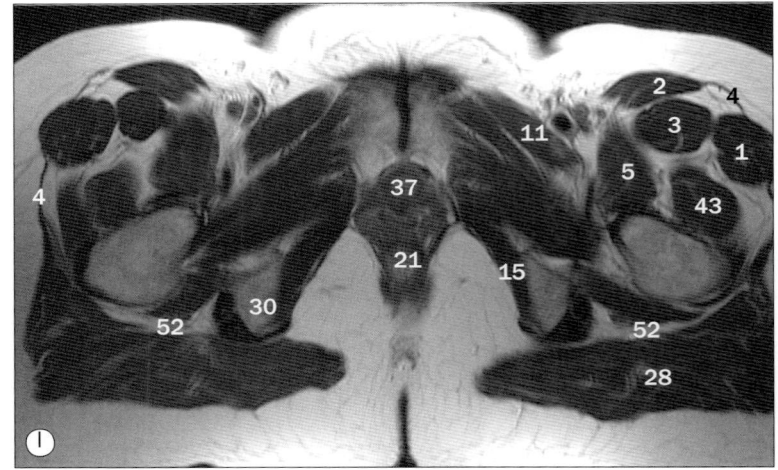

(a)–(p) Sequential axial T2w MR images of the female pelvis, from superior to inferior.

1 Tensor fasciae latae muscle	11 Pectineus	21 Vagina
2 Sartorius muscle	12 Greater trochanter of femur	22 Rectum
3 Rectus femoris muscle	13 Superior pubic ramus	23 Ischio-anal fossa
4 Fascia lata	14 Obturator vessels	24 Pudendal neurovascular bundle (Alcock's
5 Iliopsoas muscle	15 Obturator internus muscle	canal)
6 Femoral nerve branches	16 Rectus abdominis muscle	25 Puborectalis muscle
7 Common femoral artery	17 Inguinal ligament	26 Femoral head
8 Common femoral vein	18 Bladder base	27 Femoral neck
9 Round ligament of the uterus	19 Bladder neck	28 Gluteus maximus muscle
10 Femoral canal	20 Extraperitoneal fat (cave of Retzius)	29 Ischium

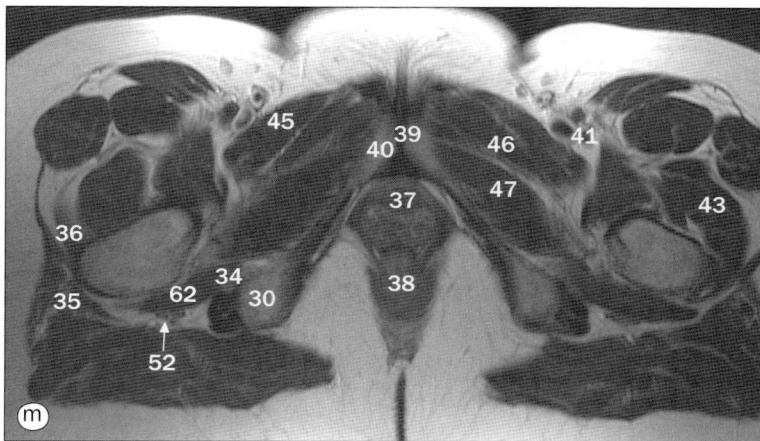

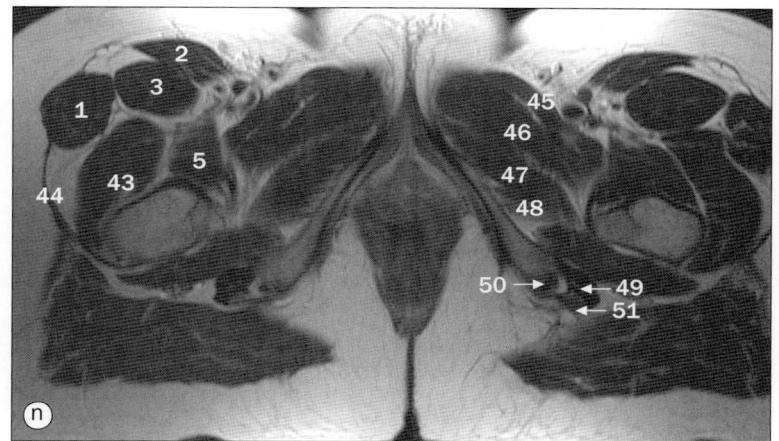

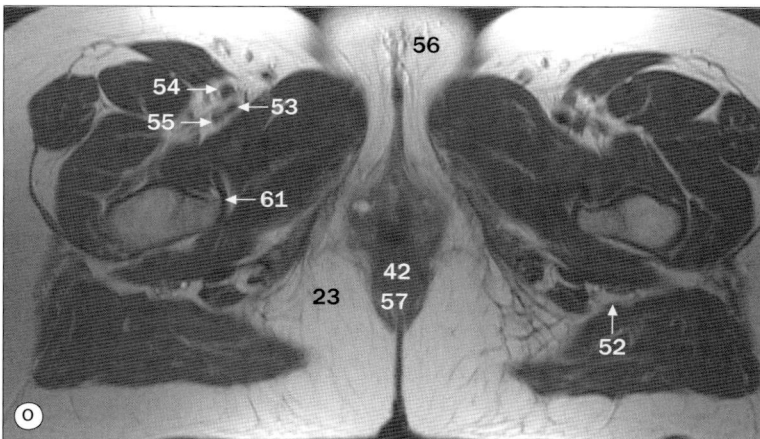

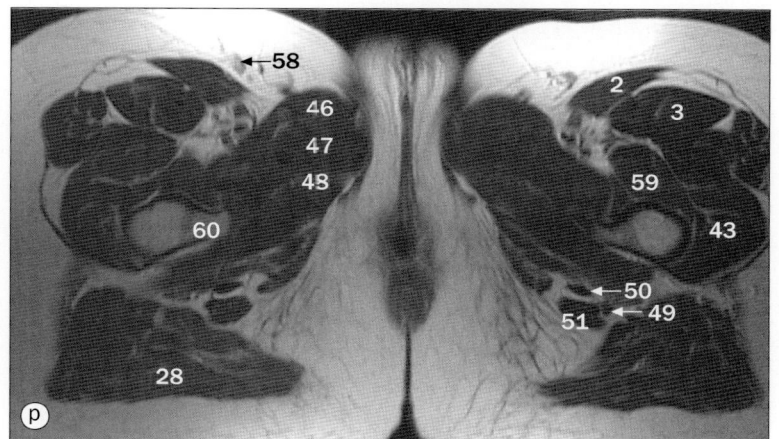

(a)–(p) Sequential axial T2w MR images of the female pelvis, from superior to inferior.

30 Ischial tuberosity	41 Profunda femoris artery	52 Sciatic nerve
31 Ureter	42 Perineal body	53 Superficial femoral vein
32 Vesico-ureteric junction	43 Vastus lateralis muscle	54 Superficial femoral artery
33 Trigone of bladder	44 Iliotibial tract	55 Profunda femoris vessels
34 Obturator externus muscle	45 Pectineus muscle	56 Labium majorum
35 Gluteus medius muscle	46 Adductor longus muscle	57 Anal canal
36 Gluteus minimis muscle (tendinous	47 Adductor brevis muscle	58 Long saphenous vein
insertion)	48 Adductor magnus muscle	59 Vastus intermedius muscle
37 Urethra	49 Semimembanosus muscle	60 Lesser trochanter of femur
38 Anorectal junction	50 Semitendinosus muscle	61 Iliopsoas insertion
39 Symphysis pubis	51 Biceps femoris muscle	62 Quadratus femoris muscle
40 Pubic body		

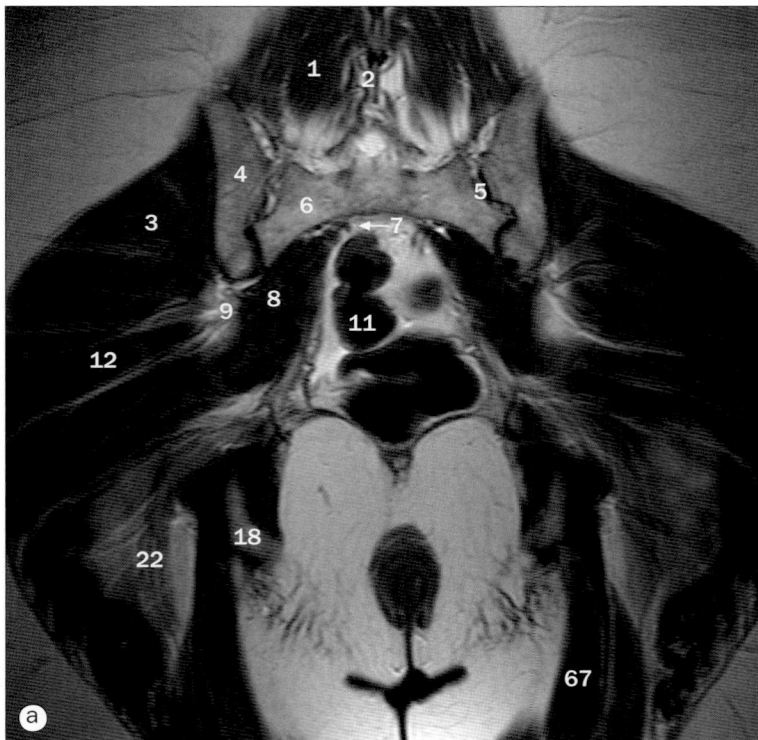

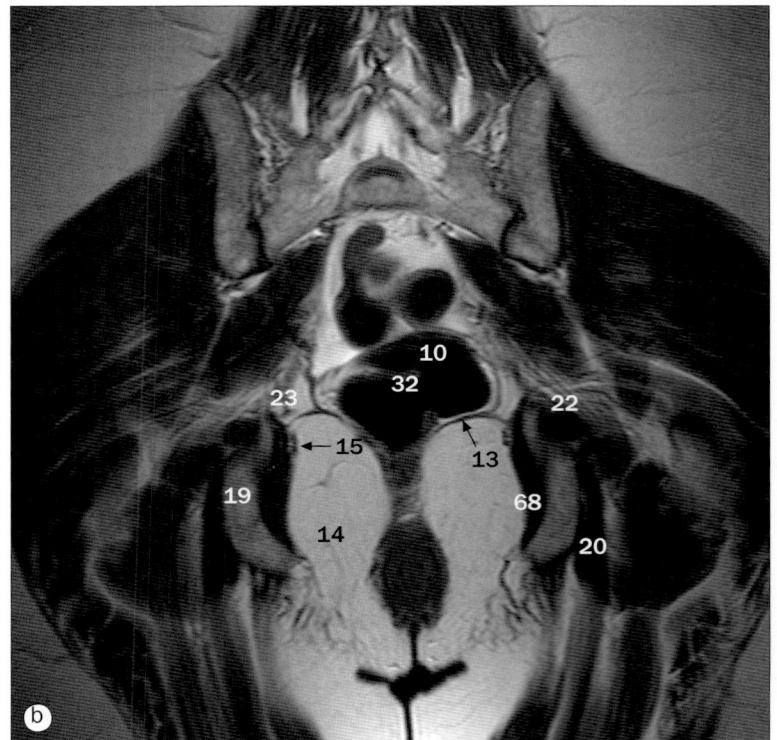

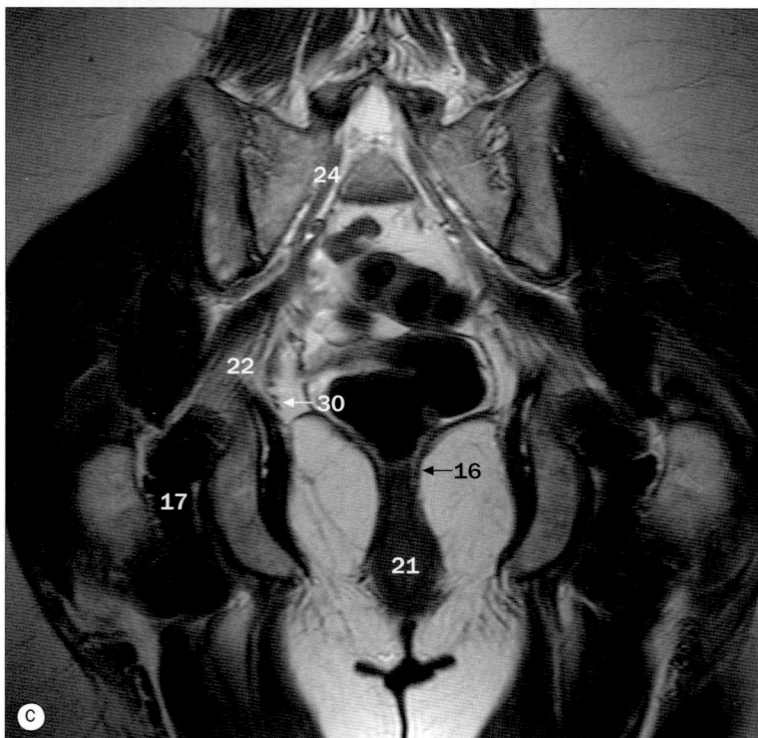

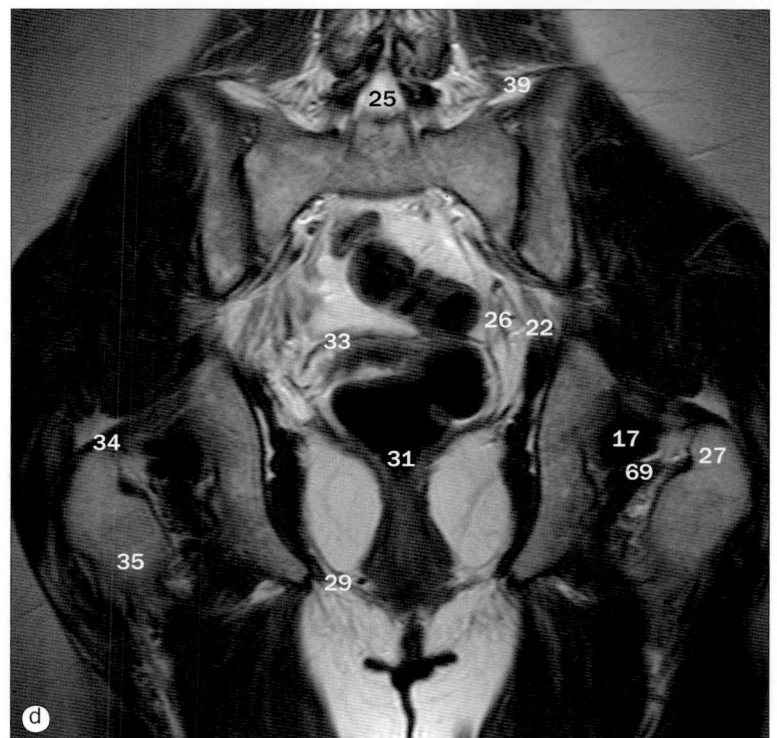

(a)–(p) Coronal T2w MR images of the female pelvis, from posterior to anterior.

1 Erector spinae muscle	13 Levator ani muscle
2 Spinous process L5	14 Ischio-anal fossa
3 Gluteus maximus muscle	15 Internal pudendal neurovascular bundle
4 Ilium	(Alcock's canal)
5 Sacro-iliac joint	16 External anal sphincter
6 Sacral ala	17 Obturator externus muscle
7 Lumbosacral trunk	18 Ischial tuberosity
8 Piriformis muscle	19 Ischium
9 Superior gluteal vessels	20 Common hamstring origin
10 Rectum	21 Anal canal
11 Rectosigmoid junction	22 Sciatic nerve
12 Gluteus medius muscle	23 Inferior gluteal vessels

24 Sacral nerve (S1)
25 Thecal sac
26 Superior rectal vessels
27 Greater trochanter of femur
28 Acetabulum
29 Urogenital diaphragm
30 Obturator neurovascular bundle
31 Rectal ampulla
32 Transverse rectal fold (of Houston)
33 Middle rectal vessels
34 Piriformis muscle (insertion)
35 Intertrochanteric part of femur

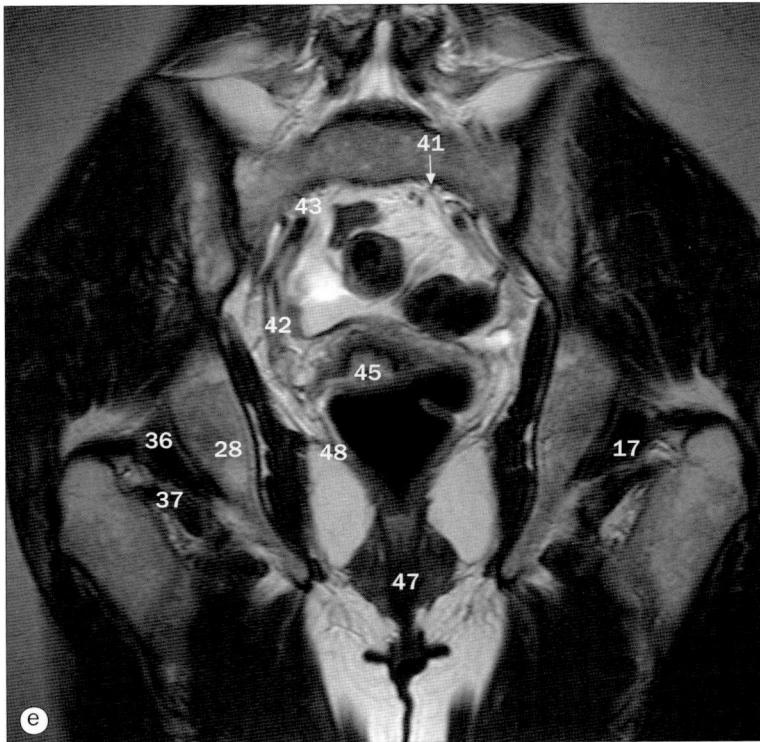

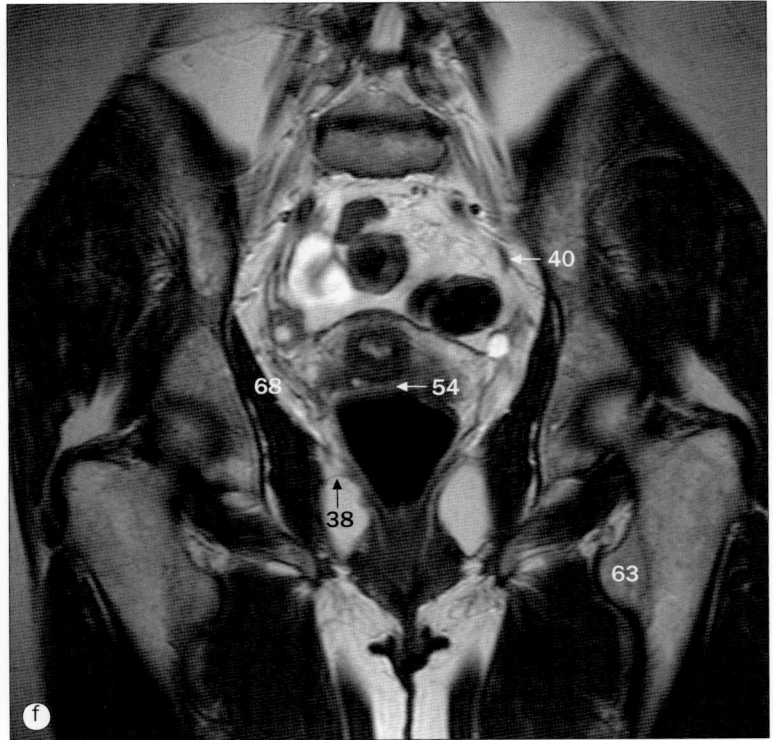

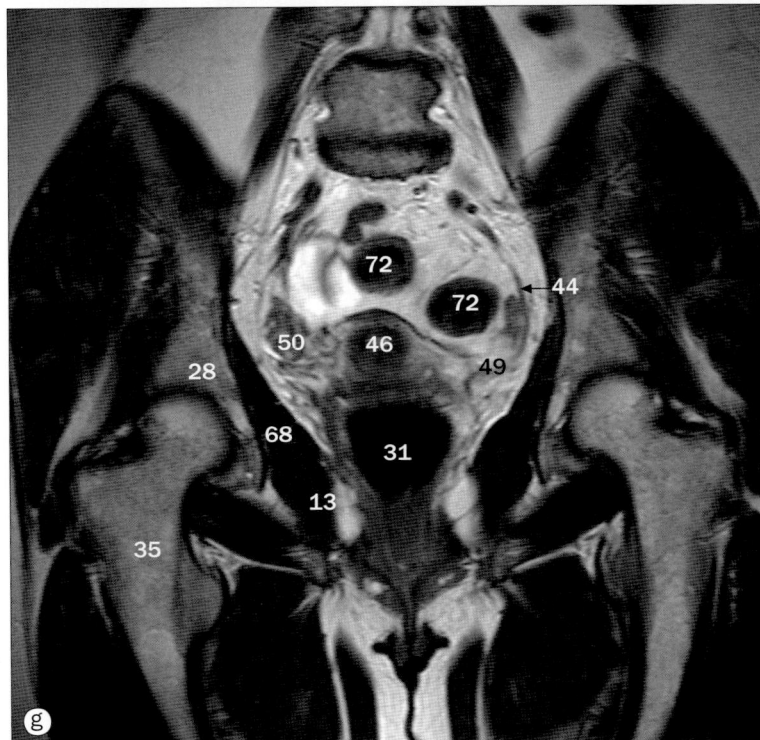

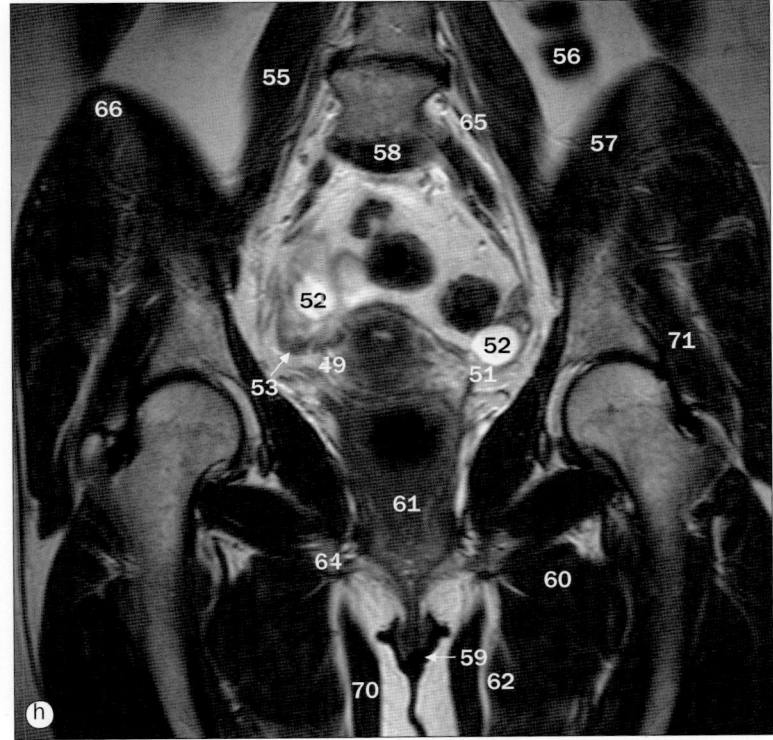

(a)–(p) Coronal T2w MR images of the female pelvis, from posterior to anterior.

36 Obturator externus muscle
37 Gemelli muscle
38 Inferior rectal neurovascular bundle
39 Iliolumbar ligament
40 Ureter
41 Sympathetic chain
42 Internal iliac vessel branches
43 Common iliac vessel bifurcation
44 Gonadal vessels
45 Cervix of uterus
46 Uterine cavity
47 Perineal body
48 Puborectalis muscle

49 Broad ligament of uterus
50 Right ovary
51 Left ovary
52 Physiological cyst of ovary (corpus luteum)
53 Uterine tube
54 Recto-uterine pouch (of Douglas)
55 Psoas major muscle
56 Descending colon
57 Iliacus muscle
58 Intervertebral disc at L5/S1
59 Labium minorum
60 Adductor brevis muscle

61 Vagina (posterior wall)
62 Adductor longus muscle
63 Lesser trochanter of femur
64 Inferior pubic ramus
65 Lumbar plexus
66 Iliac crest
67 Biceps femoris muscle
68 Obturator internus muscle
69 Quadratus femoris muscle
70 Gracilis muscle
71 Gluteus minimis muscle
72 Sigmoid colon

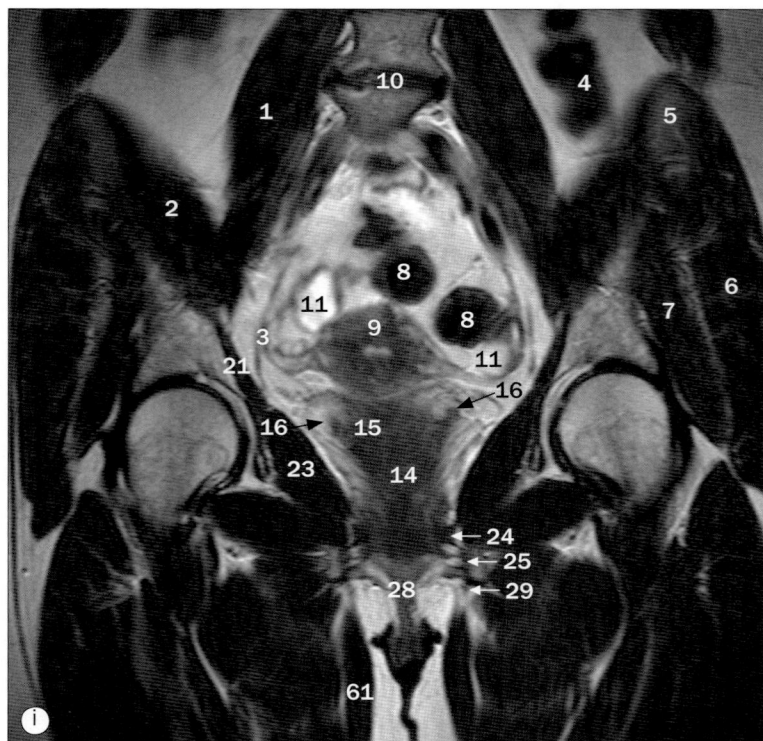

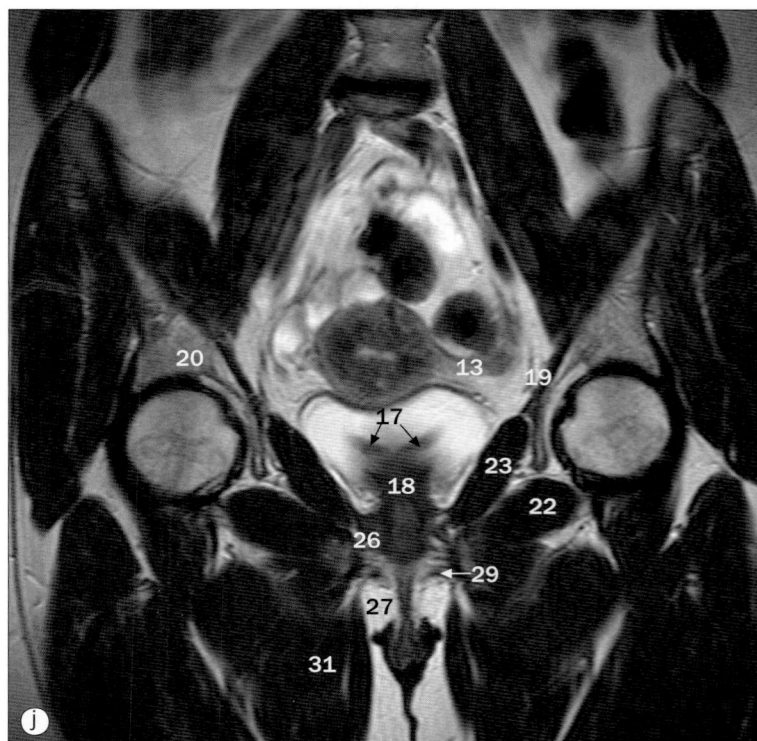

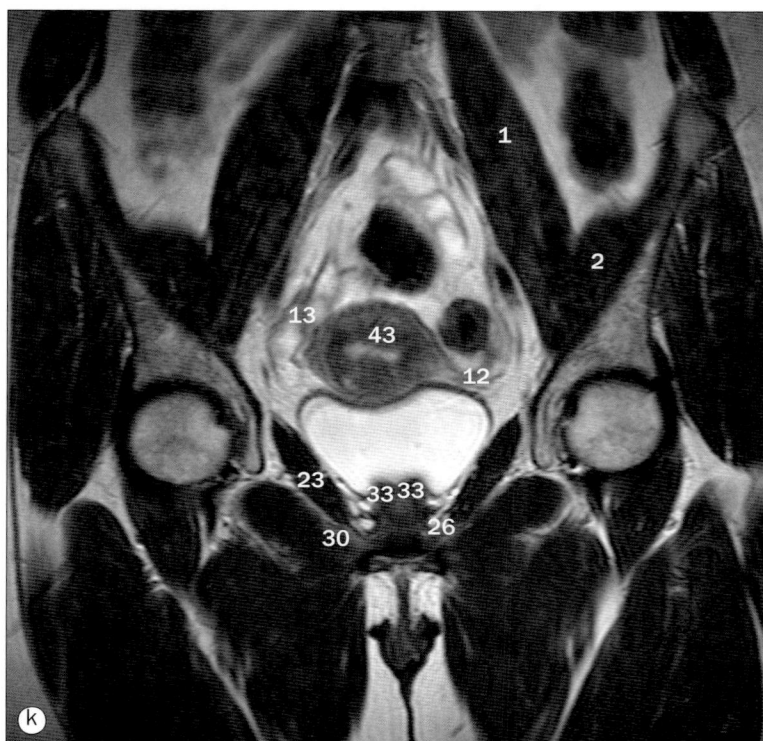

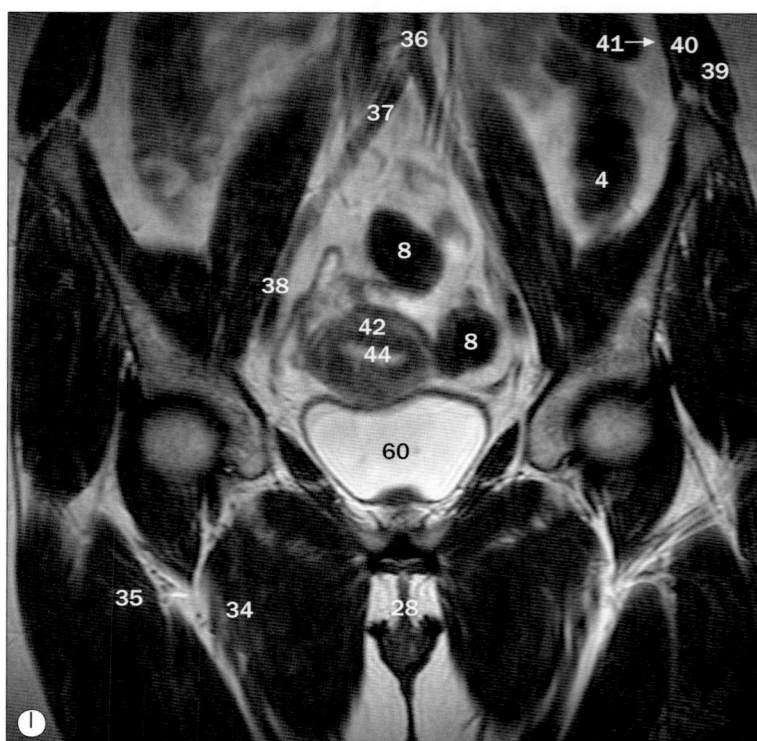

(a)–(p) Coronal T2w MR images of the female pelvis, from posterior to anterior.

1 Psoas major muscle	11 Ovaries (corpora luteal cysts)	21 Obturator internus muscle
2 Iliacus muscle	12 Broad ligament of uterus	22 Obturator externus muscle
3 Internal iliac artery branches	13 Uterine tubes	23 Levator ani muscle
4 Descending colon	14 Vagina	24 Pubovaginalis muscle
5 Iliac crest	15 Posterior fornix of vagina	25 Transverse perineii (urogenital diaphragm)
6 Gluteus medius muscle	16 Ureter	26 Deep perineal pouch
7 Gluteus minimis muscle	17 Ureteric orifice	27 Superficial perineal pouch
8 Sigmoid colon	18 Trigone of bladder	28 Urethra
9 Uterine myometrium	19 Obturator neurovascular bundle	29 Sphincter urethralis
10 Intervertebral disc at L4/5	20 Acetabular roof	30 Inferior pubic ramus

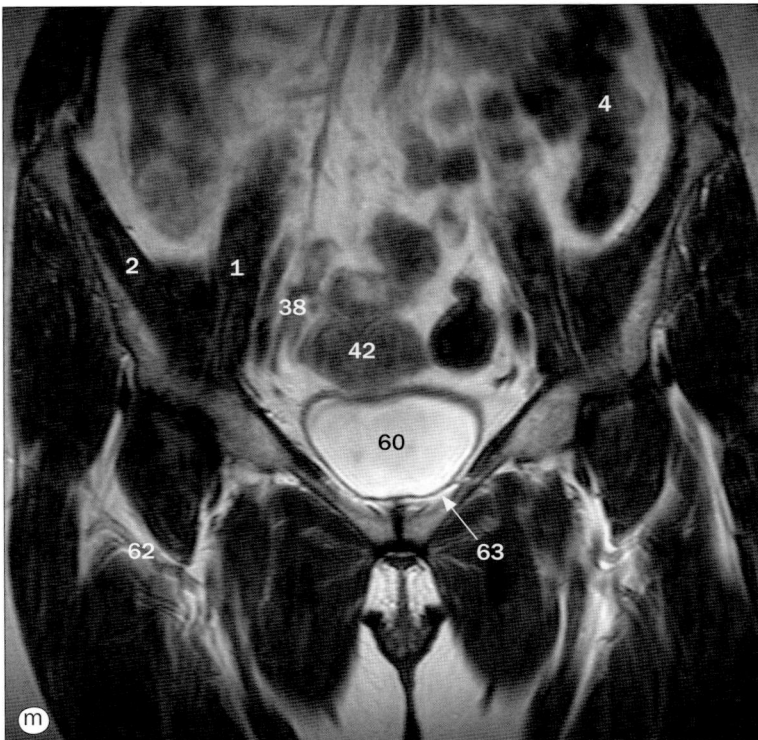

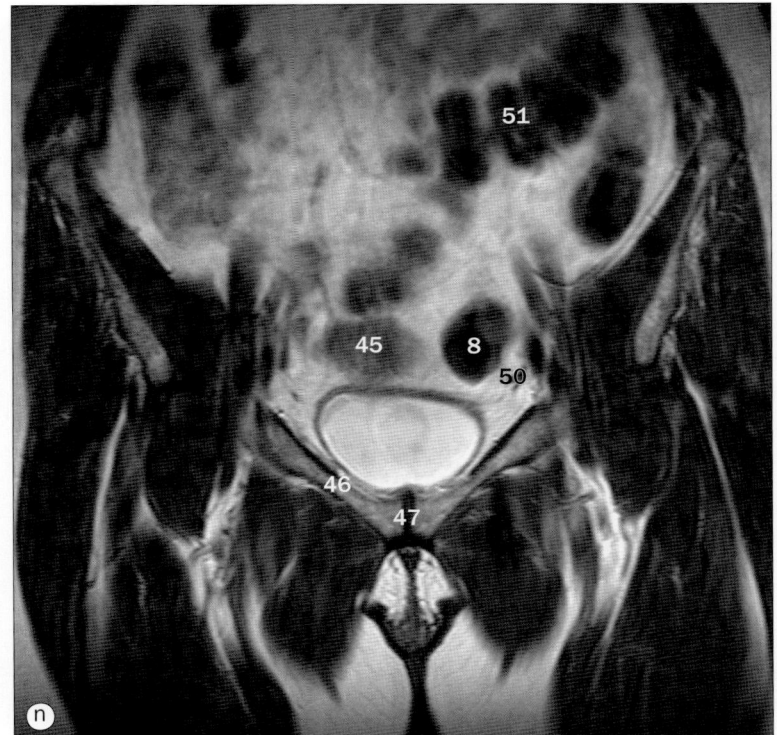

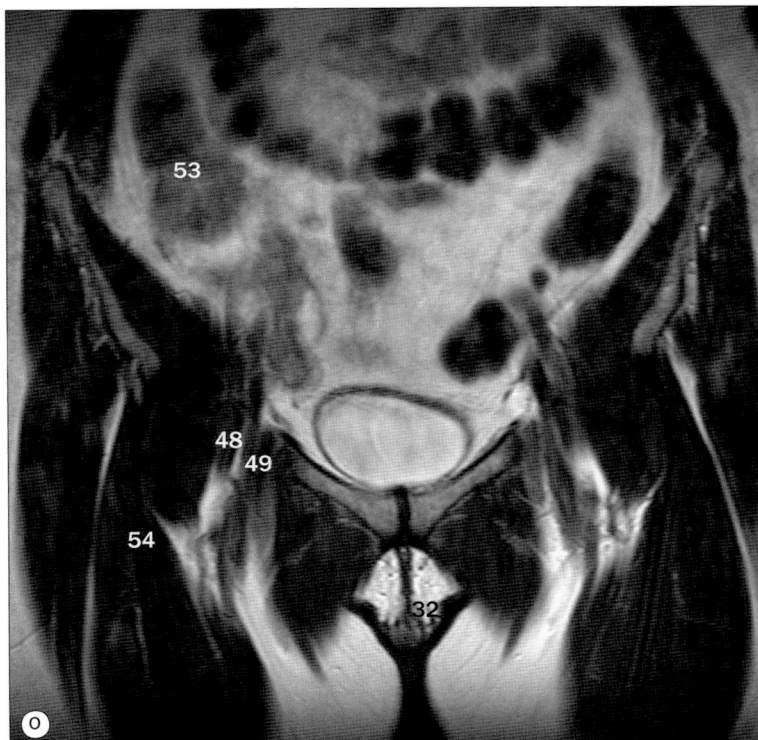

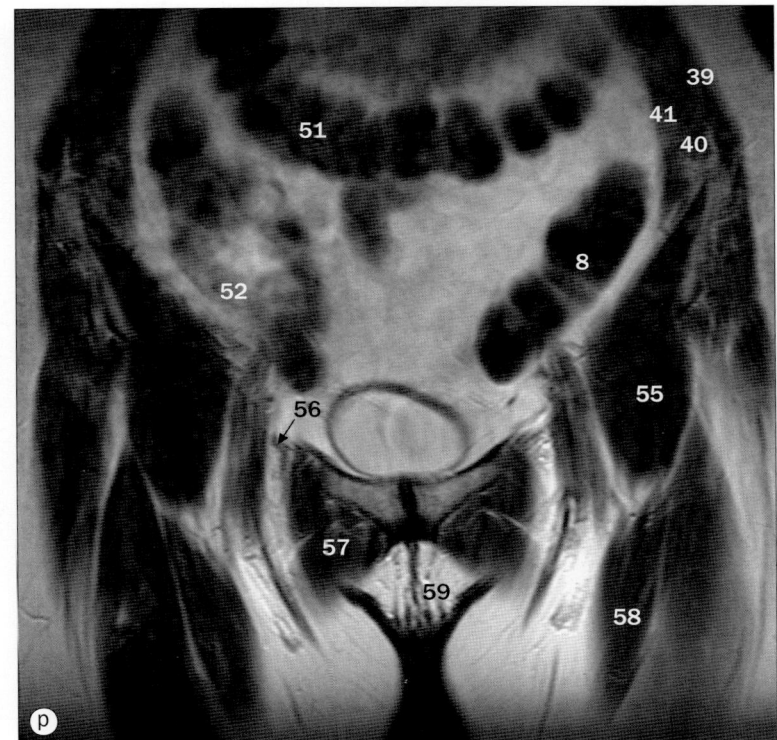

(a)–(p) Coronal T2w MR images of the female pelvis, from posterior to anterior.

31 Adductor longus muscle	42 Uterine myometrium	53 Caecum
32 Labia minora	43 Uterine endometrium	54 Rectus femoris muscle
33 Internal sphincter of bladder	44 Uterine cavity	55 Iliopsoas muscle
34 Vastus medialis muscle	45 Uterine fundus	56 Femoral canal
35 Vastus lateralis muscle	46 Superior pubic ramus	57 Adductor brevis muscle
36 Aorta	47 Symphysis pubis	58 Sartorius muscle
37 Common iliac artery	48 Common femoral artery	59 Labius majorum
38 External iliac artery	49 Common femoral vein	60 Bladder
39 External oblique muscle	50 Superior vesical vessels	61 Gracilis muscle
40 Internal oblique muscle	51 Transverse colon	62 Circumflex femoral vessels
41 Transversus abdominis muscle	52 Small bowel	63 Retropubic cave (of Retzius)

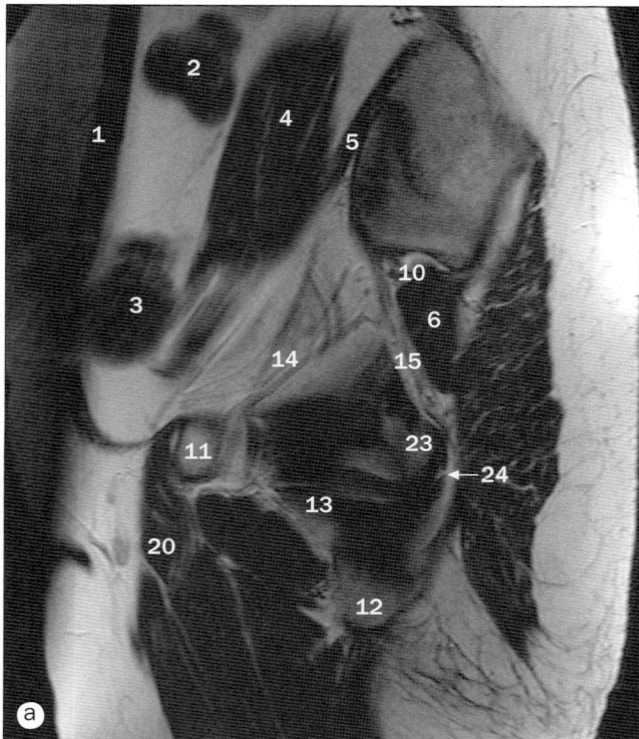

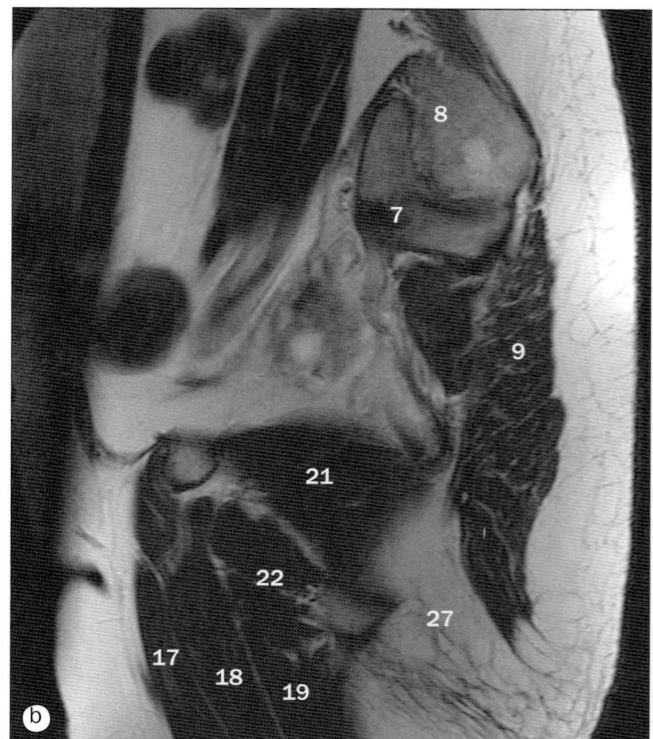

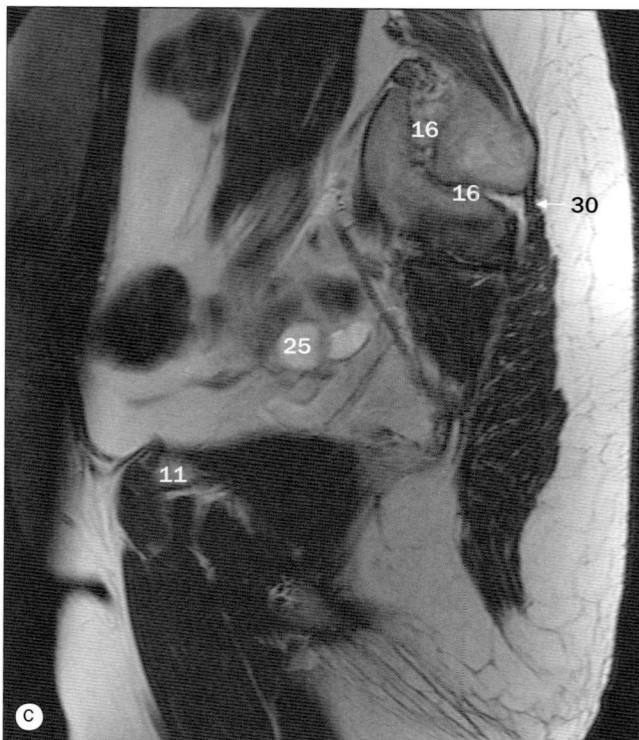

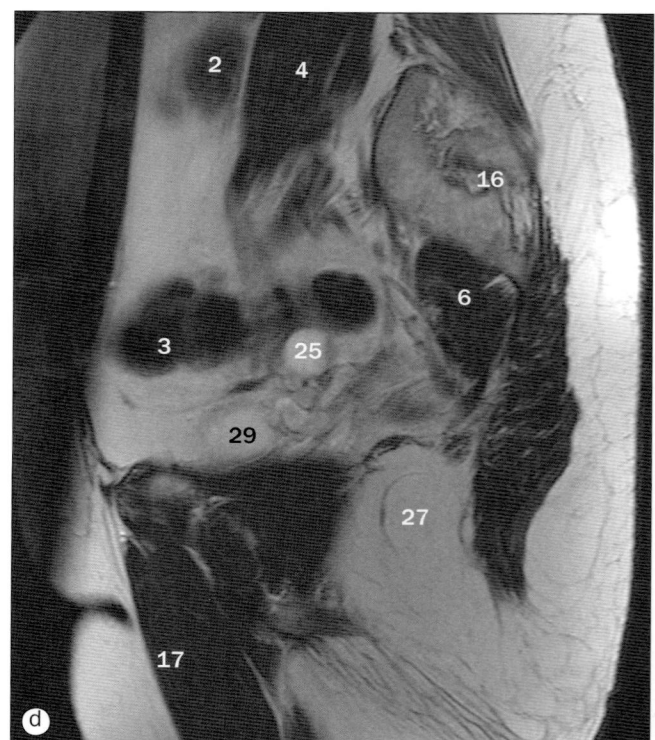

(a)–(p) Sequential sagittal T2w MR images of a female pelvis, from right to left through the midline.

1 Rectus abdominis muscle	10 Superior gluteal vessels	19 Adductor magnus muscle
2 Transverse colon	11 Superior pubic ramus	20 Iliopsoas muscle
3 Sigmoid colon	12 Inferior pubic ramus	21 Obturator internus muscle
4 Psoas major muscle	13 Obturator externus muscle	22 Pectineus muscle
5 Iliacus muscle	14 Obturator neurovascular bundle	23 Ischial tuberosity
6 Piriformis muscle	15 Sciatic nerve	24 Hamstring origin
7 Sacral ala	16 Sacro-iliac joint	25 Right ovary (corpus luteal cyst)
8 Ilium	17 Adductor longus muscle	26 Levator ani muscle
9 Gluteus maximus muscle	18 Adductor brevis muscle	27 Ischio-anal fossa

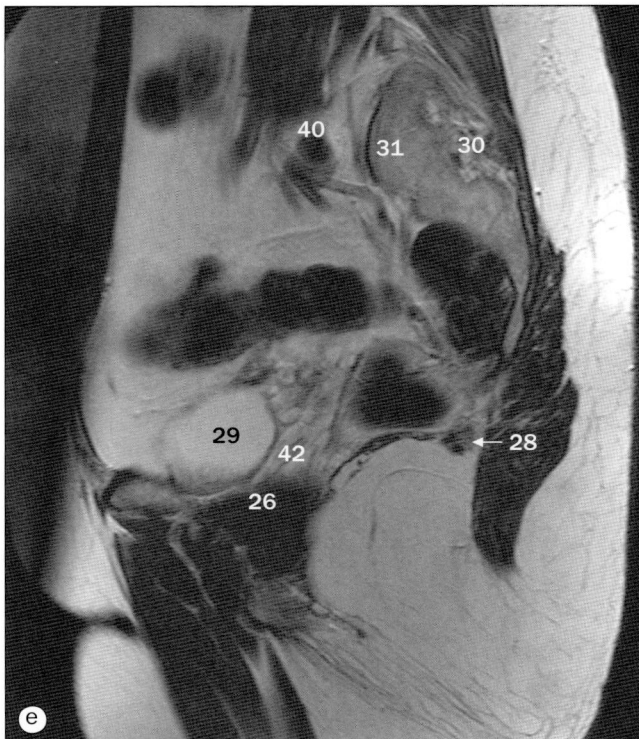

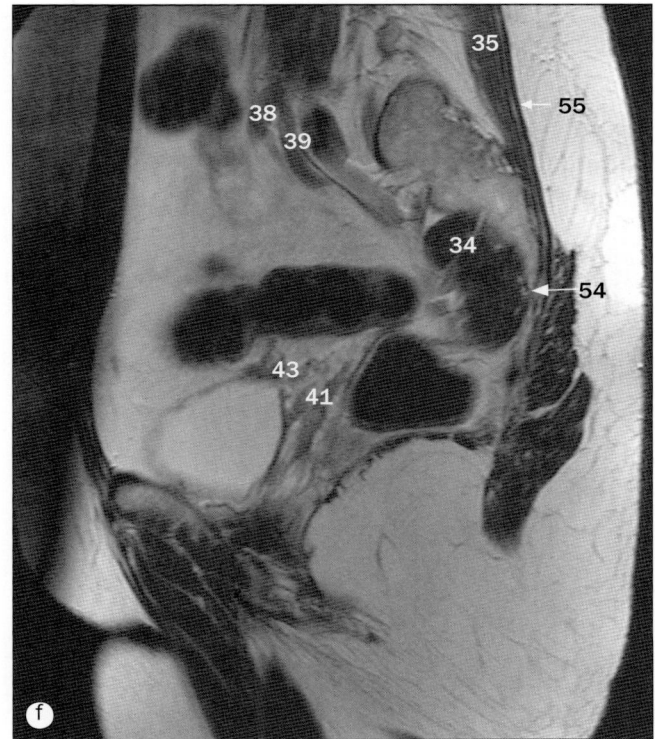

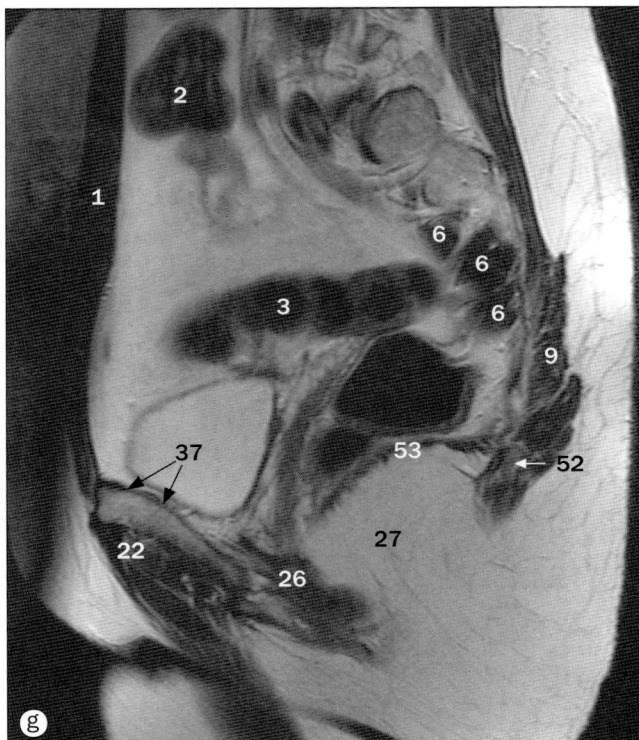

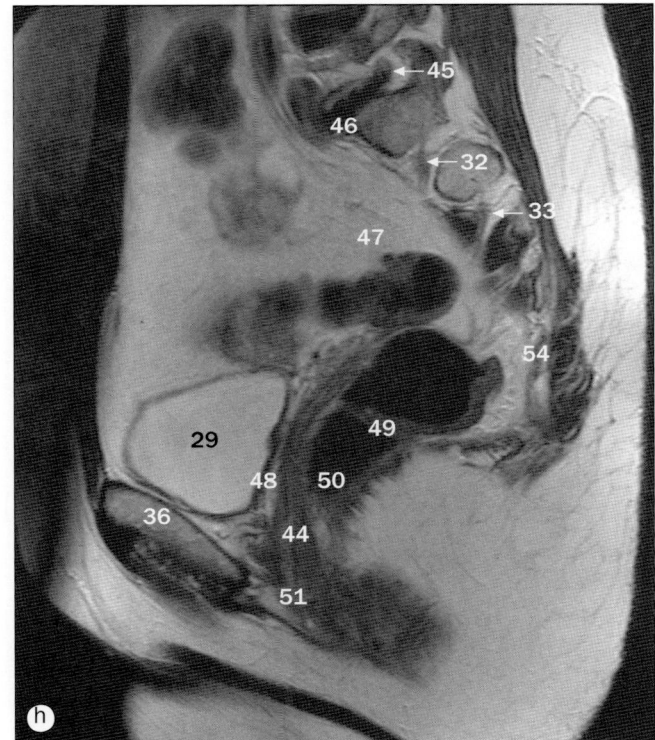

(a)–(p) Sequential sagittal T2w MR images of a female pelvis, from right to left through the midline.

28 Internal pudendal neurovascular bundle (Alcock's canal)
29 Bladder
30 Dorsal sacro-iliac ligaments
31 Sacral body
32 First sacral root
33 Second sacral root
34 Rectosigmoid junction
35 Erector spinae muscle
36 Pubic body

37 Retropubic space (cave of Retzius, extraperitoneal fat)
38 External iliac artery
39 Internal iliac artery
40 Internal iliac vein
41 Broad ligament of uterus
42 Transverse (cardinal) cervical ligament
43 Uterine tube
44 Vagina
45 Fifth lumbar root
46 Intervertebral disc at L5/S1

47 Mesosigmoid
48 Trigone of bladder
49 Transverse rectal fold (valve of Houston)
50 Rectal ampulla
51 Transverse perineii muscle (urogenital diaphragm)
52 Coccyx
53 Coccygeus muscle
54 Waldeyer's fascia
55 Thoracolumbar fascia

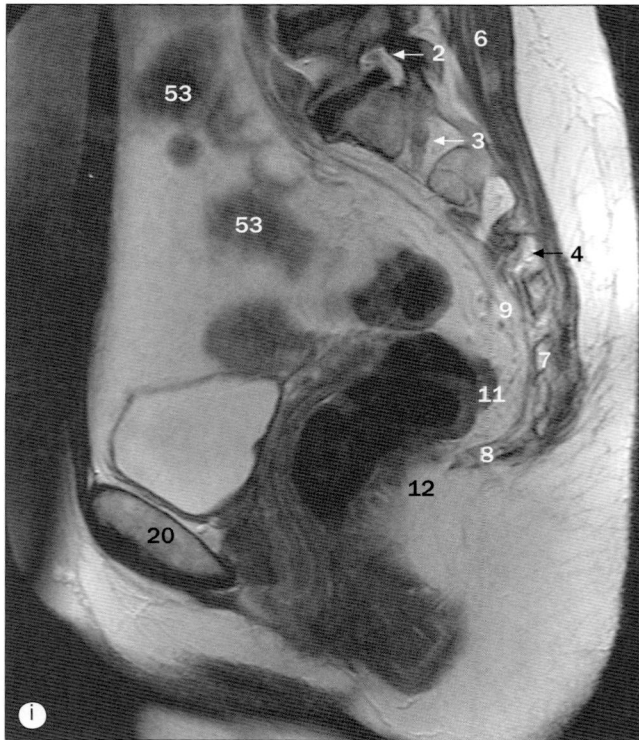

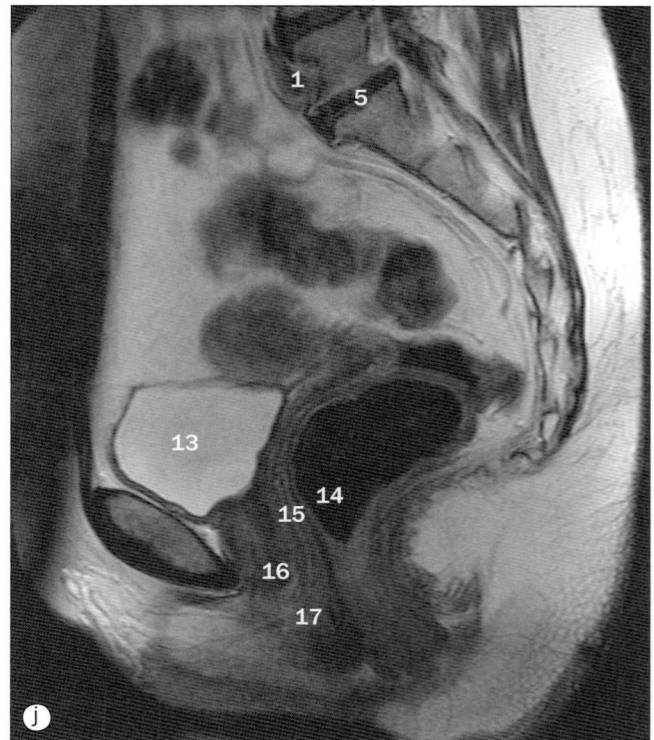

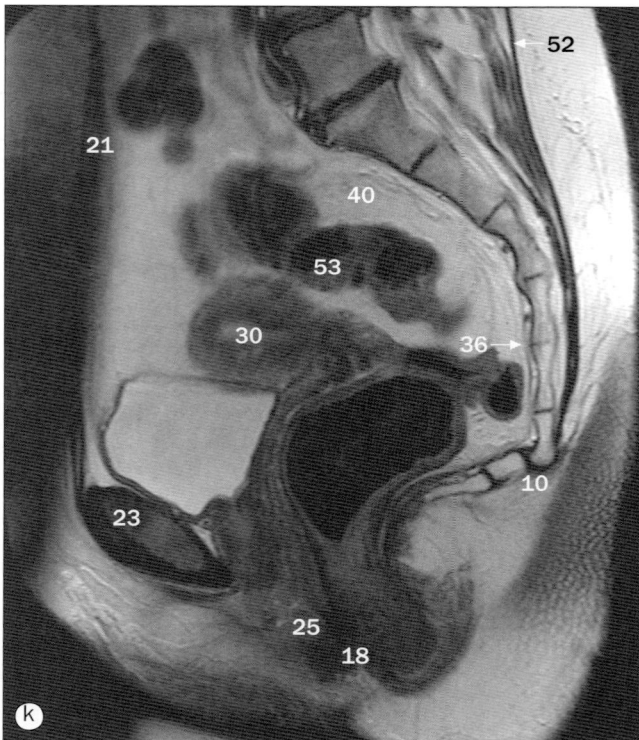

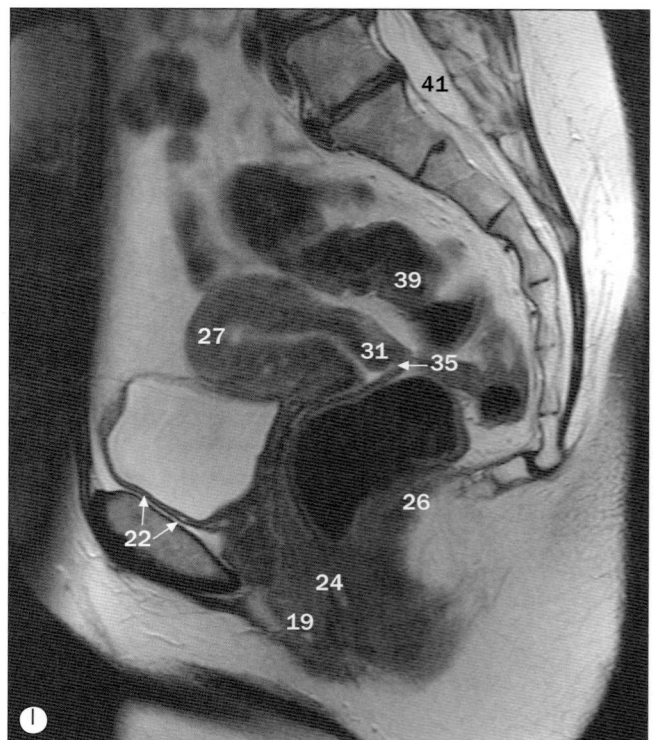

(a)–(p) Sequential sagittal T2w MR images of a female pelvis, from right to left through the midline.

1 Left common iliac vein	10 Sacro-coccygeal junction	19 External anal sphincter
2 L5 root (intervertebral foramen)	11 Levator ani muscle	20 Pubic body
3 S1 root	12 Puborectalis muscle	21 Rectus abdominis muscle
4 S3 root	13 Bladder	22 Retropubic space (extraperitoneal fat,
5 Intervertebral disc at L5/S1	14 Rectal ampulla	cave of Retzius)
6 Erector spinae muscle	15 Vagina	23 Symphysis pubis
7 Fifth sacral segment	16 Urethra	24 Anal canal
8 Coccyx	17 Vaginal introitus	25 Perineal body
9 Sacral plexus	18 Anus	26 Anococcygeal raphe

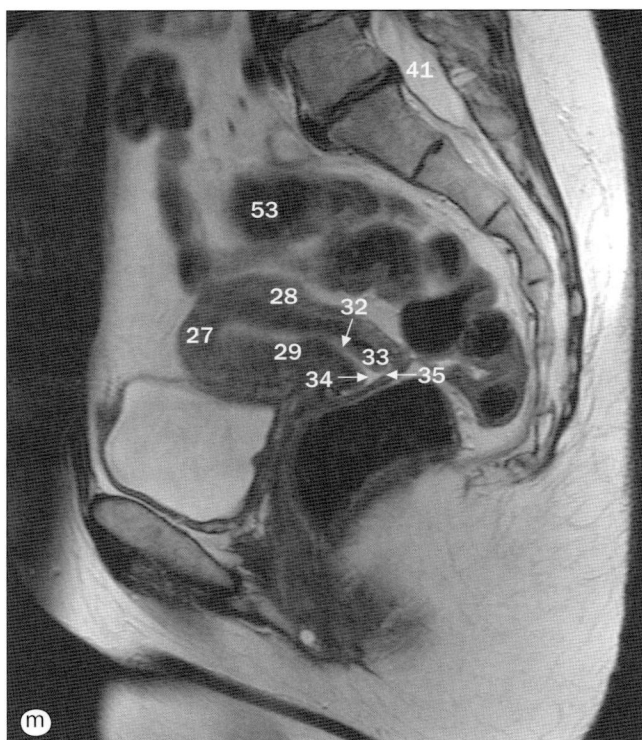

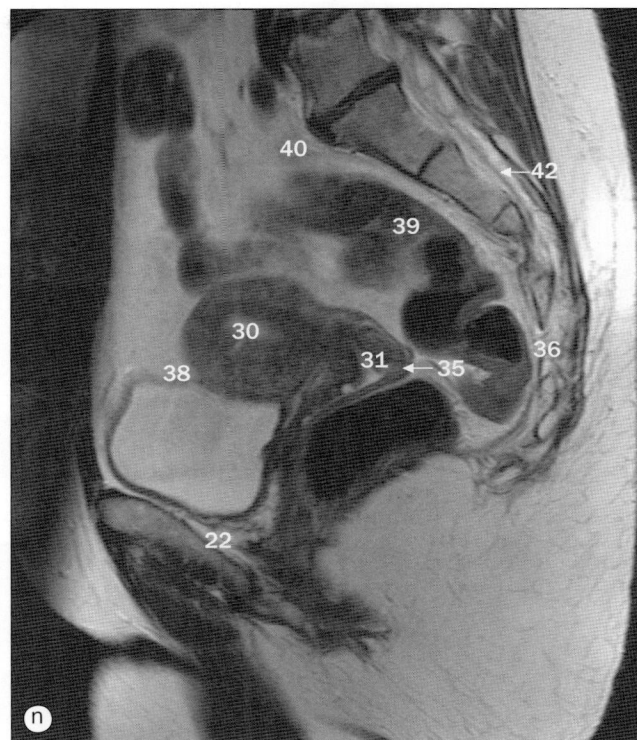

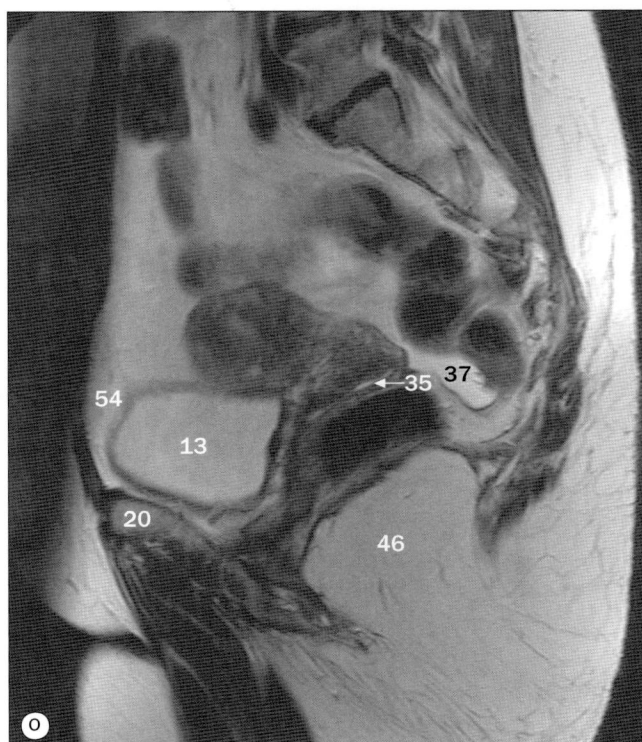

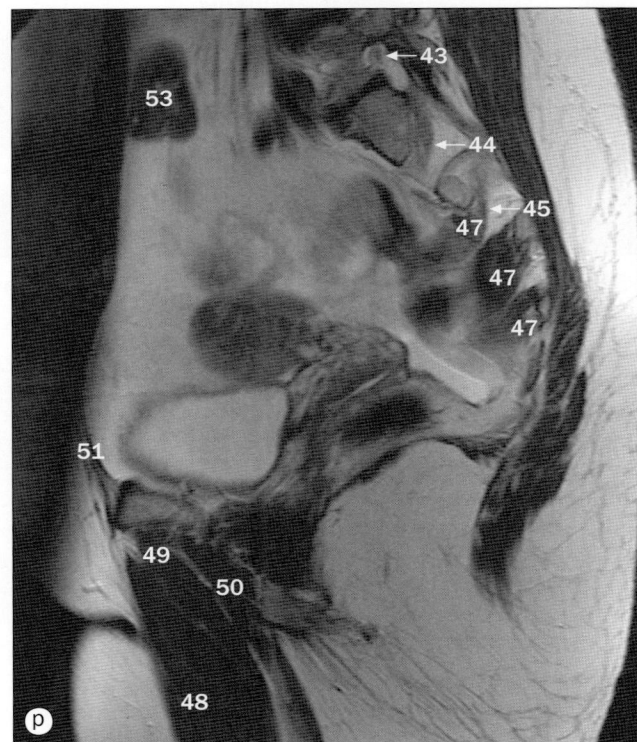

(a)–(p) Sequential sagittal T2w MR images of a female pelvis, from right to left through the midline.

27 Uterine fundus
28 Uterine myometrium
29 Uterine endometrium
30 Uterine cavity
31 Cervix
32 Internal cervical os
33 Cervical wall
34 External os of cervix
35 Posterior fornix of vagina
36 Waldeyer's fascia

37 Recto-uterine pouch (of Douglas)
38 Uterovesical pouch
39 Rectosigmoid junction
40 Mesosigmoid
41 Thecal sac
42 Filum terminale
43 Left L5 root
44 Left S1 root
45 Left S2 root

46 Ischio-anal fossa
47 Piriformis (slips of origin)
48 Adductor longus muscle
49 Adductor brevis muscle
50 Adductor magnus muscle
51 Rectus sheath
52 Thoracolumbar fascia
53 Sigmoid colon
54 Extraperitoneal fat

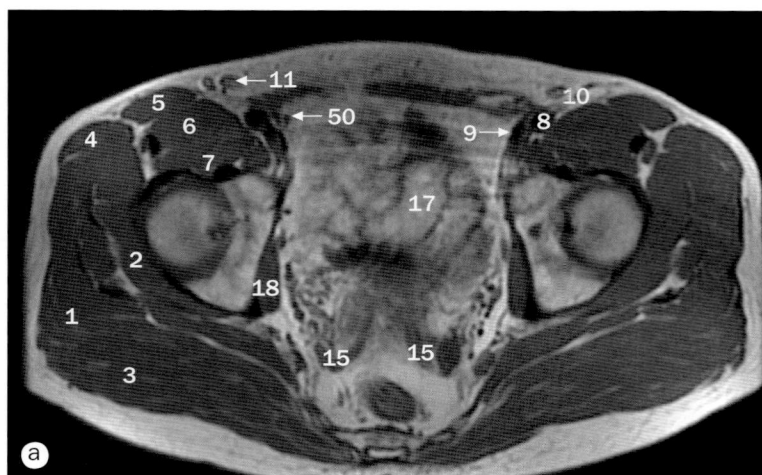

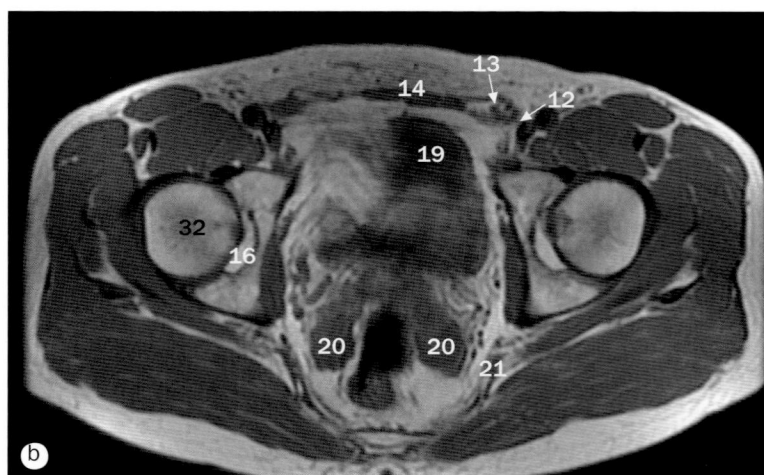

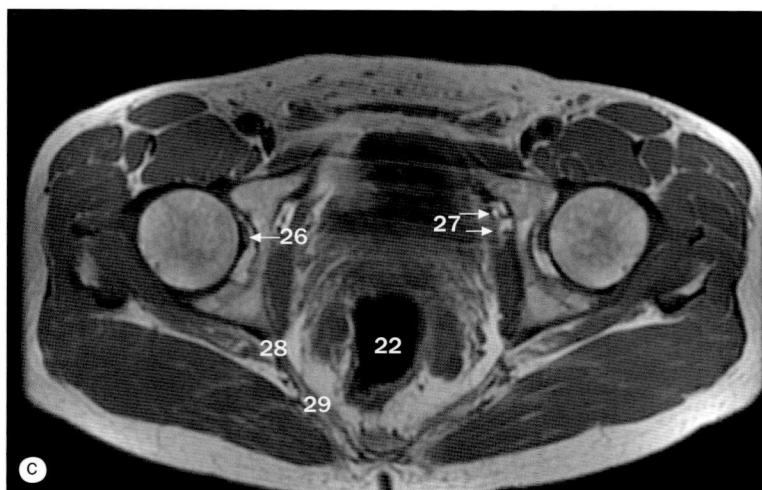

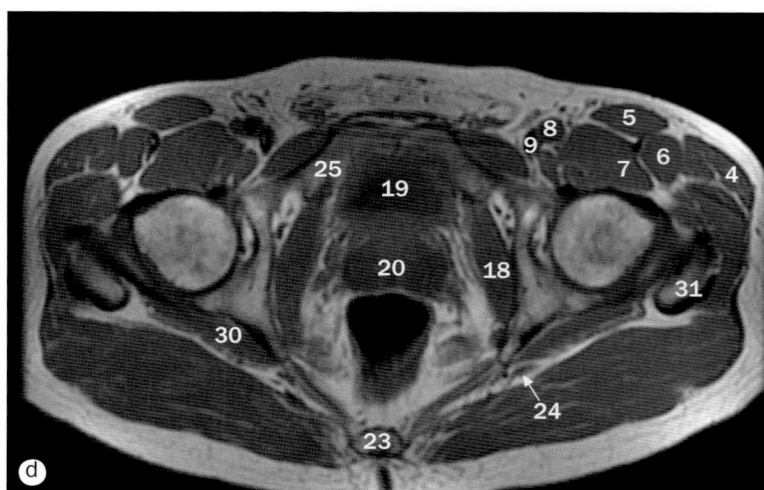

(a)–(l) Sequential axial T2w MR images of a male pelvis, from superior to inferior.

1 Gluteus medius muscle	**9** Common femoral vein	**17** Small bowel
2 Gluteus minimis muscle	**10** Femoral nerve branches	**18** Obturator internus muscle
3 Gluteus maximus muscle	**11** Long saphenous vein	**19** Bladder
4 Tensor fasciae latae muscle	**12** Femoral canal	**20** Seminal vesicle
5 Sartorius muscle	**13** Spermatic cord	**21** Inferior gluteal vessels
6 Rectus femoris muscle	**14** Rectus abdominis muscle	**22** Rectum
7 Iliopsoas muscle	**15** Ductus (vas) deferens	**23** Sacrum
8 Common femoral artery	**16** Acetabulum	**24** Sciatic nerve

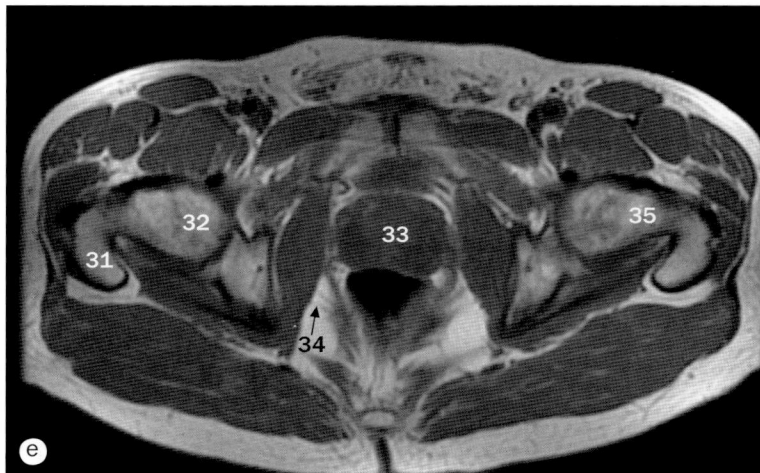

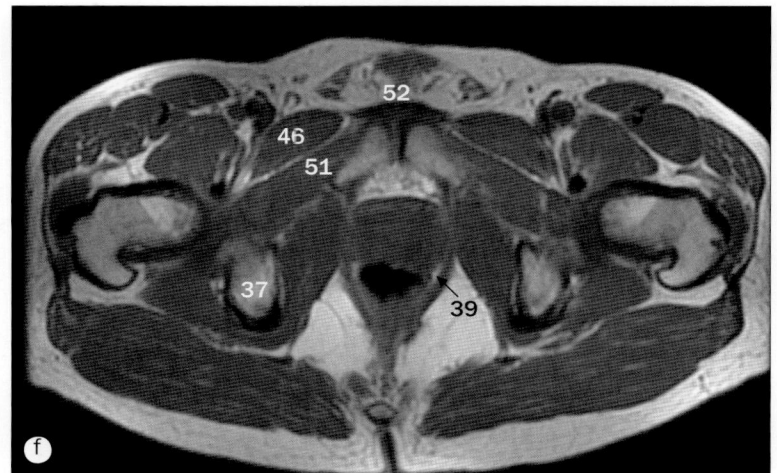

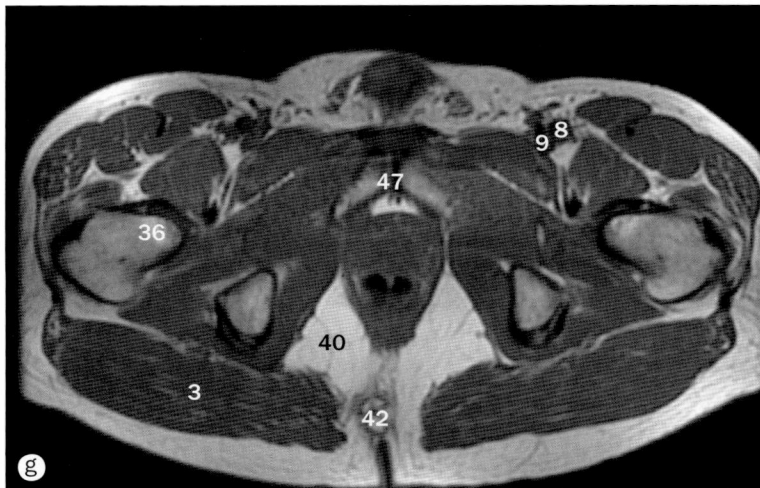

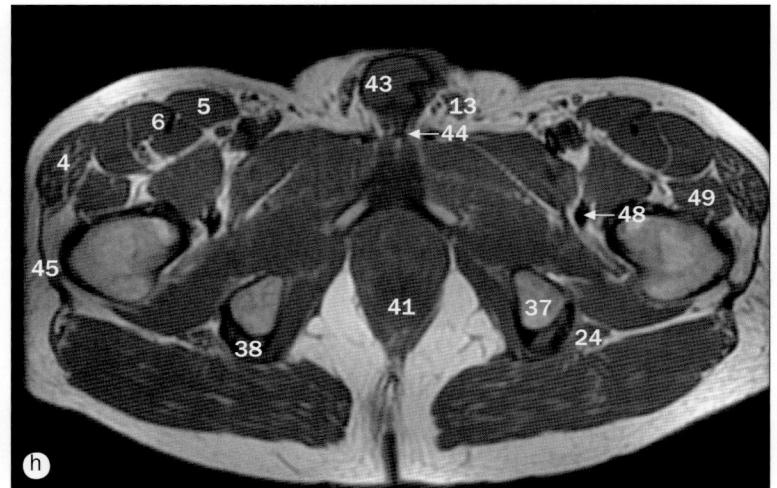

(a)–(l) Sequential axial T2w MR images of a male pelvis, from superior to inferior.

25 Superior pubic ramus
26 Ligamentum teres
27 Obturator vessels and nerve
28 Ischial spine
29 Sacrospinous ligament
30 Obturator externus muscle
31 Greater trochanter of femur
32 Femoral head
33 Prostate
34 Inferior rectal vessels and nerve

35 Femoral neck
36 Lesser trochanter of femur
37 Ischial tuberosity
38 Hamstrings (common tendinous origin)
39 Levator ani muscle (puborectalis)
40 Ischio-anal fossa
41 Anorectal junction
42 Coccyx
43 Corpus cavernosum

44 Dorsal penile vessels
45 Fascia lata
46 Pectineus muscle
47 Symphysis pubis
48 Iliopsoas tendon
49 Vastus lateralis muscle
50 Inferior epigastric vessels
51 Adductor longus muscle
52 Transverse pubic ligament

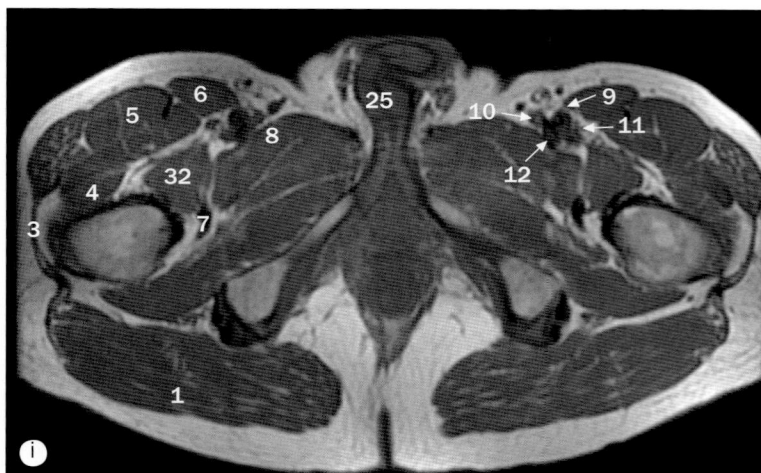

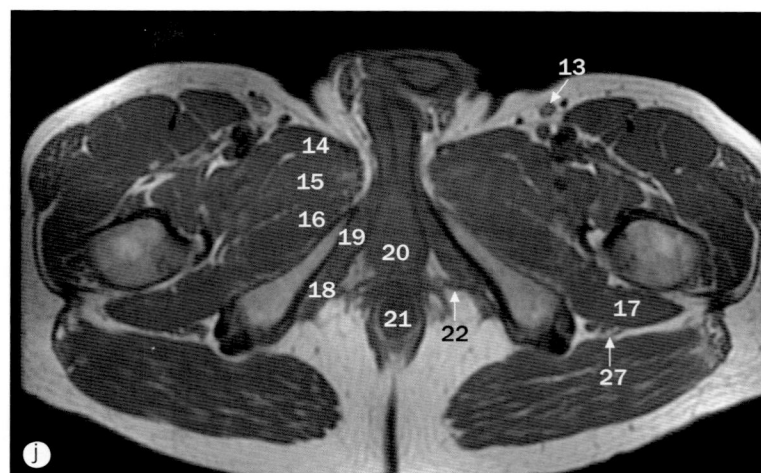

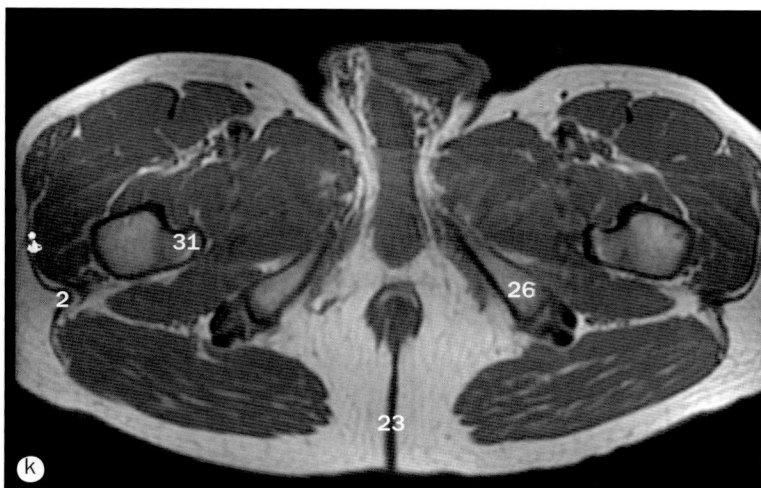

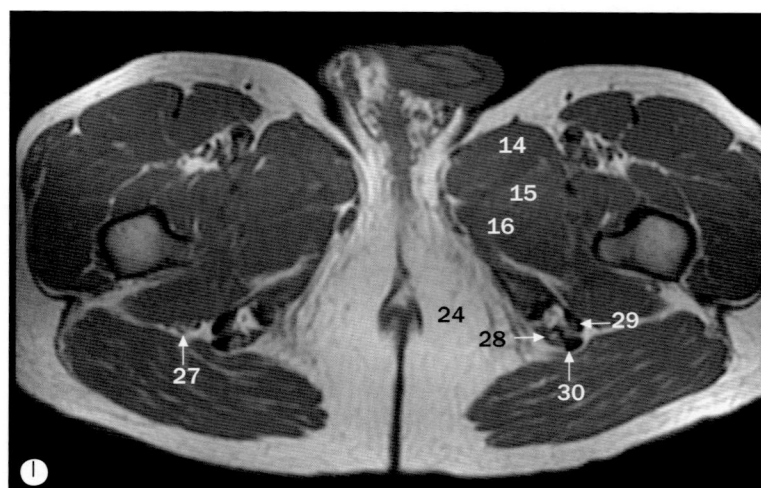

(a)–(l) Sequential axial T2w MR images of a male pelvis, from superior to inferior.

1 Gluteus maximus muscle	12 Profunda femoris vein	23 Natal cleft
2 Fascia lata	13 Long saphenous vein	24 Ischio-anal fossa
3 Iliotibial tract	14 Adductor longus muscle	25 Corpus cavernosum
4 Vastus lateralis muscle	15 Adductor brevis muscle	26 Ischial tuberosity
5 Rectus femoris muscle	16 Adductor magnus muscle	27 Sciatic nerve
6 Sartorius muscle	17 Quadratus femoris muscle	28 Semitendinosus tendinous origin
7 Iliopsoas tendon	18 Ischiocavernosus muscle	29 Semimembranosus tendinous origin
8 Pectineus muscle	19 Crus of penis	30 Biceps femoris tendinous origin
9 Superficial femoral artery	20 Bulb of penis	31 Lesser trochanter of femur
10 Superficial femoral vein	21 Anus	32 Iliopsoas muscle
11 Profunda femoris artery	22 Inferior rectal neurovascular bundle	

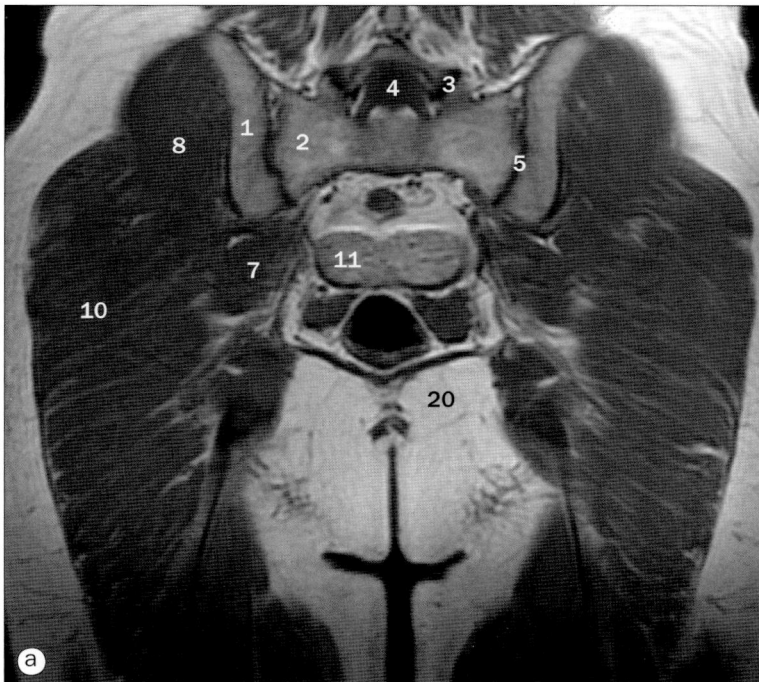

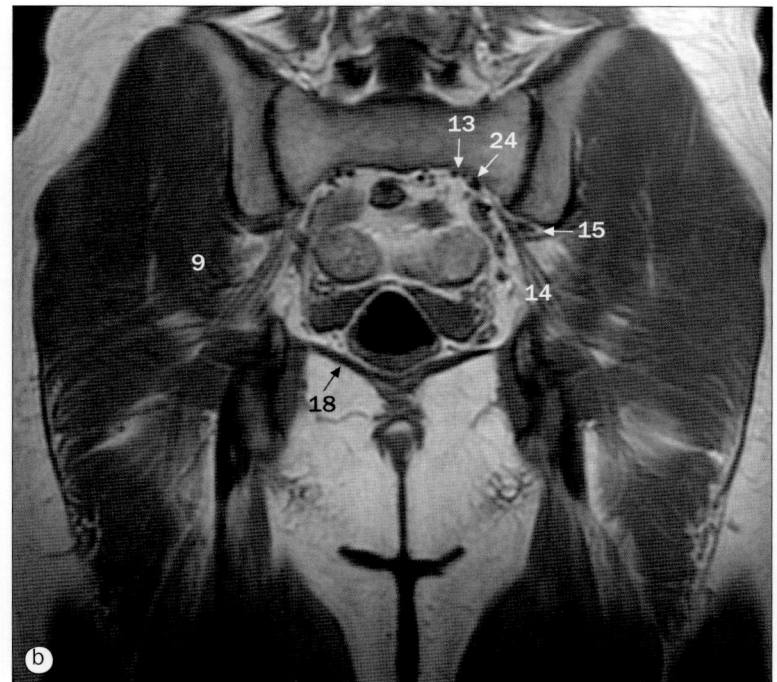

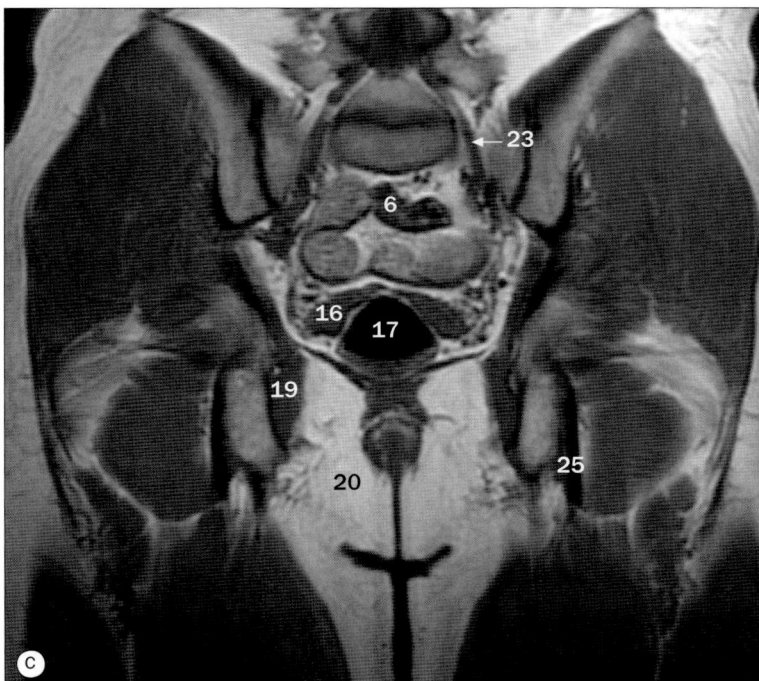

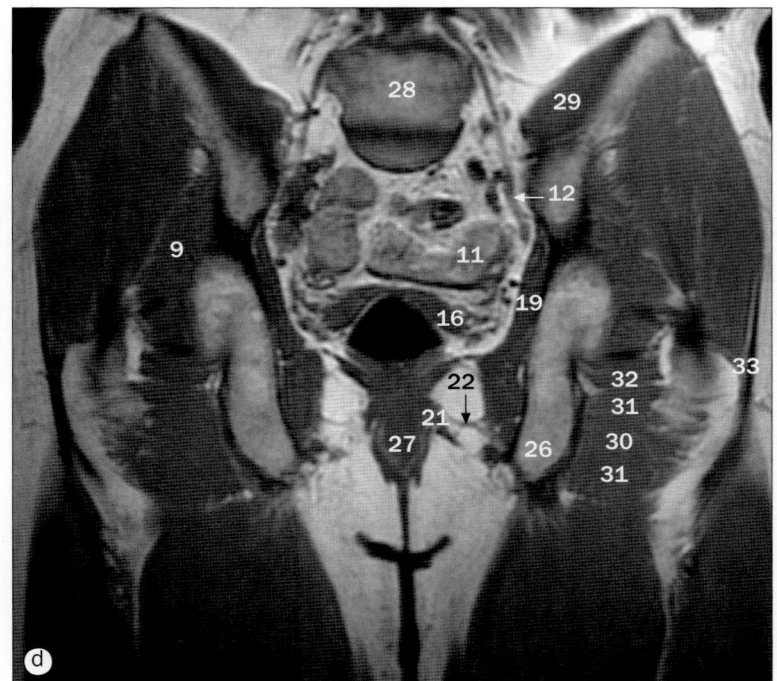

(a)–(p) Sequential coronal T2w MR images of a male pelvis, from posterior to anterior.

1 Ilium	12 Ureter	23 Fifth lumbar root
2 Sacral ala	13 Gonadal vessels	24 Lumbosacral trunk
3 Facet joint (L5/S1)	14 Sciatic nerve	25 Common hamstring origin
4 Thecal sac	15 Superior gluteal vessels	26 Ischial tuberosity
5 Sacro-iliac joint	16 Seminal vesicle	27 Anal canal
6 Rectosigmoid junction	17 Rectal ampulla	28 L5 vertebral body
7 Piriformis muscle	18 Levator ani muscle	29 Iliacus muscle
8 Gluteus medius muscle	19 Obturator internus muscle	30 Quadratus femoris muscle
9 Gluteus minimis muscle	20 Ischio-anal fossa	31 Gemelli muscles (superior and inferior)
10 Gluteus maximus muscle	21 External anal sphincter	32 Obturator externus muscle
11 Small bowel	22 Inferior rectal neurovascular bundle	33 Fascia lata

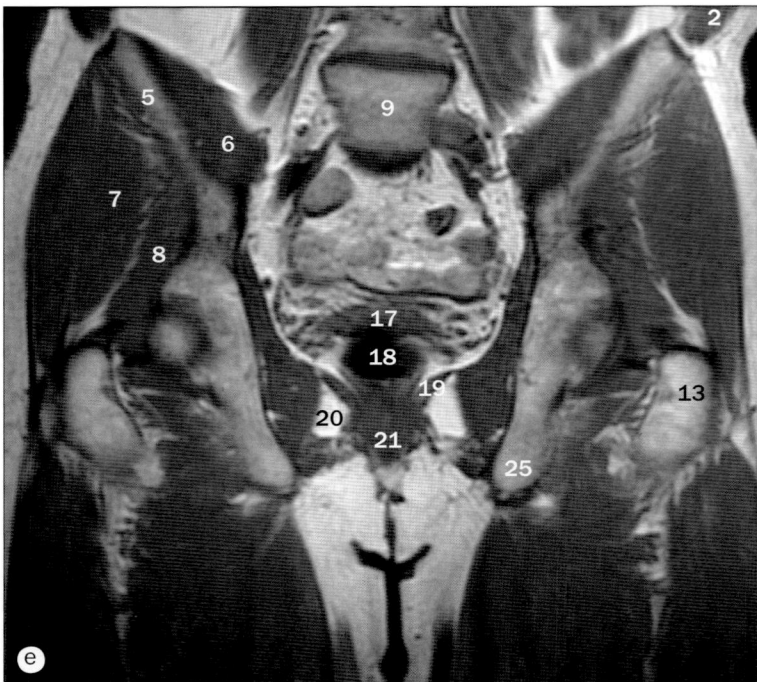

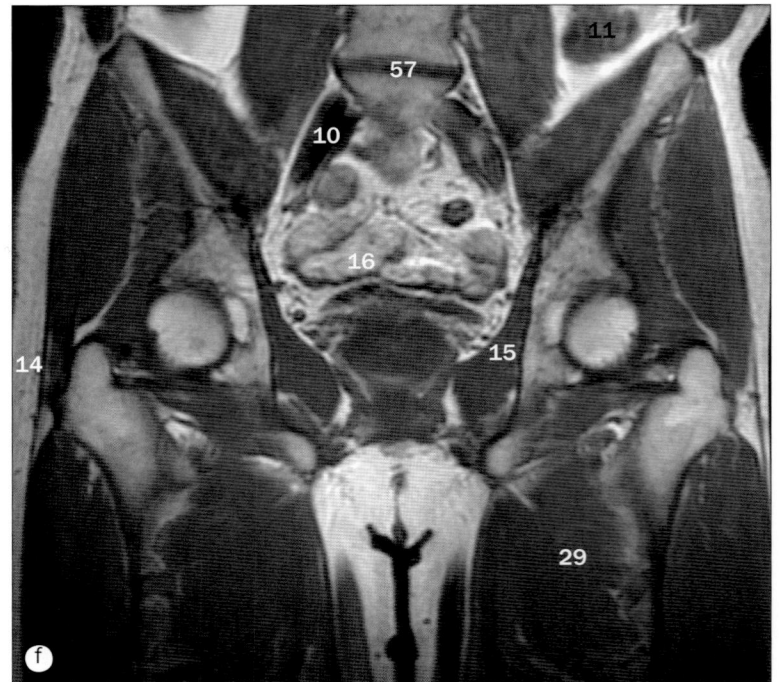

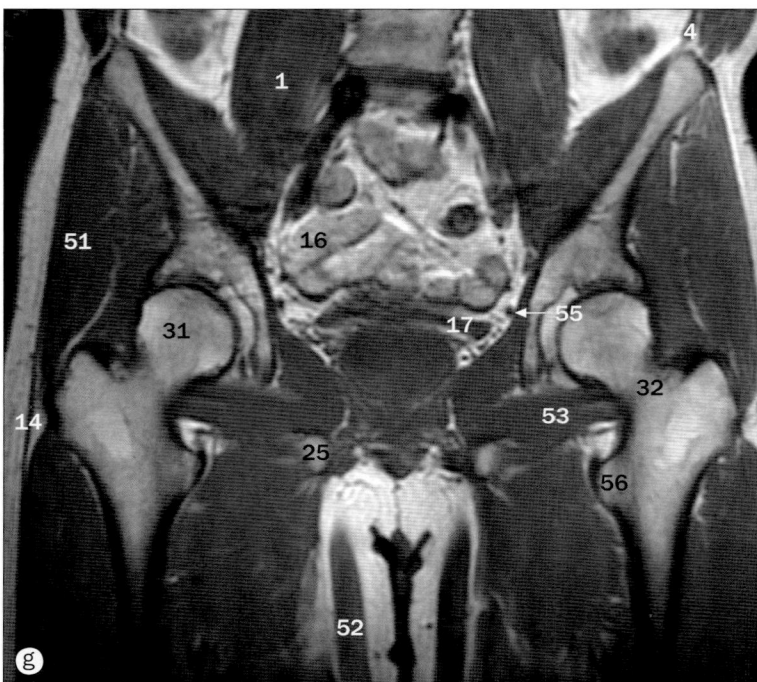

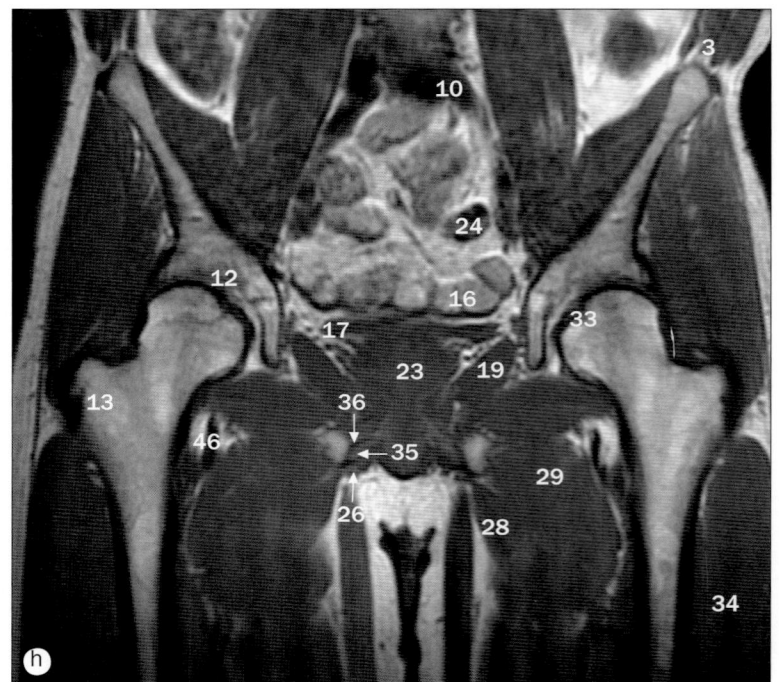

(a)–(p) Sequential coronal T2w MR images of a male pelvis, from posterior to anterior.

1 Psoas major muscle	9 Fifth lumbar vertebral body	17 Seminal vesicle
2 External oblique muscle	10 Common iliac vessels	18 Rectum
3 Internal oblique muscle	11 Descending colon	19 Levator ani muscle
4 Transversus abdominis muscle	12 Acetabulum	20 Ischio-anal fossa
5 Ilium	13 Greater trochanter of femur	21 Anal canal
6 Iliacus muscle	14 Fascia lata	22 Bladder
7 Gluteus medius muscle	15 Obturator internus muscle	23 Prostate
8 Gluteus minimis muscle	16 Small bowel	24 Sigmoid colon

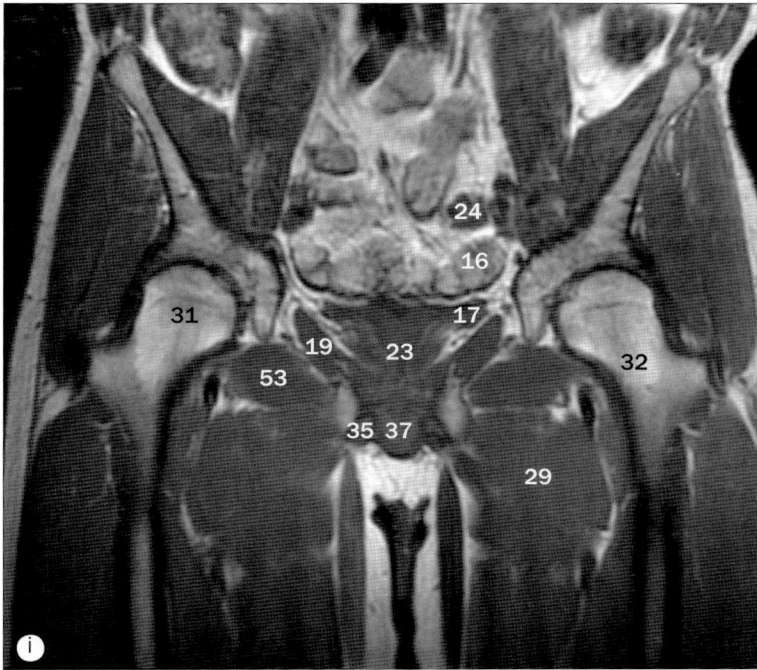

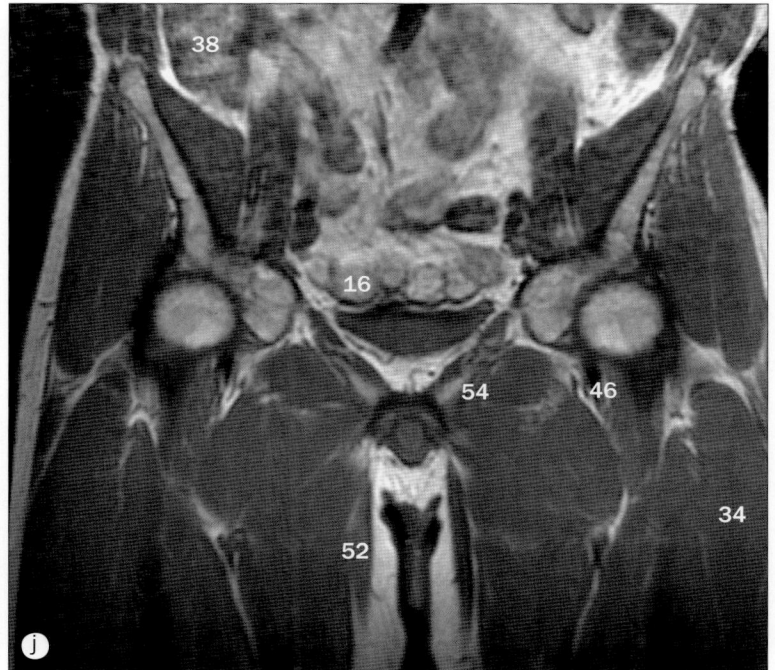

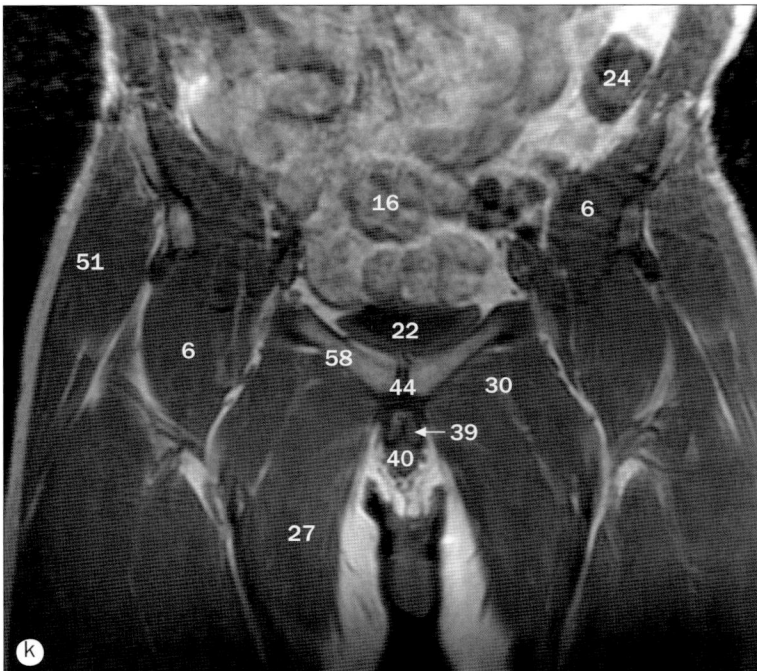

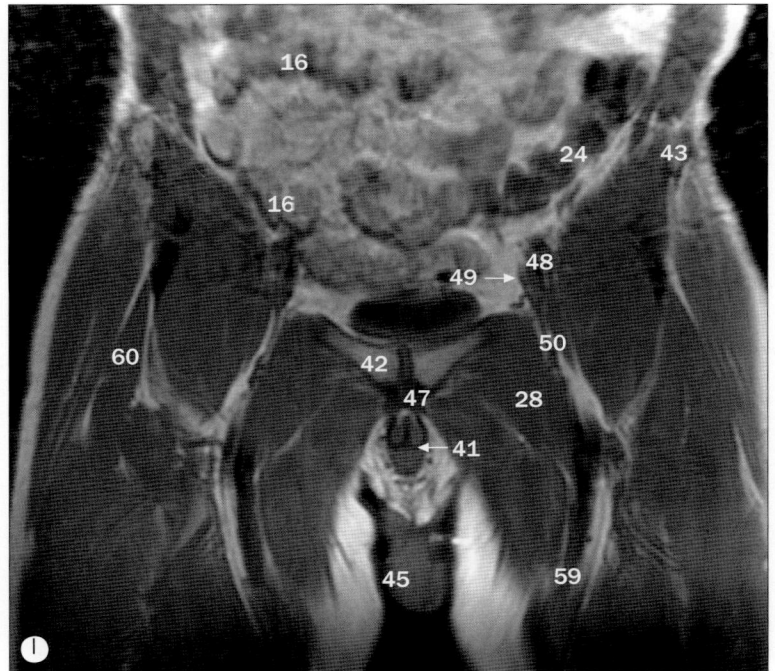

(a)–(p) Sequential coronal T2w MR images of a male pelvis, from posterior to anterior.

25 Ischium
26 Transverse perineii muscle
27 Adductor longus muscle
28 Adductor brevis muscle
29 Adductor magnus muscle
30 Pectineus muscle
31 Femoral head
32 Femoral neck
33 Fovea capitalis of femur
34 Vastus lateralis muscle
35 Crus of penis
36 Ischiocavernosus

37 Bulb of penis
38 Caecum
39 Corpus cavernosus
40 Corpus spongiosus
41 Penile (spongy) urethra
42 Pubic body
43 Anterior superior iliac spine
44 Symphysis pubis
45 Testicle
46 Profunda femoris vessels
47 Suspensory ligament of penis
48 External iliac artery

49 External iliac vein
50 Common femoral vessels
51 Gluteus maximus muscle
52 Gracilis muscle
53 Obturator externus muscle
54 Inferior pubic ramus
55 Obturator neurovascular bundle
56 Lesser trochanter of femur
57 Intervertebral disc at L4/5
58 Superior pubic ramus
59 Superficial femoral vessels
60 Tensor fasciae latae muscle

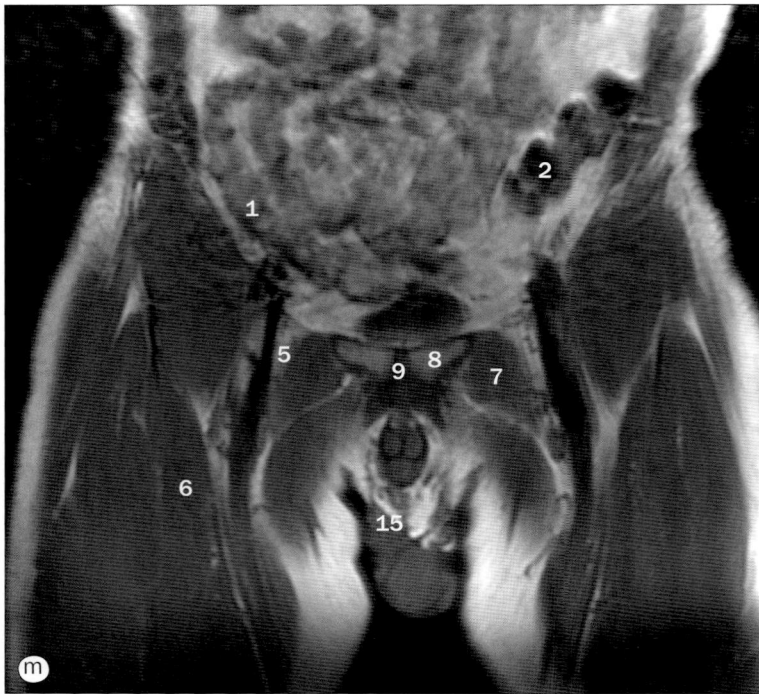

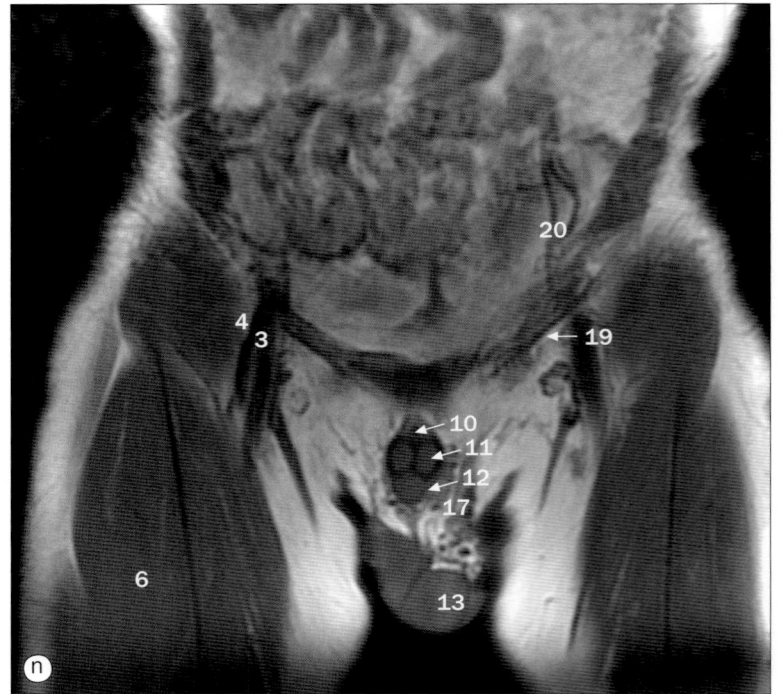

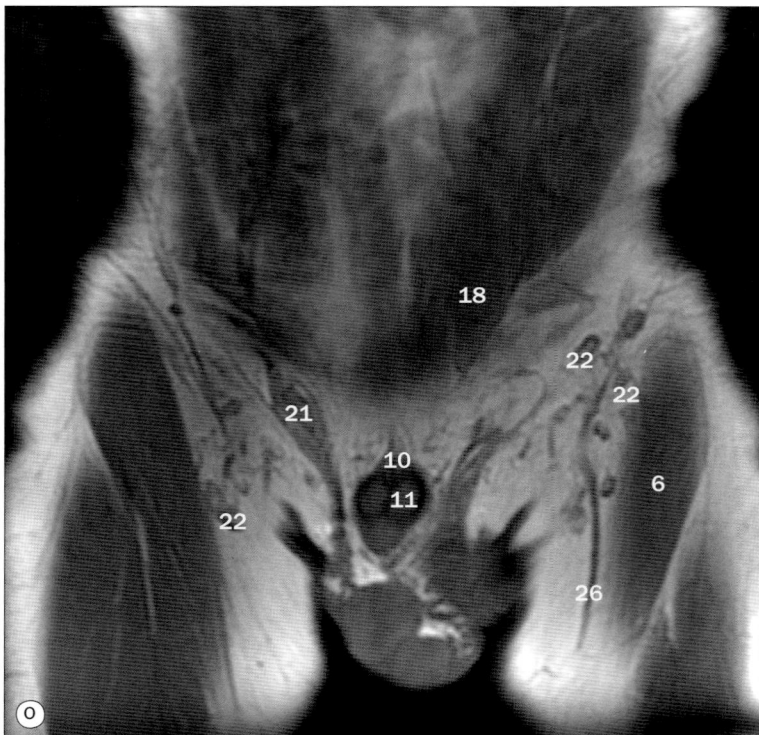

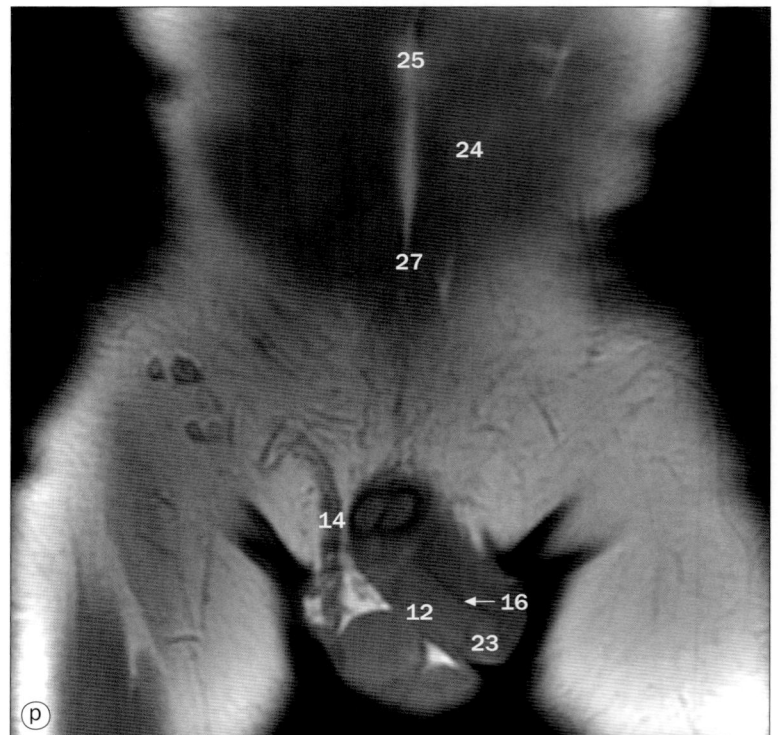

(a)–(p) Sequential coronal T2w MR images of a male pelvis, from posterior to anterior.

1 Small bowel	10 Suspensory ligament of penis	19 Inguinal ligament
2 Sigmoid colon	11 Corpus cavernosum of penis	20 Inferior epigastric vessels
3 Common femoral vein	12 Corpus spongiosum of penis	21 Inguinal canal (external ring)
4 Common femoral artery	13 Testicle	22 Superficial inguinal lymph nodes
5 Femoral canal	14 Spermatic cord	23 Glans penis
6 Rectus femoris muscle	15 Epididymal head	24 Rectus abdominis muscle
7 Pectineus muscle	16 Penile (spongy) urethra	25 Umbilicus
8 Pubic body	17 Pampiniform plexus	26 Long saphenous vein
9 Symphysis pubis	18 External oblique muscle	27 Linea alba

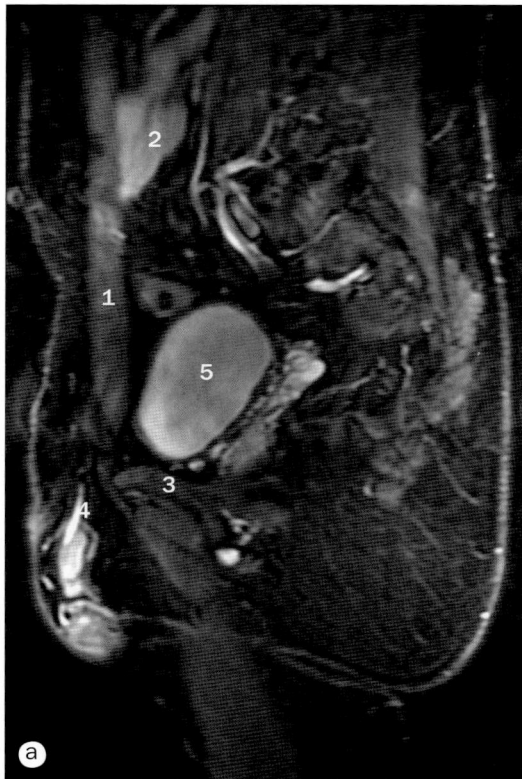

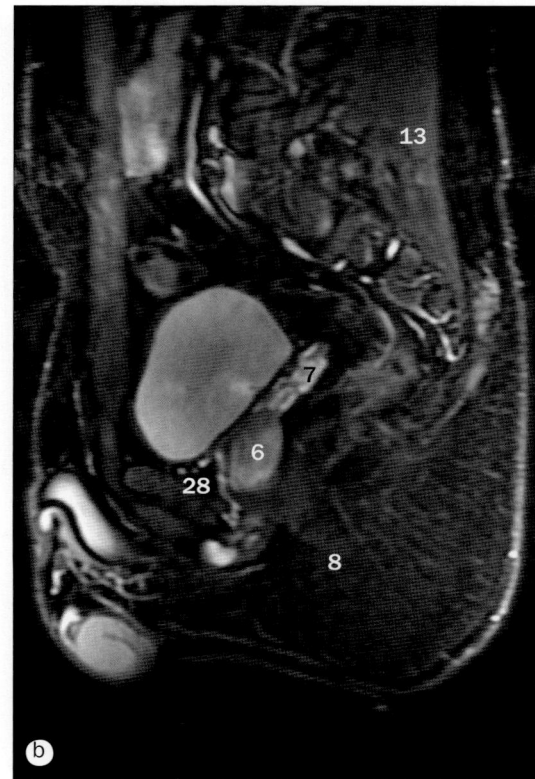

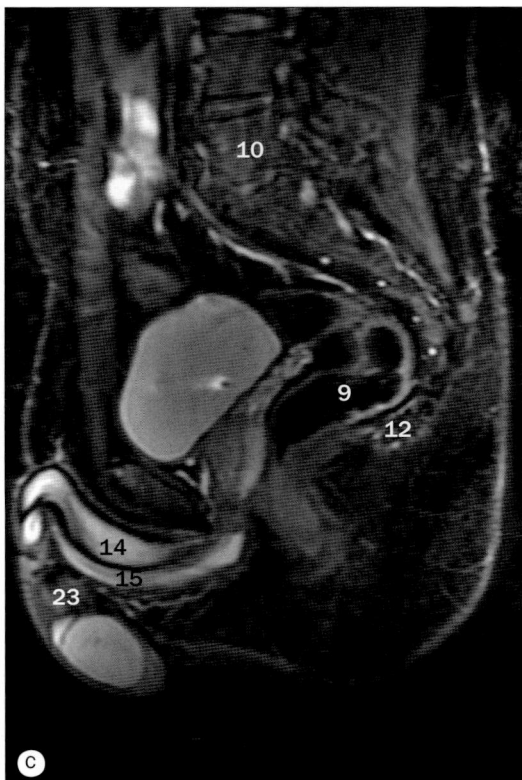

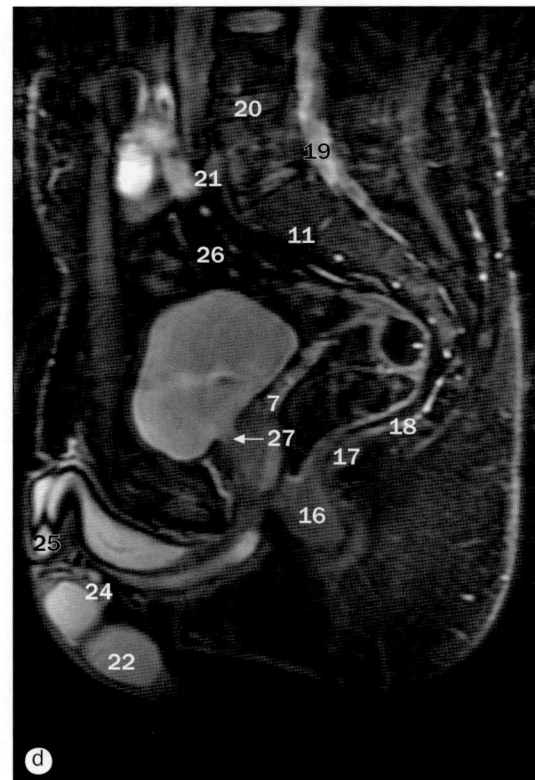

(a)–(h) Sequential sagittal MR images of a male pelvis, from right to left, through the midline (T2 Fat Sat images).

1 Rectus abdominis muscle
2 Small bowel
3 Pubic body
4 Spermatic cord
5 Bladder
6 Prostate
7 Seminal vesicle
8 Ischio-anal fossa

9 Rectum
10 Fifth lumbar vertebra
11 Sacrum
12 Coccyx
13 Erector spinae muscle
14 Corpus cavernosum
15 Corpus spongiosum

16 Anal canal
17 Puborectalis muscle
18 Anococcygeal raphe
19 Thecal sac
20 Intervertebral disc (L4/5)
21 Common iliac vein
22 Testicle

23 Epididymal head
24 Epididymal body
25 Glans penis
26 Sigmoid colon
27 Prostatic urethra
28 Retropubic space (cave of Retzius)

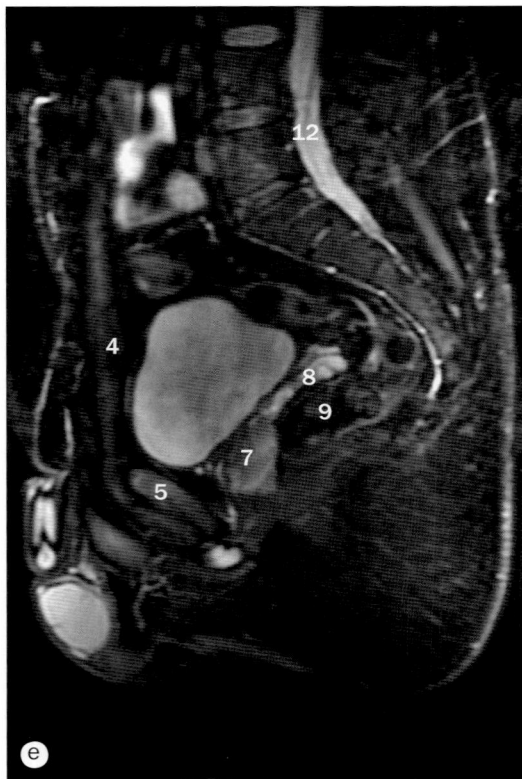

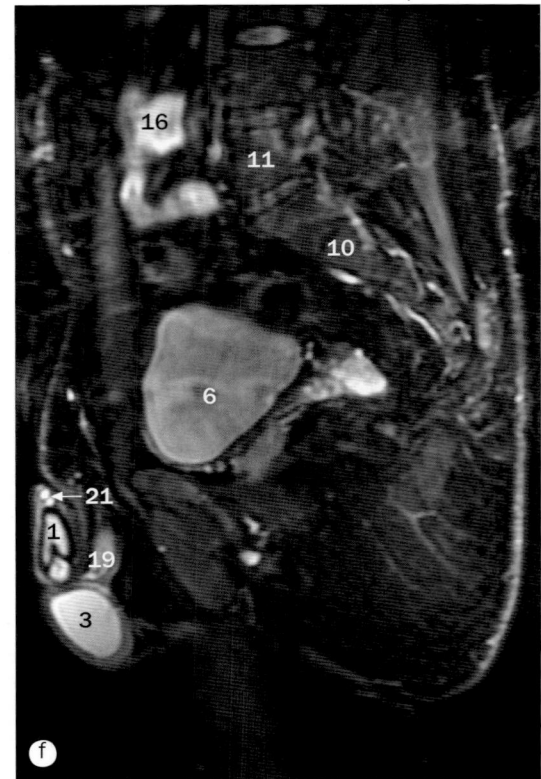

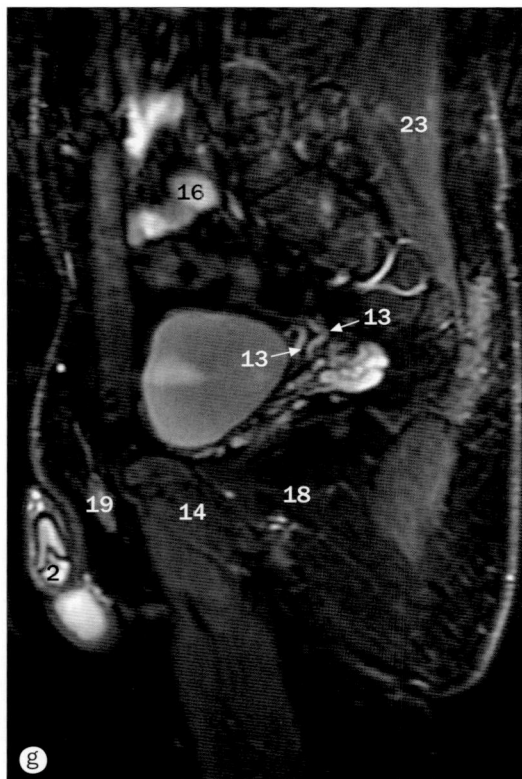

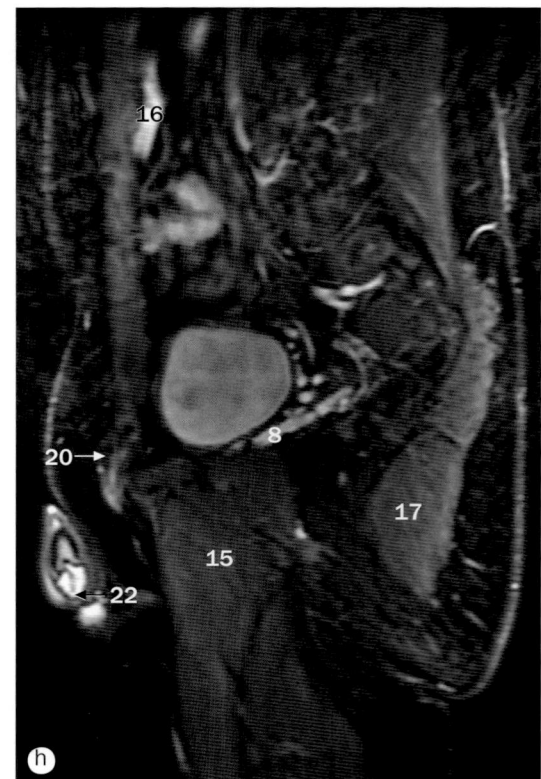

(a)–(h) Sequential sagittal MR images of a male pelvis, from right to left, through the midline (T2 Fat Sat images).

1 Corpus cavernosum	**7** Prostate	**13** Ductus (vas) deferens	**19** Spermatic cord
2 Glans penis	**8** Seminal vesicle	**14** Pectineus muscle	**20** Inguinal canal (external ring)
3 Testicle	**9** Rectum	**15** Adductor brevis muscle	**21** Dorsal vessels of penis
4 Rectus abdominis muscle	**10** Sacrum	**16** Small bowel	**22** External meatus of urethra
5 Pubic body	**11** Fifth lumbar vertebra	**17** Gluteus maximus muscle	**23** Erector spinae muscle
6 Bladder	**12** Thecal sac	**18** Ischio-anal fossa	

6 Abdomen and pelvis — Non cross-sectional

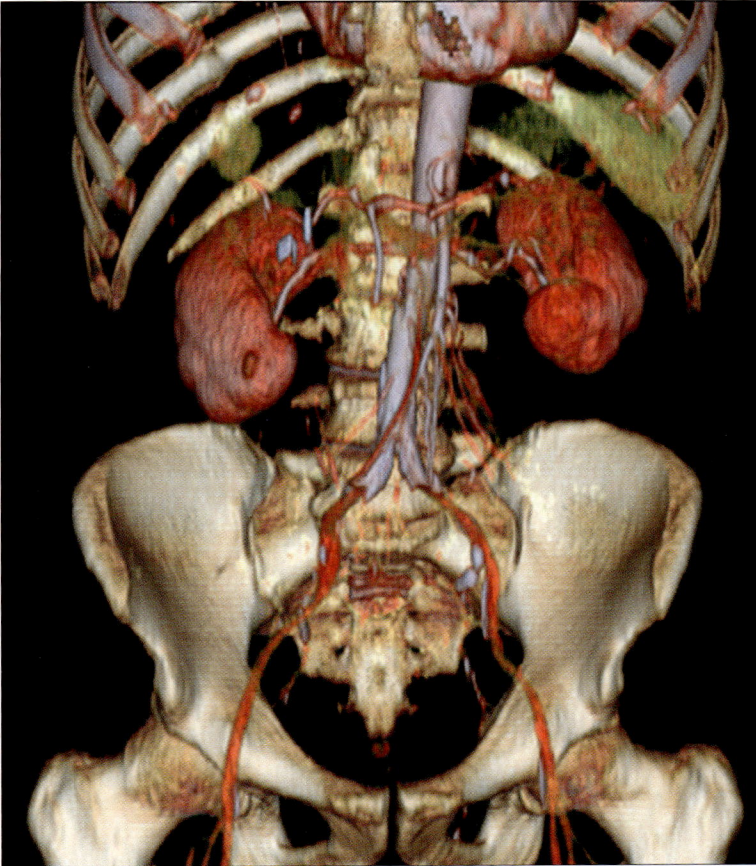

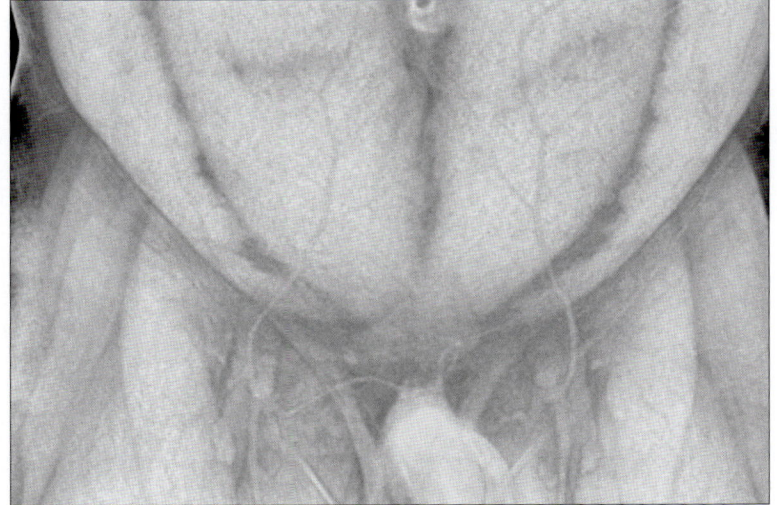

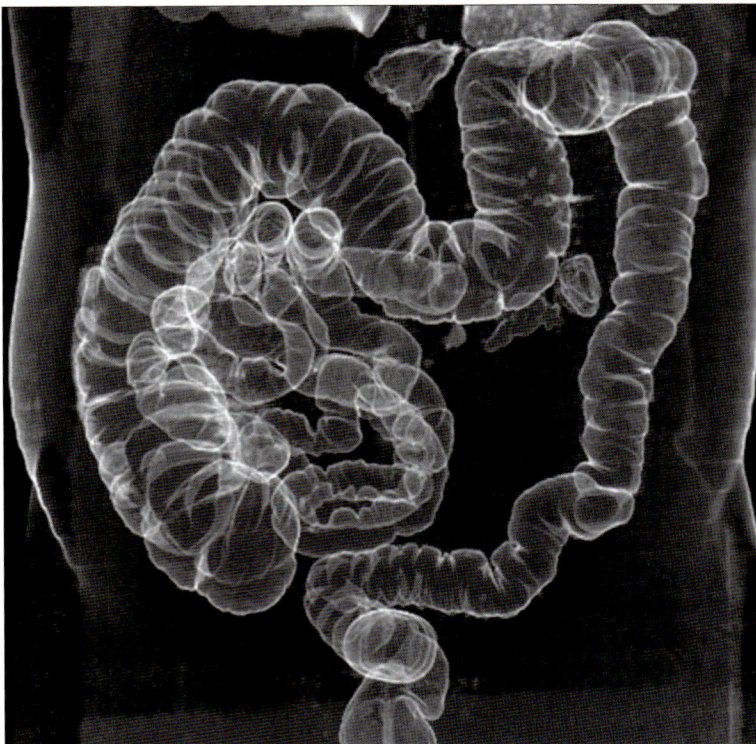

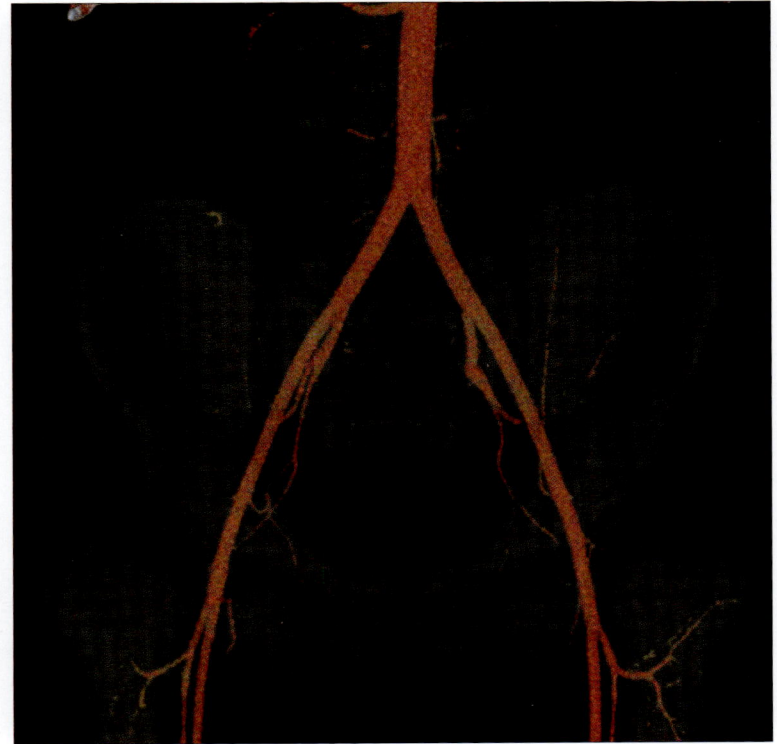

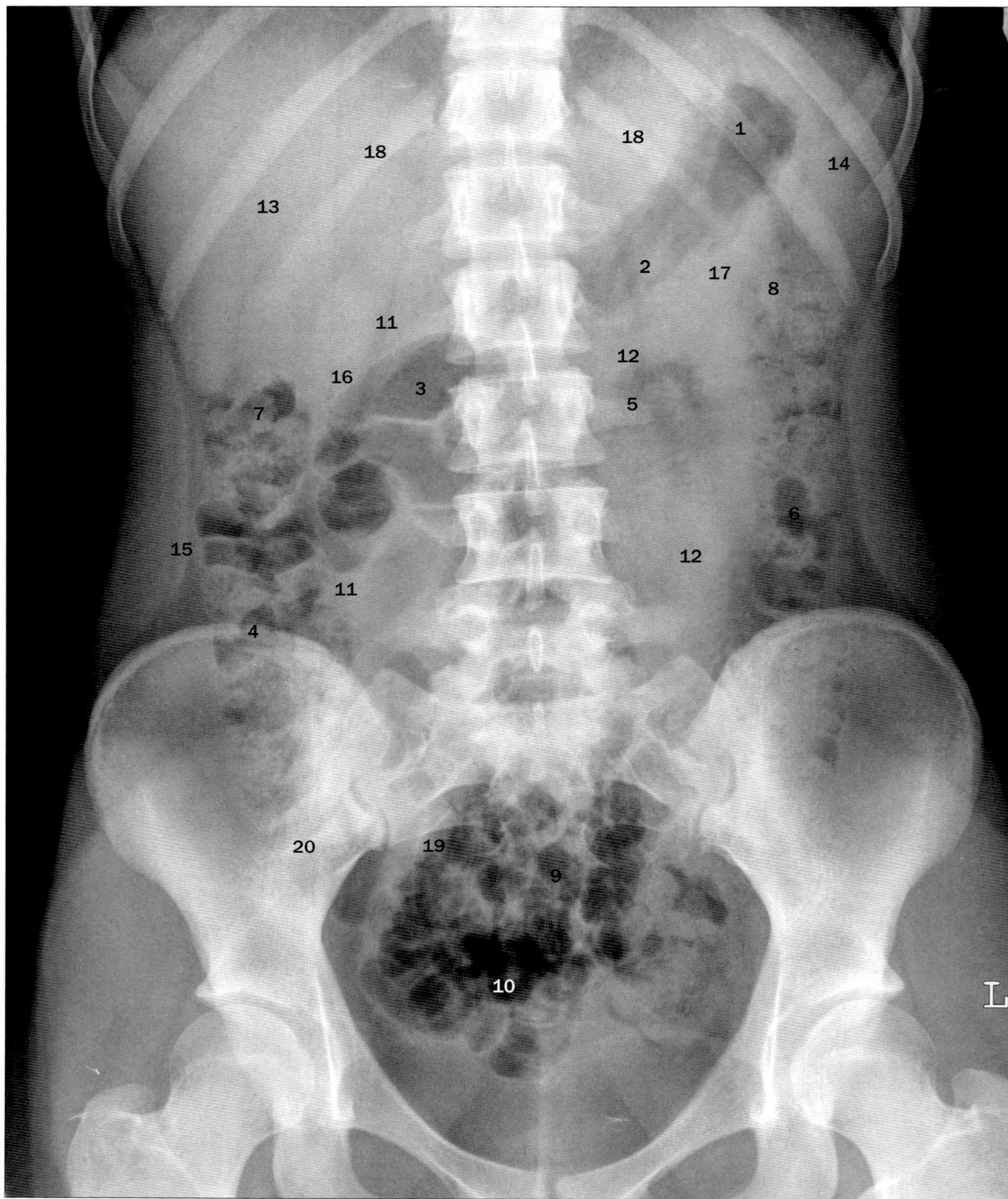

Supine abdominal radiograph.

1 Gas in fundus of stomach	**7** Hepatic flexure of colon	**14** Spleen
2 Gas in body of stomach	**8** Splenic flexure of colon	**15** Properitoneal fat line
3 Gas in first part of duodenum (duodenal cap)	**9** Sigmoid colon	**16** Right kidney
	10 Rectum	**17** Left kidney
4 Ascending colon	**11** Right psoas margin	**18** Twelfth rib
5 Transverse colon	**12** Left psoas margin	**19** Gas in ileum
6 Descending colon	**13** Liver	**20** Gas in caecum

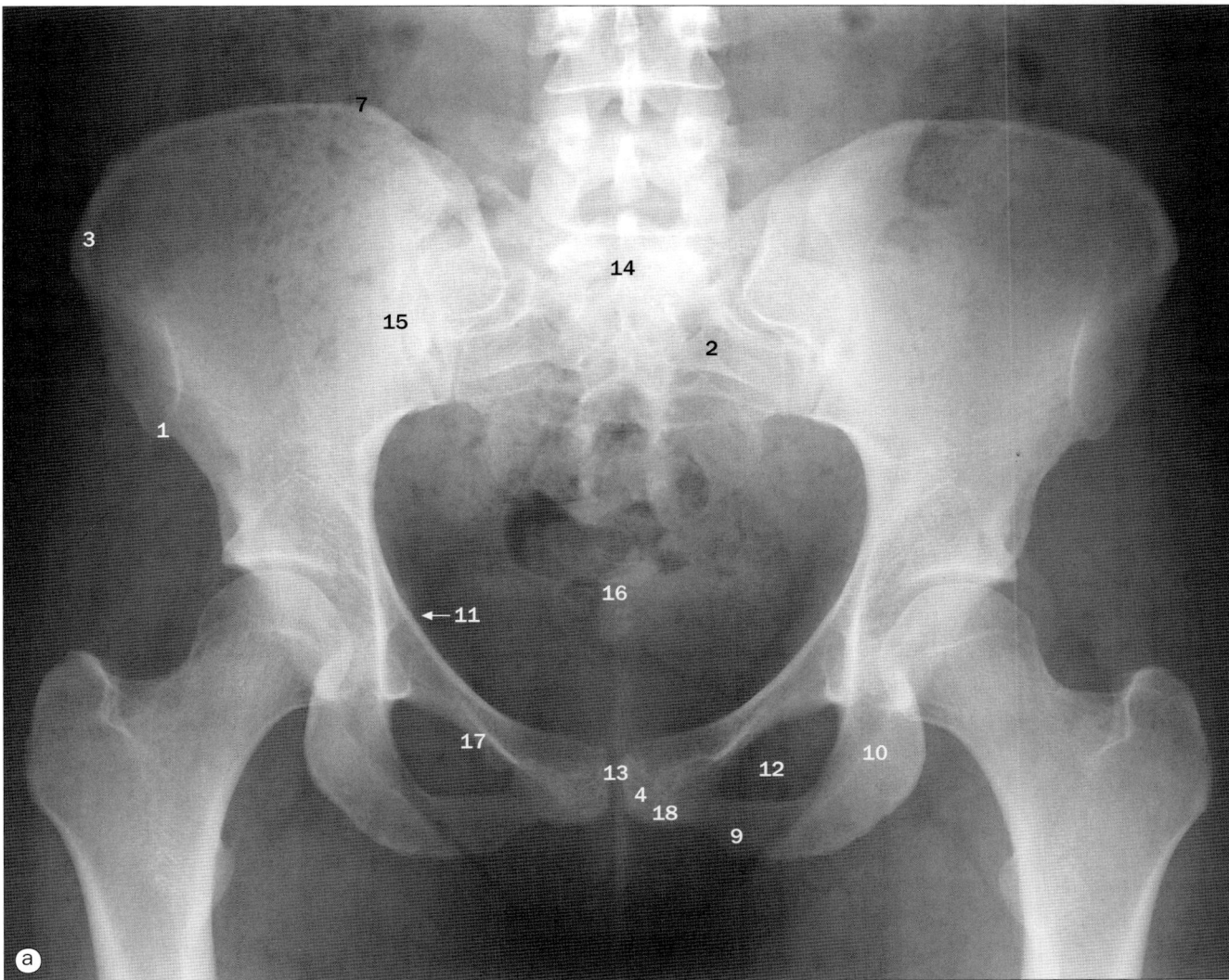

(a) Pelvis and hips of an adult female, anteroposterior projection.
(b) and (c) Pelvis of a 17-year-old male, anteroposterior projections.

1 Anterior inferior iliac spine	**7** Iliac crest	**13** Pubic symphysis
2 Anterior sacral foramen	**8** Ilium	**14** Sacral crest
3 Anterior superior iliac spine	**9** Inferior ramus of pubis	**15** Sacro-iliac joint
4 Body of pubis	**10** Ischial ramus	**16** Segment of coccyx
5 Centre for iliac crest	**11** Ischial spine	**17** Superior ramus of pubis
6 Centre for ischial tuberosity	**12** Obturator foramen	**18** Tubercle of pubis

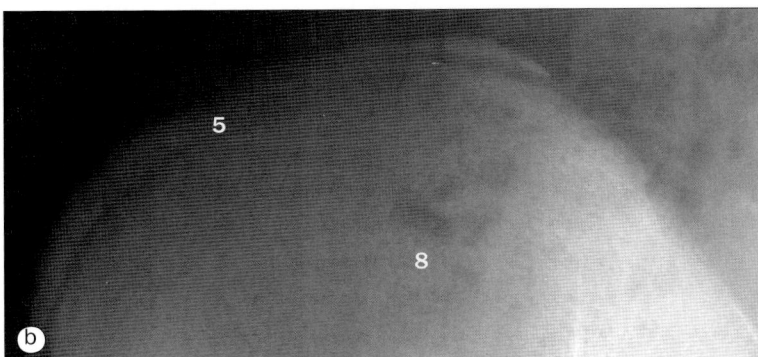

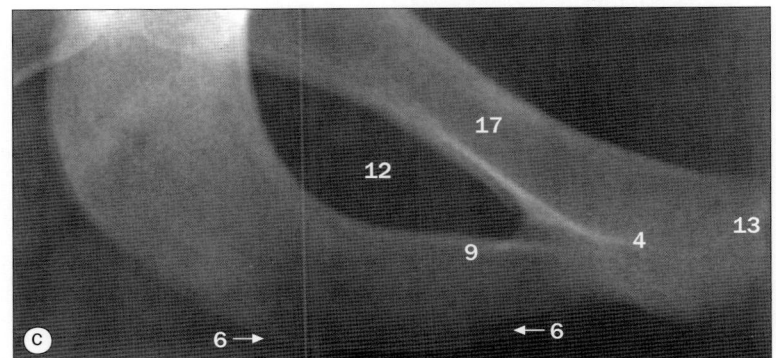

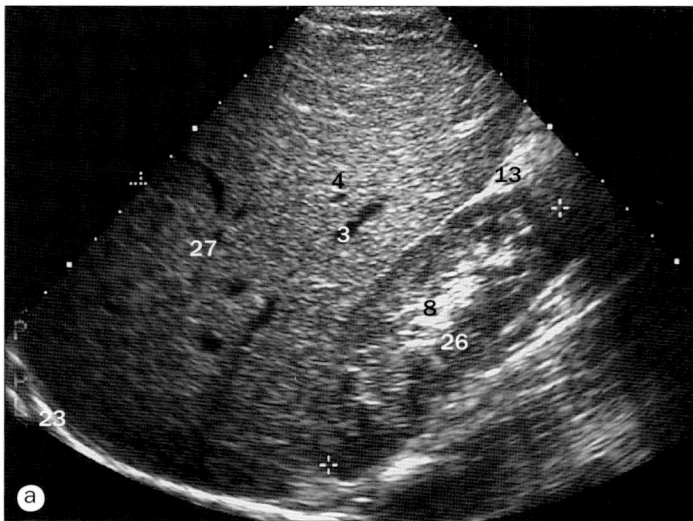

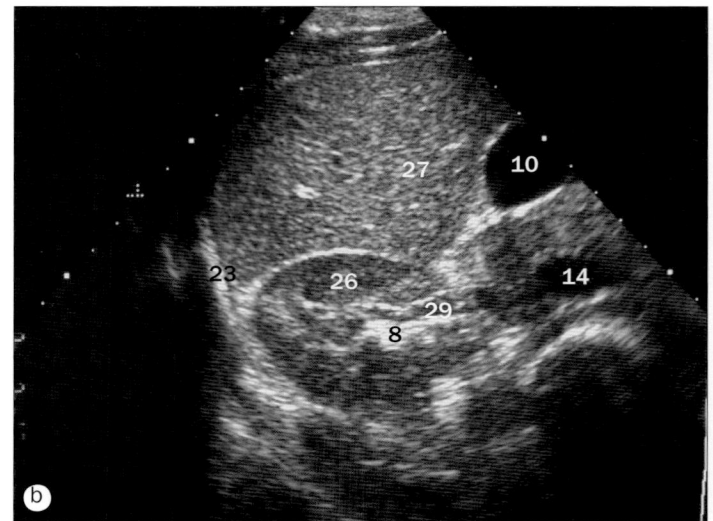

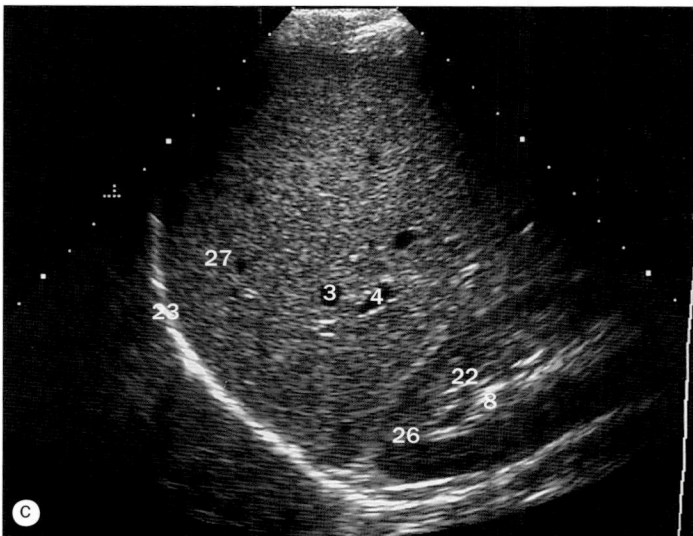

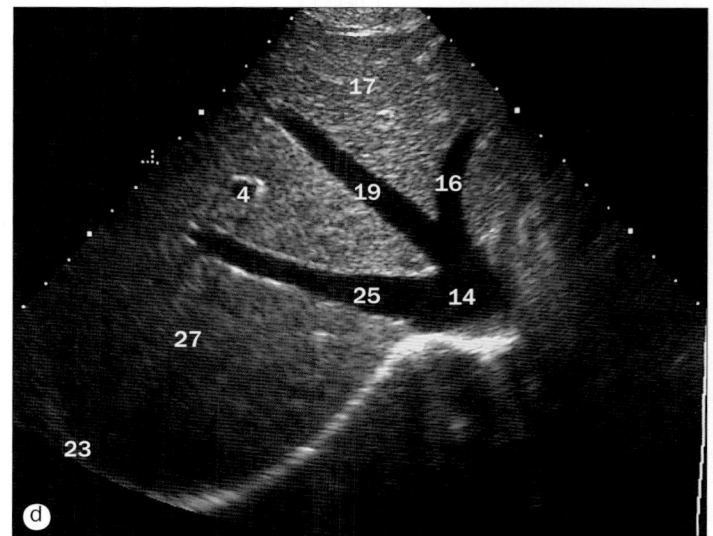

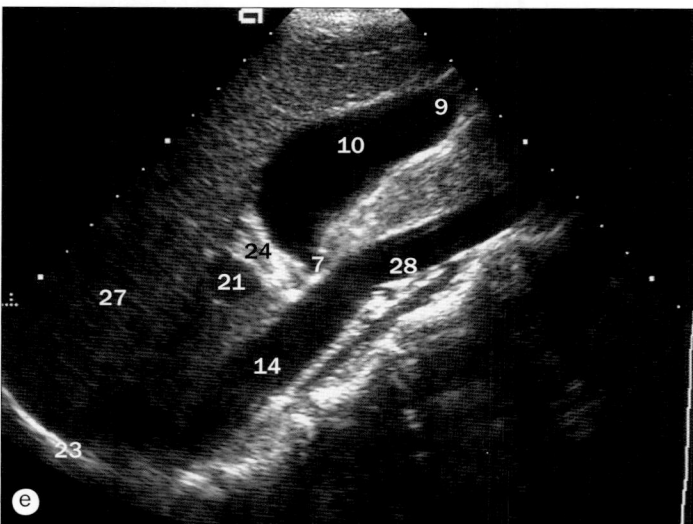

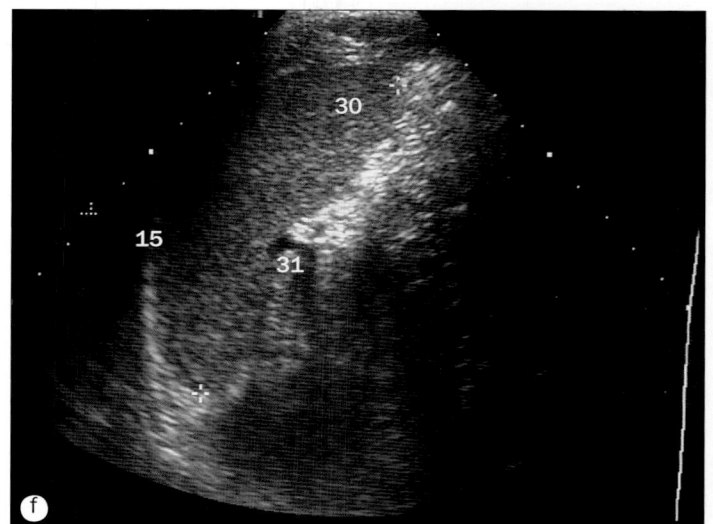

(a)–(f) Abdominal ultrasound, sagittal and parasagittal views.

1 Abdominal aorta	6 Common bile duct	11 Head of pancreas
2 Body of pancreas	7 Cystic duct	12 Hepatic artery
3 Branch of hepatic vein	8 Fat in renal sinus	13 Hepatorenal recess
4 Branch of portal vein	9 Fundus of gall bladder	14 Inferior vena cava
5 Coeliac trunk	10 Gall bladder	15 Left dome of diaphragm

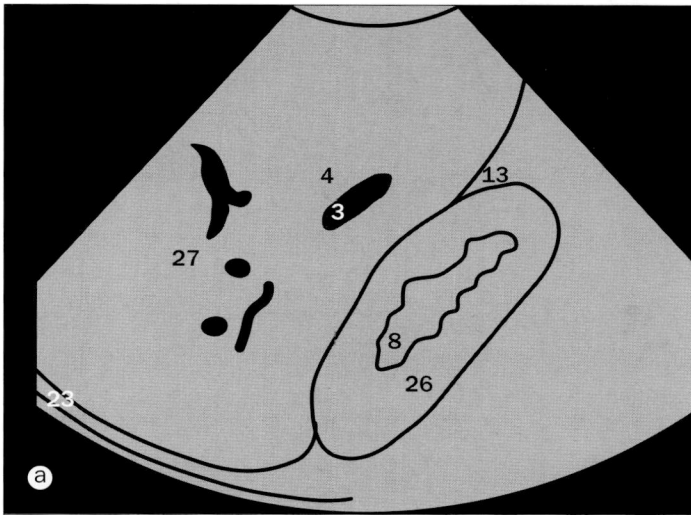

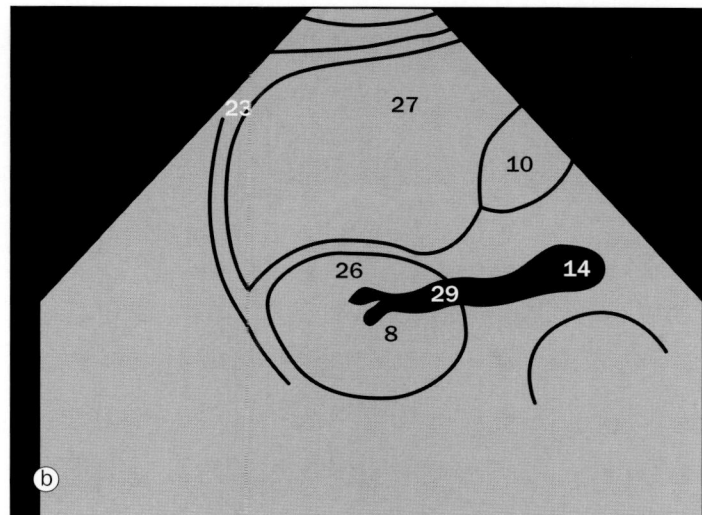

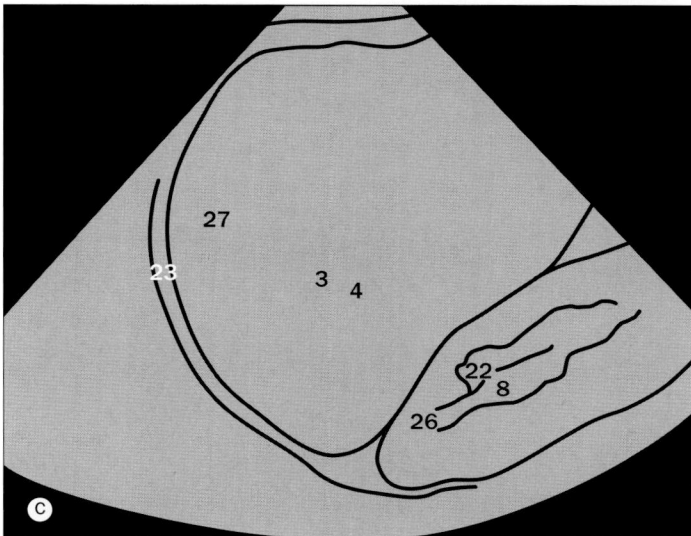

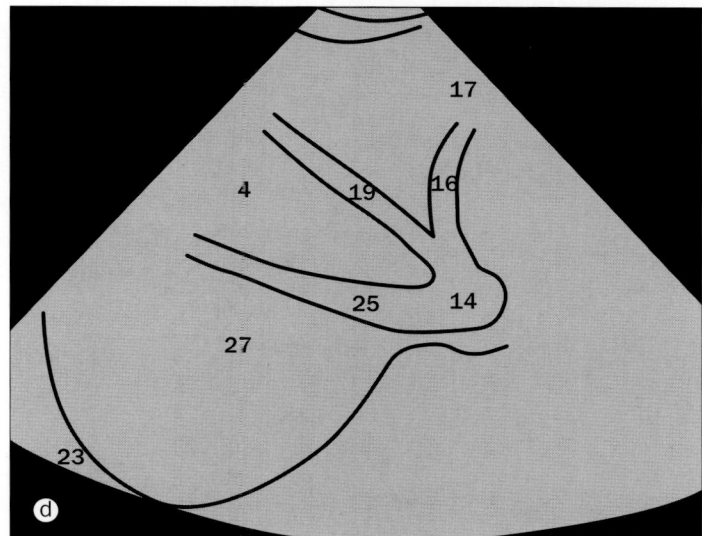

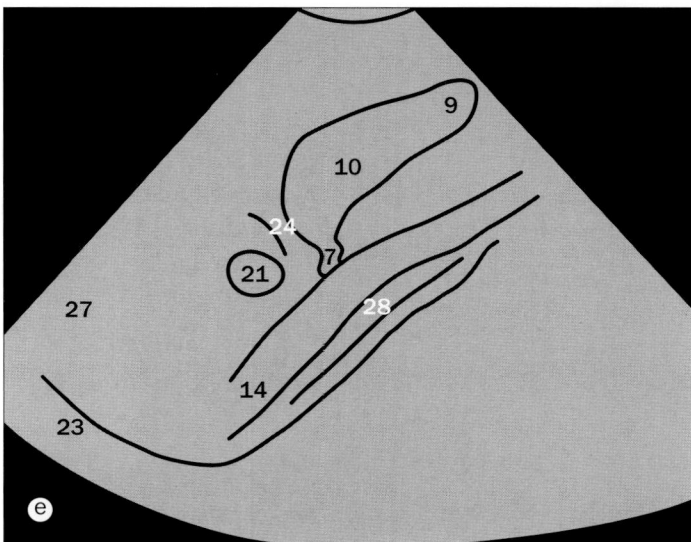

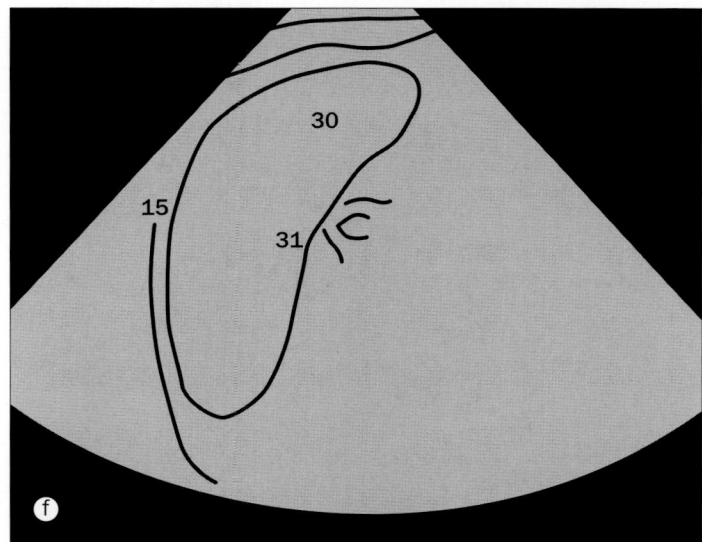

(a)–(f) Line diagrams of ultrasound images opposite.

16 Left hepatic vein	**23** Right dome of diaphragm	**30** Spleen
17 Left lobe of liver	**24** Right hepatic artery	**31** Splenic vein
18 Left renal vein	**25** Right hepatic vein	**32** Superior mesenteric artery
19 Middle hepatic vein	**26** Right kidney	**33** Superior mesenteric vein
20 Neck of pancreas	**27** Right lobe of liver	**34** Tail of pancreas
21 Portal vein	**28** Right renal artery	**35** Vertebral body
22 Renal papilla	**29** Right renal vein	

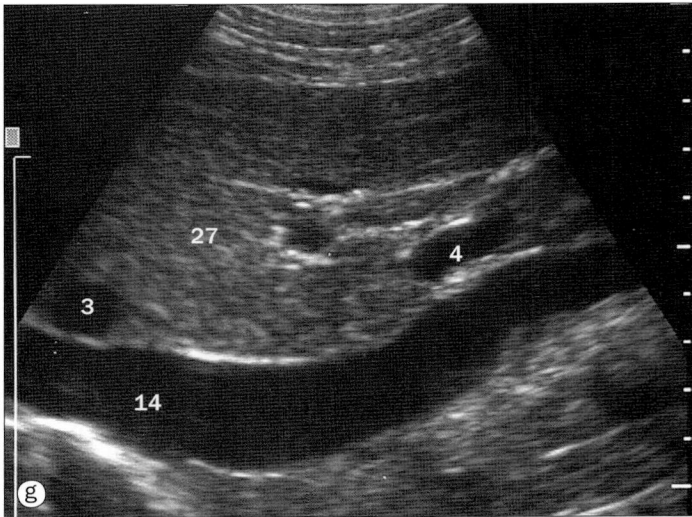

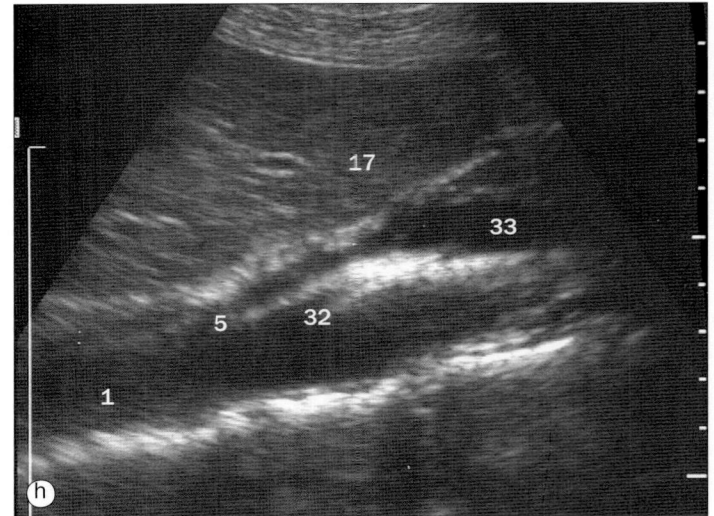

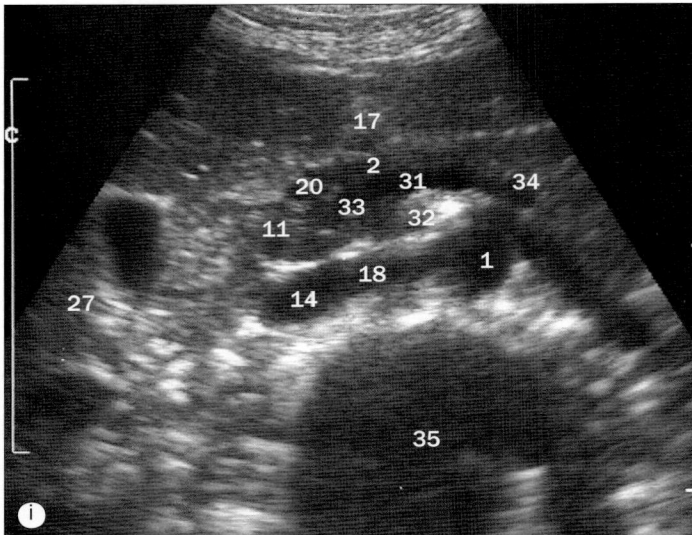

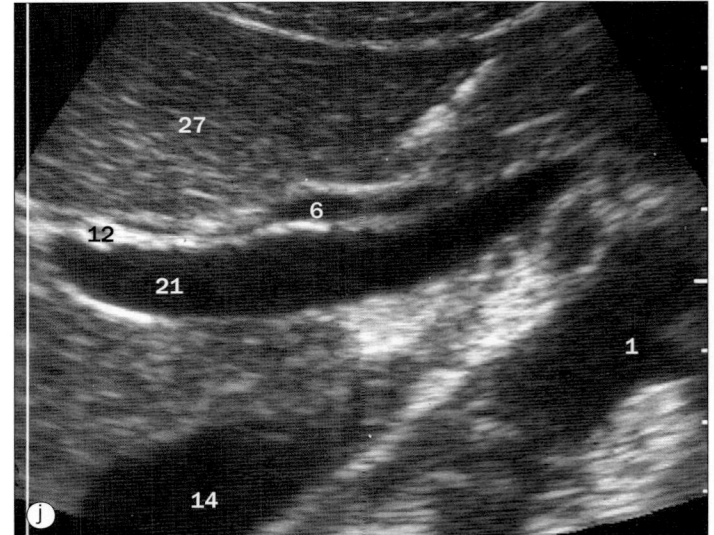

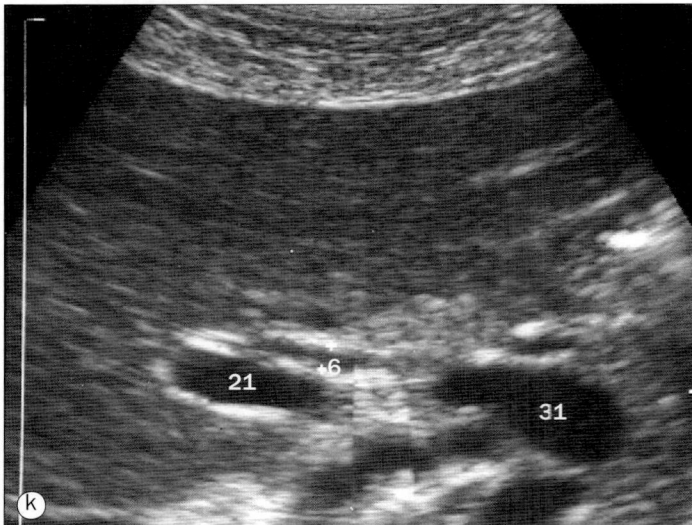

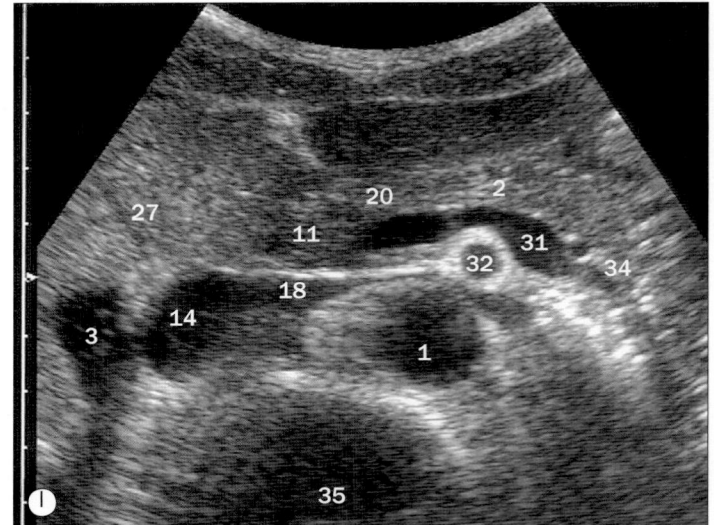

Abdominal ultrasound, (g)–(h) sagittal, (i)–(l) transverse and transverse oblique views.

1 Abdominal aorta	6 Common bile duct	11 Head of pancreas
2 Body of pancreas	7 Cystic duct	12 Hepatic artery
3 Branch of hepatic vein	8 Fat in renal sinus	13 Hepatorenal recess
4 Branch of portal vein	9 Fundus of gall bladder	14 Inferior vena cava
5 Coeliac trunk	10 Gall bladder	15 Left dome of diaphragm

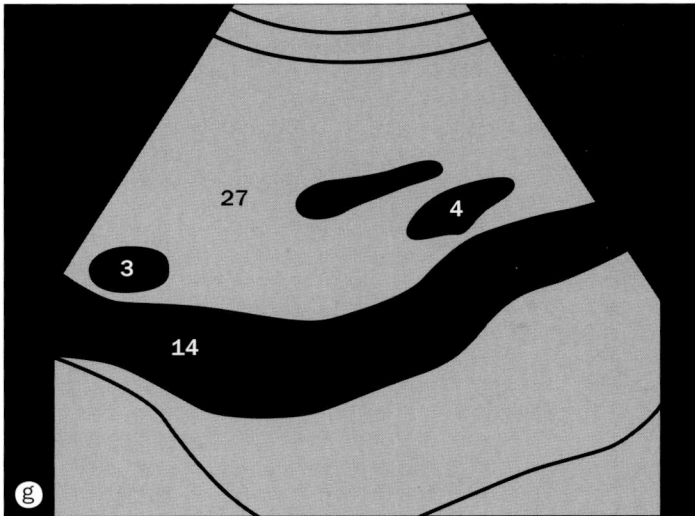

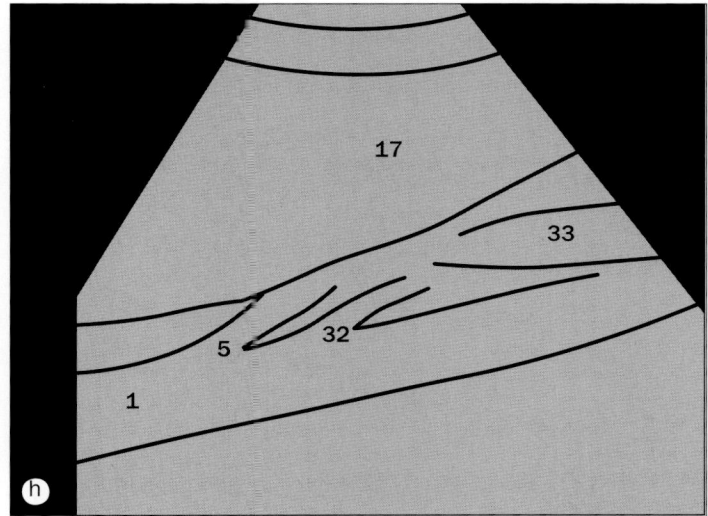

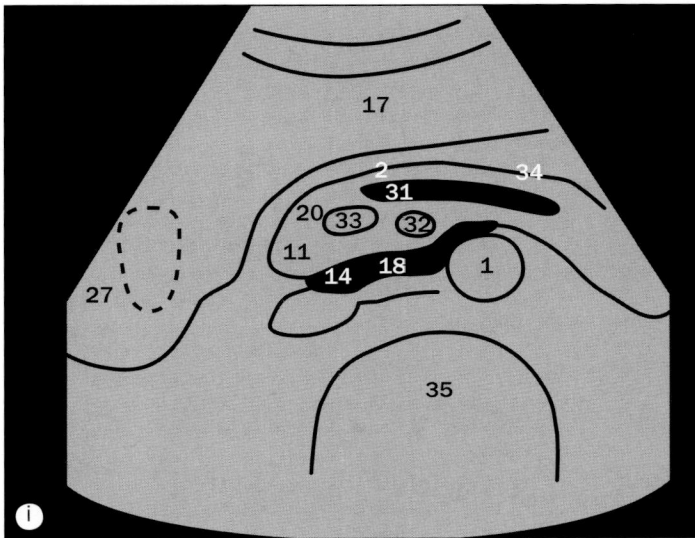

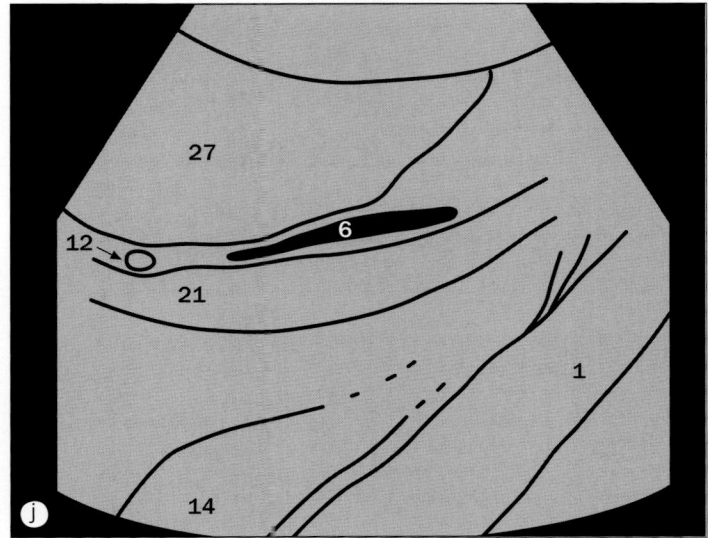

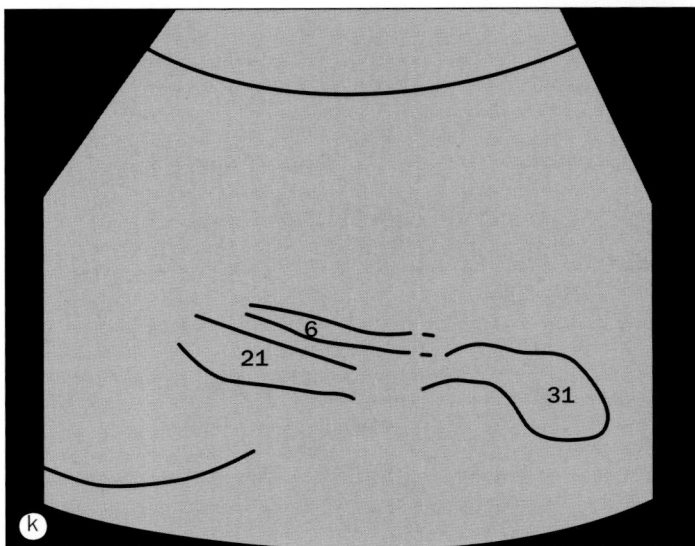

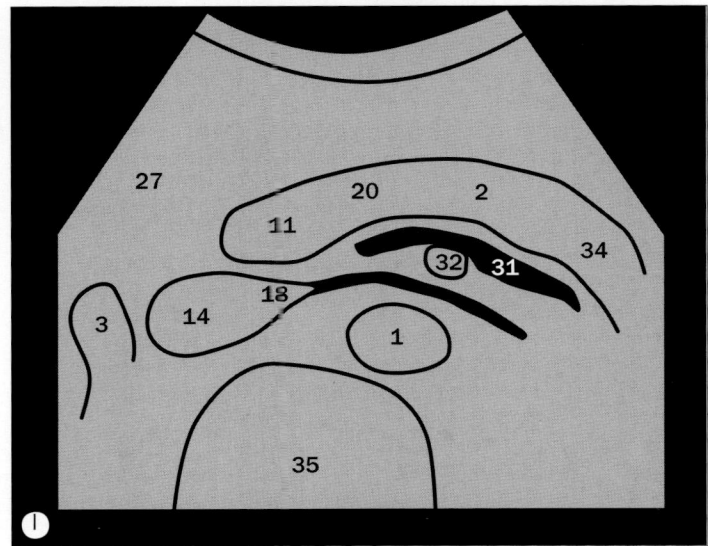

(g)–(l) Line diagrams of ultrasound images opposite.

16 Left hepatic vein	**23** Right dome of diaphragm	**30** Spleen
17 Left lobe of liver	**24** Right hepatic artery	**31** Splenic vein
18 Left renal vein	**25** Right hepatic vein	**32** Superior mesenteric artery
19 Middle hepatic vein	**26** Right kidney	**33** Superior mesenteric vein
20 Neck of pancreas	**27** Right lobe of liver	**34** Tail of pancreas
21 Portal vein	**28** Right renal artery	**35** Vertebral body
22 Renal papilla	**29** Right renal vein	

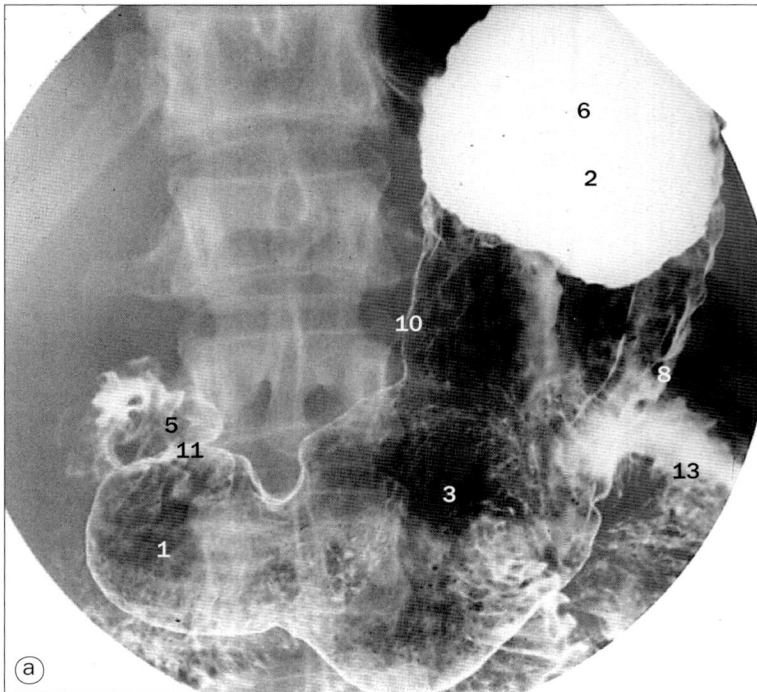

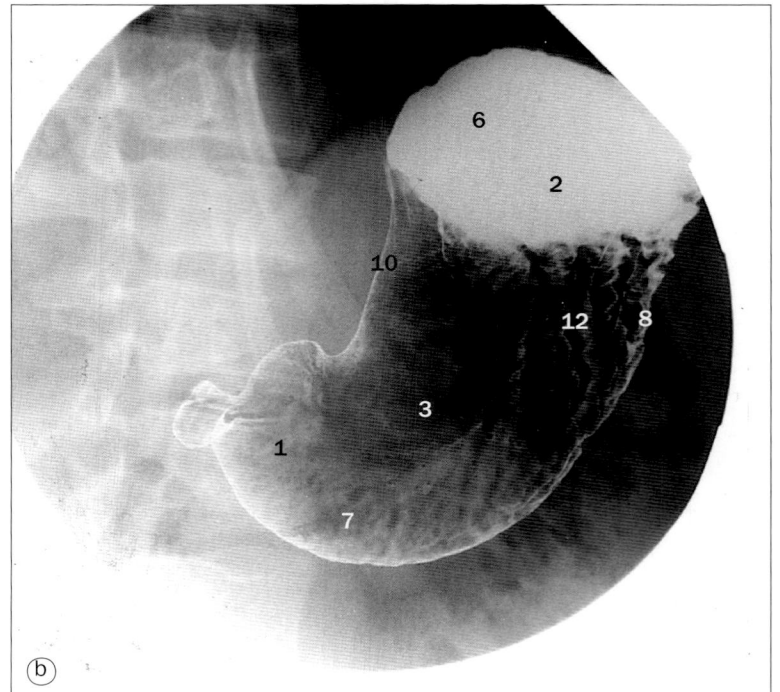

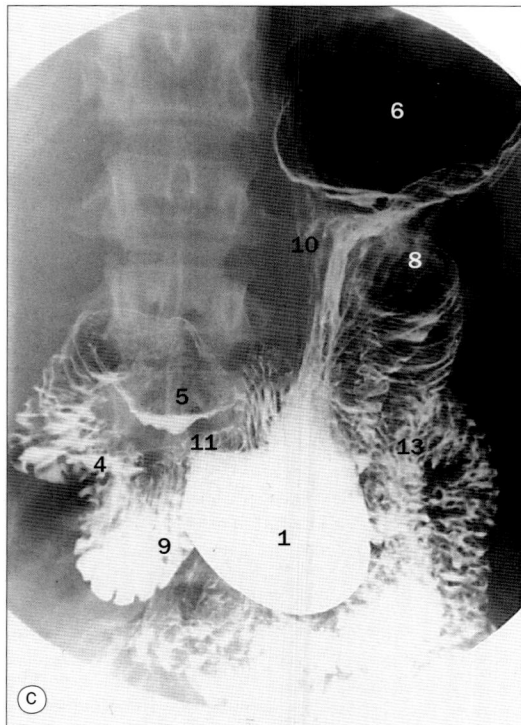

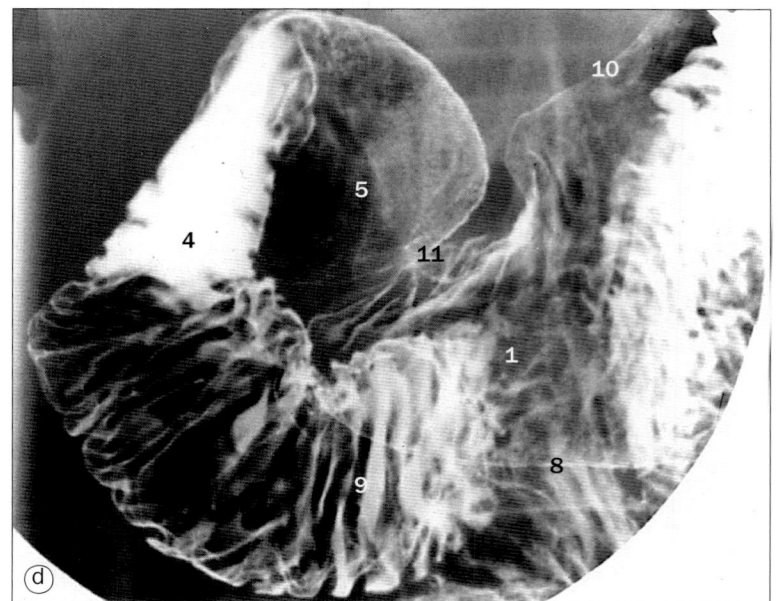

Abdomen. Double-contrast barium meals of stomach and duodenum, **(a)** and **(b)** with the patient supine (to show the mucosa of the stomach), **(c)** with the patient erect, **(d)** with the patient in a supine oblique position (to show the duodenum).

1 Antrum of stomach
2 Barium pooling in fundus of stomach
3 Body of stomach
4 Descending (second) part of duodenum
5 Duodenal cap (superior or first part of duodenum)
6 Fundus of stomach
7 Gas bubbles
8 Greater curvature of stomach
9 Horizontal (third) part of duodenum
10 Lesser curvature of stomach
11 Region of pyloric canal
12 Rugae of stomach
13 Small bowel

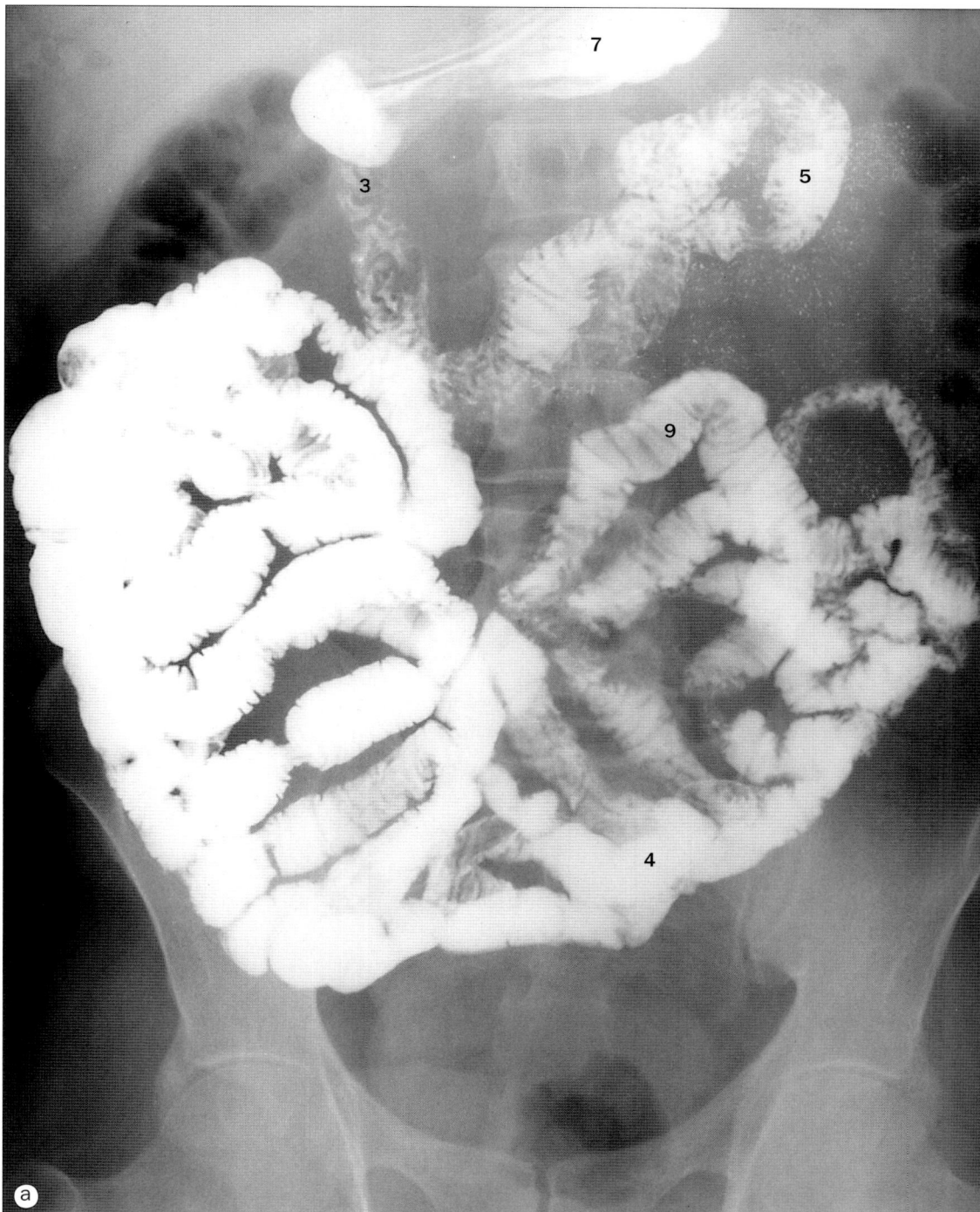

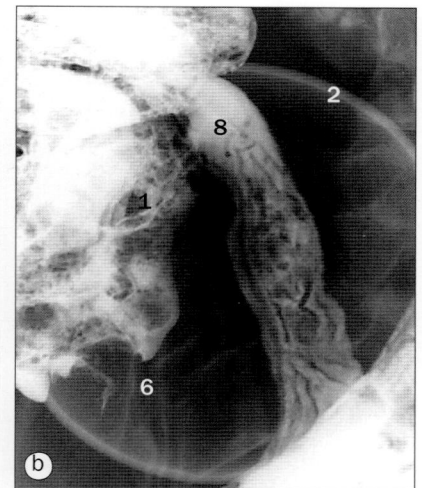

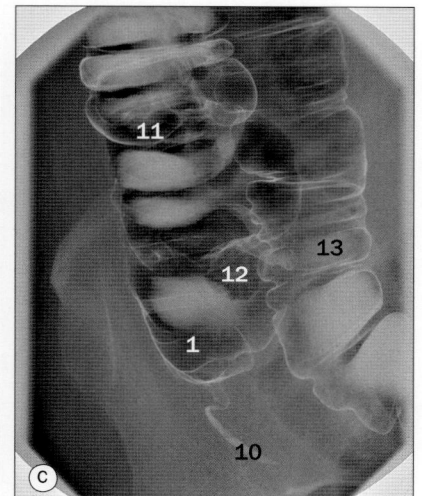

Abdomen, barium follow-throughs, (a) with the patient supine, (b) showing a localised view of the terminal ileum and (c) ileocaecal valve. Anteroposterior radiographs.

1 Caecum
2 Compression device
3 Descending (second) part of duodenum
4 Proximal ileum
5 Proximal jejunum
6 Right sacro-iliac joint
7 Stomach
8 Terminal ileum
9 Valvulae conniventes (plicae circulares) of jejunum
10 Appendix
11 Ascending colon
12 Ileocaecal valve
13 Transverse colon

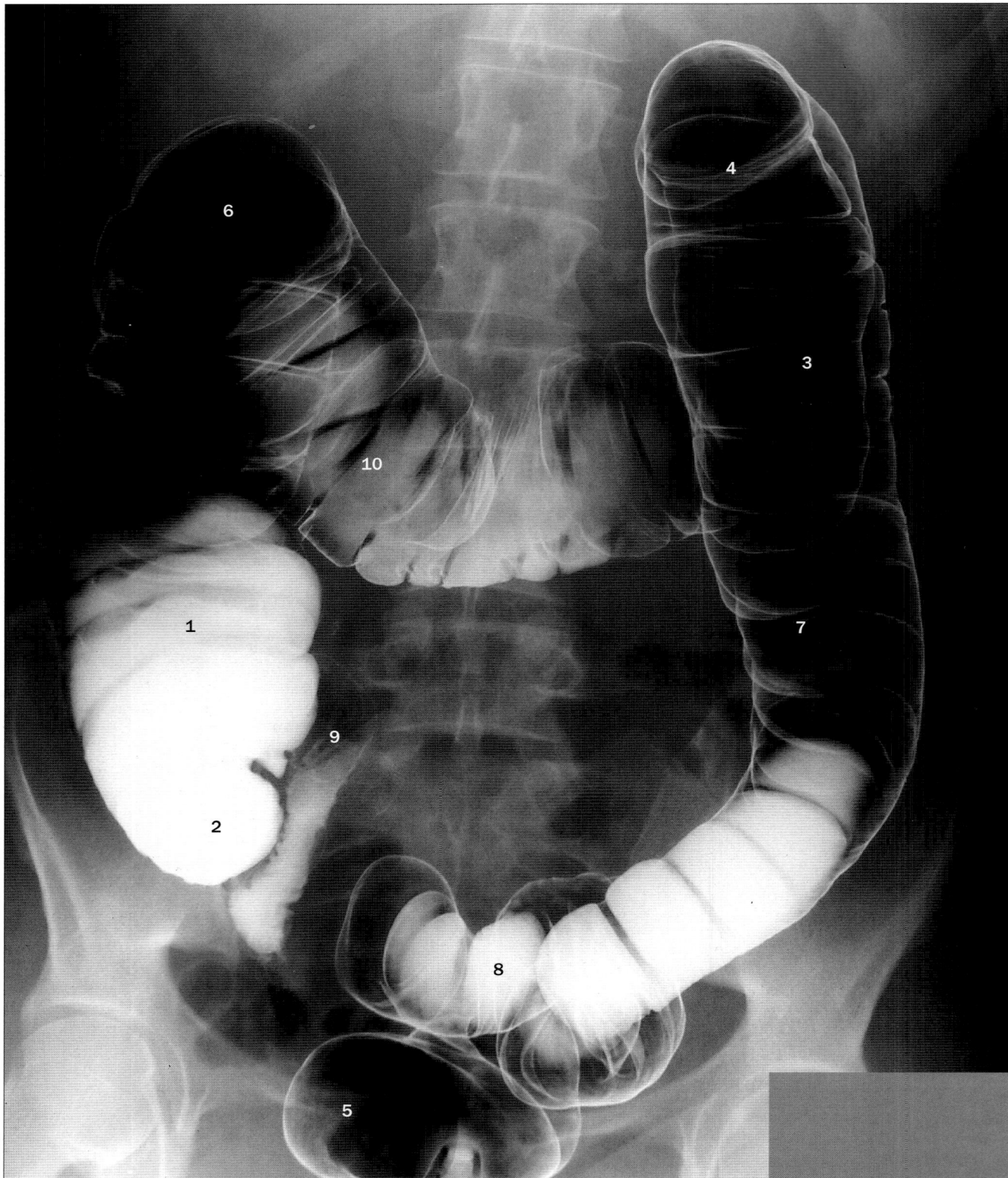

Abdomen, double-contrast barium enema of the large bowel (colon).

1 Ascending portion of colon	6 Right colic (hepatic) flexure of colon
2 Caecum	7 Sacculations (haustrations) of colon
3 Descending portion of colon	8 Sigmoid colon
4 Left colic (splenic) flexure of colon	9 Terminal ileum
5 Rectum	10 Transverse portion of colon

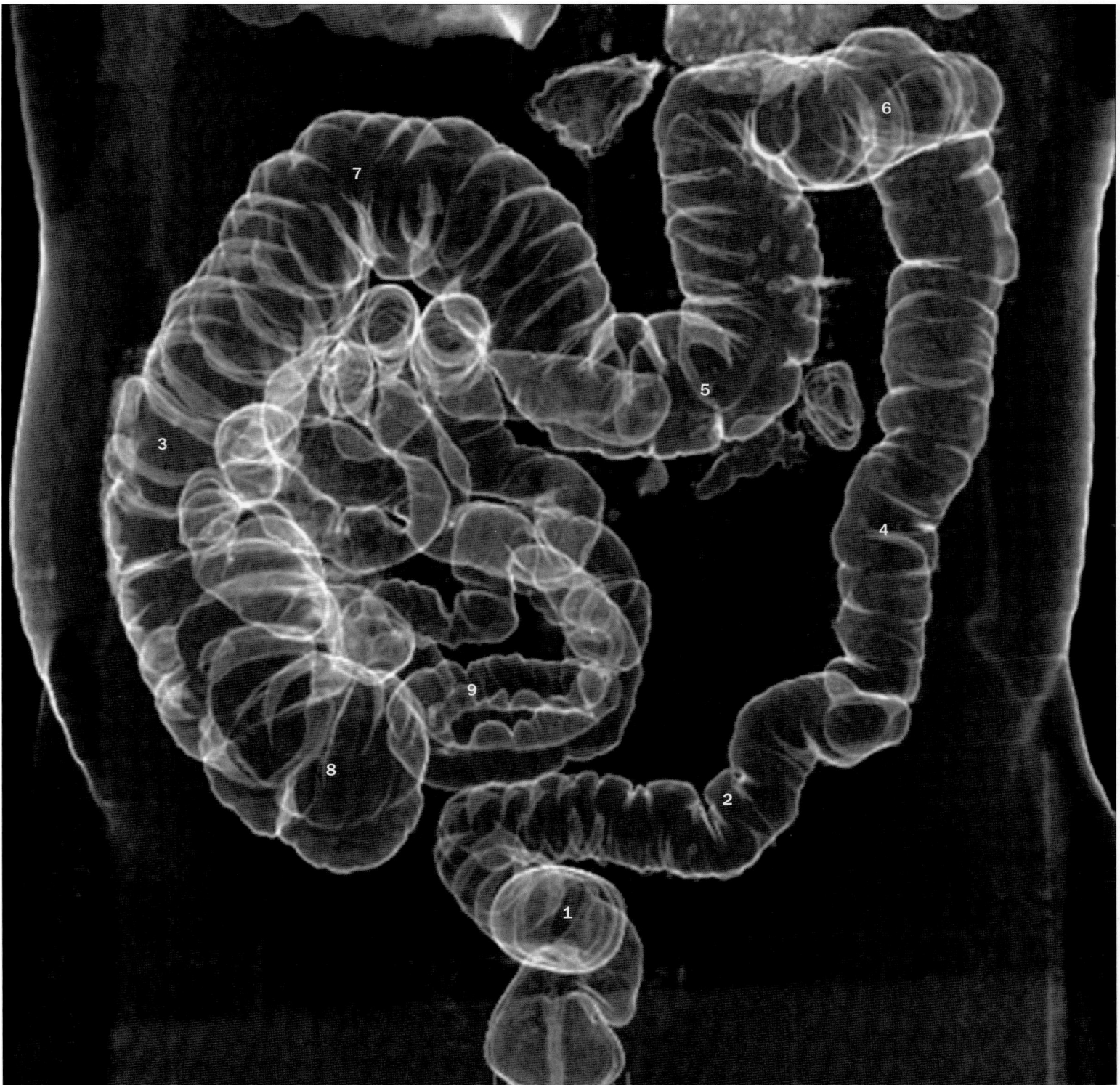

CT colonography.

1	Rectum	**6**	Splenic flexure (left colic)
2	Sigmoid colon	**7**	Hepatic flexure (right colic)
3	Ascending colon	**8**	Caecum
4	Descending colon	**9**	Terminal ileum
5	Transverse colon		

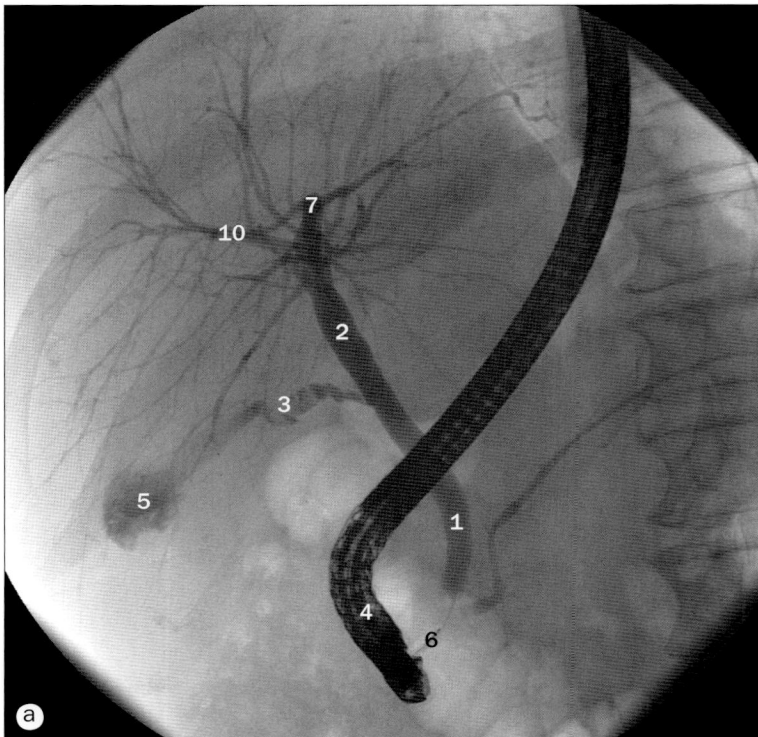

(a) Endoscopic retrograde cholangiopancreatogram (ERCP).

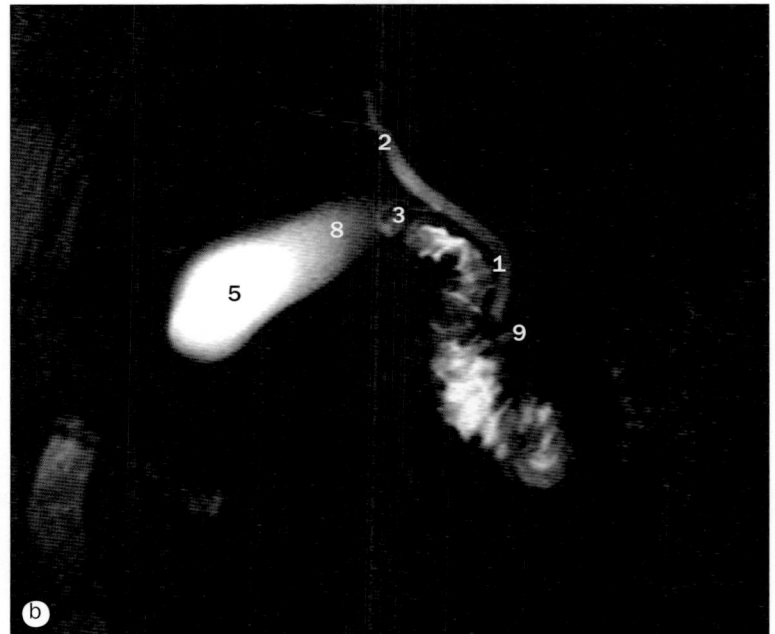

(b) Magnetic cholangiopancreatogram (MRCP).

1 Common bile duct
2 Common hepatic duct
3 Cystic duct
4 Endoscope in duodenum

5 Gall bladder
6 Hepatopancreatic (Vater's) ampulla
7 Left hepatic duct

8 Neck of gall bladder
9 Pancreatic duct
10 Right hepatic duct

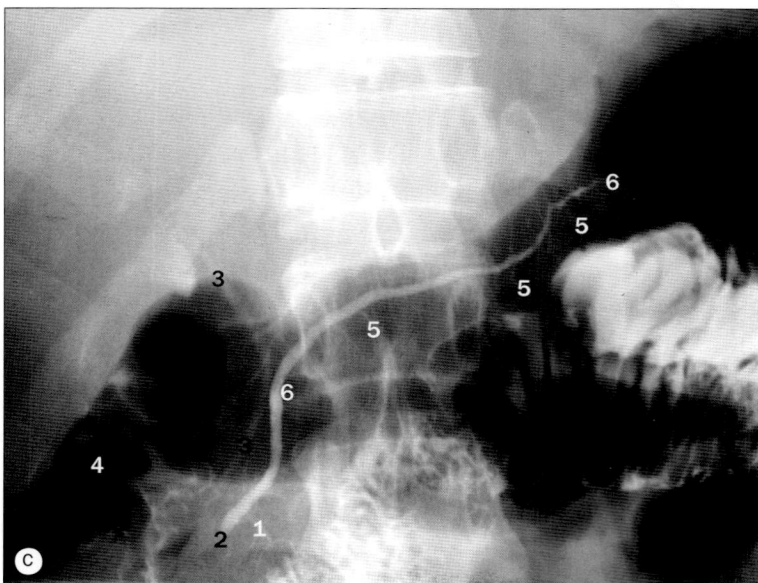

(c) ERCP.

1 Accessory pancreatic duct (Santonni's)
2 Ampullary part of pancreatic duct
3 Common bile duct
4 Contrast and gas in descending (second) part of duodenum
5 Intralobular ducts
6 Main pancreatic duct

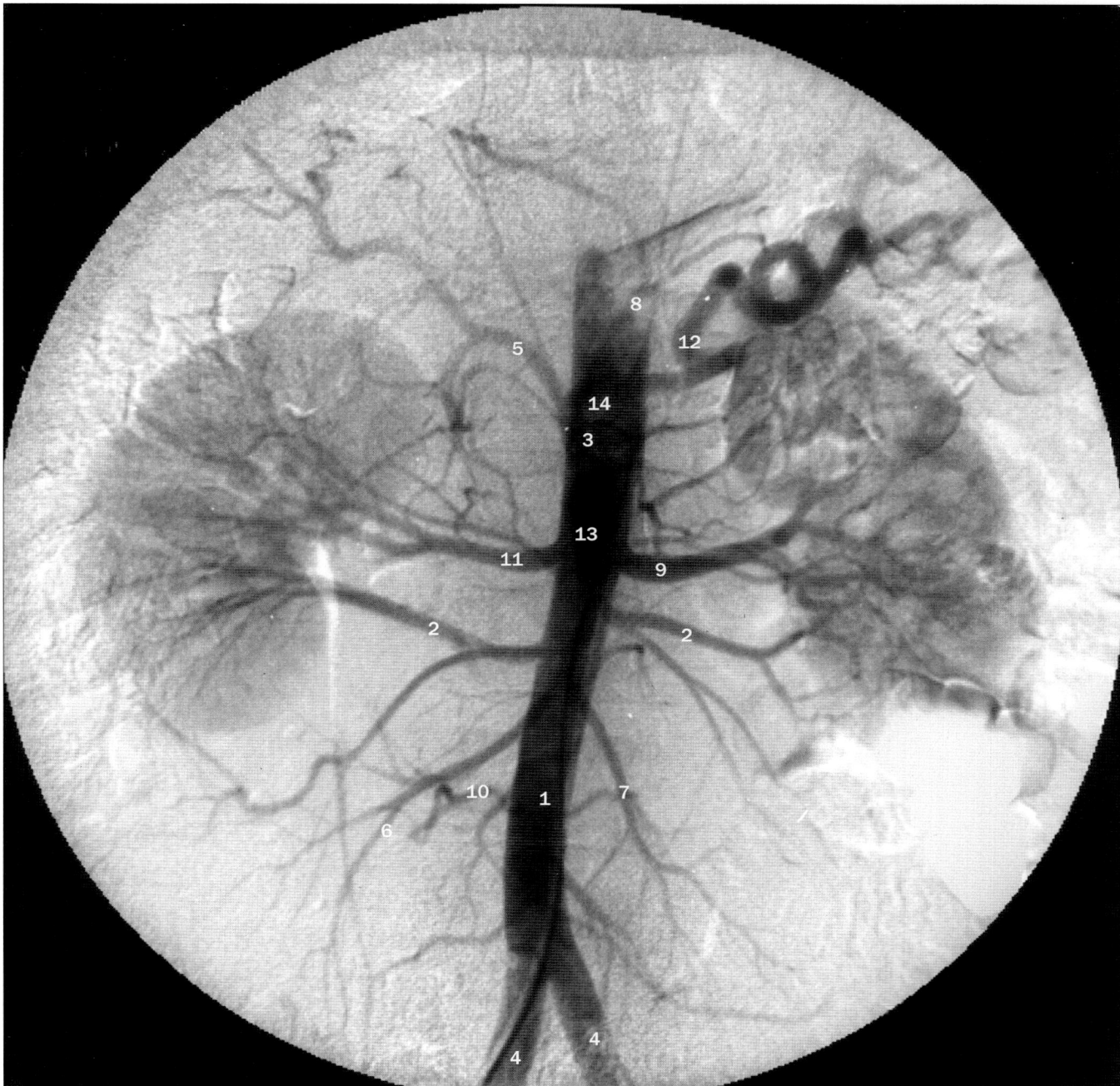

Abdominal aortogram.

1 Abdominal aorta
2 Accessory renal arteries
3 Coeliac trunk
4 Common iliac arteries
5 Hepatic artery
6 Ileocolic artery
7 Jejunal branches of superior mesenteric artery
8 Left gastric artery
9 Left renal artery
10 Lumbar arteries
11 Right renal artery
12 Splenic artery
13 Superior mesenteric artery
14 Tip of pigtail catheter in abdominal aorta

(a) and (b) Subtracted coeliac trunk arteriograms.

1 Dorsal pancreatic artery
2 Gastroduodenal artery
3 Hepatic artery
4 Left gastric artery
5 Left gastro-epiploic artery
6 Left hepatic artery
7 Pancreatica magna artery
8 Phrenic artery
9 Right gastro-epiploic artery
10 Right hepatic artery
11 Splenic artery
12 Superior pancreatico-duodenal artery
13 Tip of catheter in coeliac trunk
14 Transverse pancreatic artery

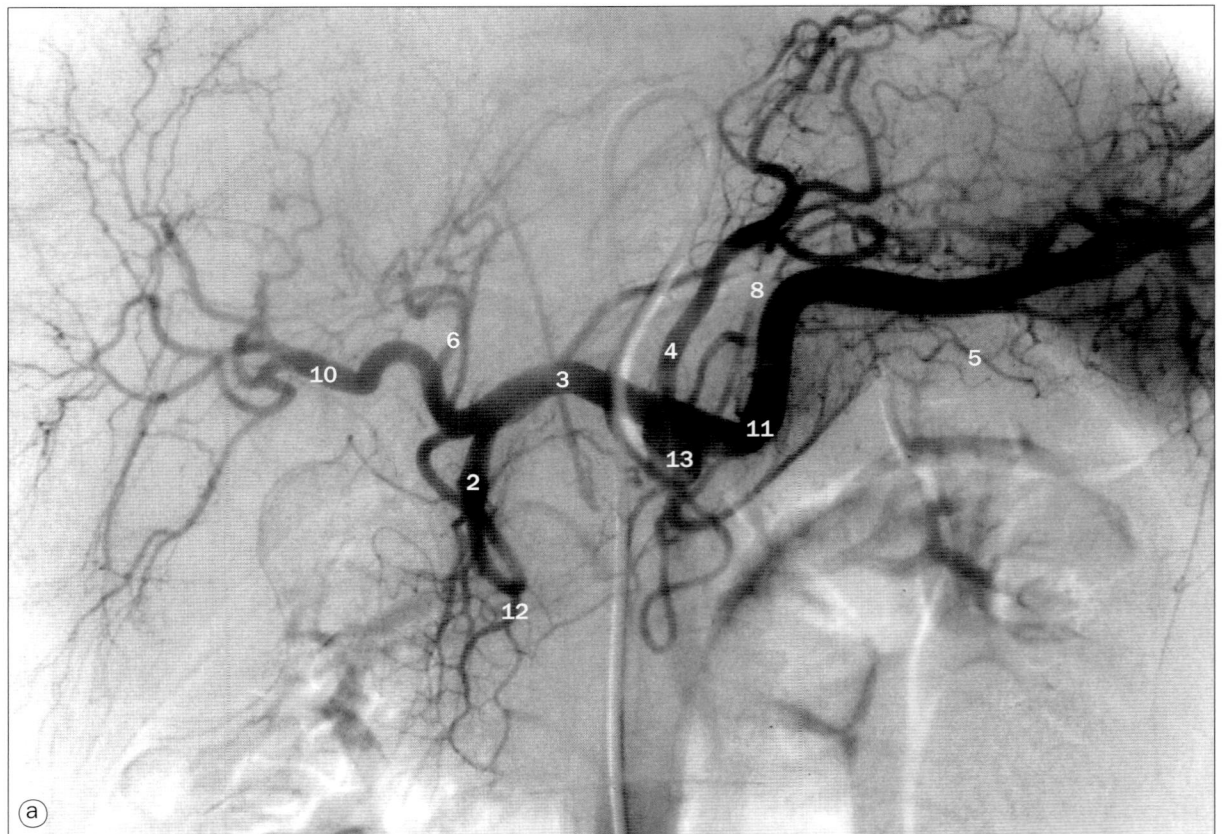

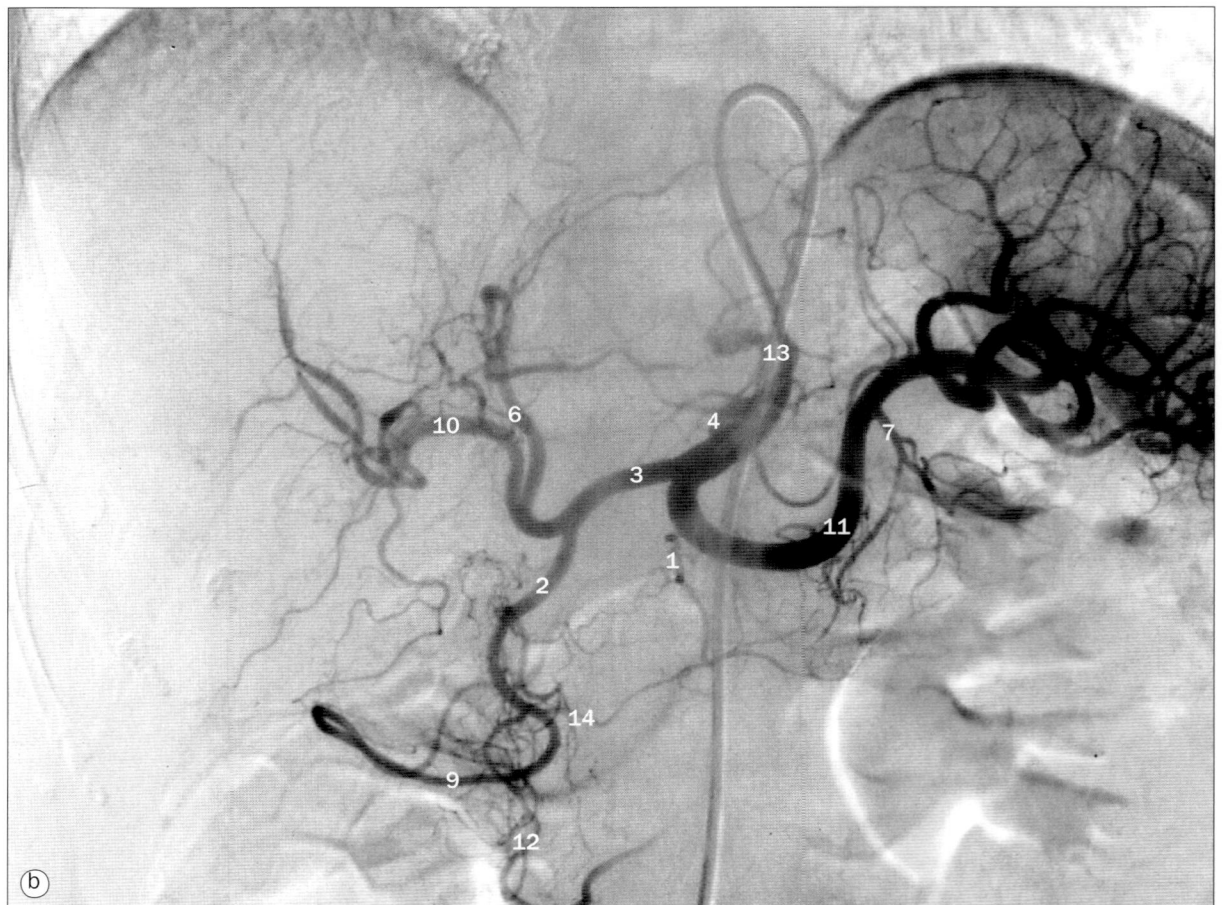

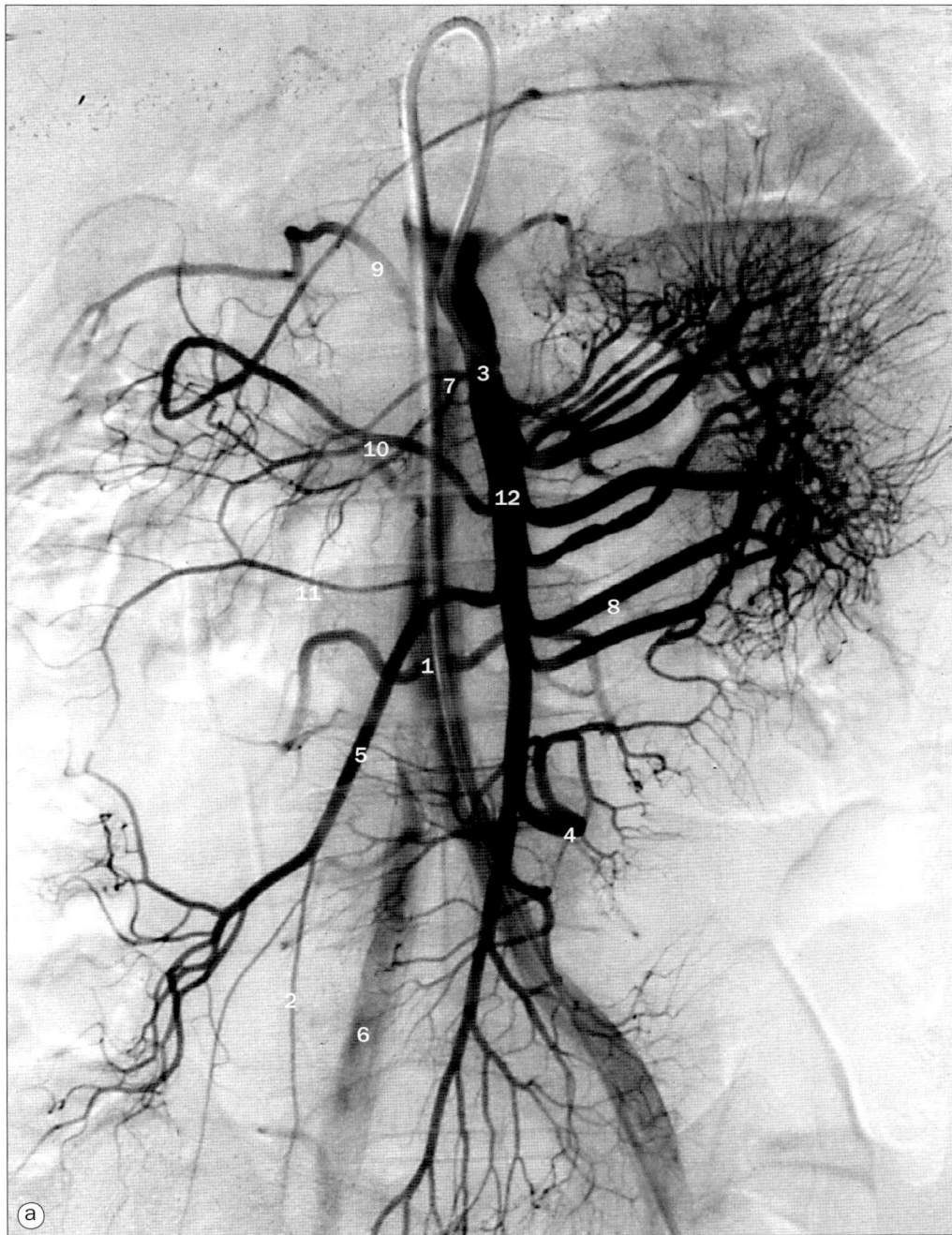

(a) Subtracted superior mesenteric arteriogram.

1 Aorta
2 Appendicular artery
3 Catheter with tip selectively in superior mesenteric artery
4 Ileal branches of superior mesenteric artery
5 Ileocolic artery
6 Iliac artery
7 Inferior pancreaticoduodenal artery
8 Jejunal branches of superior mesenteric artery
9 Lumbar arteries arising from abdominal aorta
10 Middle colic artery
11 Right colic artery
12 Superior mesenteric artery

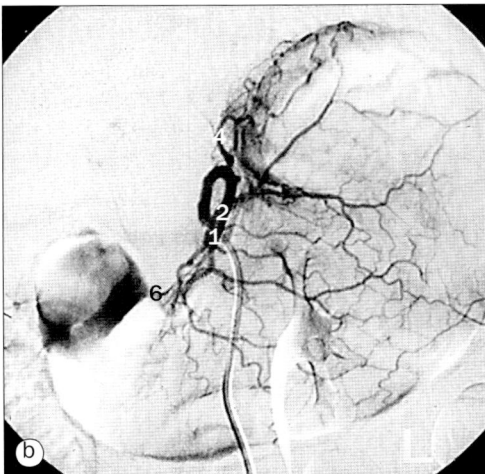

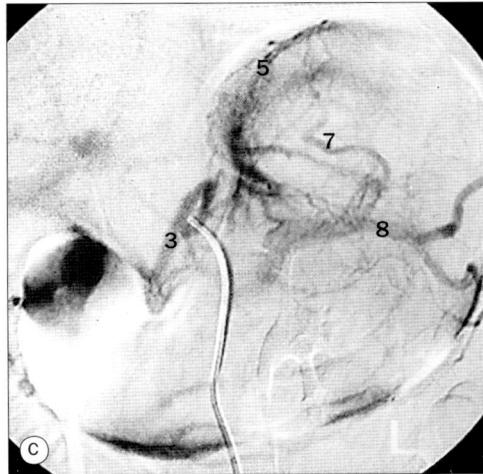

(b) Gastric arteries, (c) gastric veins.

1 Catheter in origin of left gastric artery
2 Left gastric artery
3 Left gastric vein
4 Oesophageal branch of left gastric artery
5 Oesophageal branches of left gastric vein
6 Right gastric artery
7 Short gastric veins
8 Splenic vein

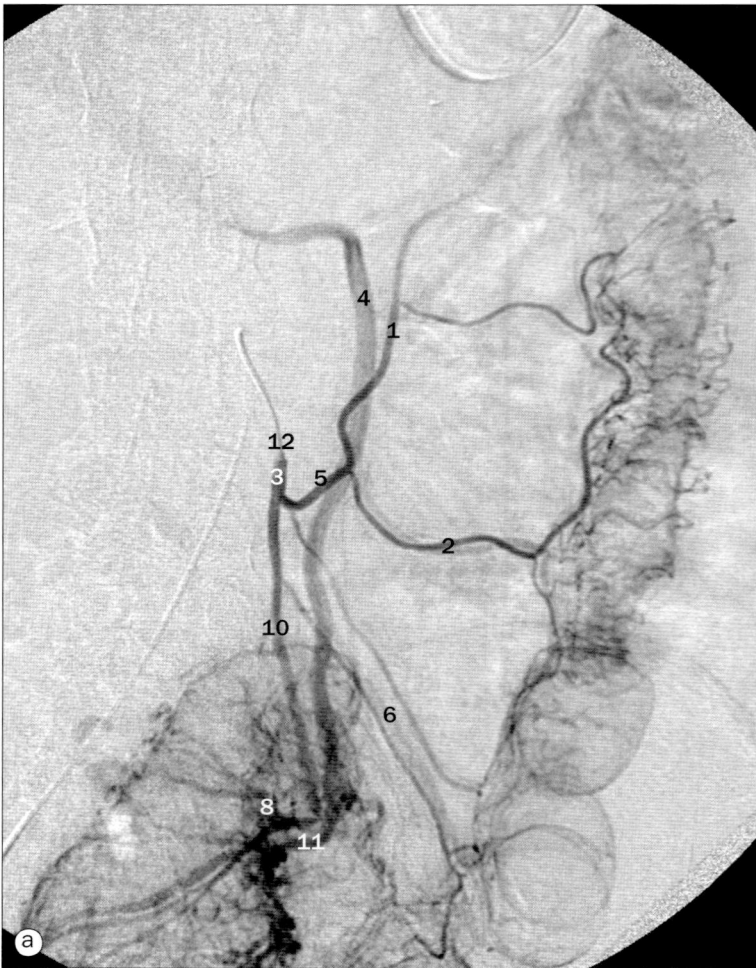

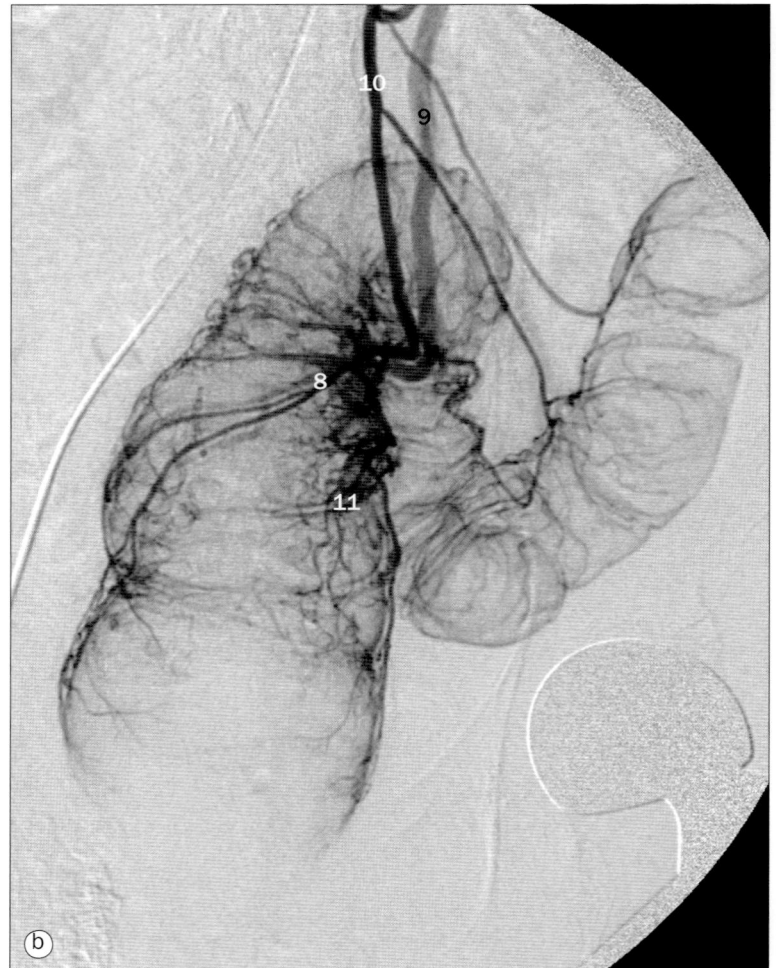

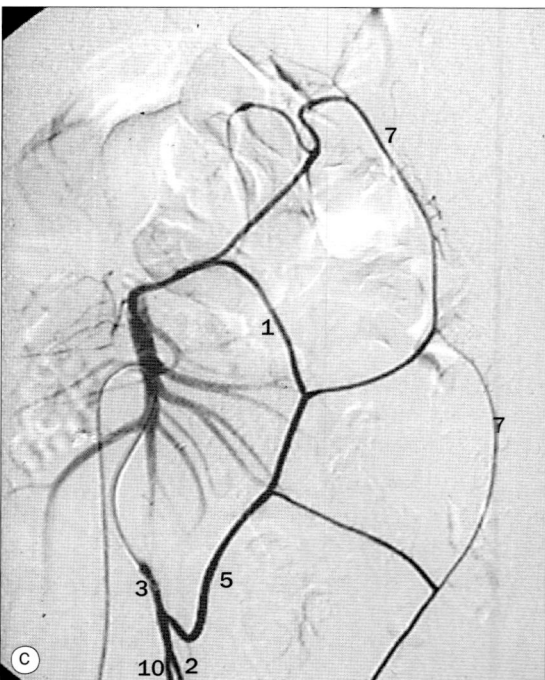

1 Ascending branch of left colic artery
2 Descending branch of left colic artery
3 Inferior mesenteric artery
4 Inferior mesenteric vein
5 Left colic artery
6 Left colic vein
7 Marginal artery of Drummond
8 Sigmoid arteries
9 Sigmoid vein
10 Superior rectal artery
11 Superior rectal vein
12 Tip of catheter in inferior mesenteric artery

(a)–(c) Inferior mesenteric arteriograms.

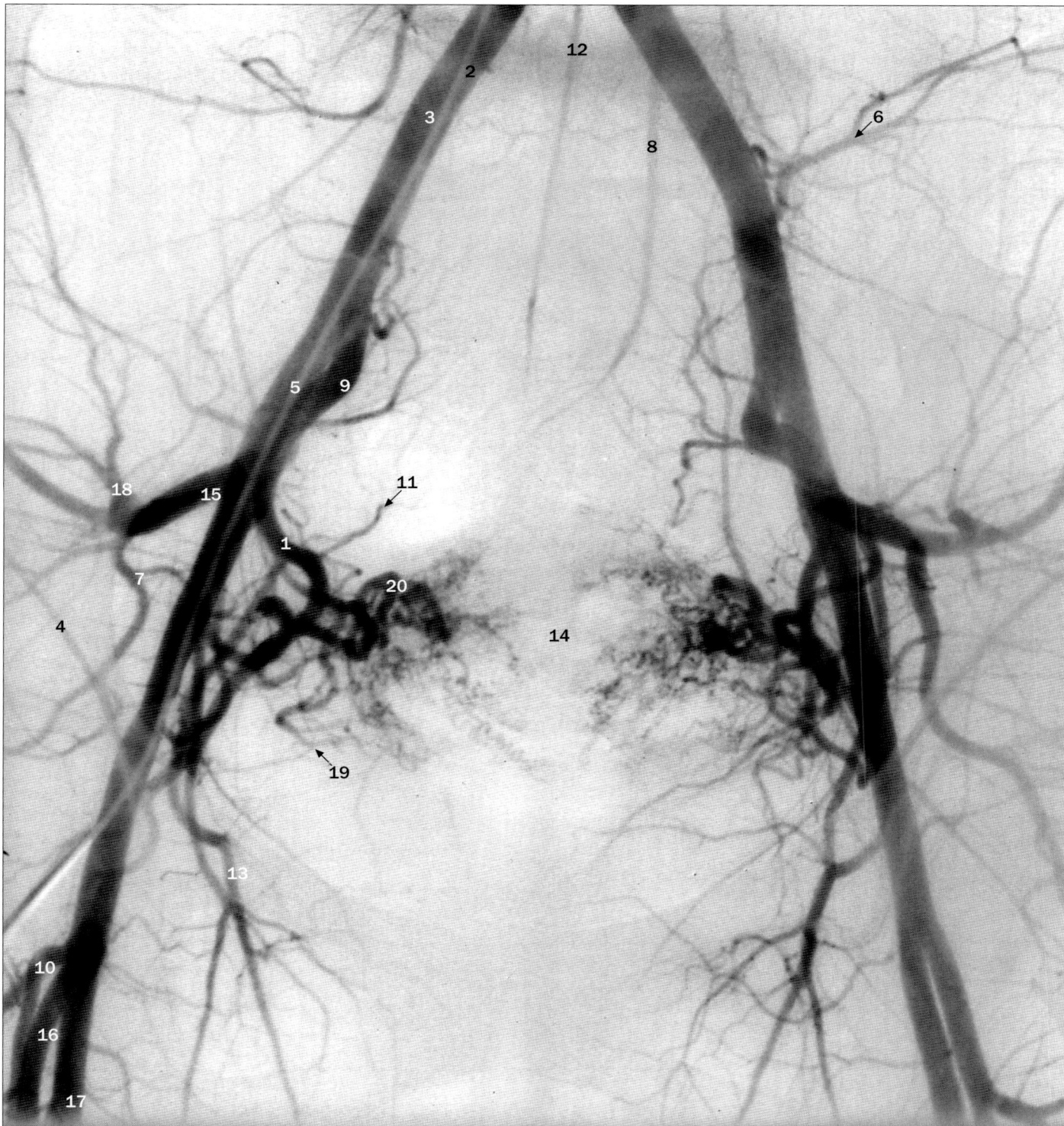

Subtracted pelvic arteriogram.

This anteroposterior film of the pelvis demonstrates both the internal and the external iliac arteries and their branches. Many of the vessels are superimposed: to see them more clearly oblique projections could be obtained. The contrast medium injected into the arteries is excreted by the kidneys, and a full bladder may obscure the branches. Selective catheterisation of the internal and external iliac arteries using a preshaped catheter gives better detail without superimposition of the vessels.

1	Anterior trunk of internal iliac artery	10 Lateral circumflex femoral artery
2	Catheter introduced into distal abdominal aorta via right femoral artery	11 Lateral sacral artery
3	Common iliac artery	12 Median sacral artery
4	Deep circumflex iliac artery	13 Obturator artery
5	External iliac artery	14 Position of uterus
6	Iliolumbar artery	15 Posterior trunk of internal iliac artery
7	Inferior gluteal artery	16 Profunda femoris artery
8	Inferior mesenteric artery	17 Superficial femoral artery
9	Internal iliac artery	18 Superior gluteal artery
		19 Superior vesical artery
		20 Uterine artery

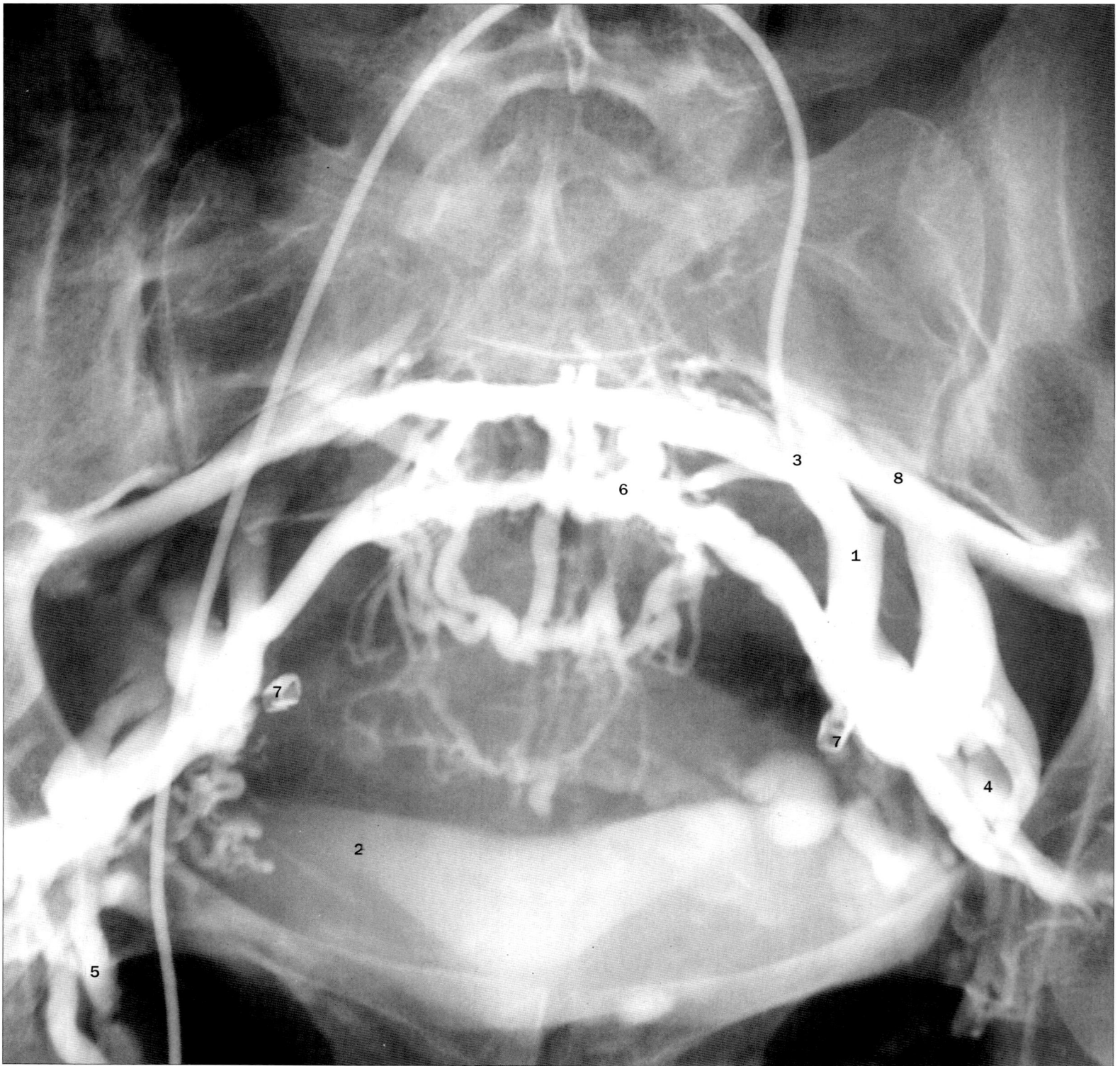

Female pelvic venogram.

1 Anterior division of internal iliac vein
2 Bladder containing contrast medium
3 Catheter introduced via right femoral vein, with tip in left internal iliac vein
4 Inferior gluteal veins
5 Obturator veins
6 Sacral plexus of veins
7 Sterilisation clips
8 Superior gluteal veins

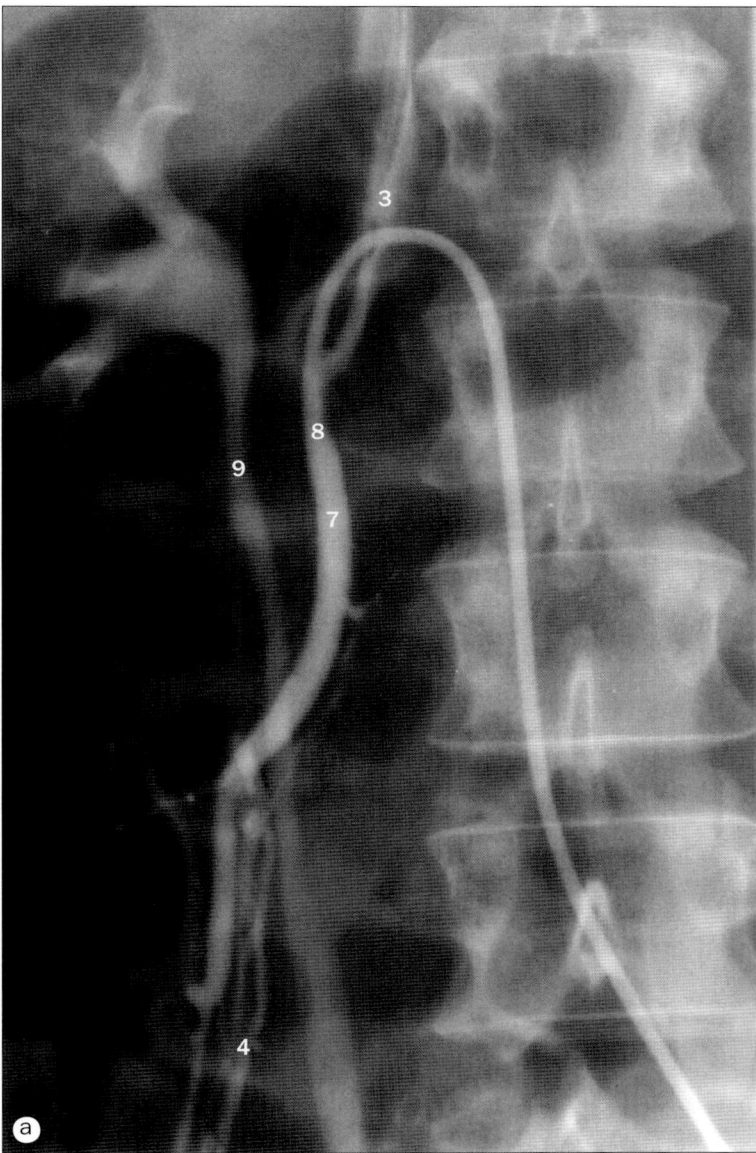

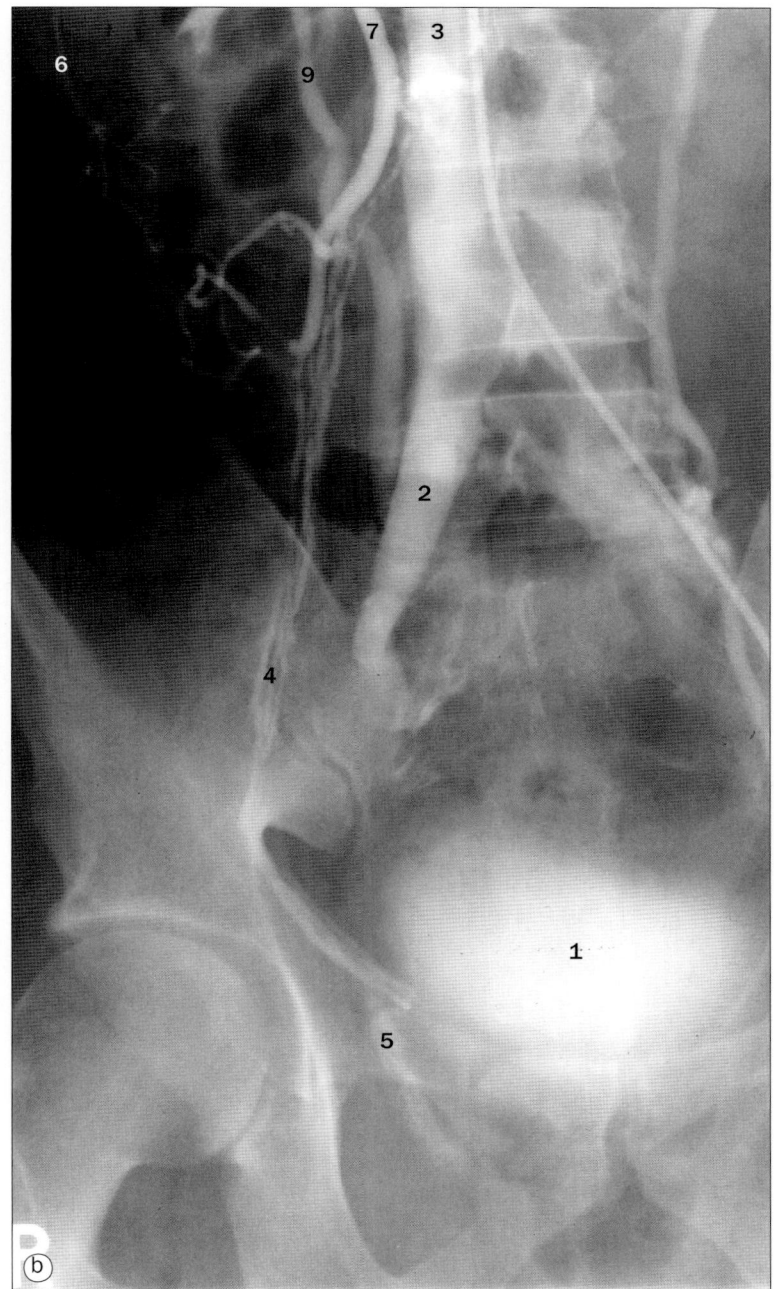

(a) and (b) Right testicular venograms.

The gonadal veins drain into one or two main veins via a venous plexus. On the left, the main vein drains into the left renal vein. It may occasionally communicate with the inferior mesenteric vein and drain into the portal venous system. On the right, the main vein usually drains into the inferior vena cava directly (as in the case illustrated), but it can drain into the right renal vein.

1 Bladder
2 Common iliac veins
3 Inferior vena cava
4 Pampiniform plexus of veins
5 Pampiniform plexus of veins (undescended testis in inguinal canal)
6 Renal capsular veins
7 Right testicular vein
8 Tip of catheter in right testicular vein, introduced via left femoral vein
9 Ureter

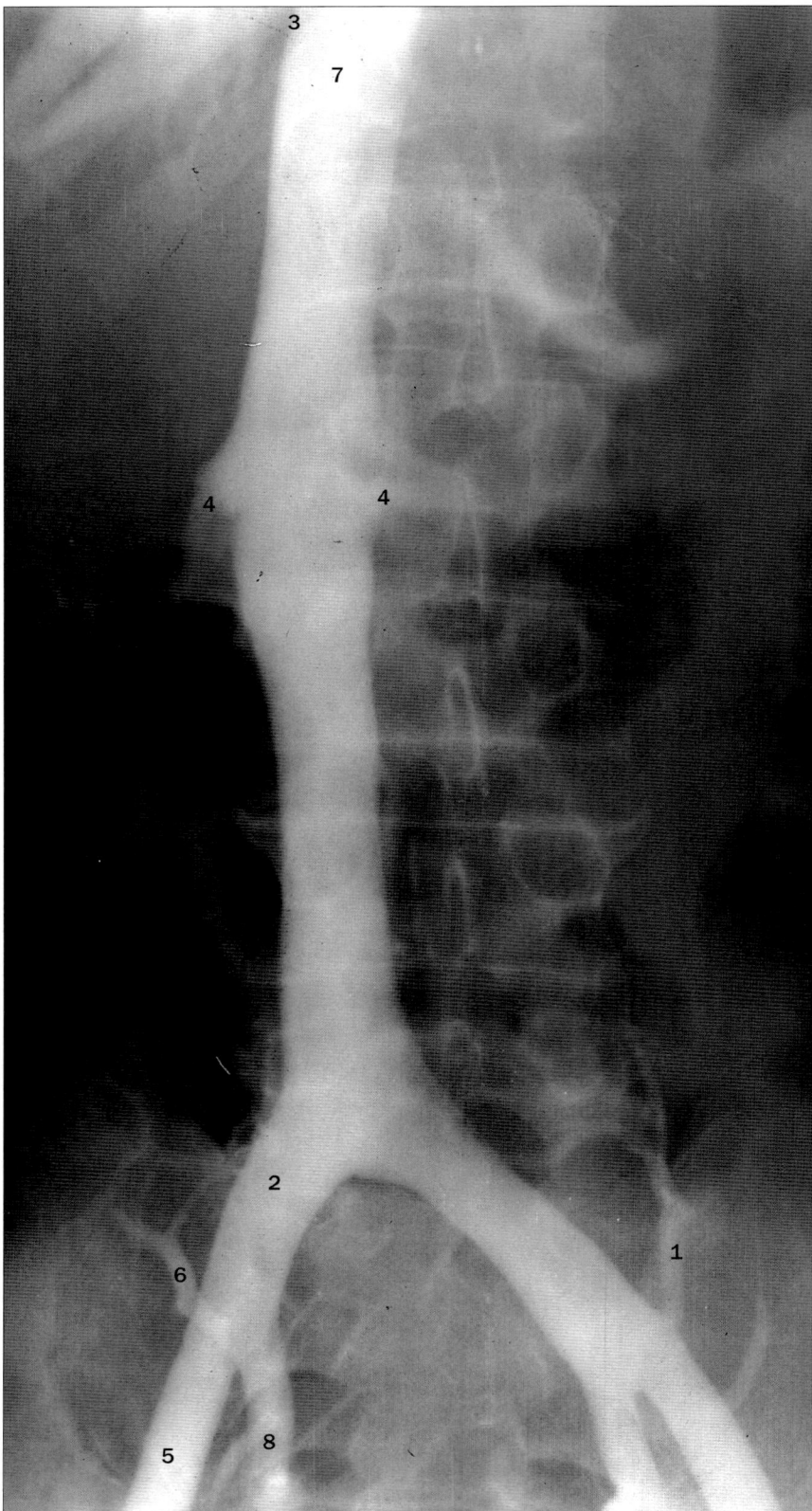

Inferior vena cavogram.

1 Ascending lumbar vein
2 Common iliac vein
3 Entrance of hepatic veins
4 Entrance of renal veins
5 External iliac vein
6 Iliolumbar vein
7 Inferior vena cava
8 Internal iliac vein

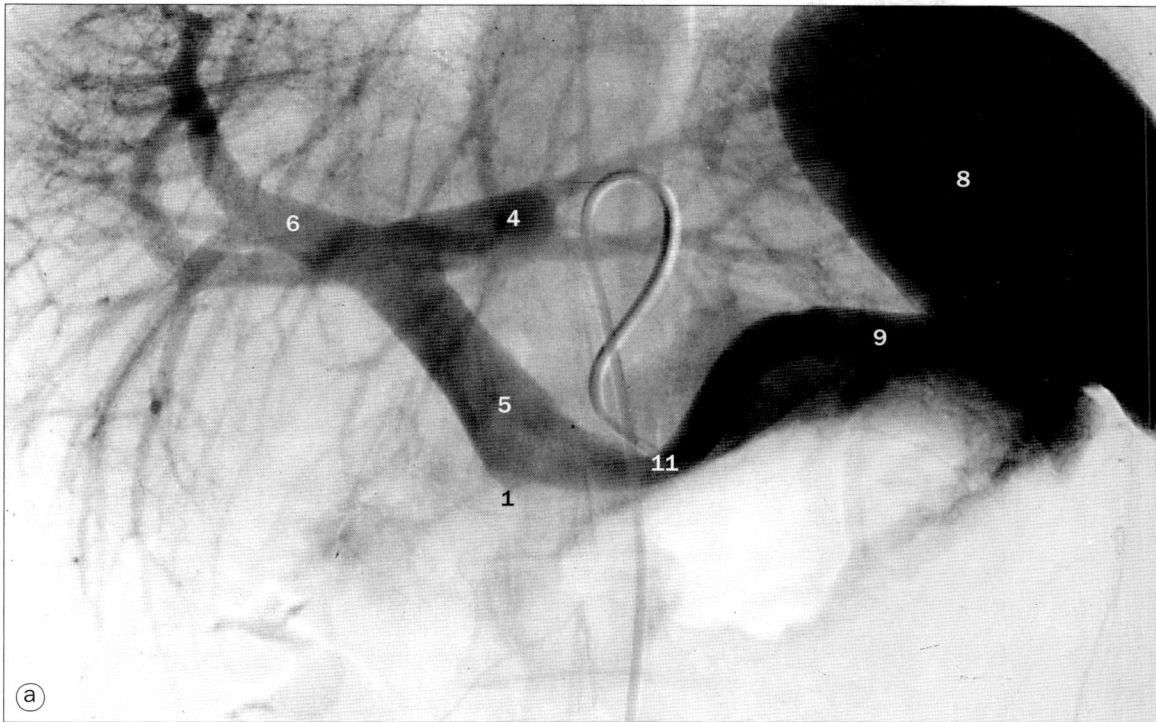

(a) Indirect splenoportogram.

(b) and (c) Venous phase of superior mesenteric arteriogram.

1 Entry of superior mesenteric vein
2 Ileocolic vein
3 Jejunal vein
4 Left branch of portal vein
5 Portal vein
6 Right branch of portal vein
7 Site of entry of splenic vein
8 Spleen
9 Splenic vein
10 Superior mesenteric vein
11 Tip of catheter in splenic artery
12 Tip of catheter in superior mesenteric artery

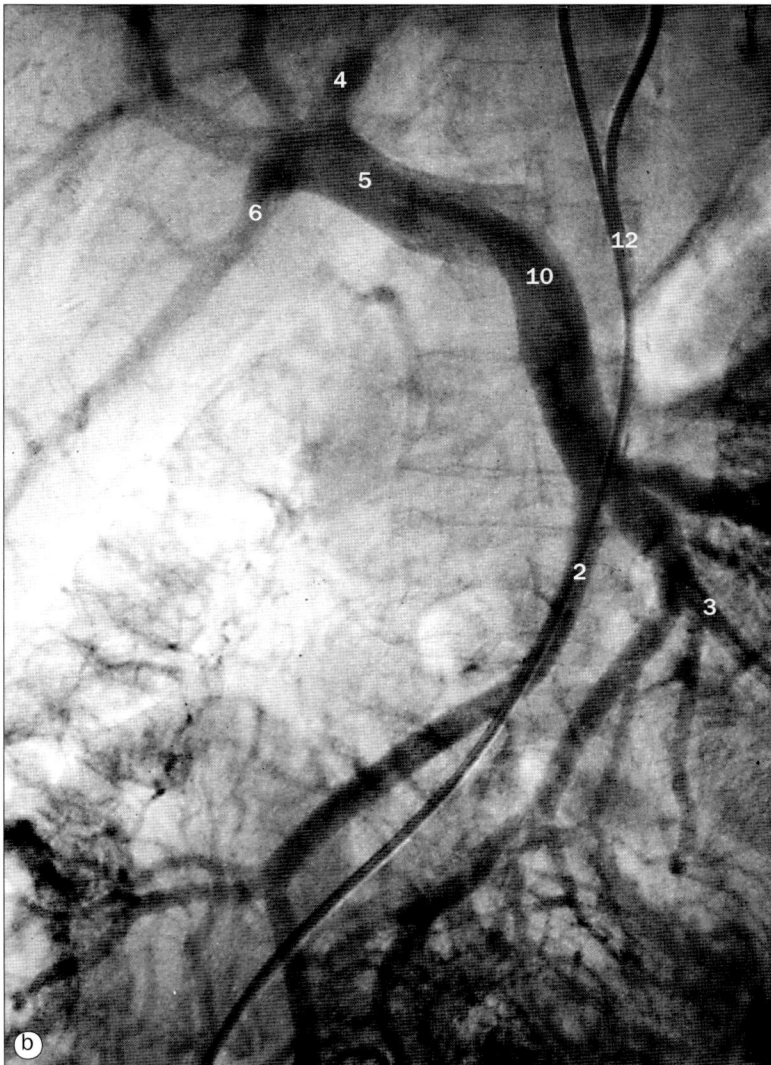

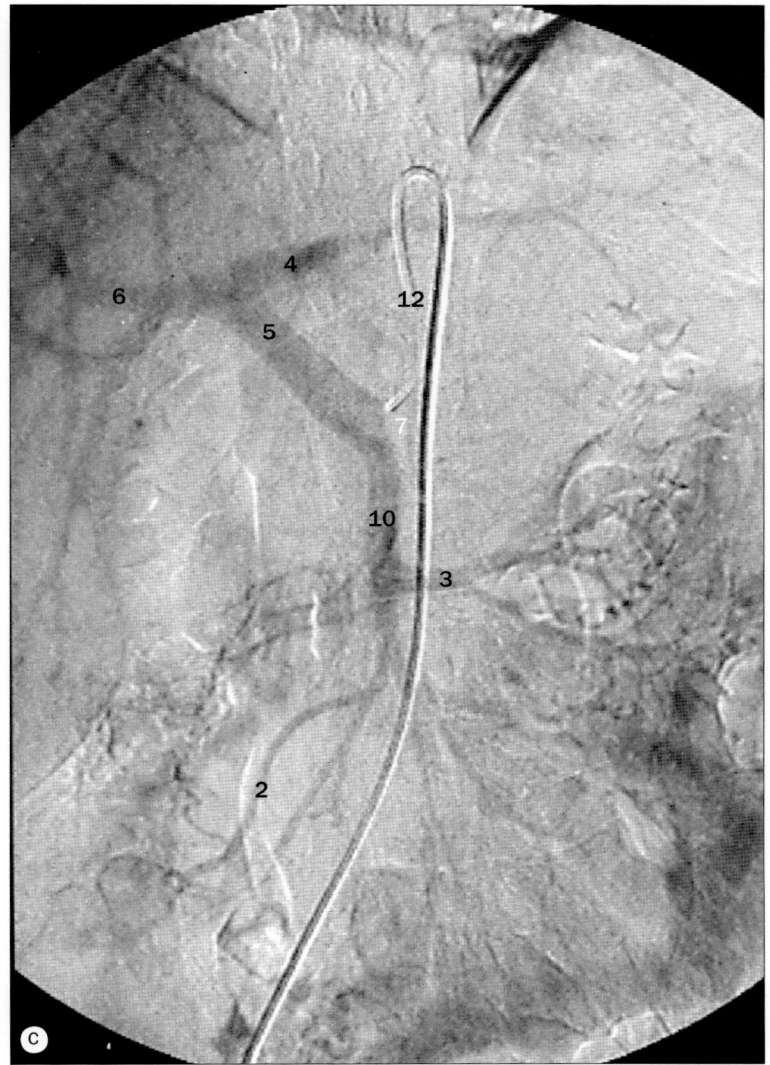

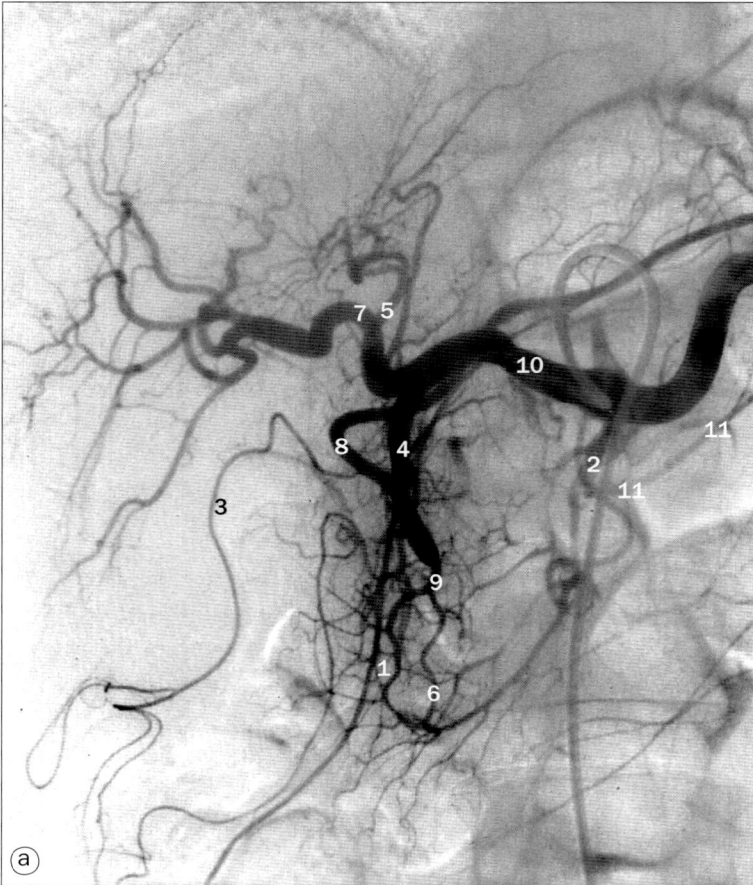

(a) Subtracted hepatic arteriogram.

1 Anterior branch of inferior pancreaticoduodenal artery
2 Dorsal pancreatic artery
3 Epiploic artery
4 Gastroduodenal artery
5 Left branch of hepatic artery
6 Posterior branch of superior pancreaticoduodenal artery
7 Right branch of hepatic artery
8 Right gastro-epiploic artery
9 Superior pancreaticoduodenal artery
10 Tip of catheter in hepatic artery
11 Transverse pancreatic artery

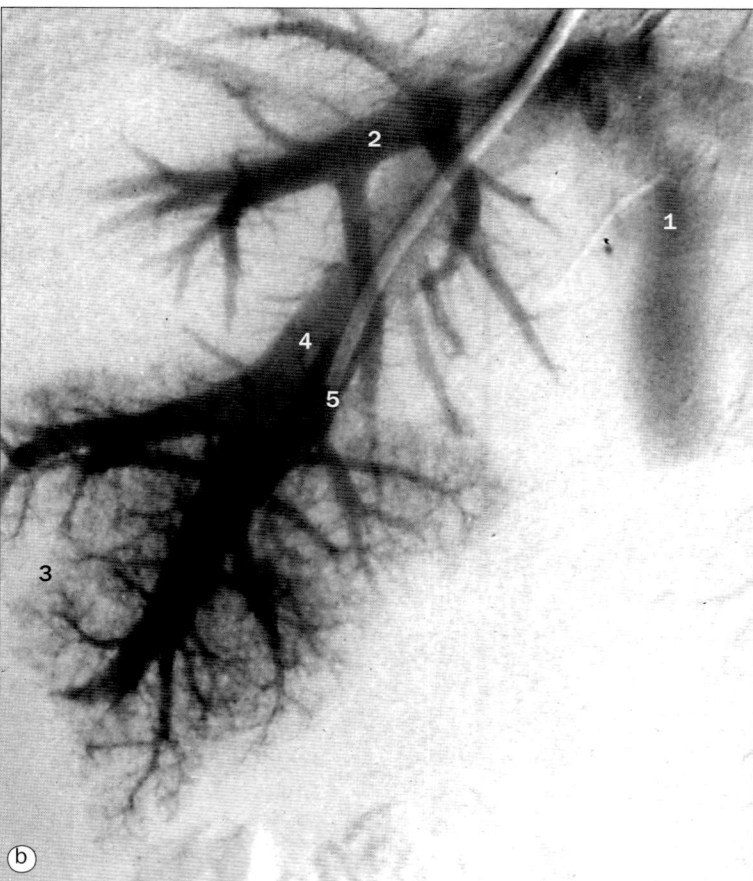

(b) Subtracted hepatic venogram.

1 Inferior vena cava
2 Middle hepatic vein
3 Parenchyma of liver
4 Right hepatic vein
5 Tip of catheter in hepatic vein

(a) Selective gastroduodenal arteriogram.

(b) Subtracted pancreatic arteriogram.

1 Anterior branch of inferior pancreaticoduodenal artery
2 Anterior branch of superior pancreaticoduodenal artery
3 Gastroduodenal artery
4 Left gastro-epiploic artery
5 Posterior branch of inferior pancreaticoduodenal artery
6 Posterior branch of superior
   pancreatico-duodenal artery
7 Right gastro-epiploic artery
8 Superior mesenteric artery
9 Tip of catheter in dorsal pancreatic
   artery
10 Transverse pancreatic artery

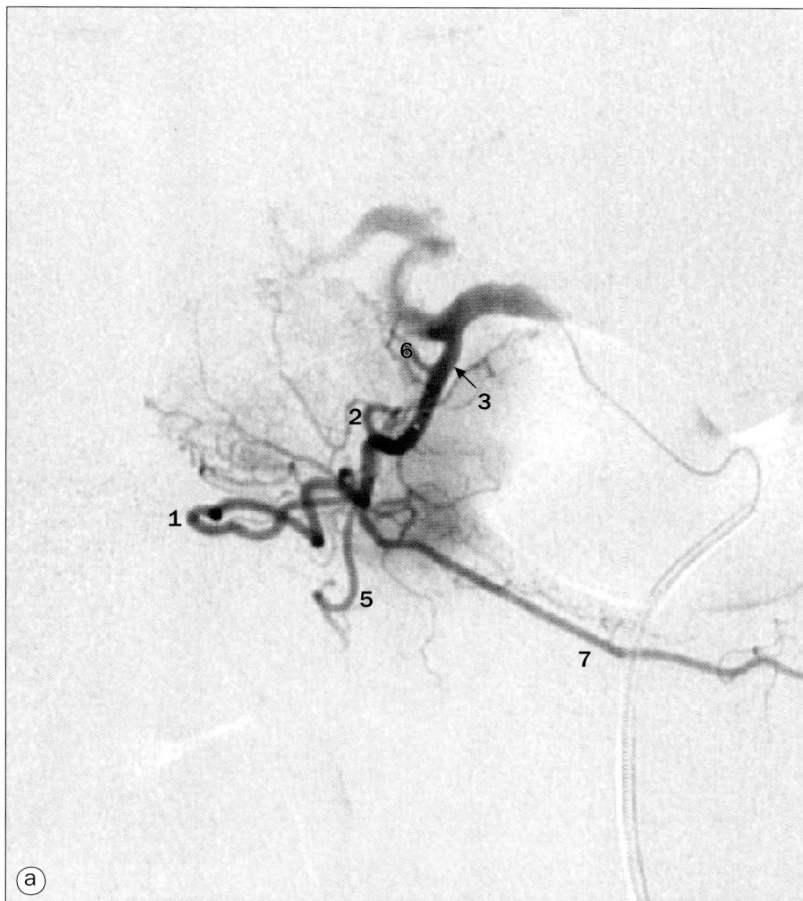

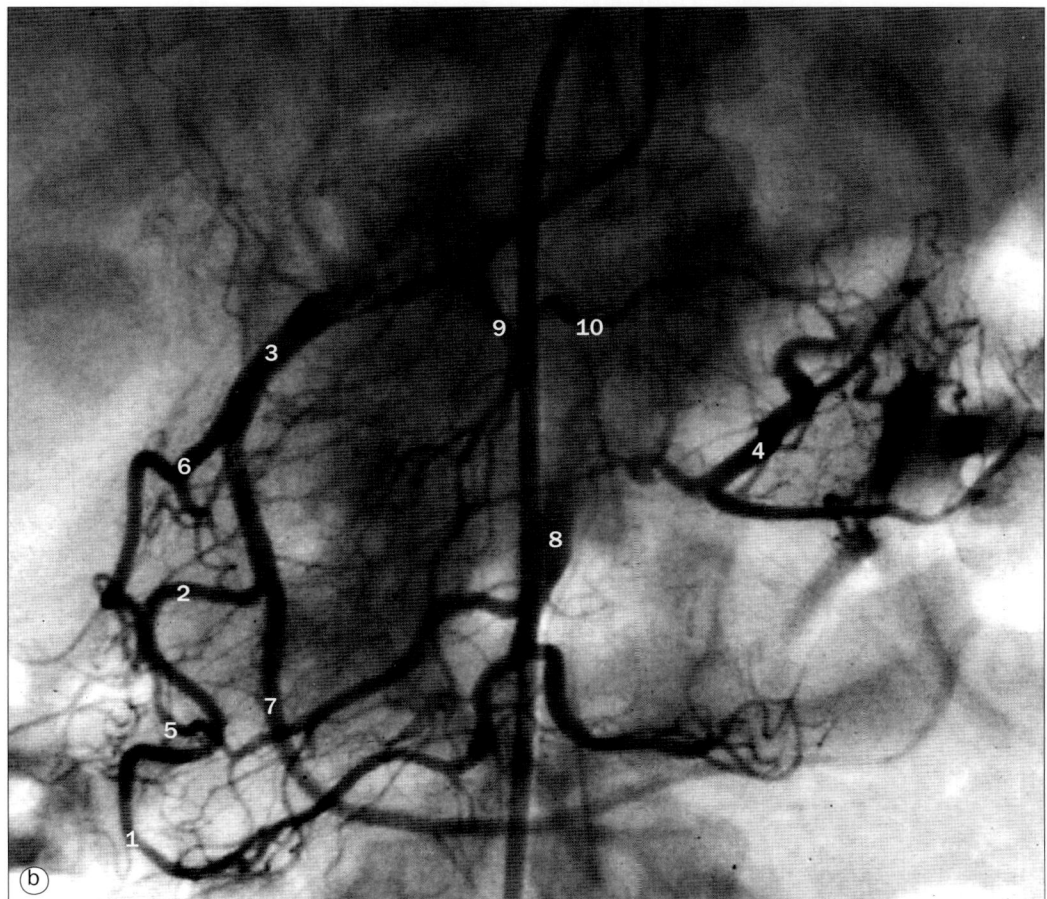

(a) Renal arteriogram.

1 Arcuate arteries
2 Interlobar arteries
3 Lobar arteries
4 Main renal artery
5 Tip of catheter in renal artery

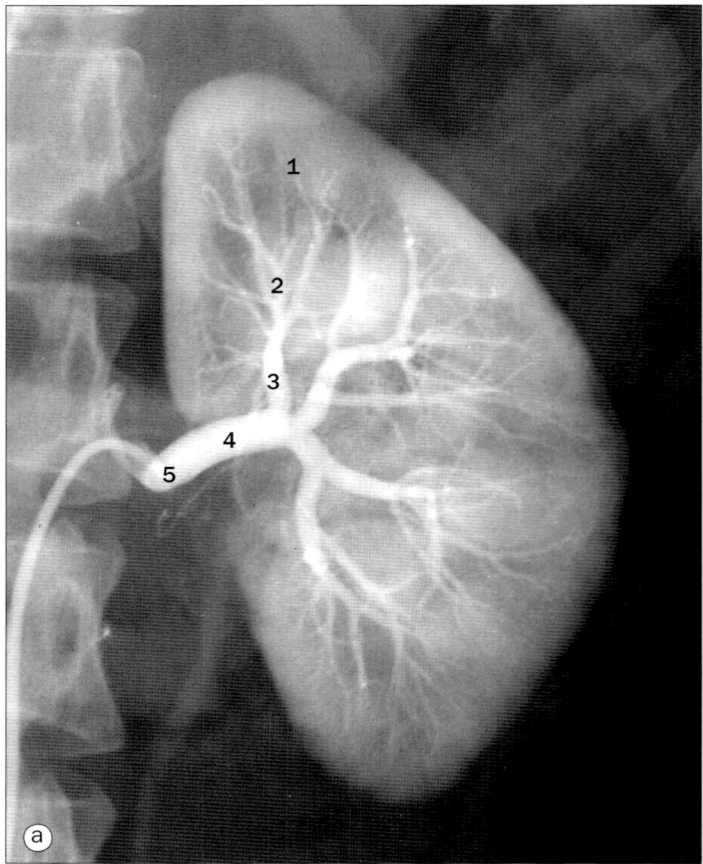

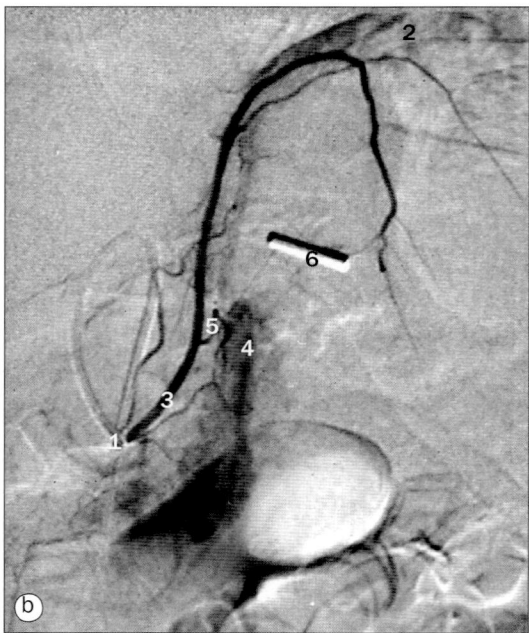

(b) Left suprarenal arteriogram.

1 Catheter in origin of inferior phrenic artery
2 Diaphragm
3 Inferior phrenic artery
4 Left suprarenal gland
5 Superior suprarenal arteries
6 Tip of nasogastric tube

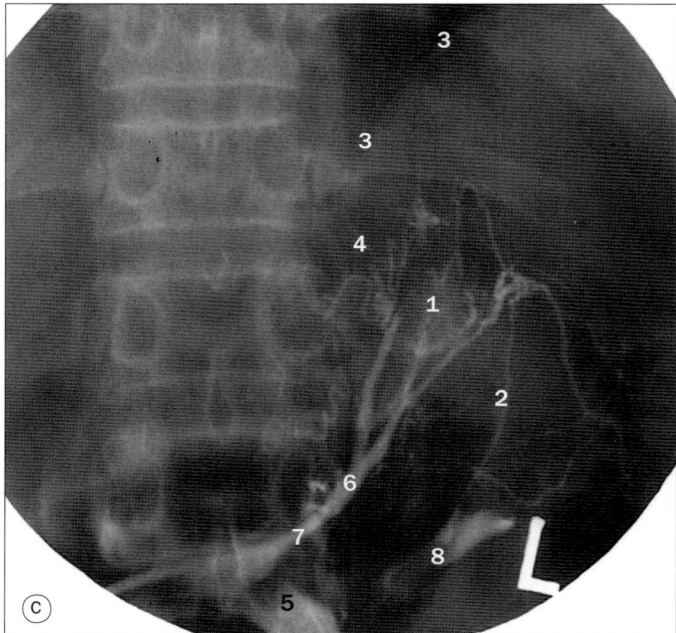

(c) Left suprarenal venogram.

1 Adenoma in suprarenal gland
2 Capsular veins
3 Diaphragm
4 Inferior phrenic vein
5 Left renal vein
6 Left suprarenal vein
7 Tip of catheter in left suprarenal vein
8 Upper pole calyx

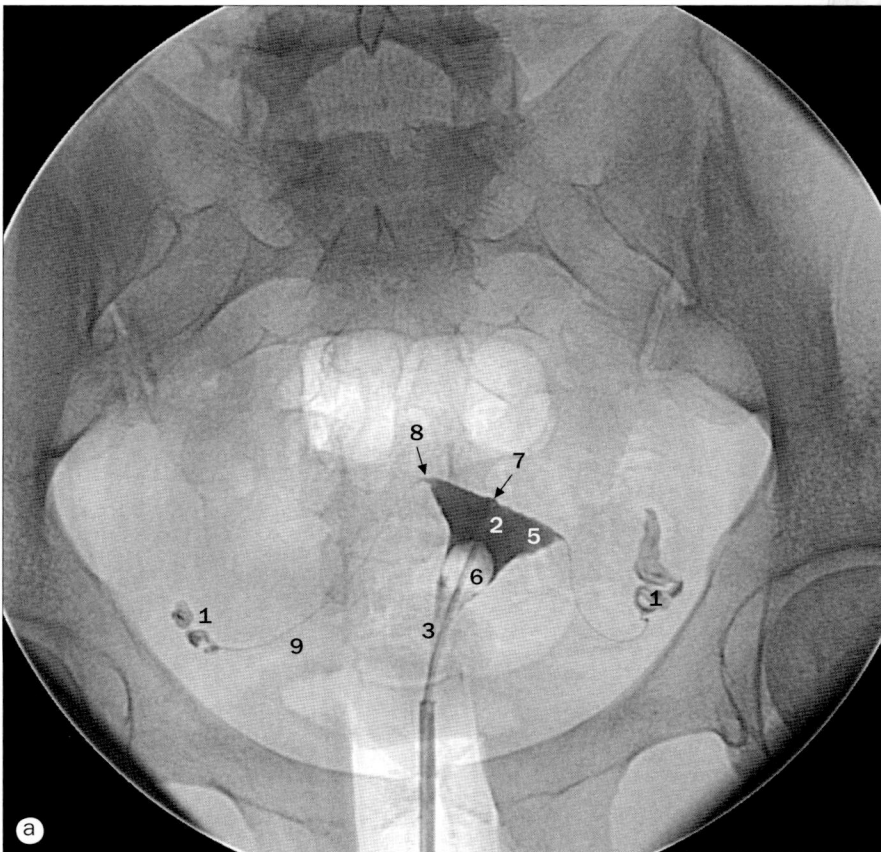

(a) Early phase of uterine filling.

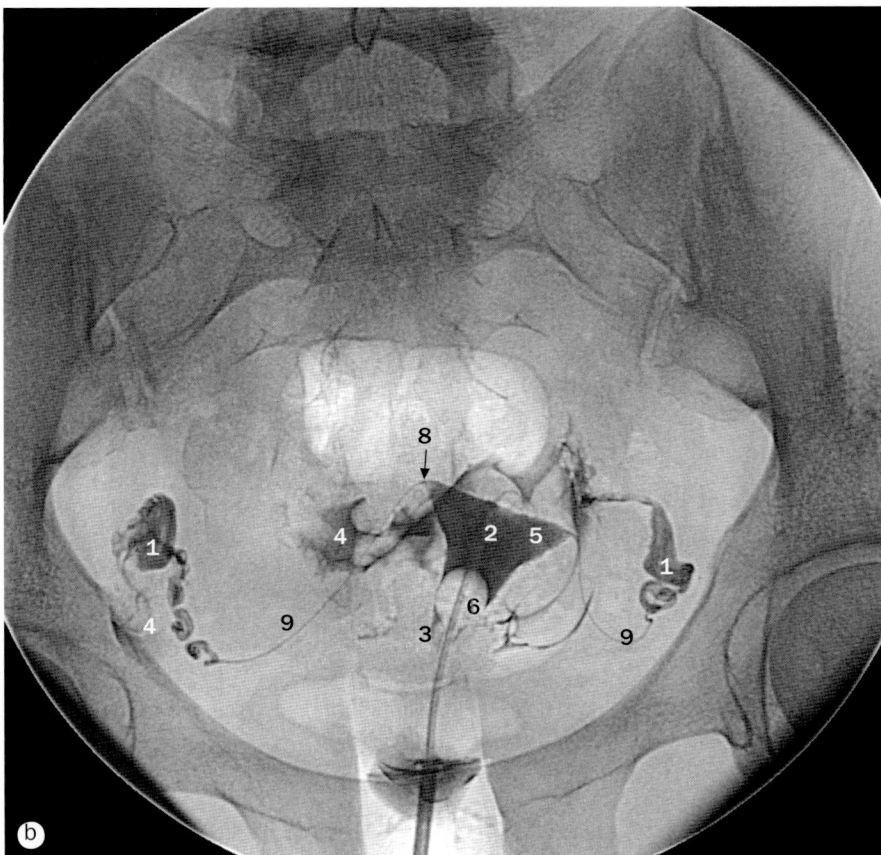

(b) Late phase with peritoneal spill.

1 Ampulla of uterine tube
2 Body of uterus
3 Cervix of uterus
4 Contrast spillage into peritoneal cavity
5 Cornu of uterus
6 Foley balloon catheter in uterus
7 Fundus of uterus
8 Isthmus of uterine tube
9 Uterine tube (fallopian tube)

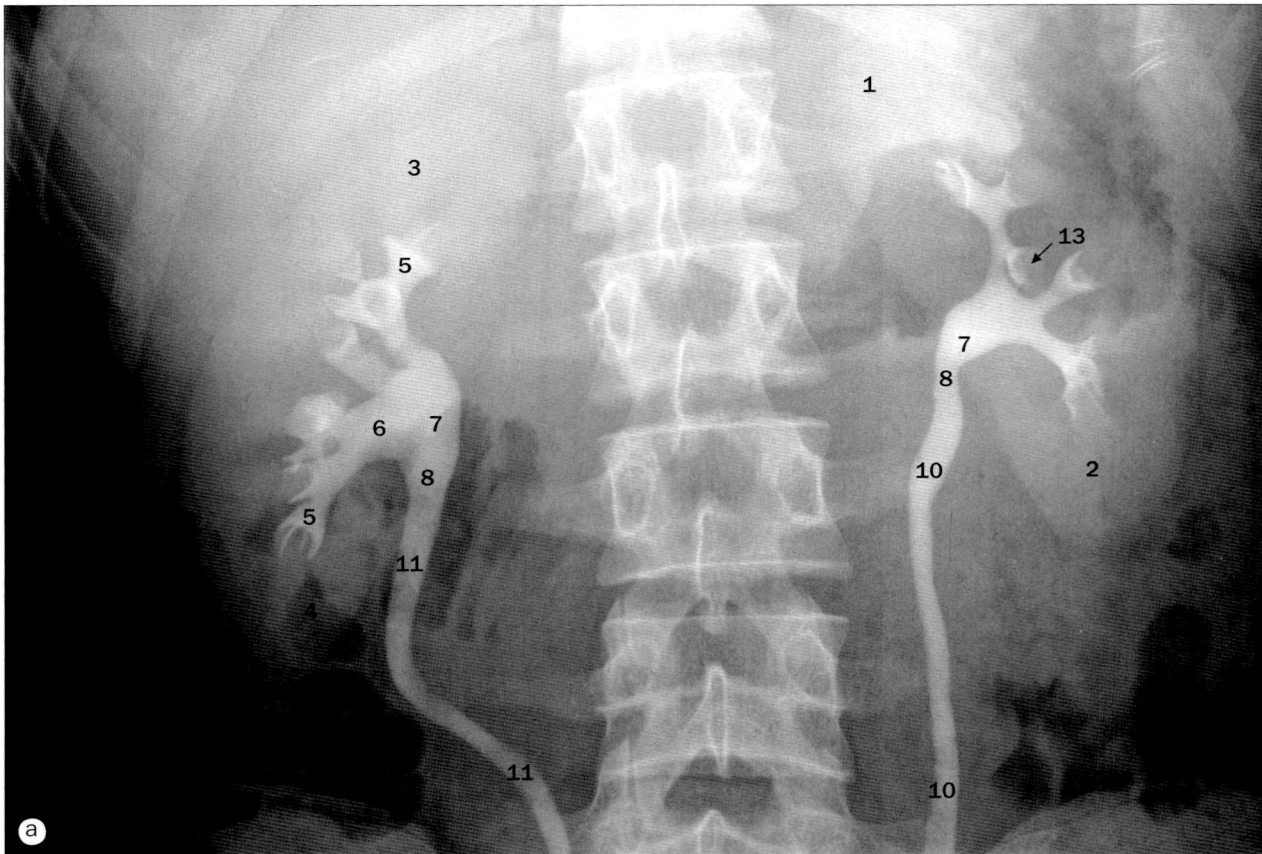

(a) 10 minutes IVU (intravenous urogram) with abdominal compression.

(b) Full length 15 minutes IVU after release of compression.

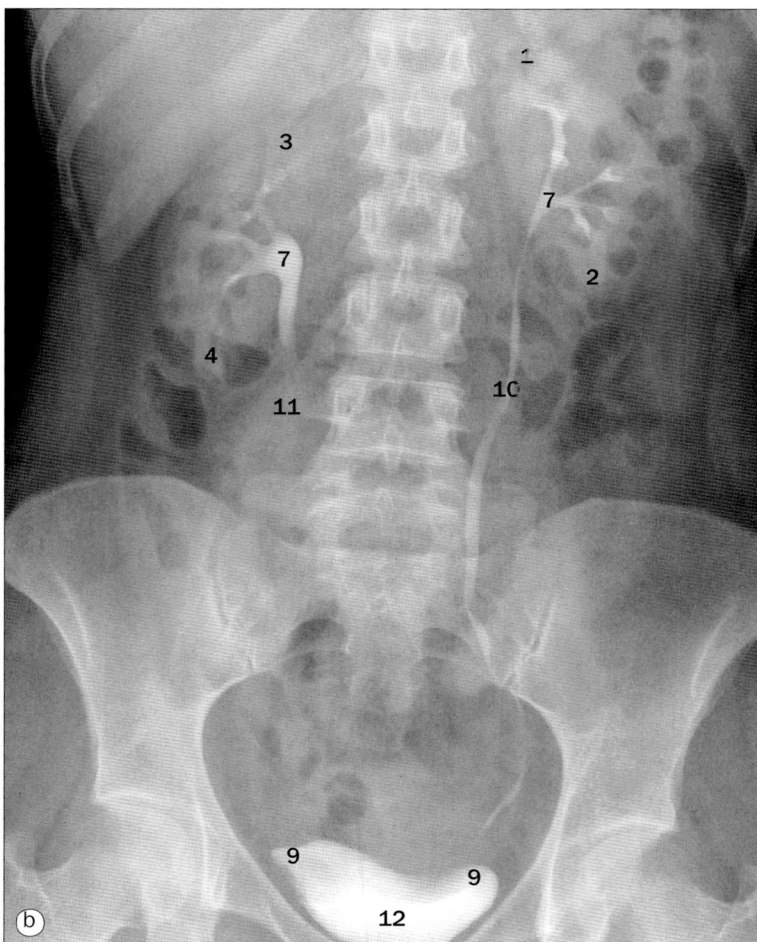

1	Upper pole of left kidney
2	Lower pole of left kidney
3	Upper pole of right kidney
4	Lower pole of right kidney
5	Minor calyx
6	Major calyx
7	Renal pelvis
8	Pelvi-ureteric junction
9	Vesico-ureteric junction
10	Left ureter
11	Right ureter
12	Urinary bladder
13	Renal papilla

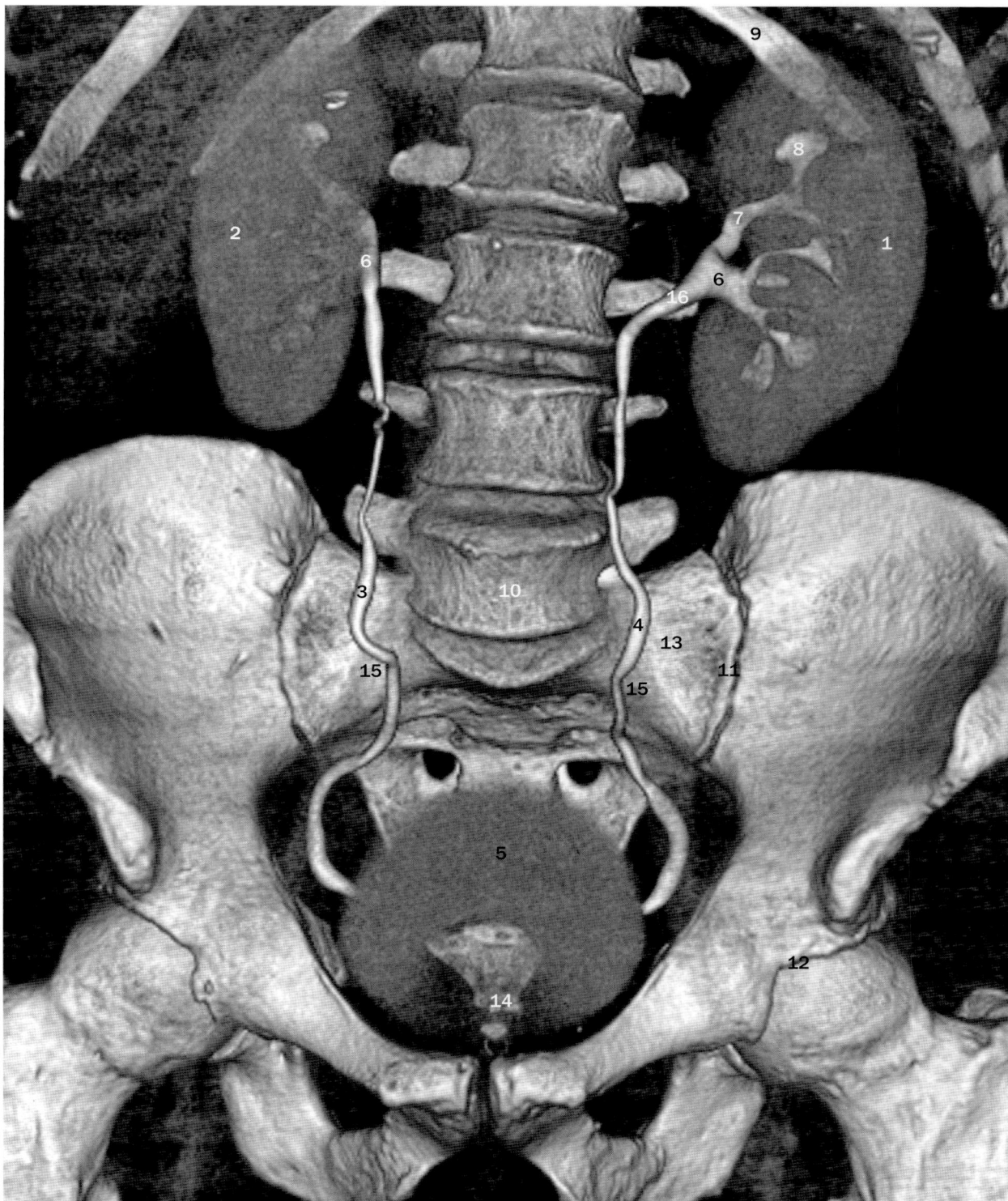

3D CT urogram at 10 minutes post intravenous injection.

1	Left kidney	
2	Right kidney	
3	Right ureter	
4	Left ureter	
5	Urinary bladder	
6	Renal pelvis	
7	Major calyx	
8	Minor calyx	
9	Twelfth rib	
10	Body of L5 vertebra	
11	Sacro-iliac joint	
12	Hip joint	
13	Sacral alum	
14	Coccyx	
15	Point of ureteric crossover cf common iliac vesse s	
16	Pelvi-ureteric junction (PUJ)	

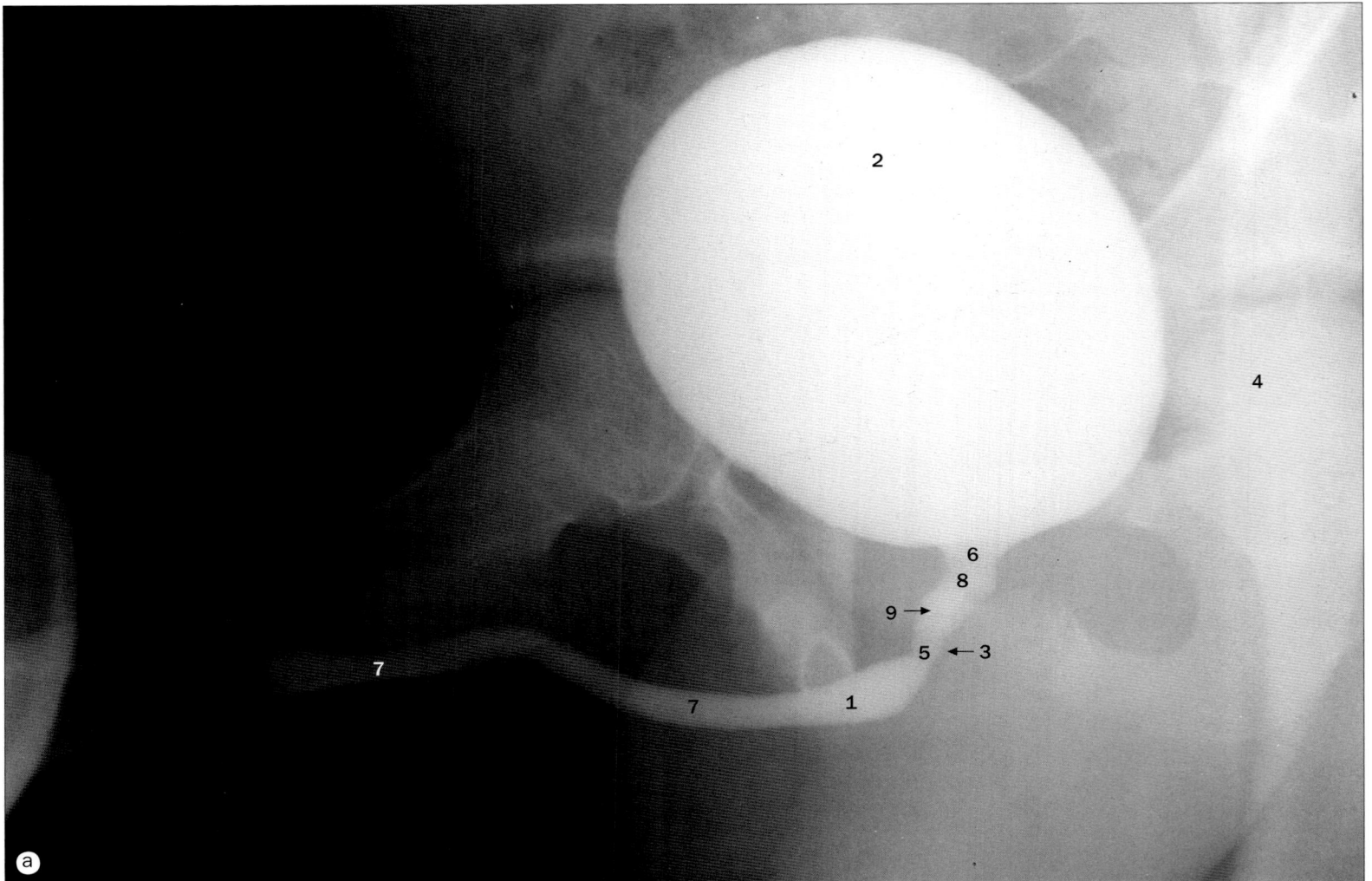

(a) Male urethrogram, oblique image.

(b) Penile arteriogram.

(c) Cavernosogram.

1 Bulbous urethra	6 Neck of urinary bladder
2 Contrast in urinary bladder	7 Penile urethra
3 External sphincter	8 Prostatic urethra
(sphincter urethrae)	9 Seminal colliculus
4 Head of femur	(verumontanum)
5 Membranous urethra	

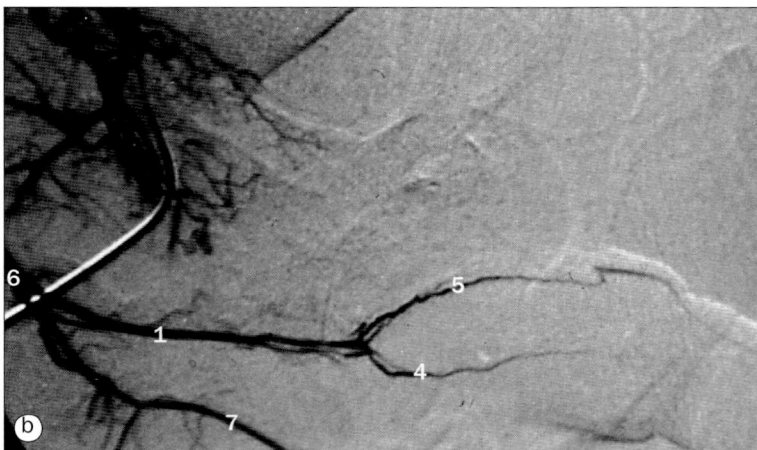

1 Artery of the penis	5 Dorsal artery of the penis
2 Corpus cavernosum	6 Internal pudendal artery
3 Crus of corpus cavernosum	7 Perineal artery
4 Deep artery of the penis	

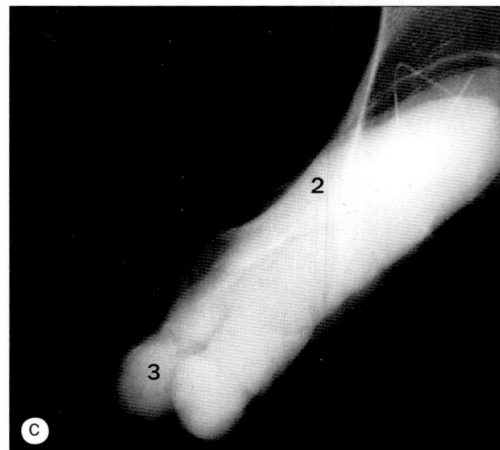

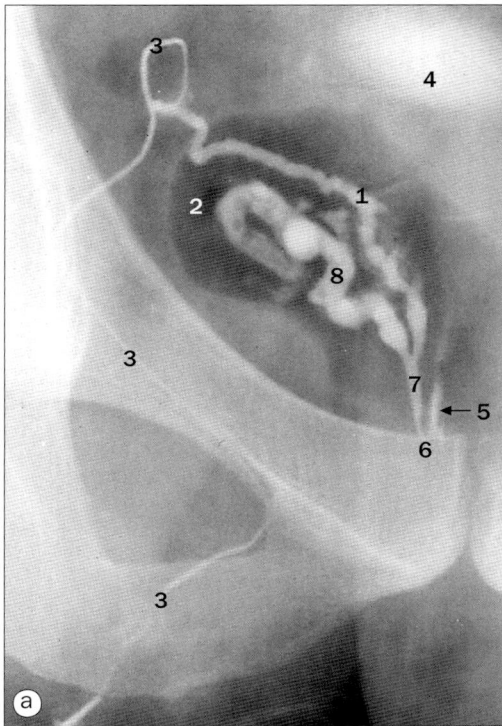

(a) Seminal vesiculogram.

1 Ampulla of ductus deferens
2 Colonic gas
3 Ductus deferens (vas deferens)
4 Full urinary bladder
5 Left ejaculatory duct
6 Position of seminal colliculus (verumontanum)
7 Right ejaculatory duct
8 Seminal vesicle

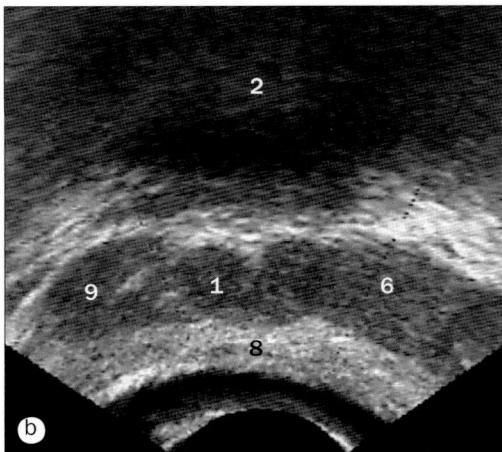

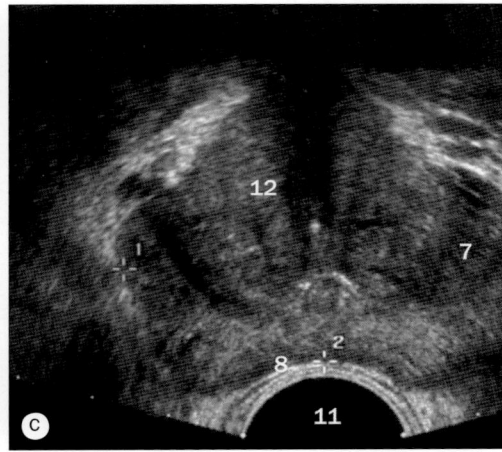

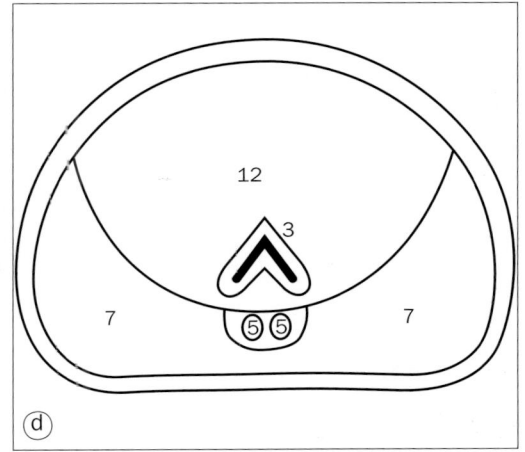

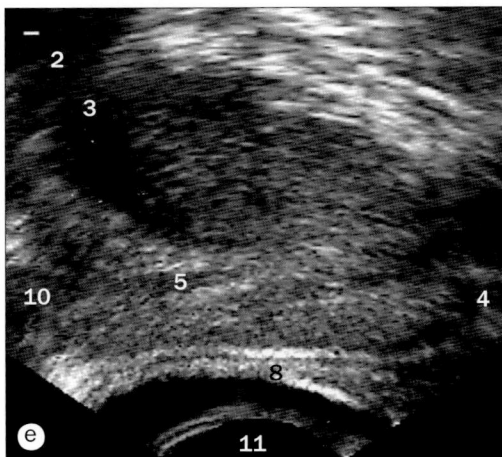

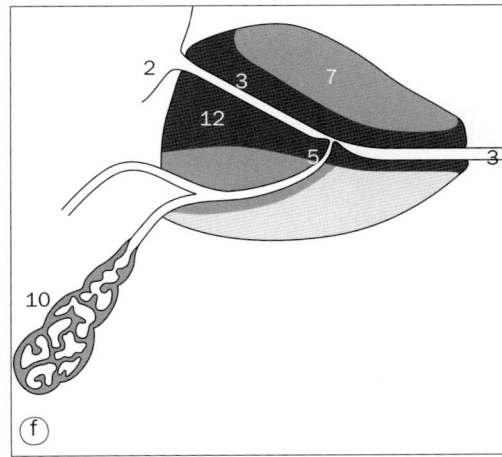

1 Ampulla of ductus deferens
2 Bladder
3 Course of urethra
4 Distal urethra
5 Ejaculatory duct
6 Left seminal vesicle
7 Peripheral zone of prostate
8 Rectal wall
9 Right seminal vesicle
10 Seminal vesicle
11 Transducer
12 Transitional zone of prostate

Rectal ultrasound of the prostate, (b) axial scan through bladder base, (c) axial scan through mid prostate, (d) line drawing of axial scan prostate, (e) sagittal midline scan, (f) line drawing of midline sagittal scan.

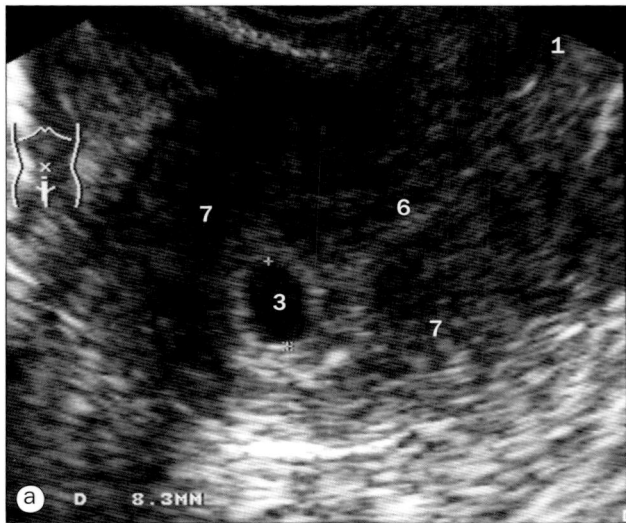

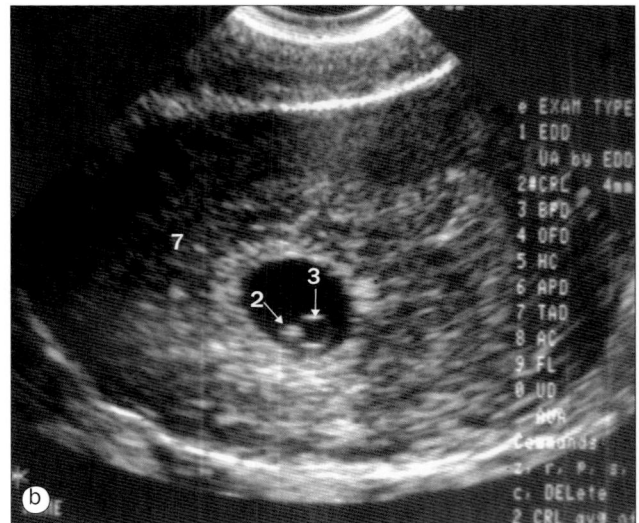

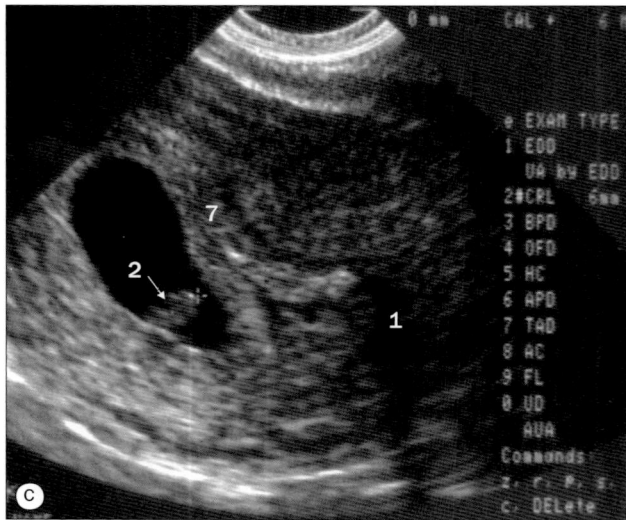

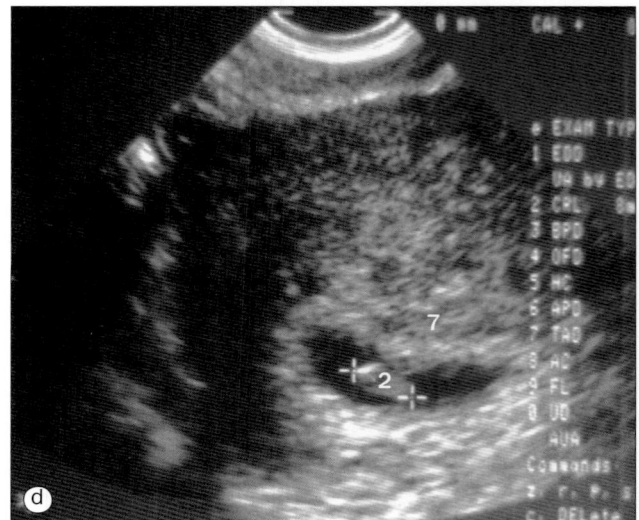

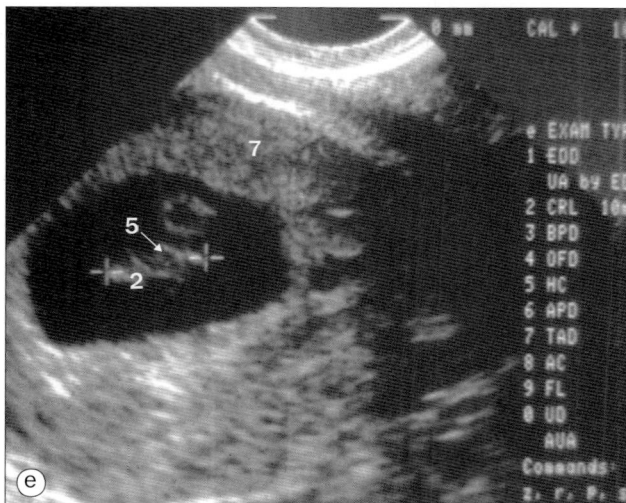

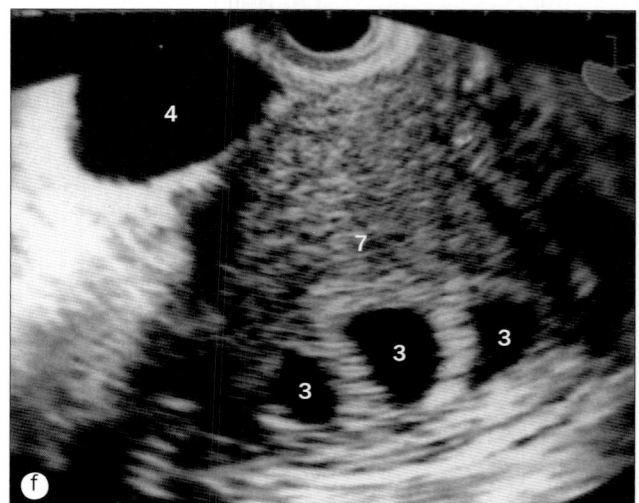

(a) Gestational sac of 8 mm = 5 weeks + 3 days gestational age, (b) CRL (crown rump length) = 4 mm = 6 weeks gestational age, (c) CRL = 6 mm = 6 weeks + 3 days gestational age, (d) CRL = 8 mm = 6 weeks + 5 days gestational age, (e) CRL = 10 mm = 7 weeks + 2 days gestational age, (f) triplets – three separate gestational sacs.

1 Cervix	3 Gestation sac	5 Position of fetal heart	7 Uterus
2 Fetus	4 Maternal bladder	6 Uterine cavity	

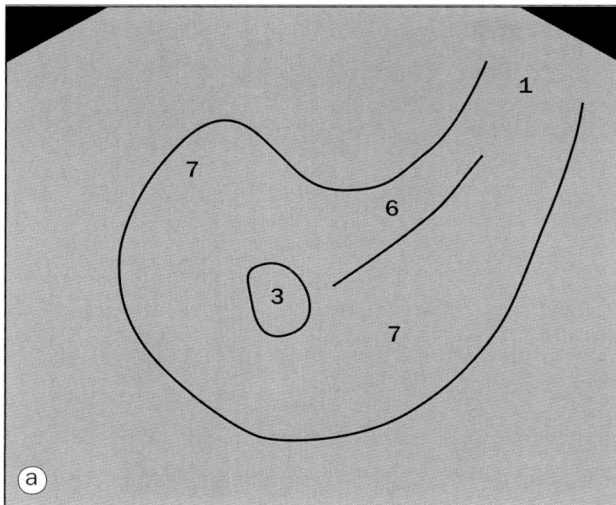

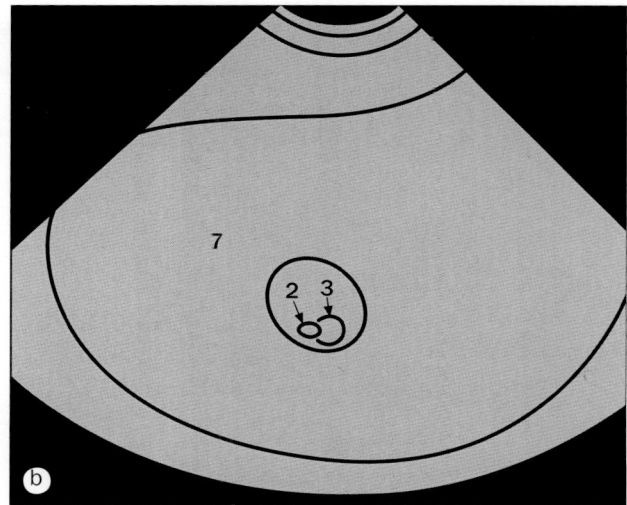

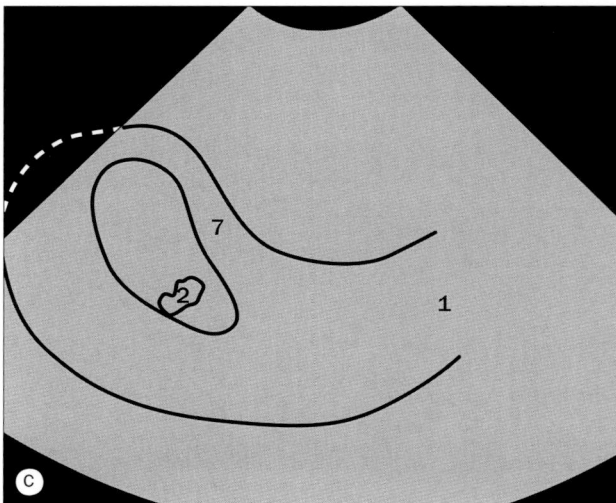

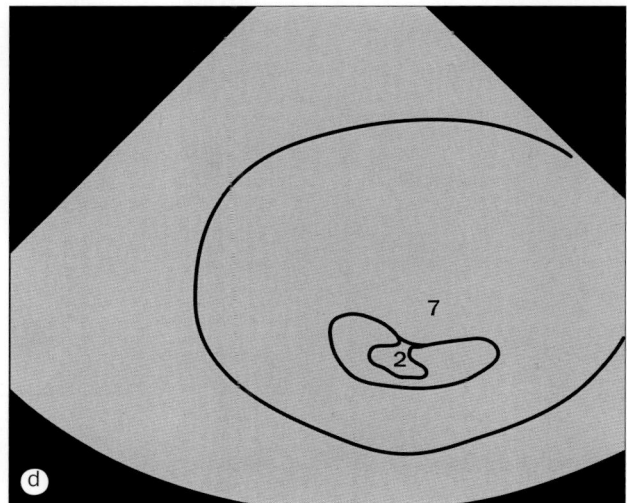

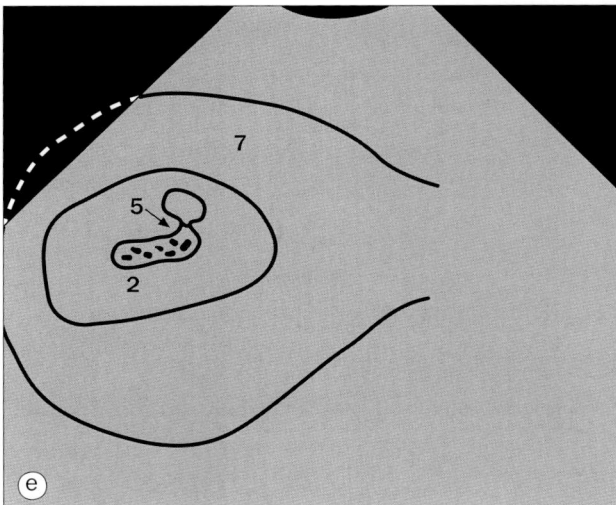

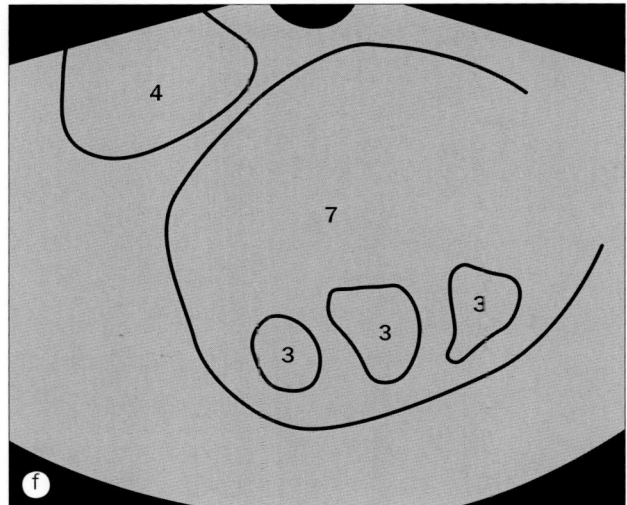

(a)–(f) Line diagrams of ultrasound images opposite.

1 Cervix	**3** Gestation sac	**5** Position of fetal heart	**7** Uterus
2 Fetus	**4** Maternal bladder	**6** Uterine cavity	

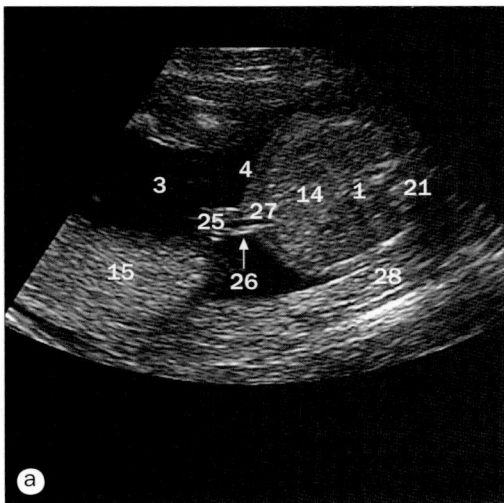

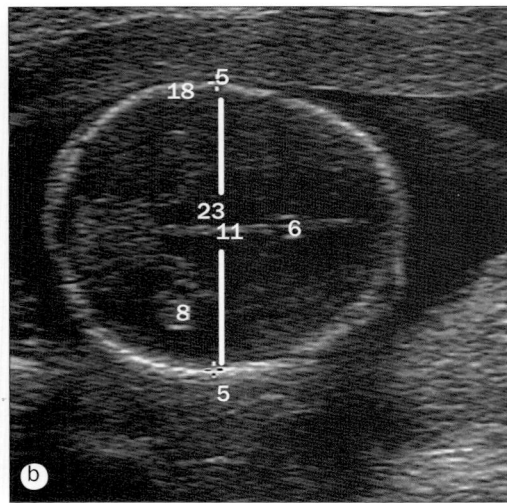

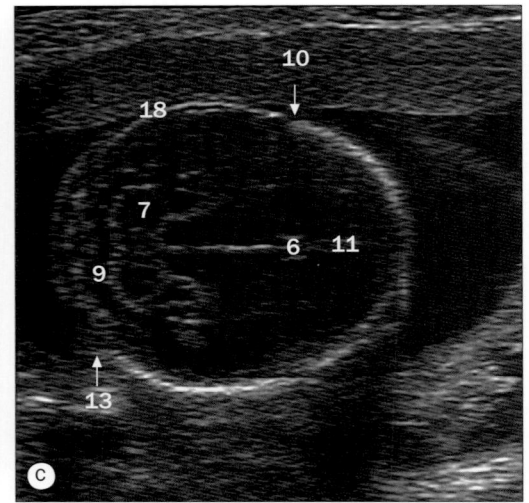

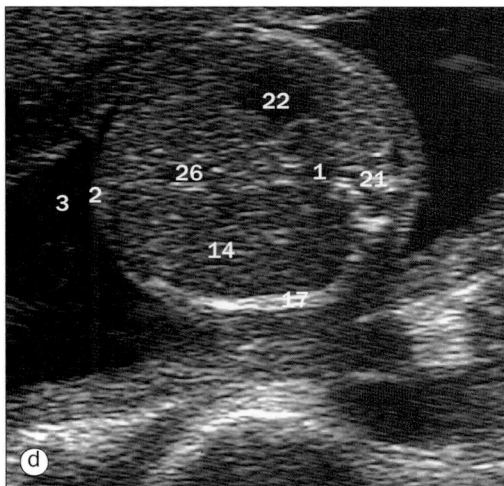

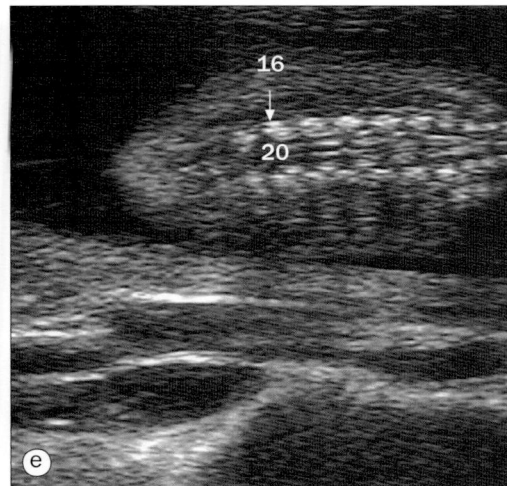

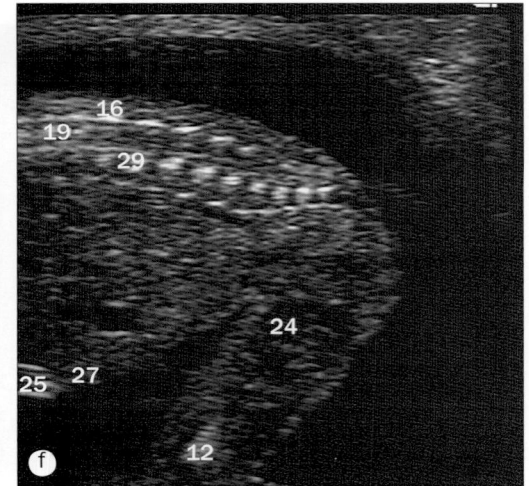

Fetal ultrasound, second trimester,
(a) cord insertion, (b) and (c) skull,
(d) abdomen, (e) and (f) spine.

1 Abdominal aorta	15 Placenta
2 Abdominal circumference measurement	16 Posterior elements of vertebrae
3 Amniotic fluid	17 Ribs
4 Anterior abdominal wall	18 Skull
5 Biparietal diameter measurement	19 Spinal canal
6 Cavum septum pellucidum	20 Spinal cord
7 Cerebellum	21 Spine
8 Choroid plexus	22 Stomach
9 Cisterna magna (cerebellomedullary cistern)	23 Thalamus
10 Coronal suture	24 Thigh
11 Falx cerebri	25 Umbilical cord
12 Femur	26 Umbilical vein
13 Lambdoid suture	27 Umbilicus
14 Liver	28 Uterine wall
	29 Vertebral body

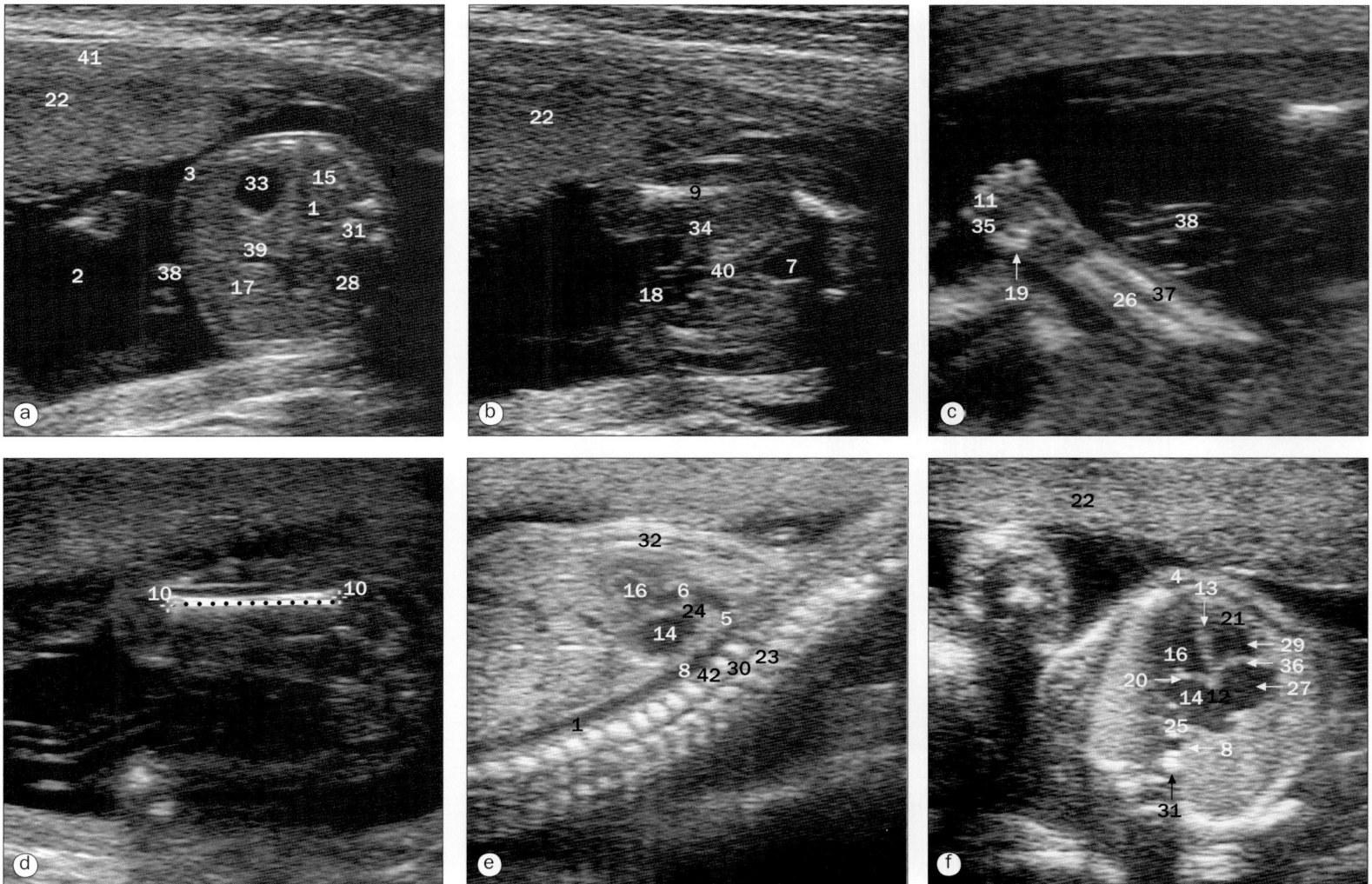

Fetal ultrasound, second trimester,
(a) abdomen, (b) pelvis, (c) forearm,
(d) femur, (e) heart and aorta,
(f) four chamber view of the heart.

1 Abdominal aorta	**22** Placenta
2 Amniotic fluid	**23** Posterior elements of vertebrae
3 Anterior abdominal wall	**24** Pulmonary artery
4 Anterior chest wall	**25** Pulmonary vein
5 Aortic arch	**26** Radius
6 Ascending aorta	**27** Right atrium
7 Bladder	**28** Right kidney
8 Descending aorta	**29** Right ventricle
9 Femur	**30** Spinal canal
10 Femur for femoral length measurement	**31** Spine
11 Finger	**32** Sternum
12 Interatrial septum	**33** Stomach
13 Interventricular septum	**34** Thigh
14 Left atrium	**35** Thumb
15 Left kidney	**36** Tricuspid valve
16 Left ventricle	**37** Ulna
17 Liver	**38** Umbilical cord
18 Male external genitalia	**39** Umbilical vein
19 Metacarpal shaft	**40** Urethra
20 Mitral valve	**41** Uterine wall
21 Moderator band	**42** Vertebral body

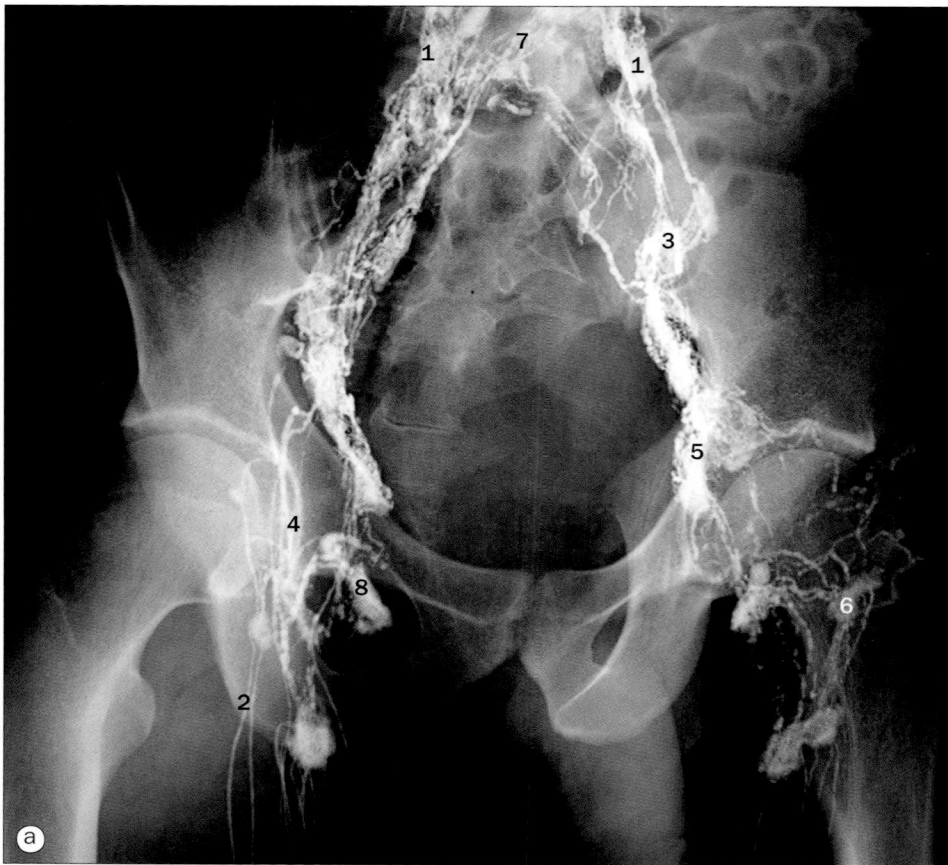

(a) Early filling phase, pelvis.

(b) Late filling phase, pelvis.

1 Ascending lumbar chains
2 Afferent inguinal lymphatics
3 Common iliac nodes
4 Efferent inguinal lymphatics
5 External iliac nodes
6 Superficial inguinal nodes
7 Lumbar crossover
8 Deep inguinal nodes

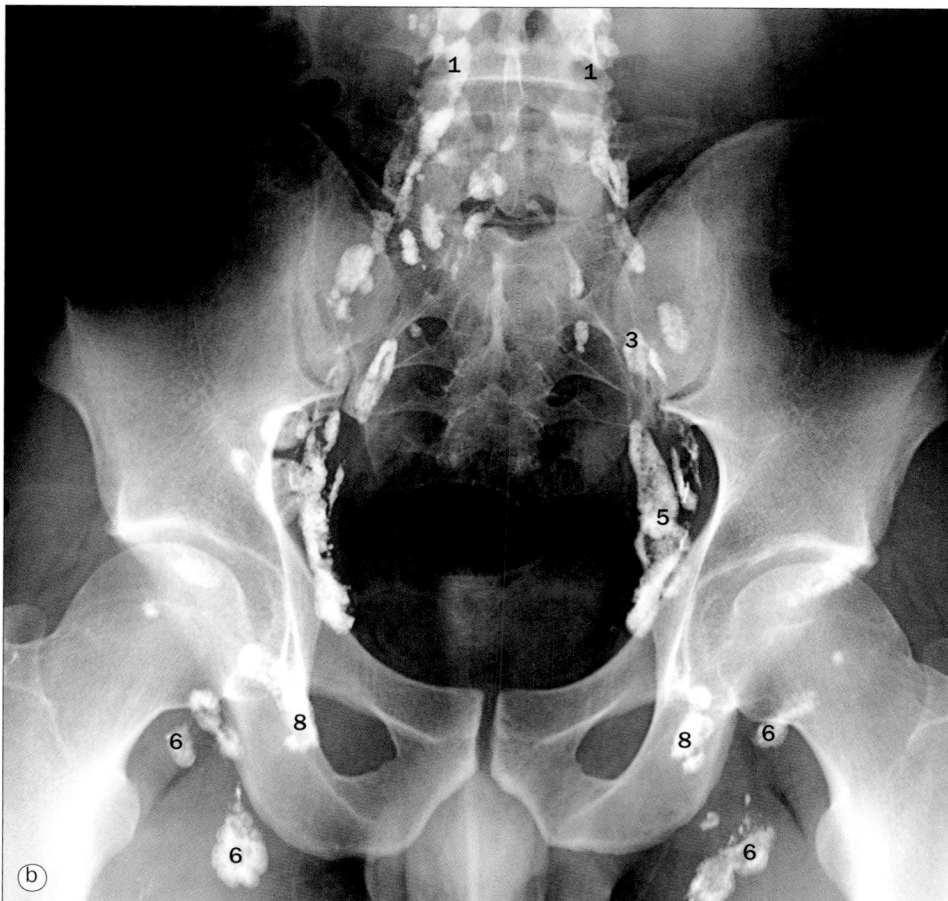

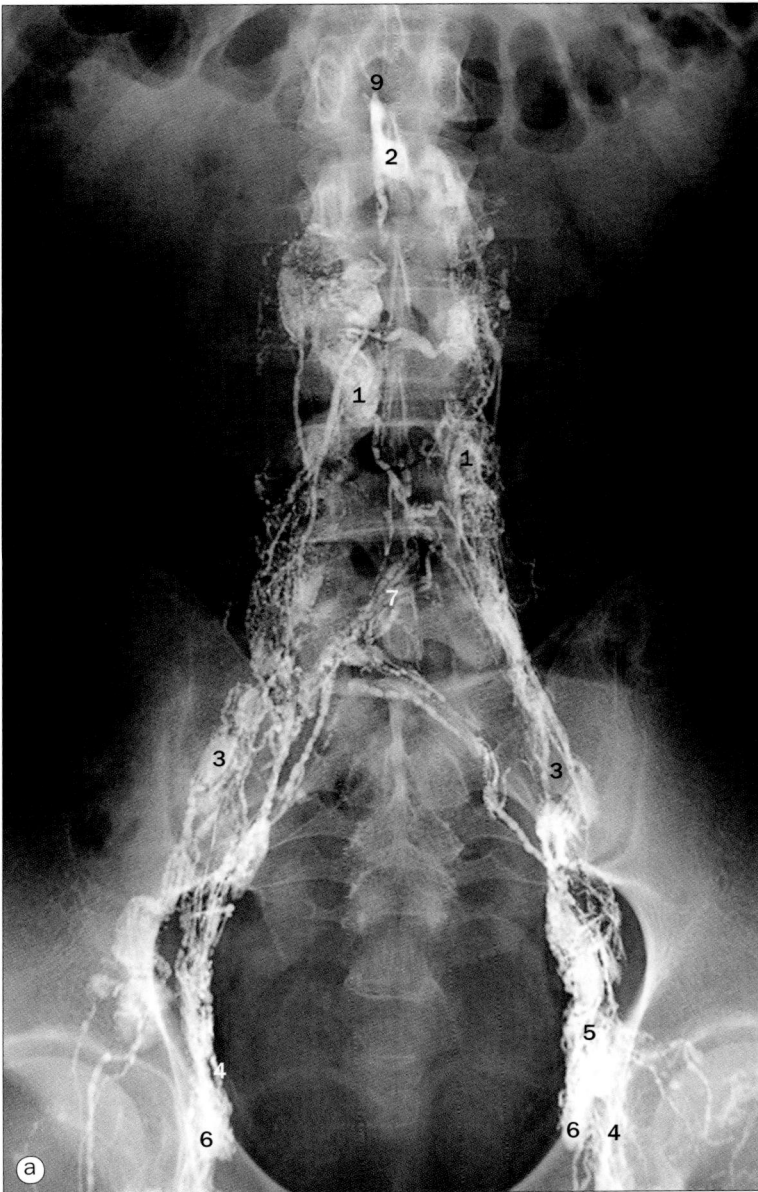

(a) Early filling phase, abdomen.

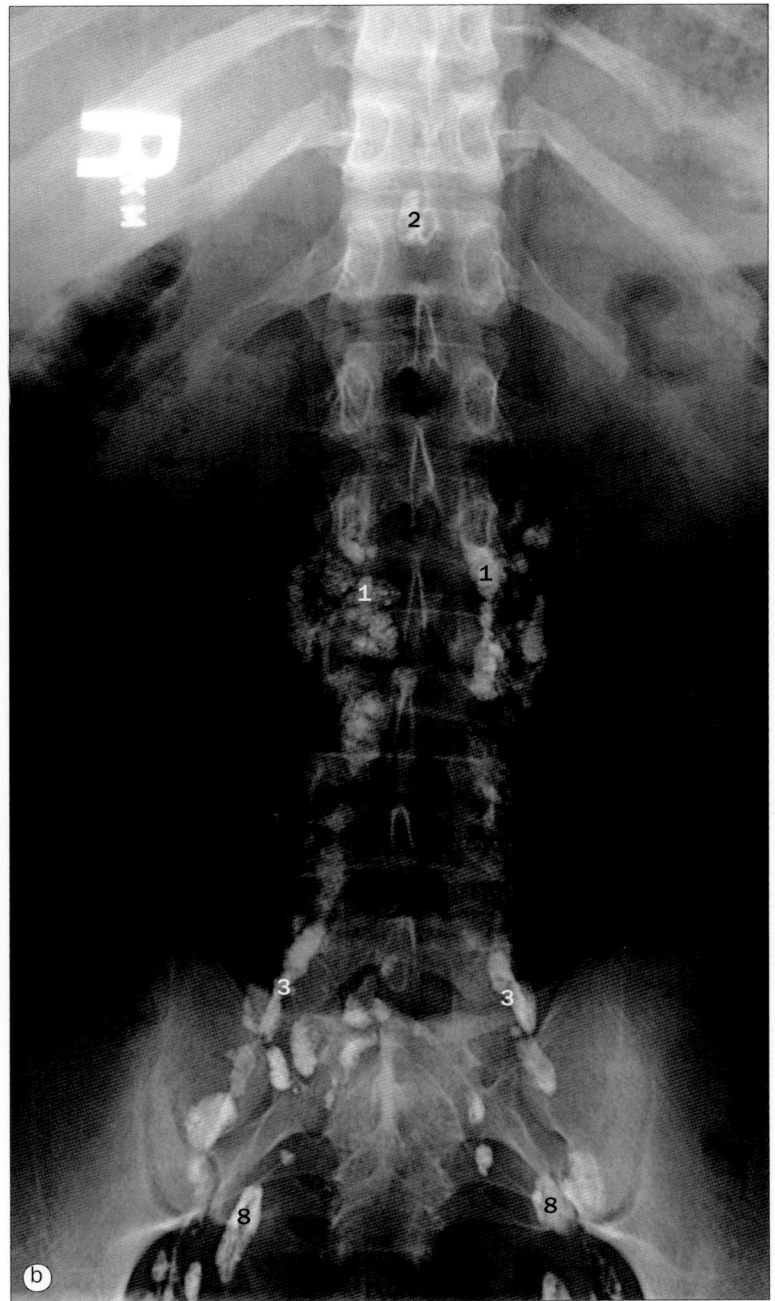

(b) Late filling phase, abdomen.

1 Ascending lumbar chains	**6** Inguinal nodes (early filling)
2 Cisterna chyli	**7** Lumbar crossover
3 Common iliac nodes	**8** Deep inguinal nodes
4 Efferent inguinal lymphatics	**9** Thoracic duct
5 External iliac nodes (early filling)	

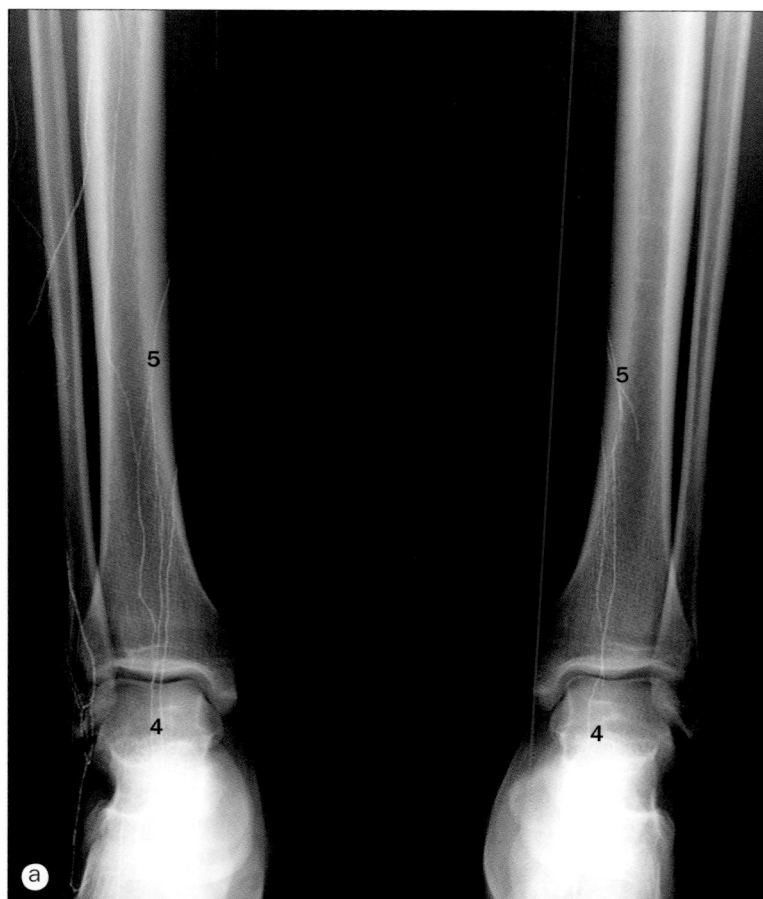

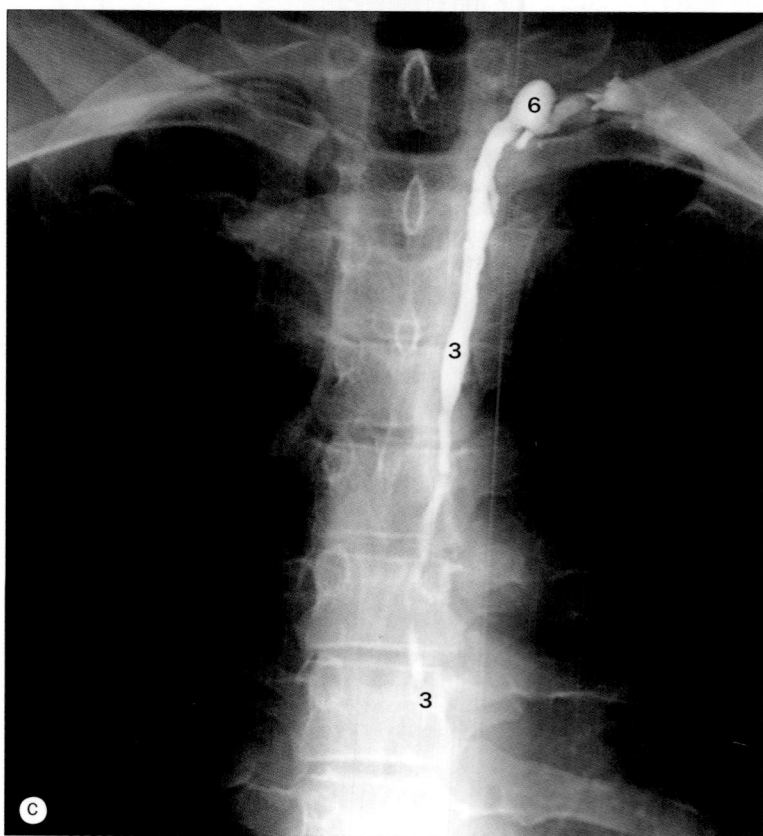

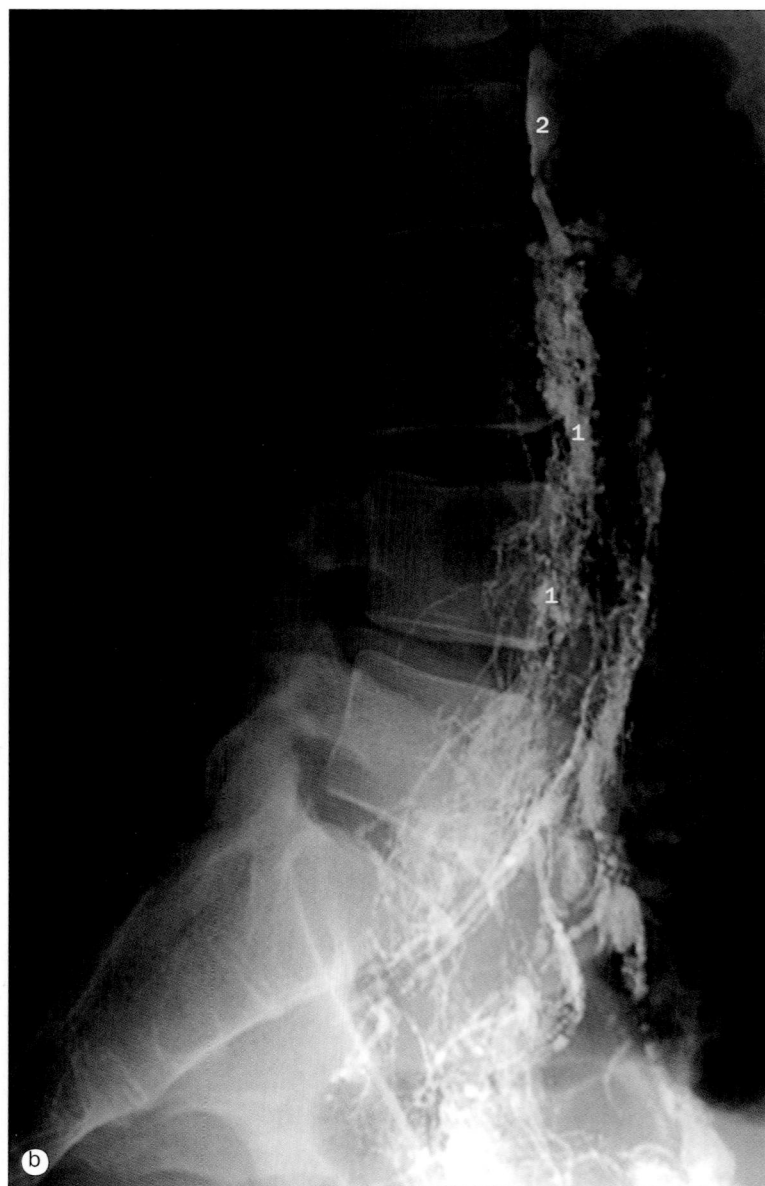

(a) Calf lymphatics following cannulation of lymphatic vessels in the feet.

(b) Lateral early phase filling in abdomen.

(c) Thoracic duct.

1 Ascending lumbar chains of lymph nodes
2 Cysterna chyli
3 Thoracic duct
4 Peripheral foot lymphatic channels
5 Peripheral lower leg lymphatic channels
6 Terminal ampulla

7 Lower limb

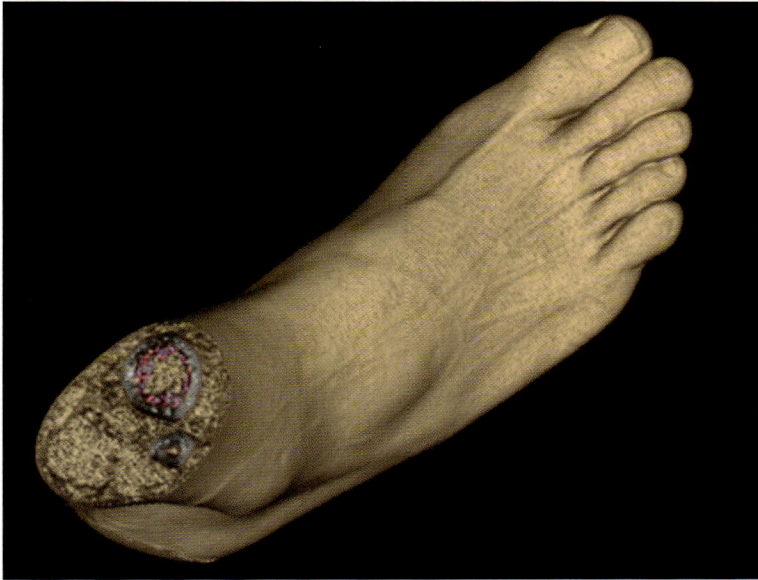

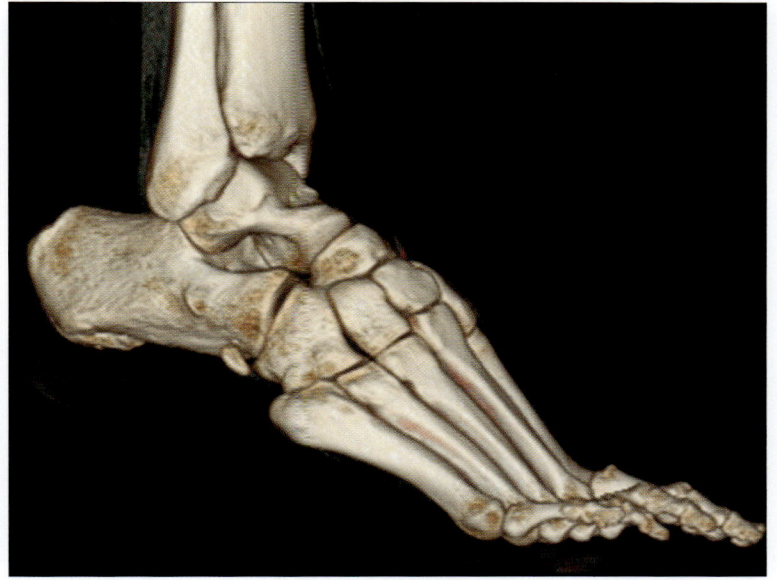

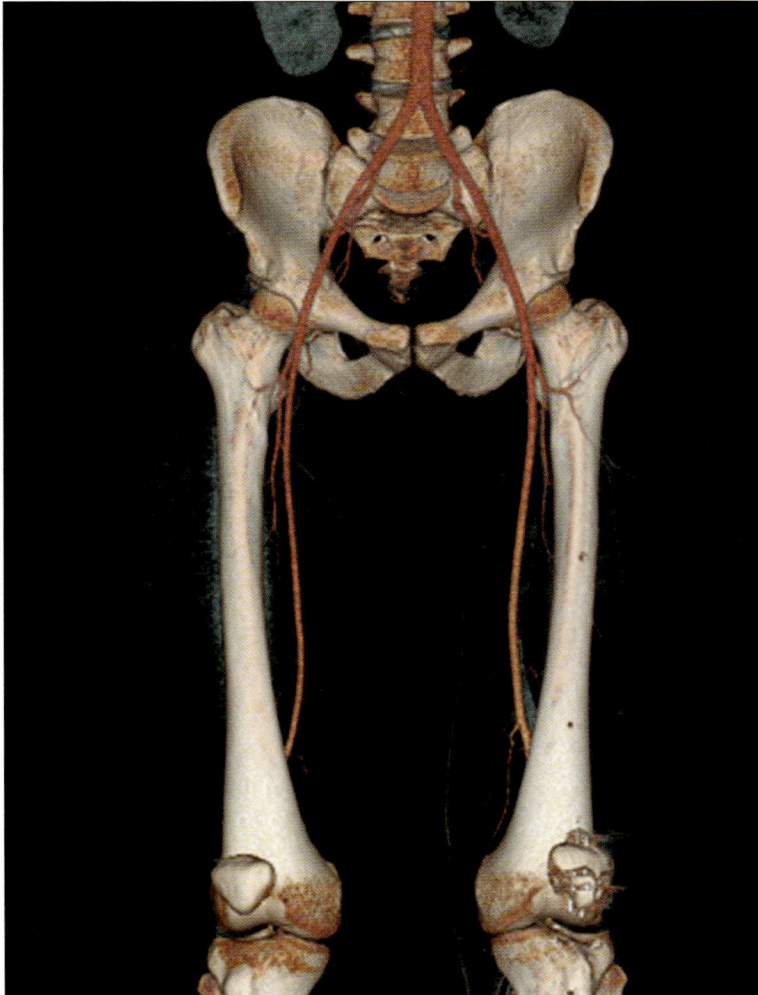

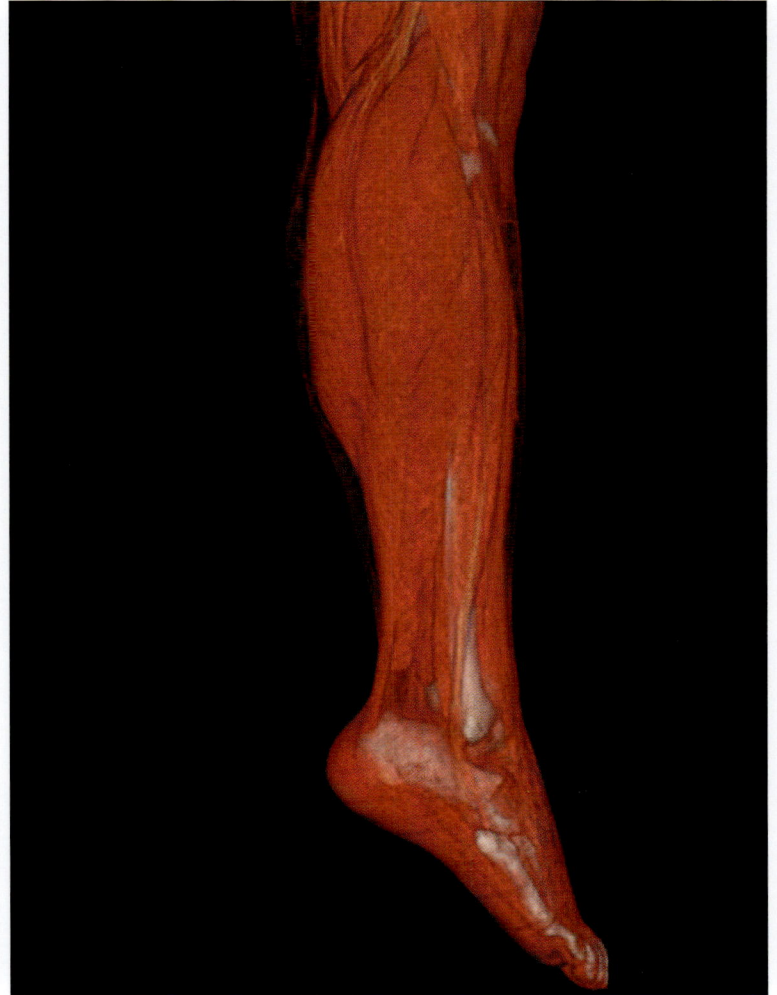

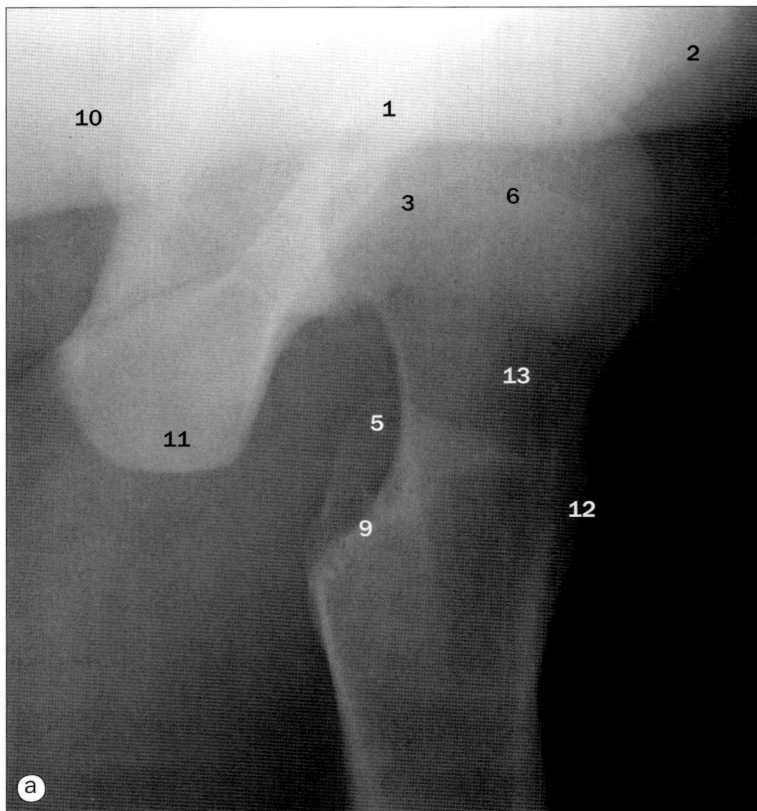

(a) Hip (for neck of femur), lateral projection.

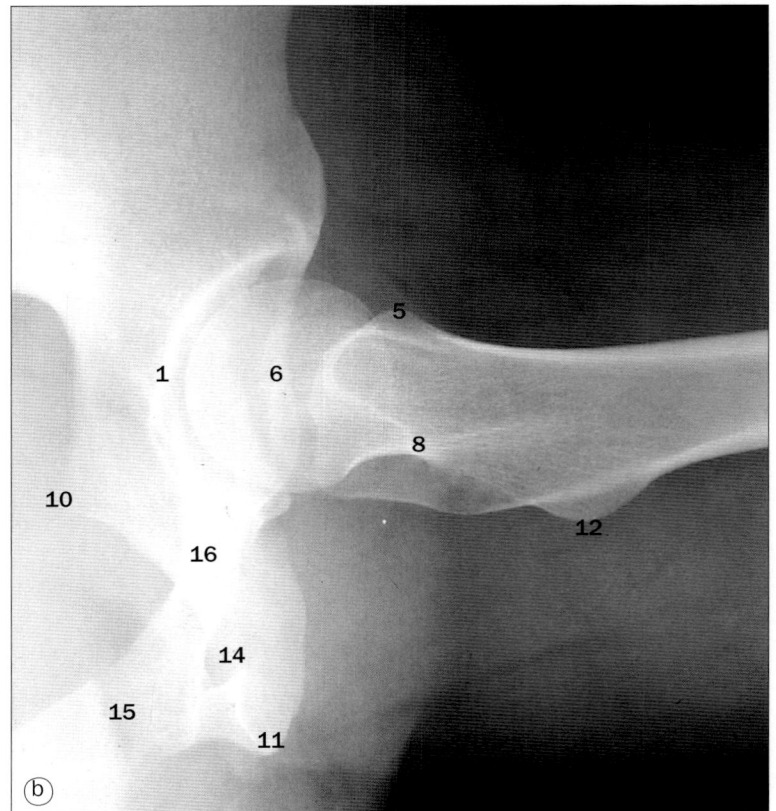

(b) Hip, lateral projection.

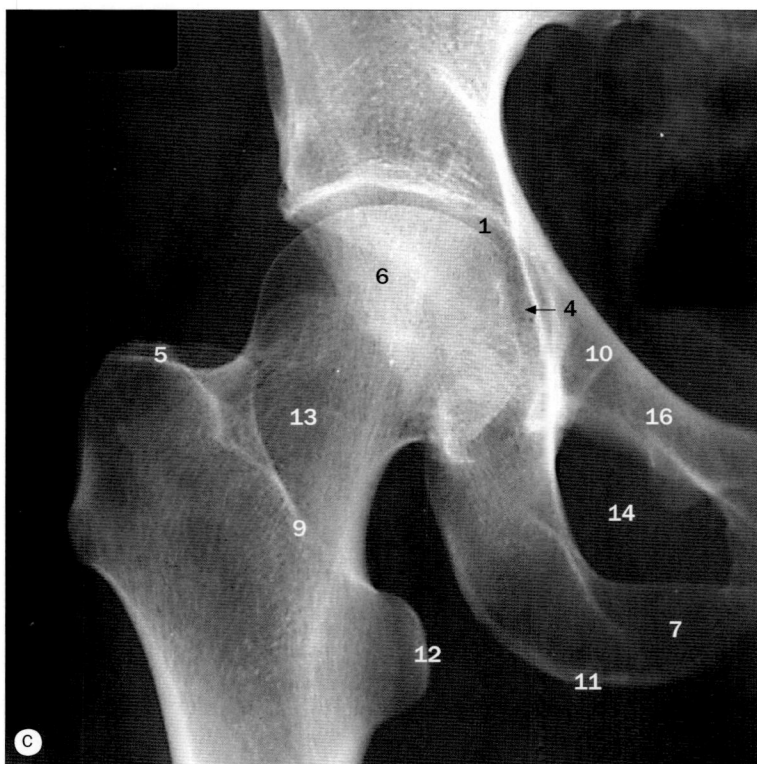

(c) Hip, anteroposterior projection.

1 Acetabulum
2 Anterior inferior iliac spine
3 Epiphysial line
4 Fovea
5 Greater trochanter of femur
6 Head of femur
7 Inferior ramus of pubis
8 Intertrochanteric crest of femur
9 Intertrochanteric line
10 Ischial spine
11 Ischial tuberosity
12 Lesser trochanter of femur
13 Neck of femur
14 Obturator foramen
15 Pubic symphysis
16 Superior ramus of pubis

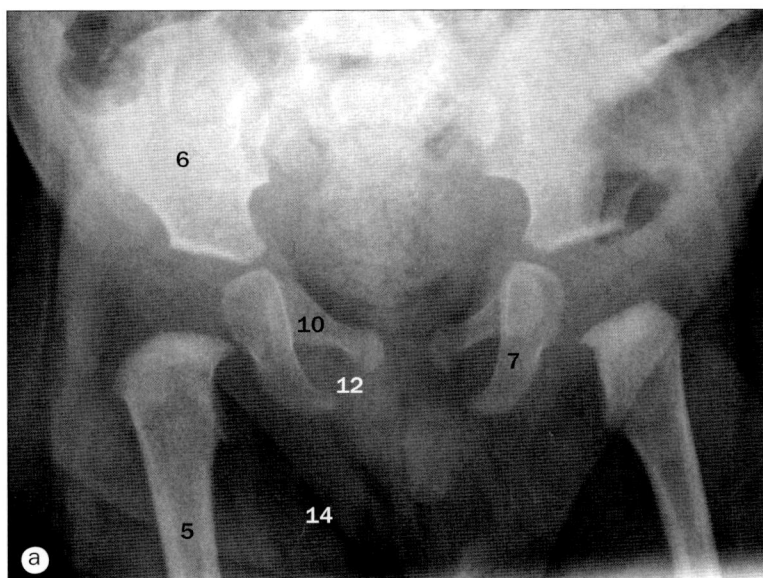

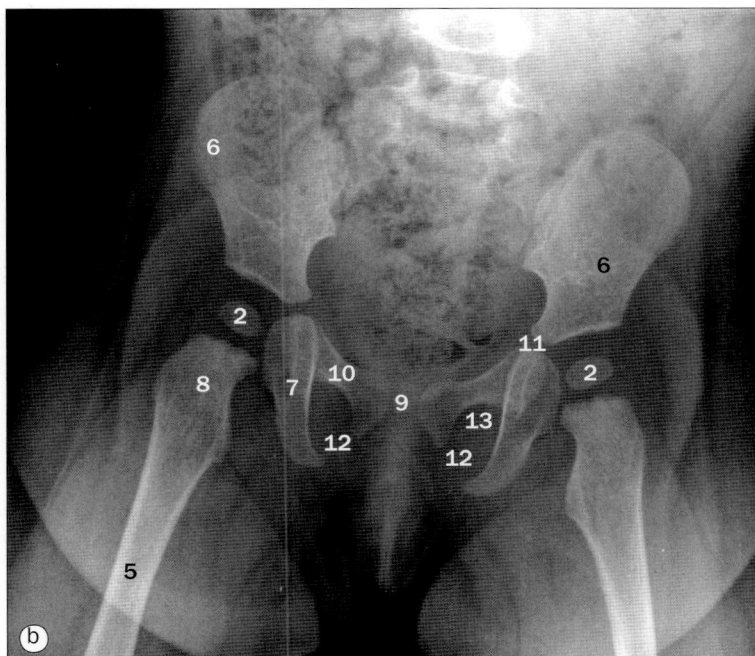

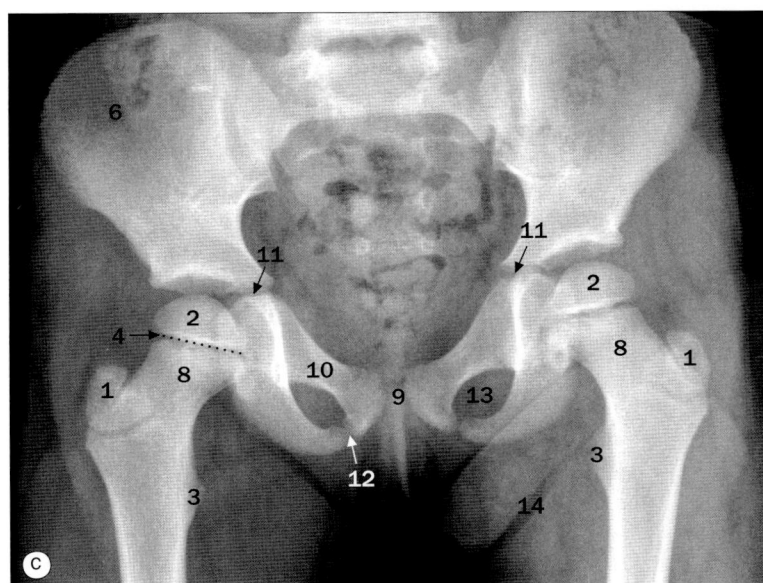

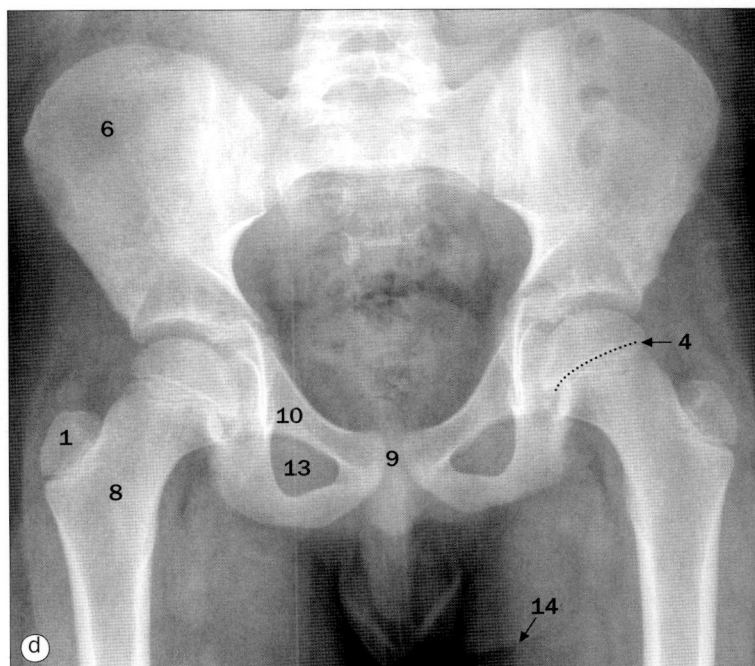

Pelvis, (a) of a 4-month-old girl, (b) of a 9-month-old girl, (c) of a 6-year-old girl, (d) of an 11-year-old girl.

1 Centre for greater trochanter
2 Centre for head of femur (femoral capital epiphysis)
3 Centre for lesser trochanter
4 Epiphysial line
5 Femur
6 Ilium
7 Ischium
8 Neck of femur
9 Pubic symphysis
10 Pubis
11 Triradiate cartilage
12 Unossified junction between ischium and pubis
13 Obturator foramen
14 Fat creases

INNOMINATE (HIP)	Appears	Fused
Ilium	2–3 miu	7–9 yrs
Ischium	4 miu	7–9 yrs
Pubis	4 miu	7–9 yrs
Acetabulum	11–14 yrs	15–25 yrs
Ant. sup. iliac spine	Puberty	15–25 yrs
Iliac crest/sup. spines	Puberty	15–25 yrs
Ischial tuberosity	Puberty +	15–25 yrs
FEMUR (c)		
Shaft	7 wiu	
Head	4–6 mths	14–18 yrs
Greater trochanter	2–4 yrs	14–18 yrs
Lesser trochanter	10–12 yrs	14–18 yrs
Distal end	9 miu	17–19 yrs

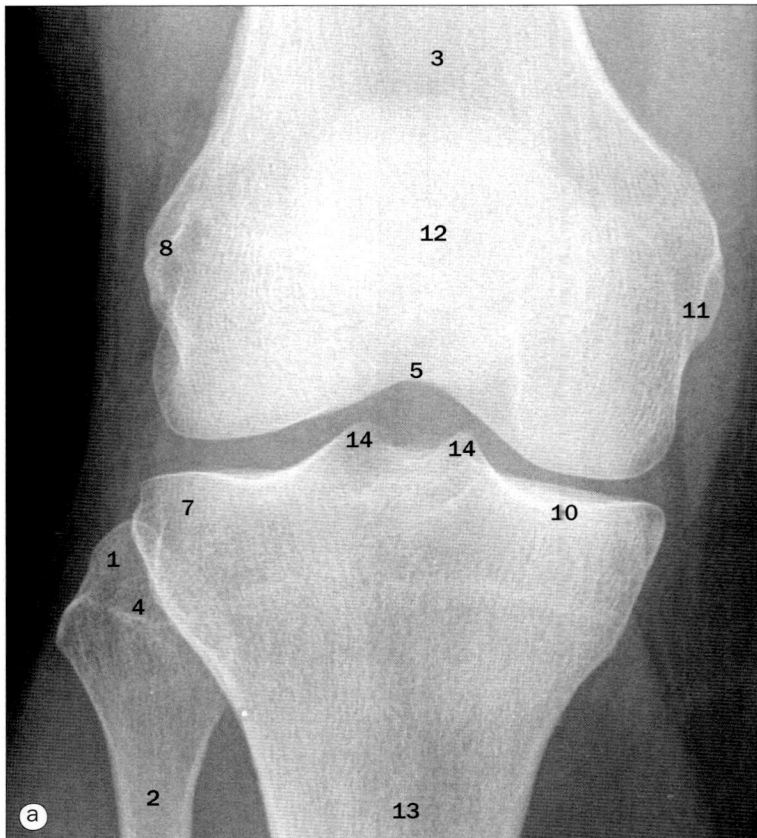

(a) Anteroposterior projection.

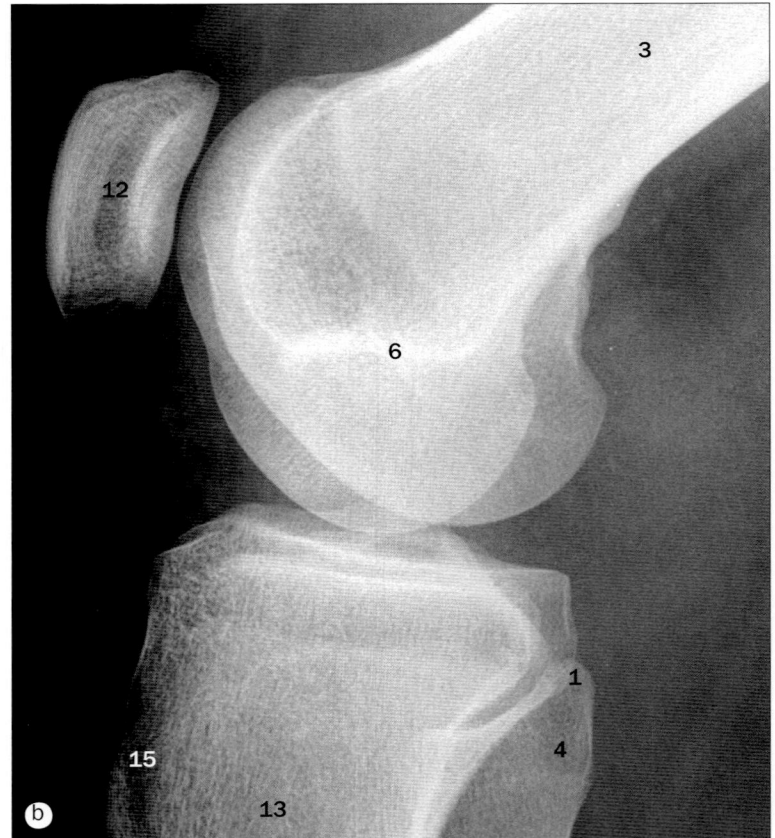

(b) Lateral projection.

 1 Apex (styloid process) of fibula
 2 Fibula neck
 3 Femur
 4 Head of fibula
 5 Intercondylar fossa
 6 Lateral condyle of femur
 7 Lateral condyle of tibia
 8 Lateral epicondyle of femur
 9 Medial condyle of femur
10 Medial condyle of tibia
11 Medial epicondyle of femur
12 Patella
13 Tibia
14 Tubercles of intercondylar eminence
15 Tuberosity of tibia

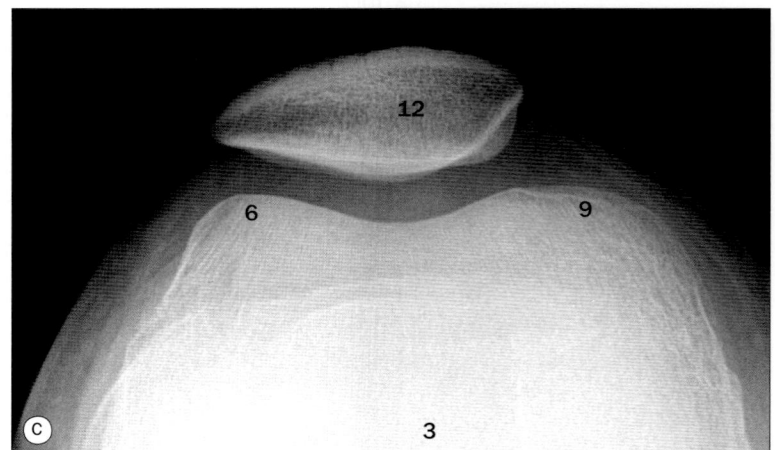

(c) Inferosuperior (skyline) projection.

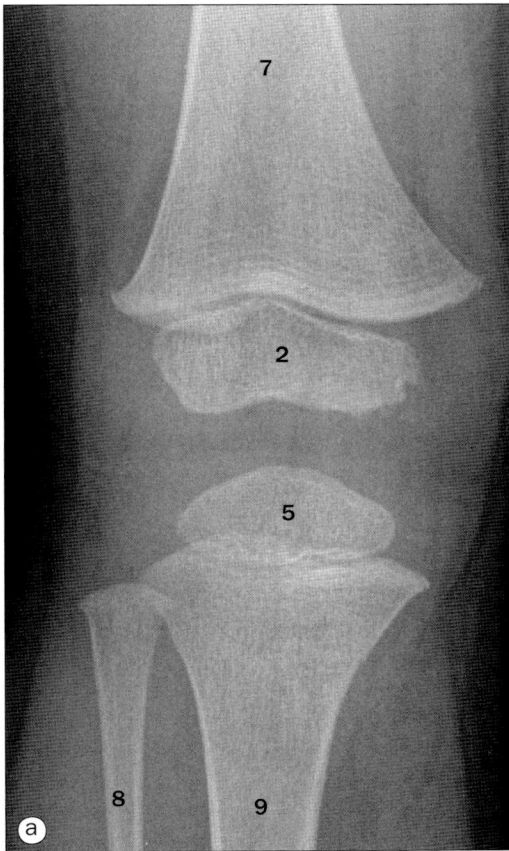

(a) 2-year-old girl.

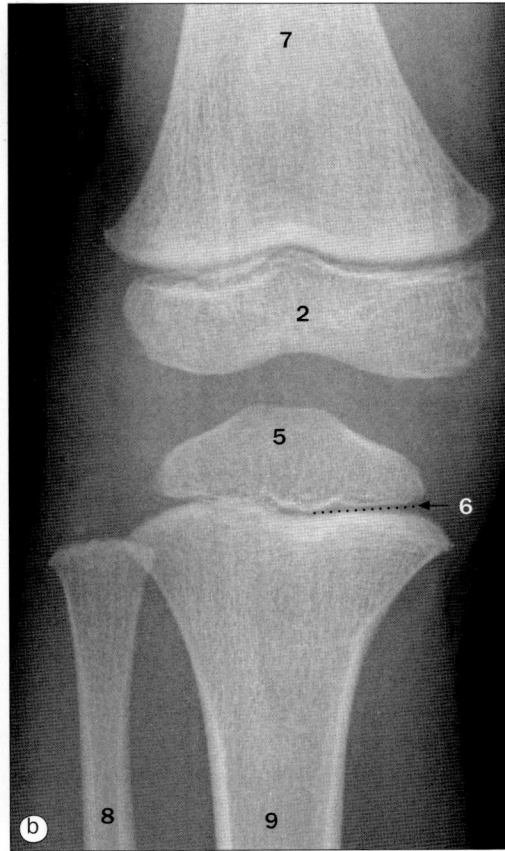

(b) and (c) 5-year-old girl.

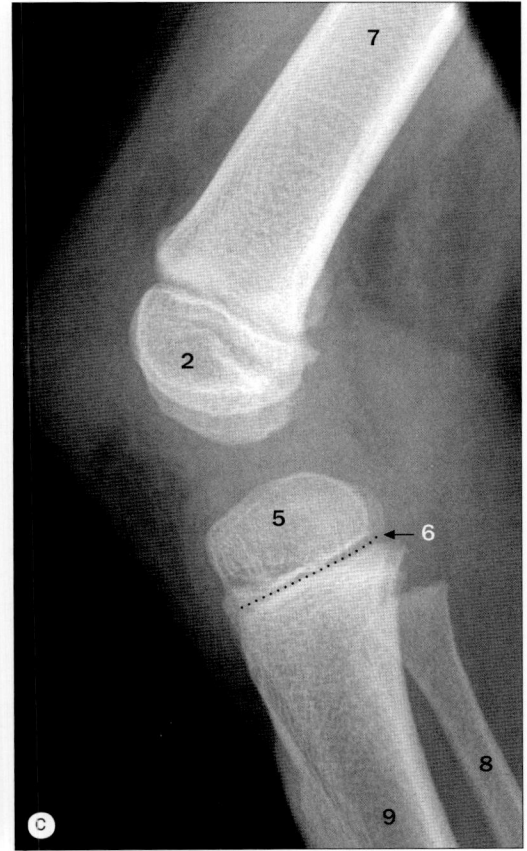

1 Antero-inferior extension of proximal
  tibial centre for tuberosity of tibia
2 Centre for distal femur
3 Centre for head of fibula
4 Patella
5 Centre for proximal tibia
6 Epiphysial line
7 Femur
8 Fibula
9 Tibia

PATELLA (c)	Appears	Fused
1–3 centres	3–5 yrs	Puberty
TIBIA (c)		
Shaft	7 wiu	
Proximal/plateau	9 miu	16–18 yrs
Tuberosity	10–12 yrs	12–14 yrs
Distal end	4 mths–1 yr	15–17 yrs
FIBULA (c)		
Shaft	8 wiu	
Proximal end/head	2–4 yrs	17–19 yrs
Distal end	6 mths–1 yr	15–17 yrs

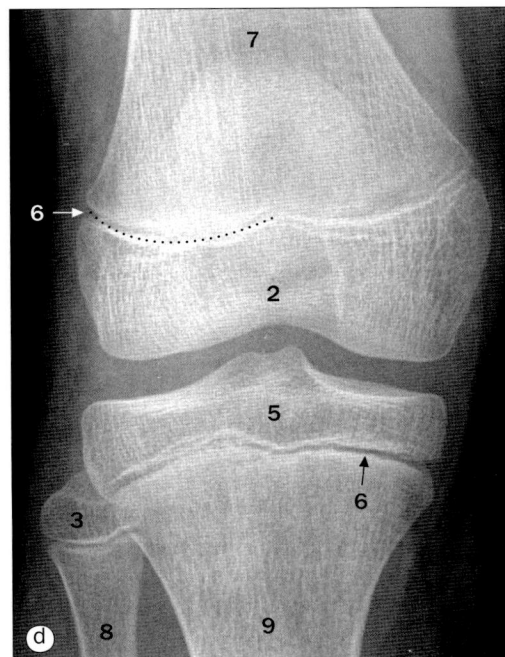

(d) and (e) 12-year-old girl.

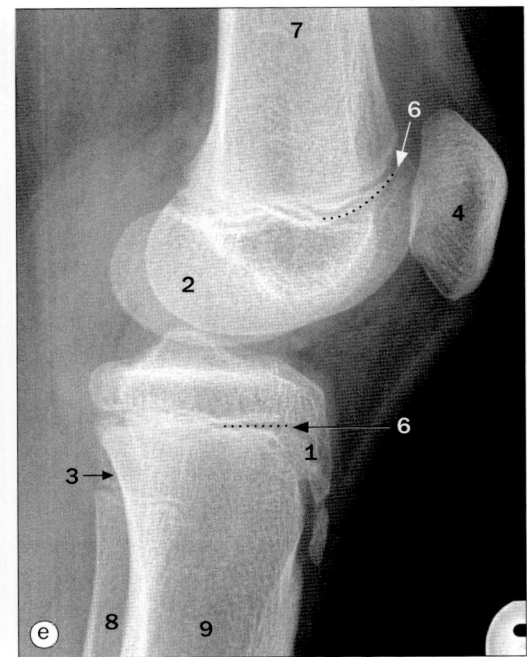

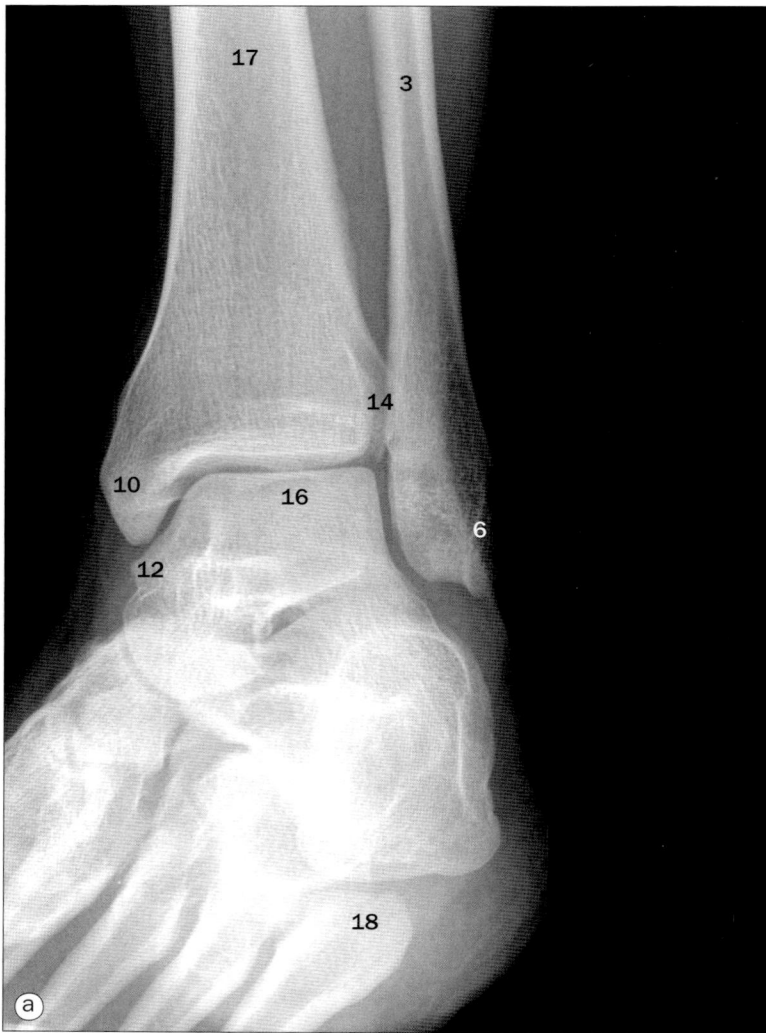

(a) Ankle joint, anteroposterior projection.

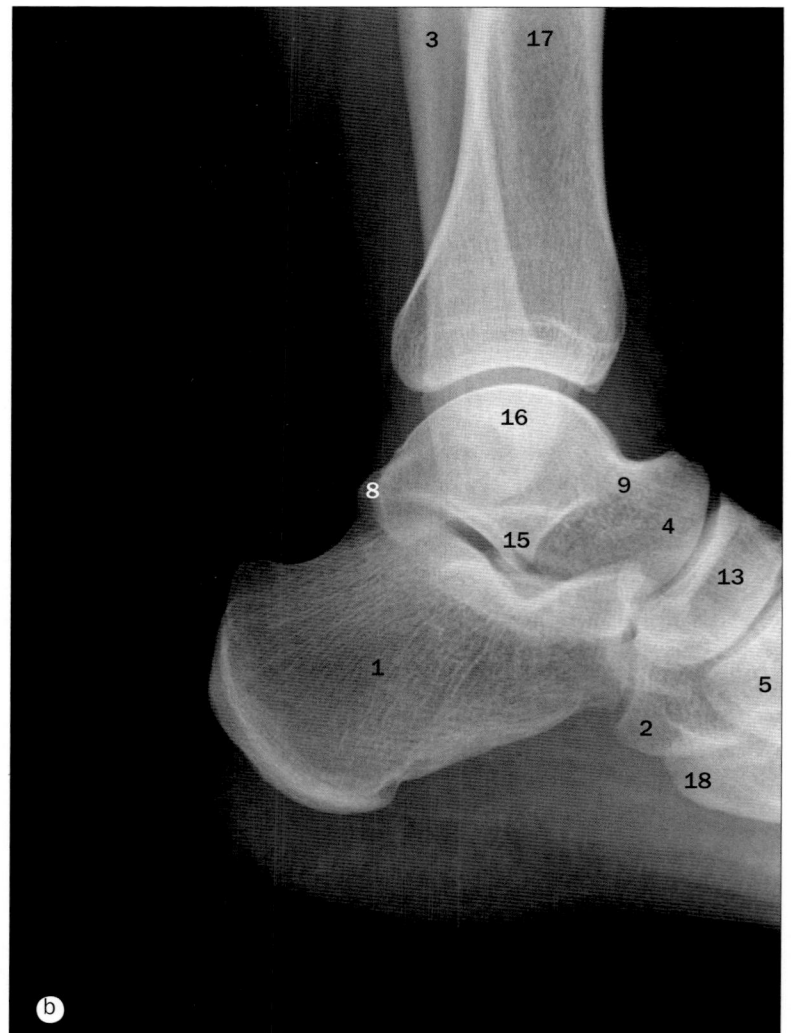

(b) Ankle joint, lateral projection.

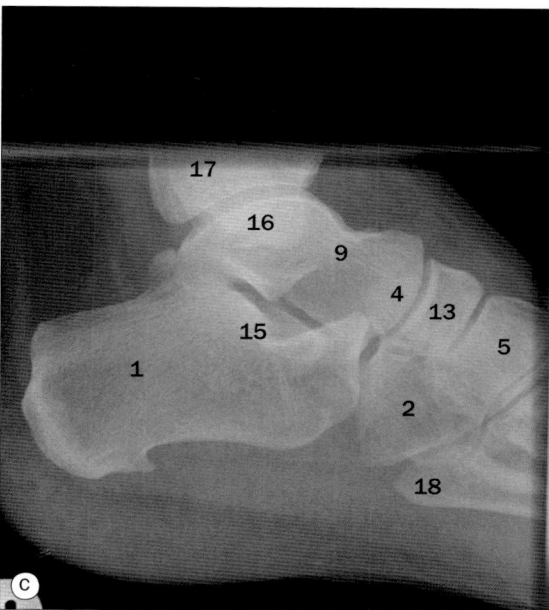

(c) Calcaneus, lateral projection.

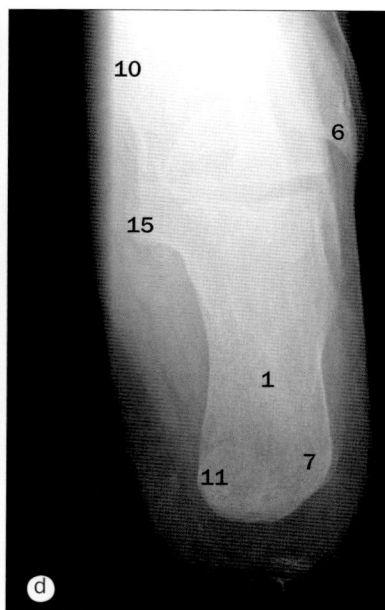

(d) Calcaneus, axial (caudo cranial) projection.

1 Calcaneus
2 Cuboid
3 Fibula
4 Head of talus
5 Lateral cuneiform
6 Lateral malleolus of fibula
7 Lateral process of calcaneus
8 Lateral tubercle of talus
9 Neck of talus
10 Medial malleolus of tibia
11 Medial process of calcaneus
12 Medial tubercle of talus
13 Navicular
14 Region of inferior tibiofibular joint
15 Sustentaculum tali of calcaneus
16 Talus
17 Tibia
18 Tuberosity of base of fifth metatarsal

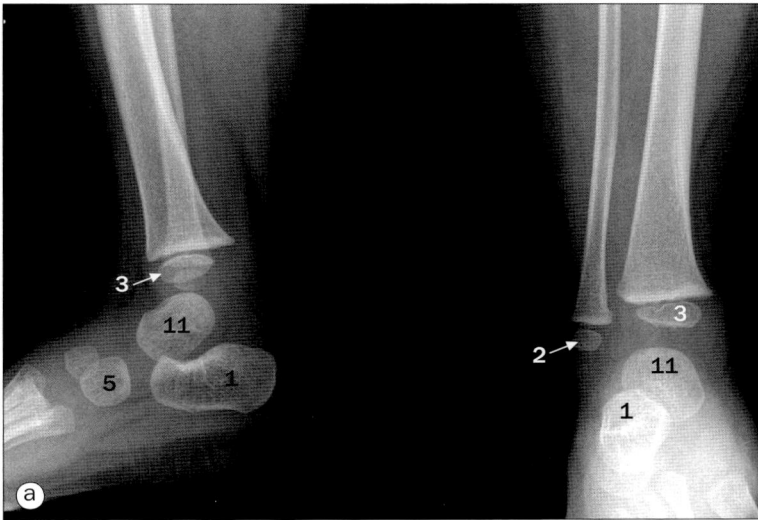

(a) Ankle of a 3-year-old girl.

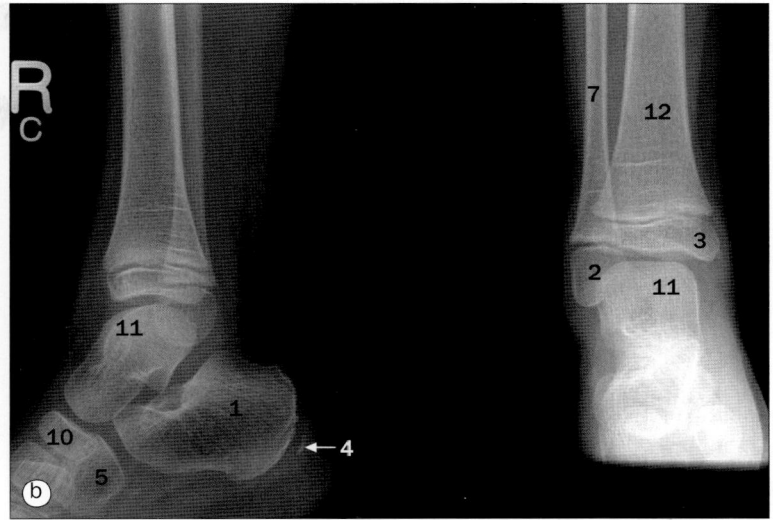

(b) Ankle of a 5-year-old girl.

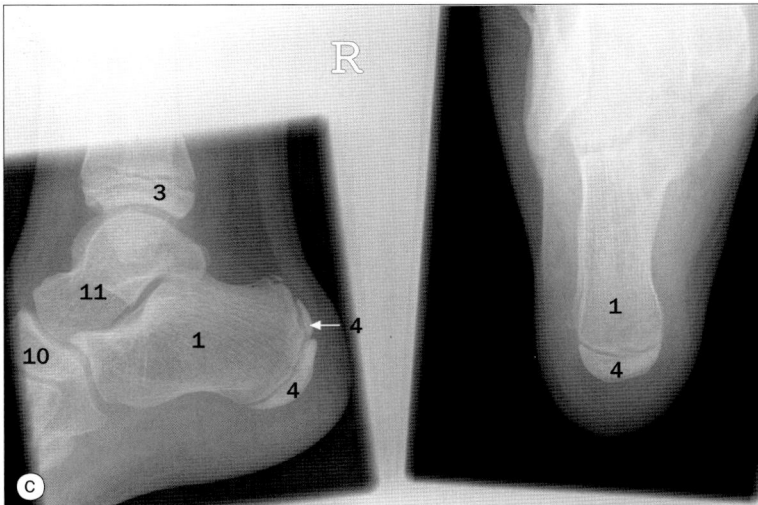

(c) Ankle of a 13-year-old girl.

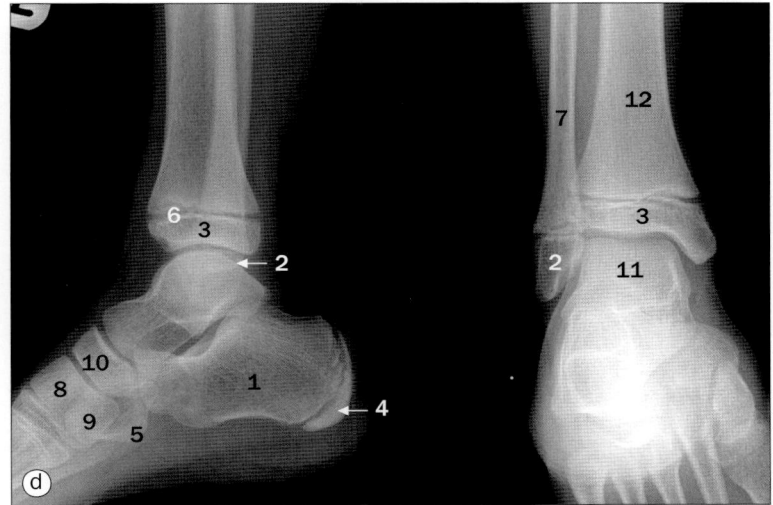

(d) Calcaneus of a 10-year-old girl.

 1 Calcaneus
 2 Centre for distal fibula
 3 Centre for distal tibia
 4 Centre for posterior aspect of calcaneus
 5 Cuboid
 6 Epiphyseal line
 7 Fibula
 8 Intermediate cuneiform
 9 Lateral cuneiform
10 Navicular
11 Talus
12 Tibia

TARSAL BONES (c)	Appears	Fused
Calcaneus	3 miu	14–16 yrs
Talus	6 miu	
Navicular	3 yrs	
Cuneiform lateral	6 mths–1 yr	
Cuneiform intermediate	2–3 yrs	
Cuneiform medial	1–2 yrs	
Cuboid	9 miu	

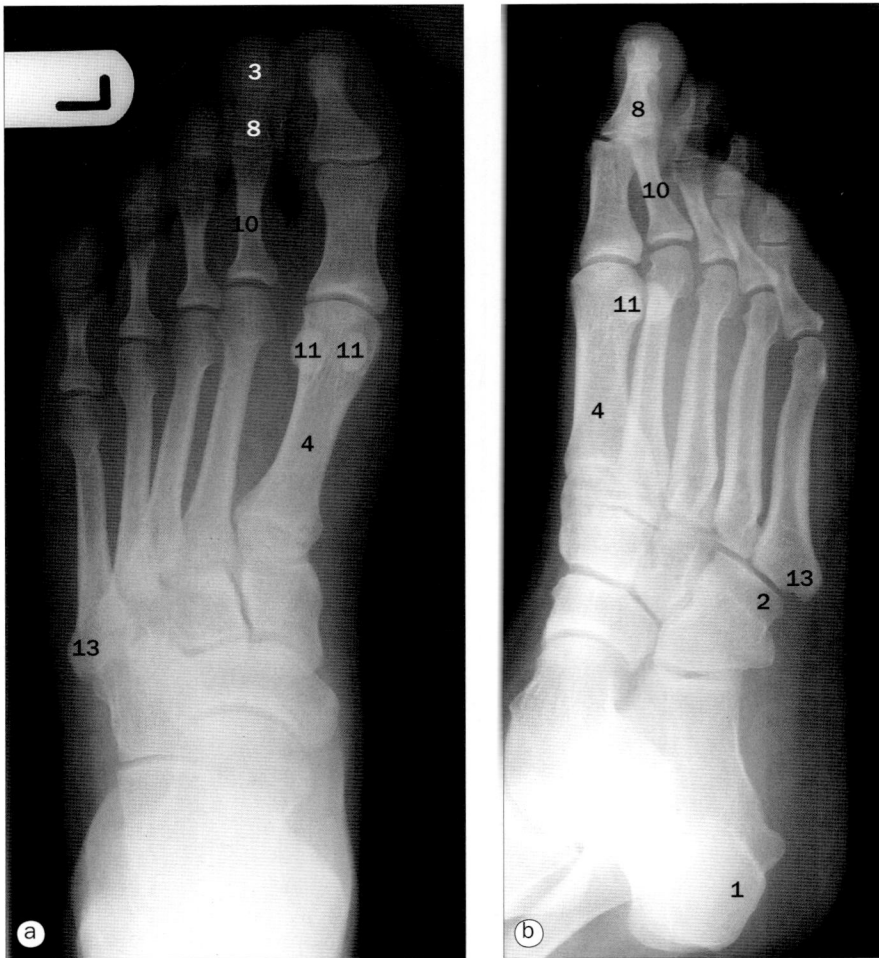

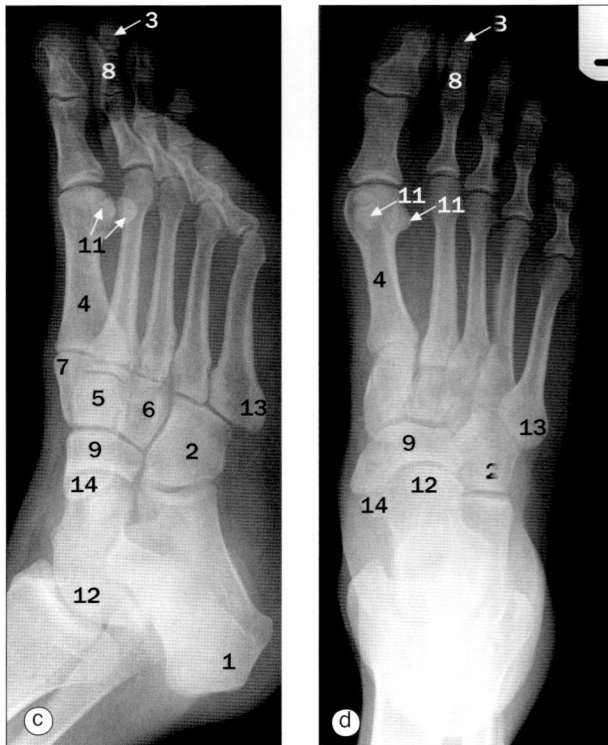

Foot, (a) dorsoplantar projection, (b) dorsoplantar oblique projection, (c) and (d) os naviculare.

1 Calcaneus
2 Cuboid
3 Distal phalanx of second toe
4 First metatarsal
5 Intermediate cuneiform
6 Lateral cuneiform
7 Medial cuneiform
8 Middle phalanx of second toe
9 Navicular
10 Proximal phalanx of second toe
11 Sesamoid bones in flexor hallucis brevis muscle
12 Talus
13 Tuberosity of base of fifth metatarsal
14 Os naviculare

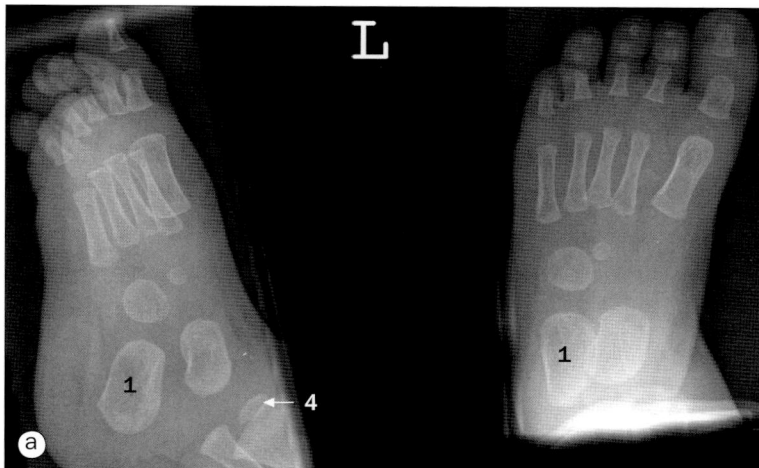

(a) Foot of an 11-month-old girl.

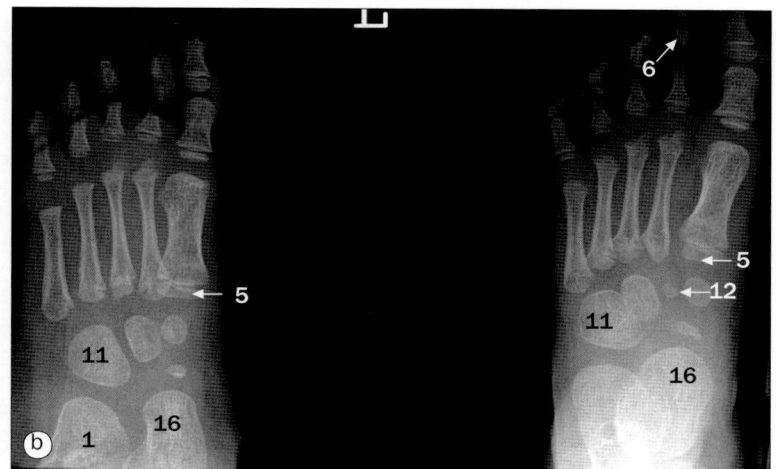

(b) Foot of a 3-year-old girl.

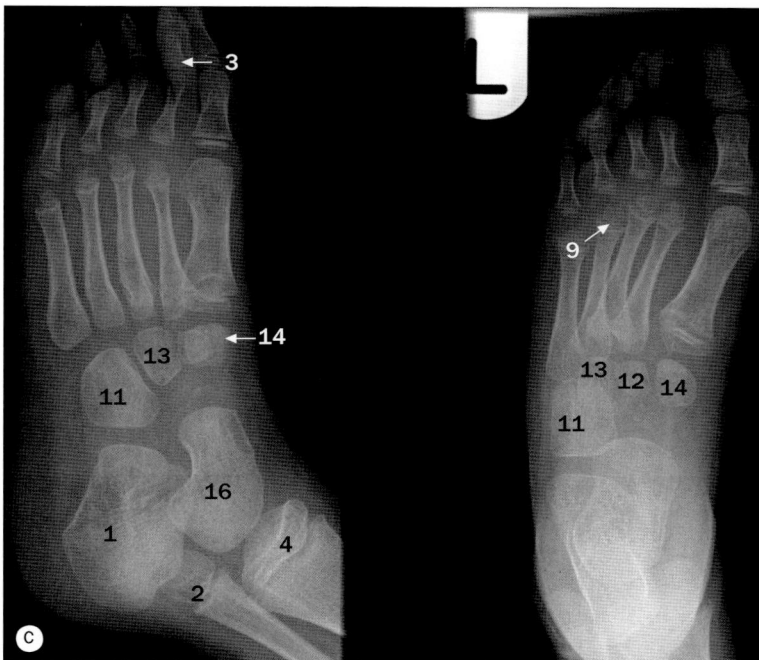

(c) Foot of a 6-year-old girl.

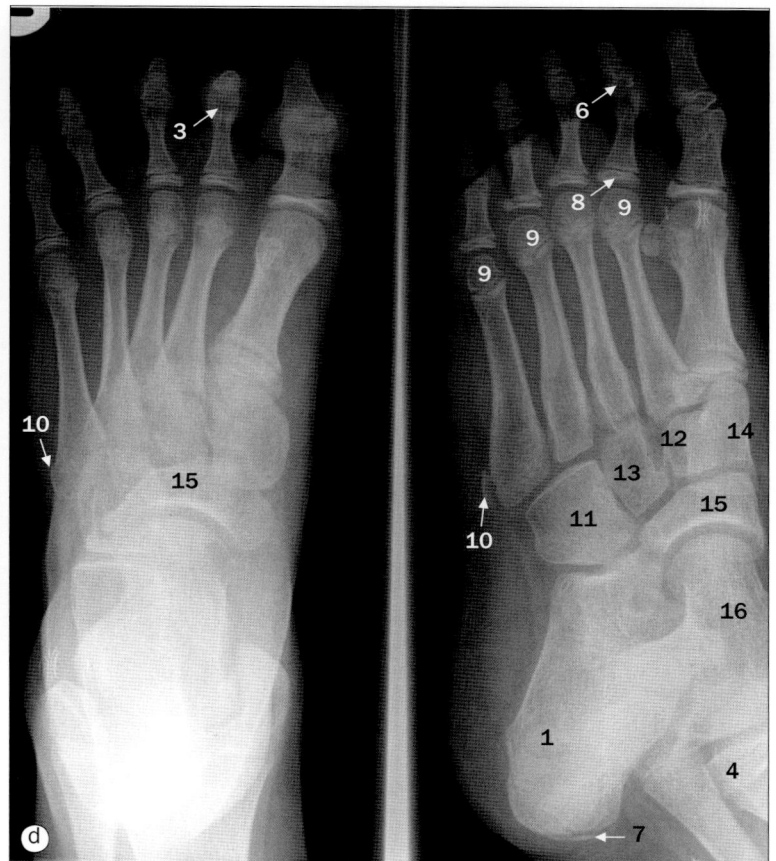

(d) Foot of a 12-year-old girl.

1 Calcaneus
2 Centre for distal fibula
3 Centre for distal phalanx of second toe
4 Centre for distal tibia
5 Centre for first metatarsal
6 Centre for middle phalanx of second toe
7 Centre for posterior aspect of calcaneus
8 Centre for proximal phalanx of second toe
9 Centre for second metatarsal (applies to second to fifth metatarsal)
10 Centre for tuberosity of base of fifth metatarsal
11 Cuboid
12 Intermediate cuneiform
13 Lateral cuneiform
14 Medial cuneiform
15 Navicular
16 Talus

METATARSALS (c)	Appears	Fused
Shafts	9 wiu	
Heads (2–5) or base (1)	3–4 yrs	17–20 yrs
Tuberosity of 5	10–12 yrs	13–15 yrs

PHALANGES (c)		
Shaft	9–12 wiu	
Bases (variable)	1–6 yrs	14–18 yrs

TARSAL BONES (c)	Appears	Fused
Calcaneus	3 miu	14–16 yrs
Talus	6 miu	
Navicular	3 yrs	
Cuneiform lateral	6 mths–1 yr	
Cuneiform intermediate	2–3 yrs	
Cuneiform medial	1–2 yrs	
Cuboid	9 miu	

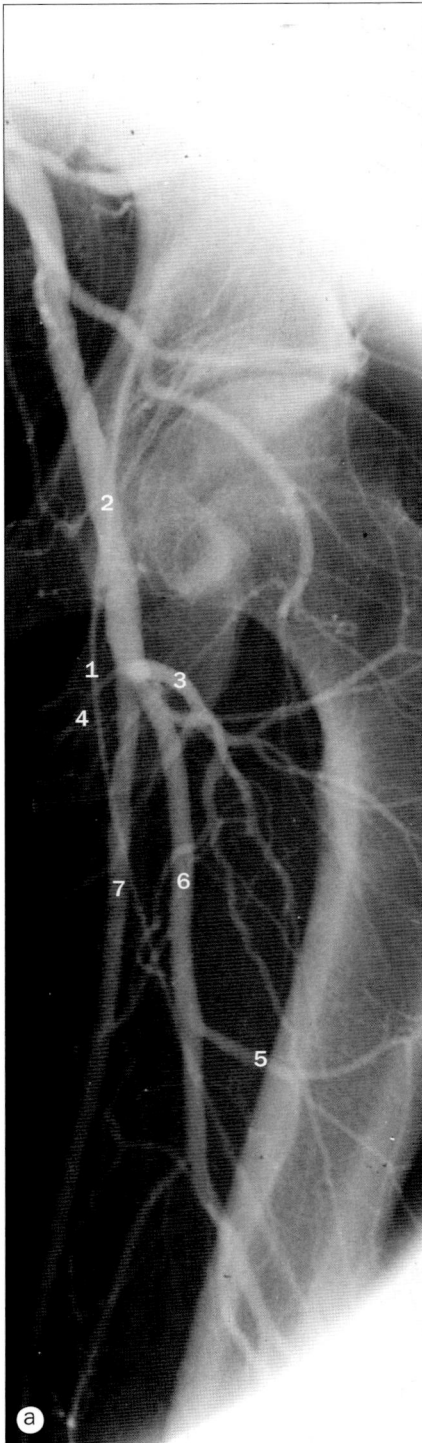

(a) Femoral arteriogram.

The femoropopliteal and tibial arteries are imaged by catheterising the distal abdominal aorta and injecting contrast medium. The column of contrast is then followed as it passes down the legs. If only one leg is to be imaged, an injection into the ipsilateral femoral artery suffices. The external iliac artery continues as the common femoral artery, which originates deep to the inguinal ligament, dividing into the superficial and deep (profunda) femoral arteries. An oblique view is often useful to image the femoral bifurcation and to identify atheroma at the origins of these vessels.

1 Catheter introduced into distal abdominal aorta via left femoral artery
2 Common femoral artery
3 Lateral circumflex femoral artery
4 Medial circumflex femoral artery
5 Perforating artery
6 Profunda femoris artery
7 Superficial femoral artery

(b) Popliteal arteriogram.

The superficial femoral artery becomes the popliteal artery as it passes through the hiatus in the adductor magnus muscle. The popliteal artery terminates at the lower border of the popliteus muscle, dividing into the anterior and posterior tibial arteries.

1 Anterior tibial artery
2 Inferior lateral genicular artery
3 Inferior medial genicular artery
4 Muscular branches of anterior tibial artery
5 Muscular branches of posterior tibial artery
6 Peroneal artery
7 Popliteal artery
8 Posterior tibial artery
9 Superior lateral genicular artery
10 Superior medial genicular artery

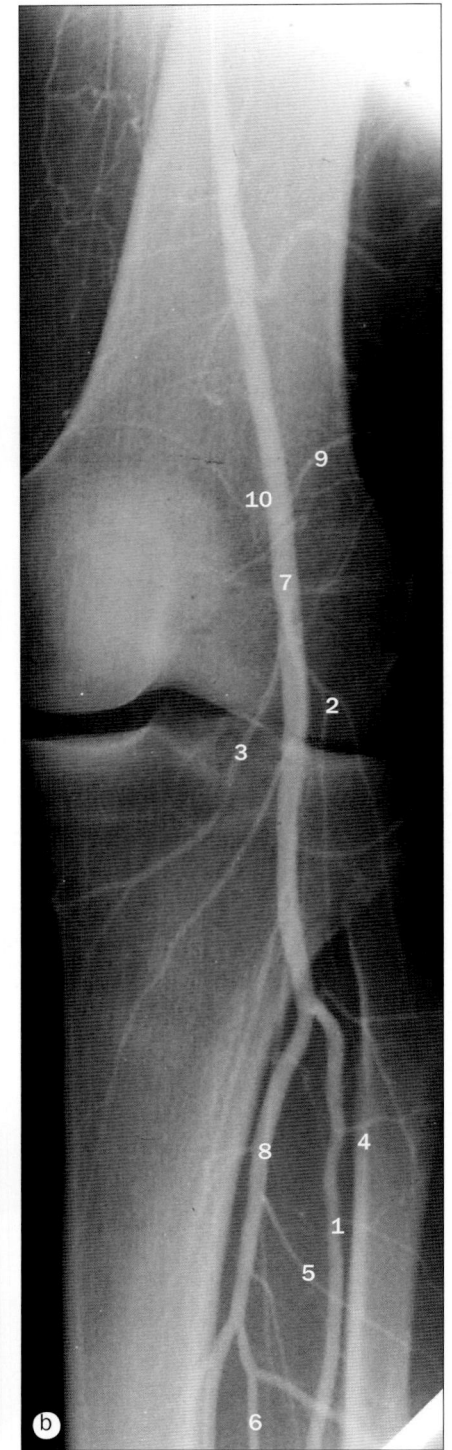

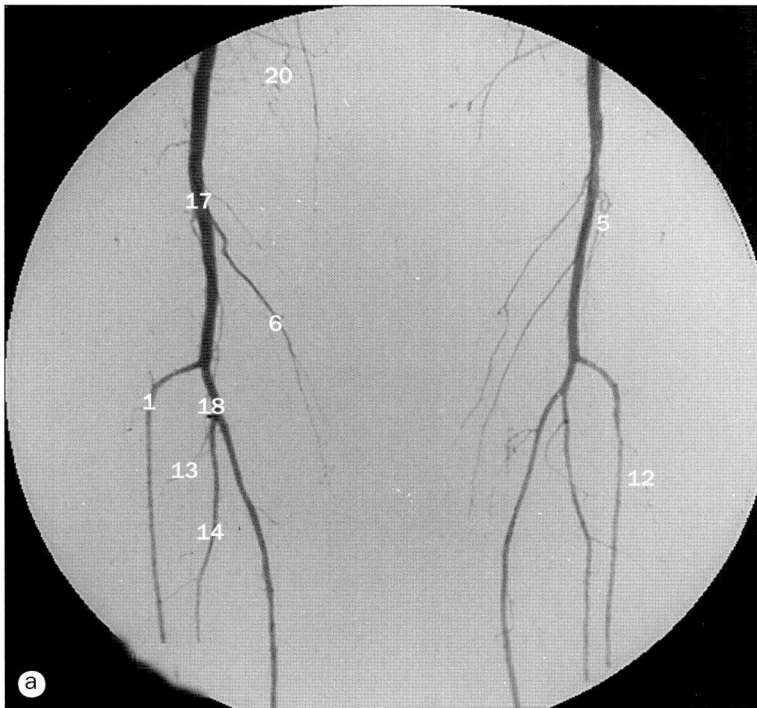

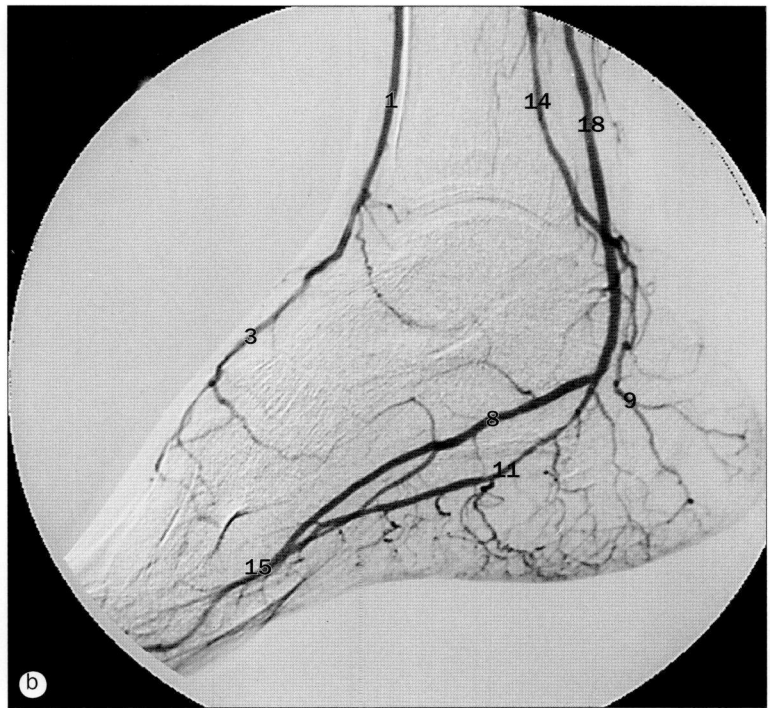

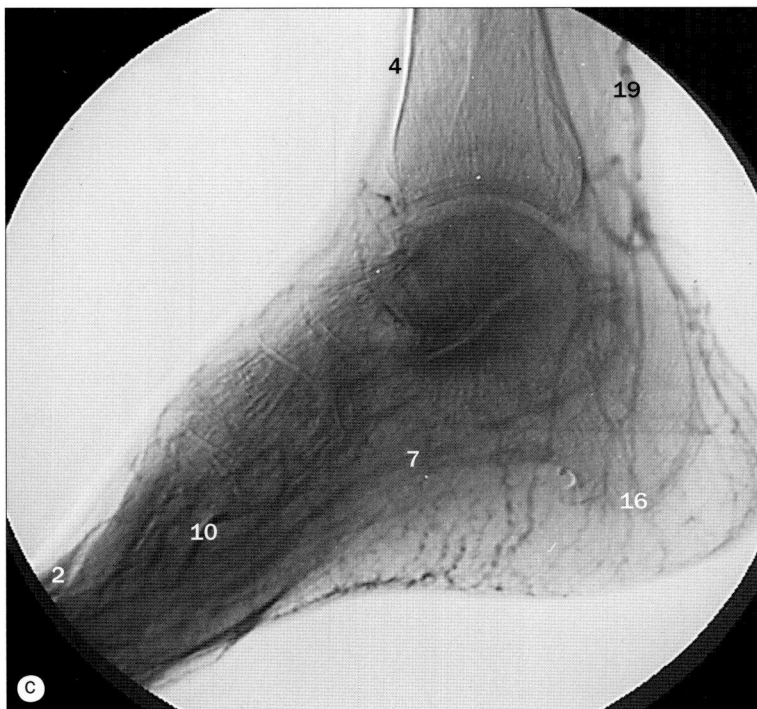

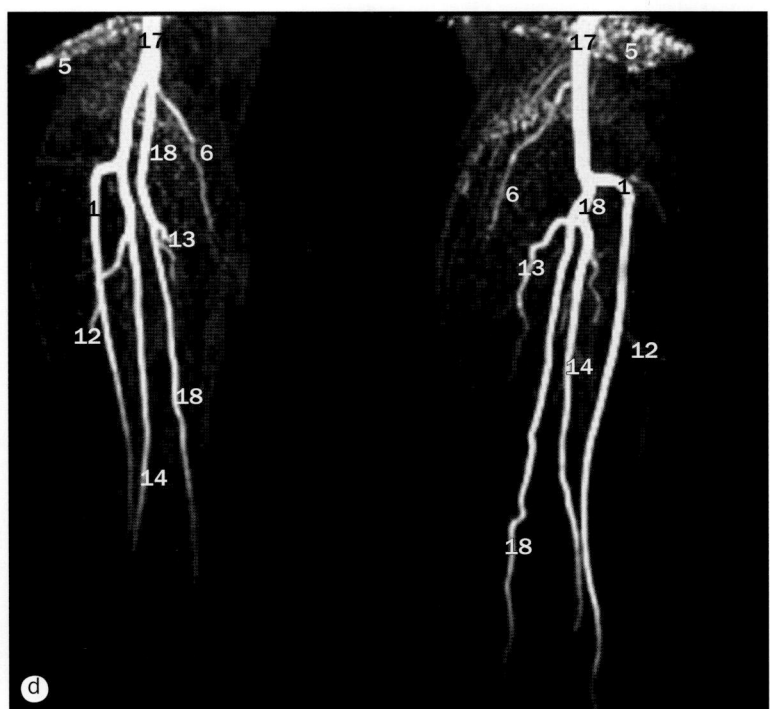

(a) Popliteal arteriogram, (b) foot arteriogram, lateral image, (c) foot venogram, (d) MR angiogram of calf arteries.

1 Anterior tibial artery	8 Lateral plantar artery	14 Peroneal artery
2 Dorsal venous arch	9 Medial calcaneal artery	15 Plantar arch
3 Dorsalis pedis artery	10 Medial marginal vein	16 Plantar cutaneous venous plexus
4 Great saphenous vein	11 Medial plantar artery	17 Popliteal artery
5 Inferior lateral genicular artery	12 Muscular branches of anterior tibial artery	18 Posterior tibial artery
6 Inferior medial genicular artery	13 Muscular branches of posterior tibial	19 Small saphenous vein
7 Lateral marginal vein	artery	20 Superior medial genicular artery

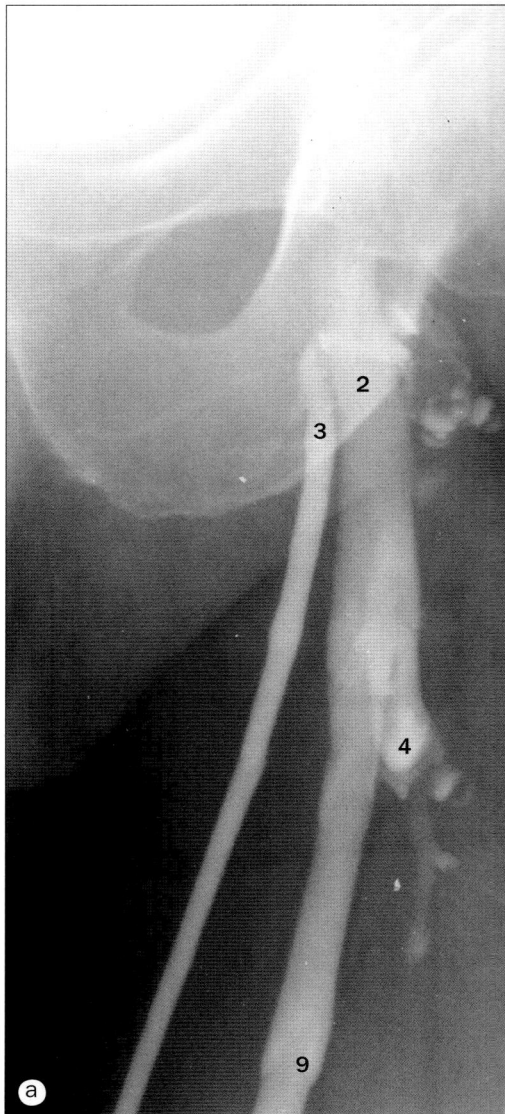

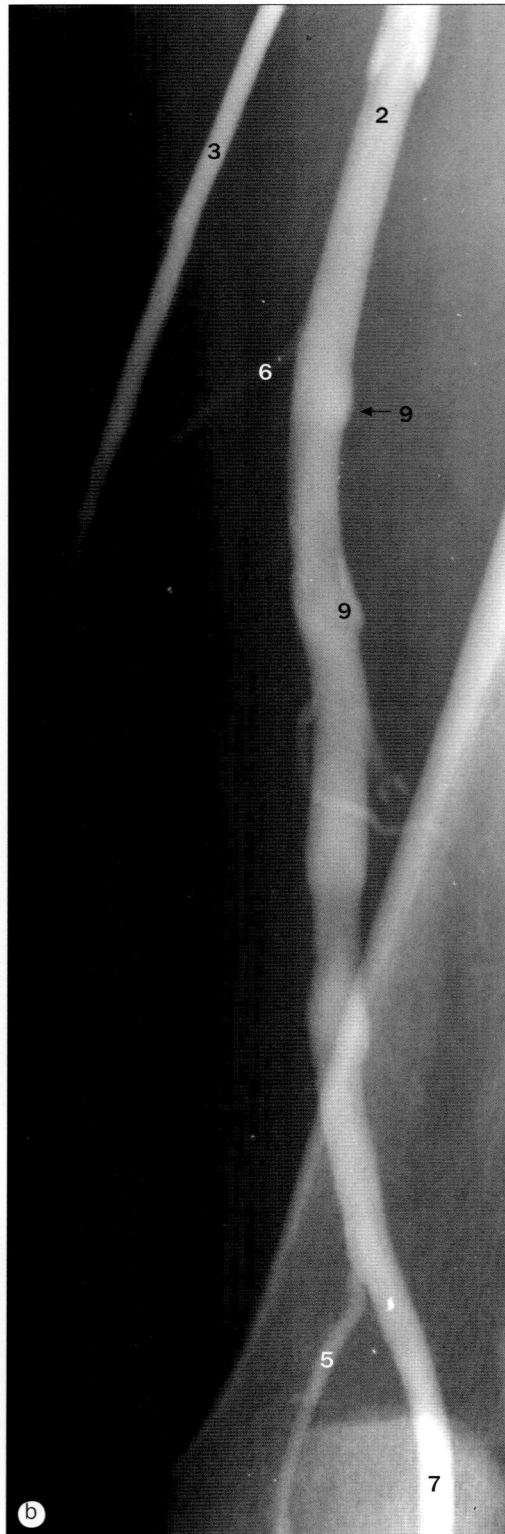

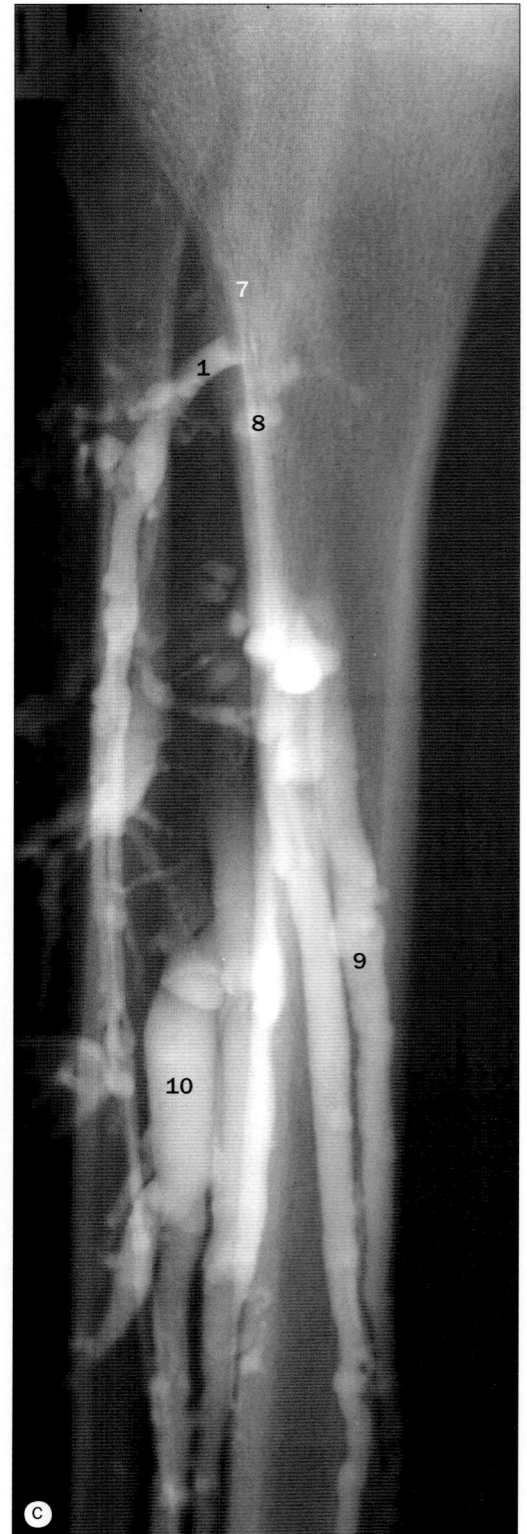

(a)–(c) Lower limb venograms.

1 Anterior tibial vein
2 Femoral vein
3 Great (long) saphenous vein
4 Lateral circumflex vein
5 Muscular tributary of femoral vein
6 Perforating vein
7 Popliteal vein
8 Posterior tibial veins
9 Venous valves
10 Venous calf plexus

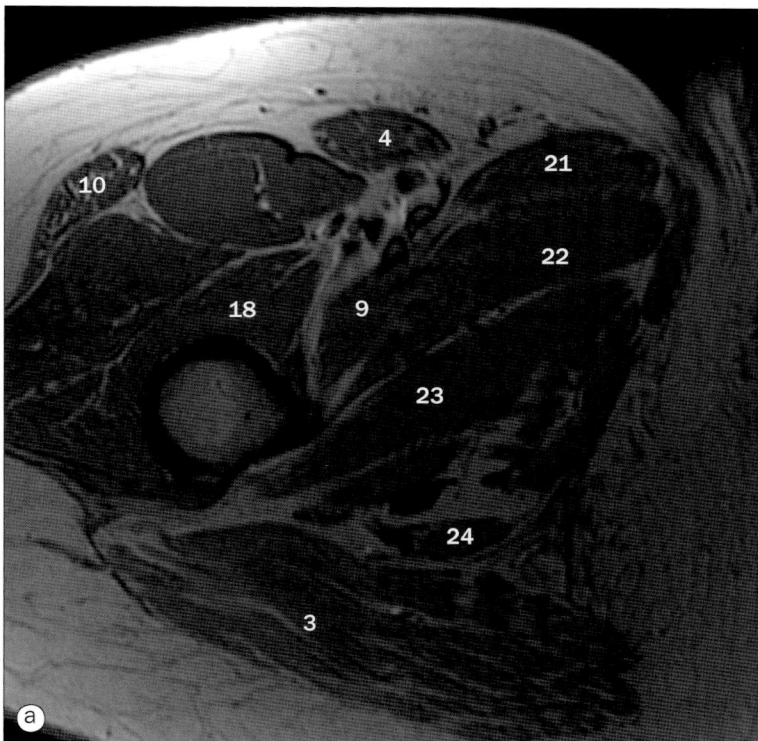

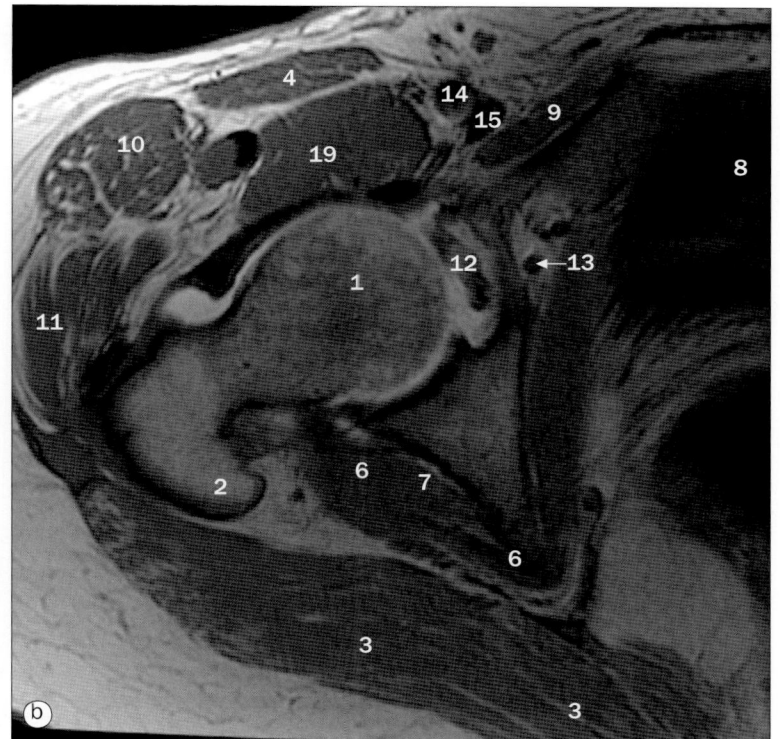

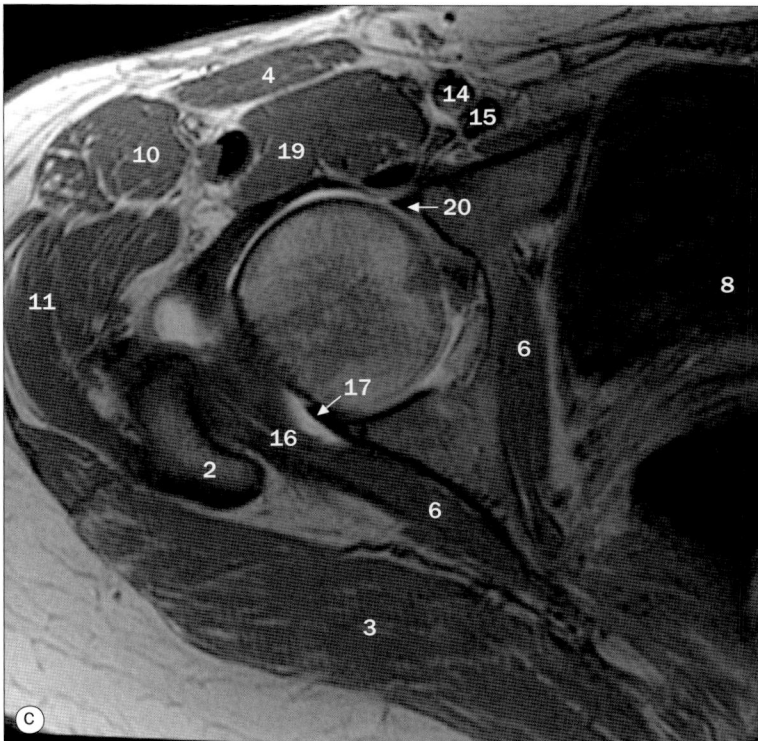

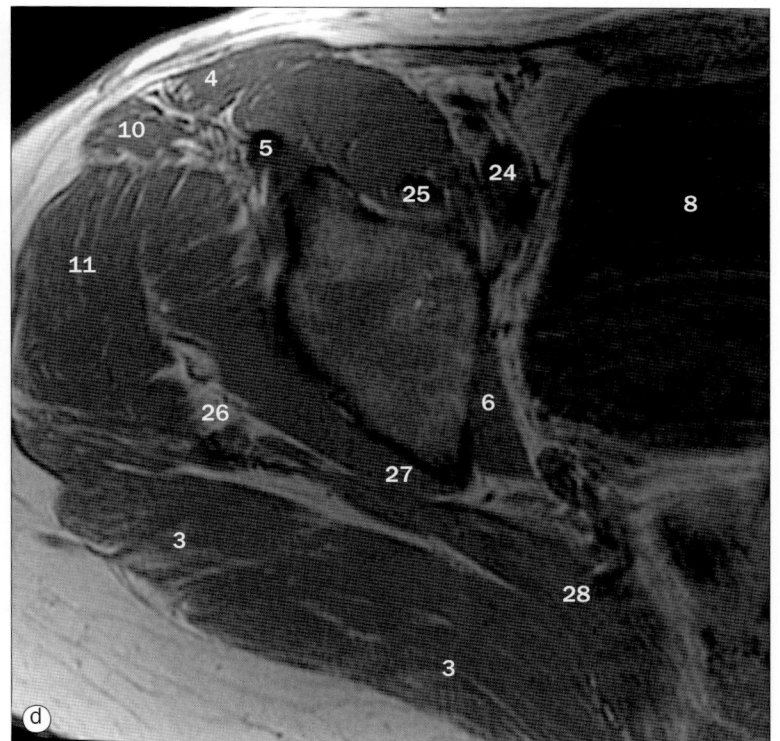

(a)–(d) Hip, axial MR images, from superior to inferior.

1 Femoral head	**8** Bladder
2 Greater trochanter	**9** Pectineus muscle
3 Gluteus maximus muscle	**10** Tensor fascia lata muscle
4 Sartorius muscle	**11** Vastus lateralis muscle
5 Tendon of rectus femoris muscle	**12** Ligamentum teres
6 Obturator internus muscle	**13** Obturator nerve
7 Superior gemellus muscle	**14** Femoral artery
	15 Femoral vein

16 Tendon of obturator internus muscle	**22** Adductor brevis muscle
17 Posterior acetabular labrum	**23** Adductor magnus muscle
18 Vastus intermedius muscle	**24** Semitendinosus muscle
19 Iliopsoas muscle	**25** Profunda femoris artery
20 Anterior acetabular labrum	**26** External iliac artery
21 Adductor longus muscle	**27** Gluteus minimus muscle
	28 Gluteus medius muscle

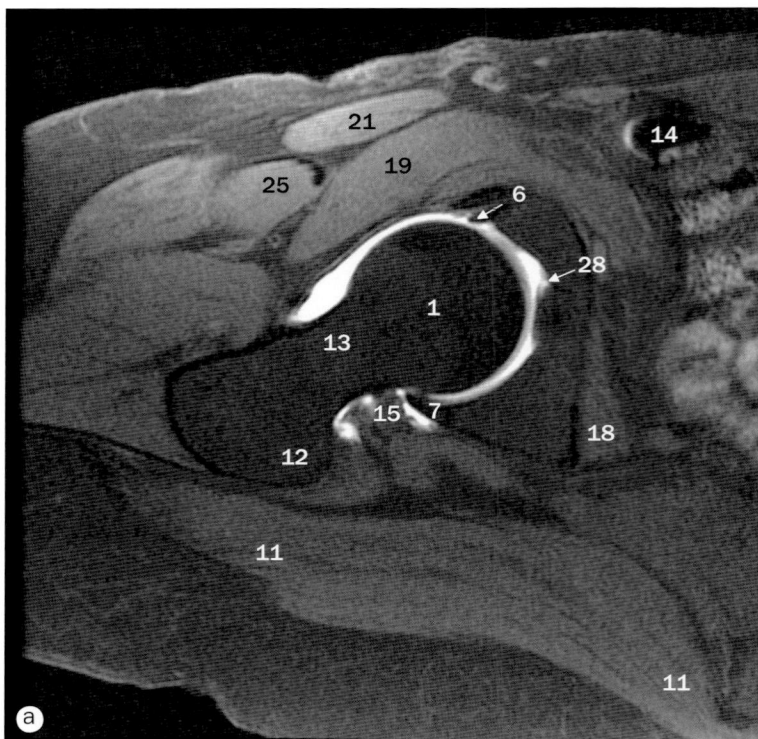

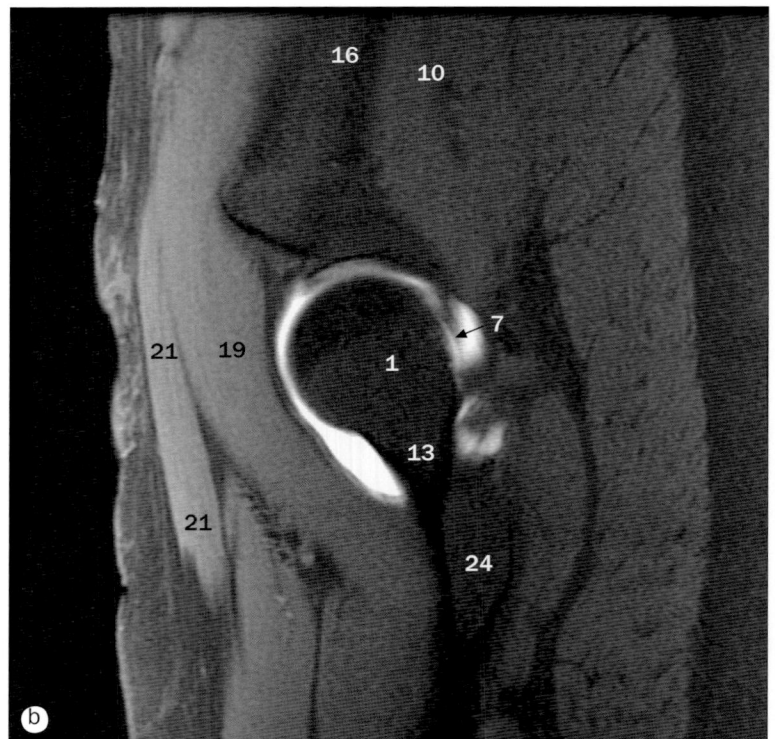

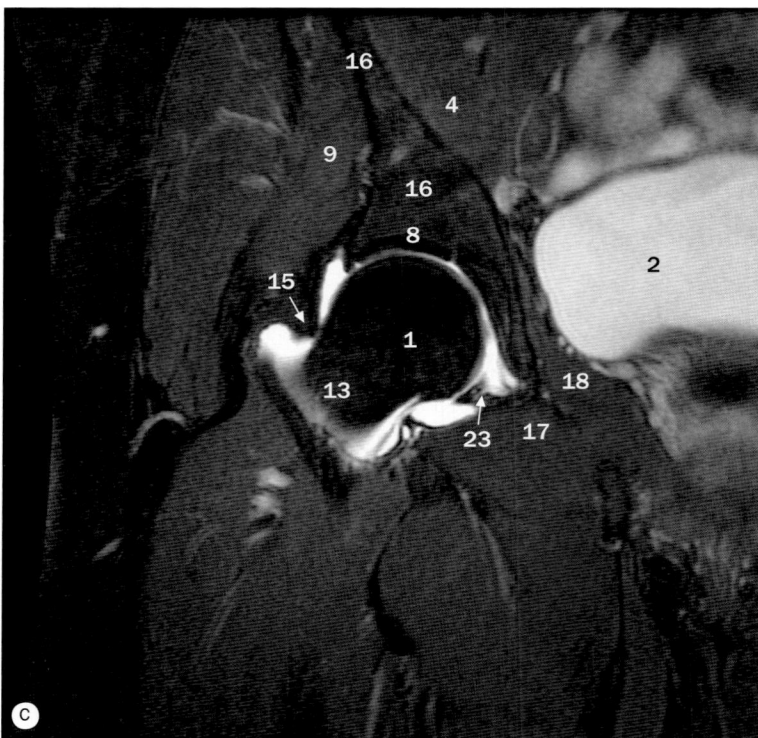

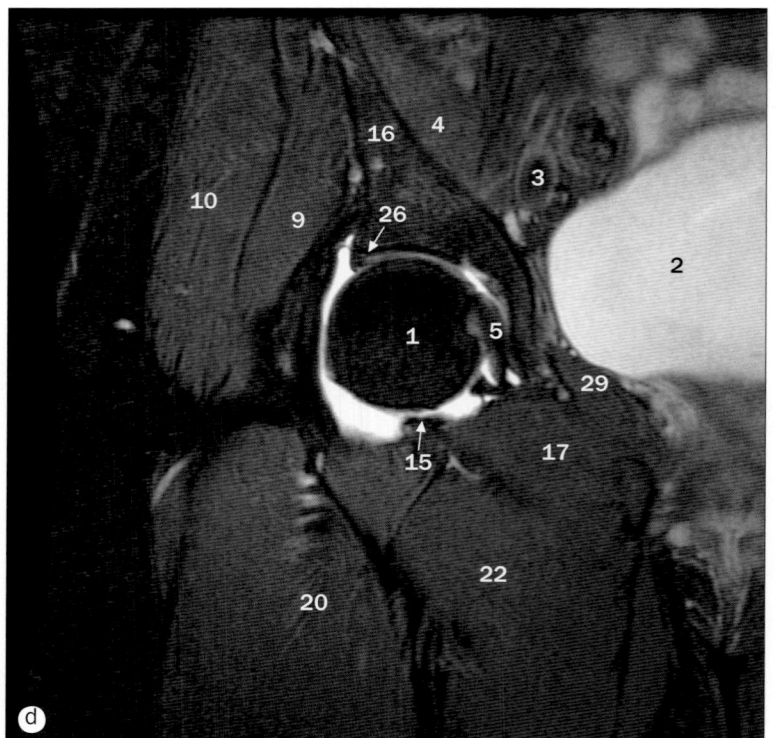

Hip, MR arthrogram images, (a) axial, (b) sagittal, (c) and (d) coronal.

1 Femoral head	11 Gluteus maximus muscle	21 Sartorius muscle
2 Bladder	12 Greater trochanter	22 Adductor longus muscle
3 External iliac artery	13 Femoral neck	23 Transverse acetabular ligament
4 Iliacus muscle	14 Femoral artery	24 Quadratus femoris muscle
5 Ligamentum teres	15 Zona orbicularis (circular fibrous capsule)	25 Rectus femoris muscle
6 Anterior acetabular labrum	16 Iliac bone	26 Superior acetabular labrum
7 Posterior acetabular labrum	17 Obturator externus muscle	27 Gemellus muscle
8 Acetabular roof	18 Obturator internus muscle	28 Acetabular notch (pulvinar)
9 Gluteus minimus muscle	19 Iliopsoas muscle	29 Pectineus muscle
10 Gluteus medius muscle	20 Vastus intermedius	

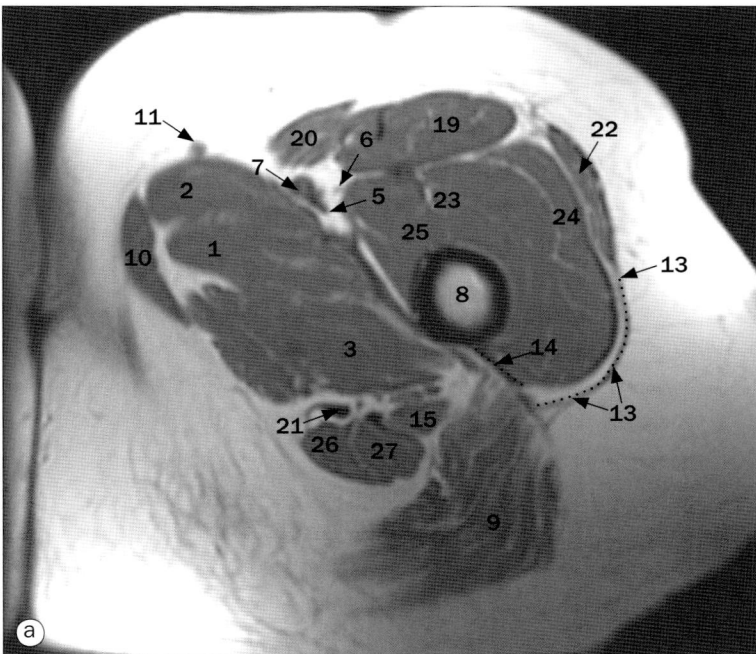

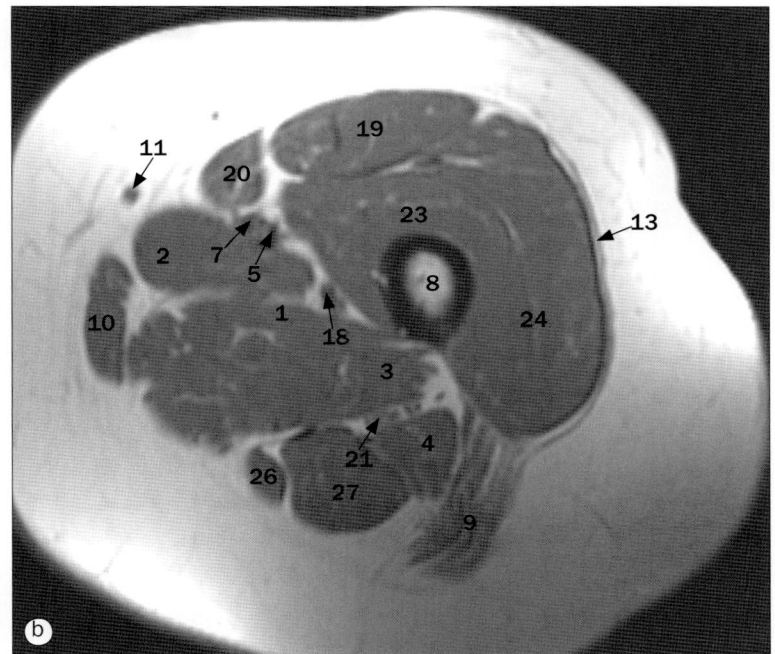

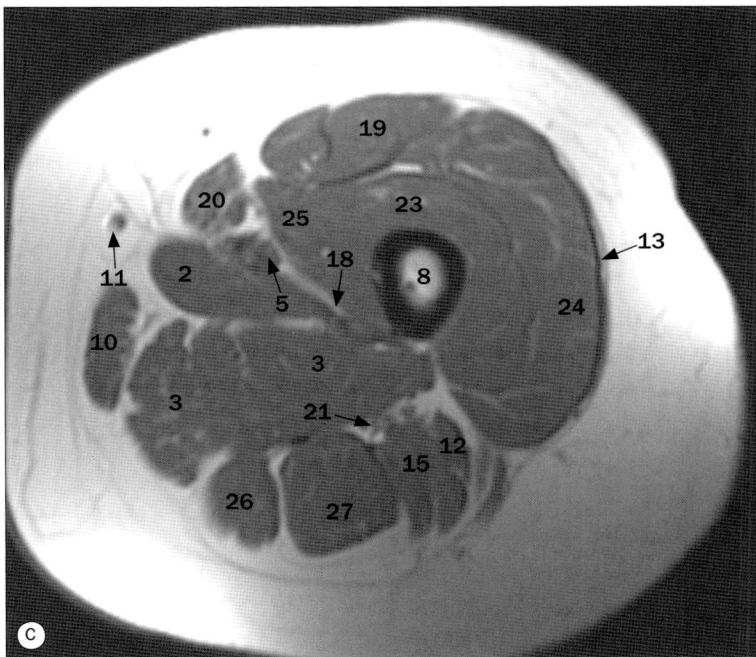

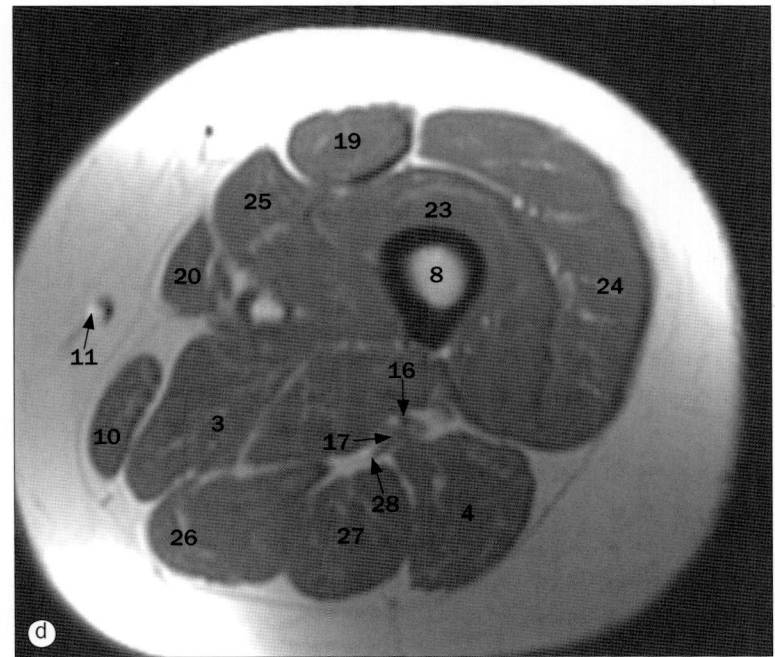

(a)–(d) Axial MR images of the thigh.

1	Adductor brevis muscle	11	Great (long) saphenous vein	21	Sciatic nerve
2	Adductor longus muscle	12	Short head of biceps femoris muscle	22	Tensor fasciae latae muscle
3	Adductor magnus muscle	13	Iliotibial tract	23	Vastus intermedius muscle
4	Biceps femoris muscle	14	Lateral intermuscular septum	24	Vastus lateralis muscle
5	Femoral artery	15	Long head of biceps femoris muscle	25	Vastus medialis muscle
6	Femoral nerve	16	Popliteal artery	26	Semimembranosus muscle
7	Femoral vein	17	Popliteal vein	27	Semitendinosus muscle
8	Femur	18	Profunda femoris artery	28	Tibial nerve
9	Gluteus maximus muscle	19	Rectus femoris muscle		
10	Gracilis muscle	20	Sartorius muscle		

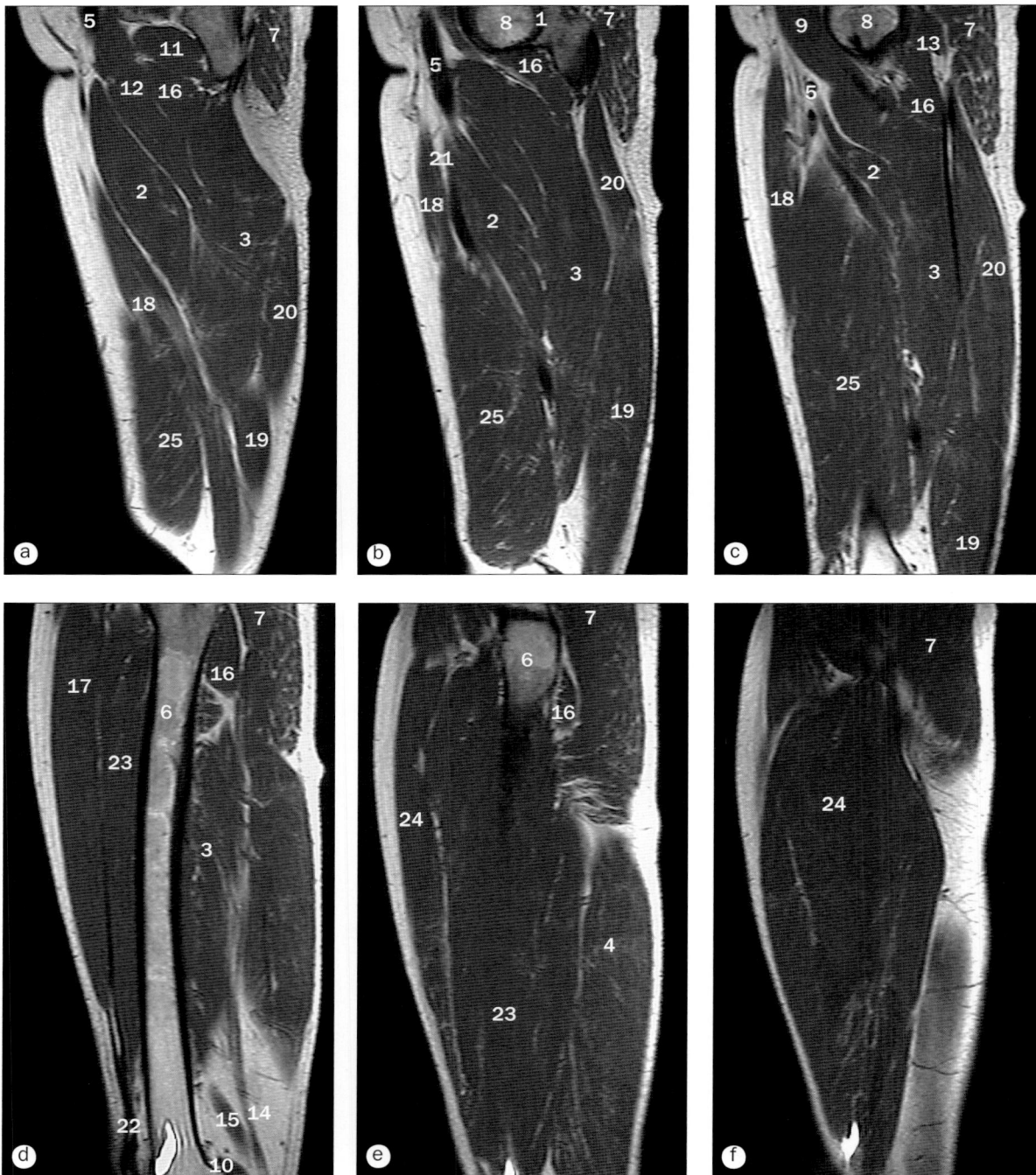

(a)–(f) Thigh, sagittal MR images.

1 Acetabulum	10 Lateral head of gastrocnemius muscle	18 Sartorius muscle
2 Adductor longus muscle	11 Obturator externus muscle	19 Semimembranosus muscle
3 Adductor magnus muscle	12 Pectineus muscle	20 Semitendinosus muscle
4 Biceps femoris muscle	13 Piriformis muscle	21 Subsartorial canal (Hunter's canal)
5 Femoral artery	14 Popliteal artery	22 Tendon of quadriceps muscle
6 Femur	15 Popliteal vein	23 Vastus intermedius muscle
7 Gluteus maximus muscle	16 Quadratus femoris muscle	24 Vastus lateralis muscle
8 Head of femur	17 Rectus femoris muscle	25 Vastus medialis muscle
9 Iliopsoas muscle		

(a)–(f) Thigh, coronal MR images.

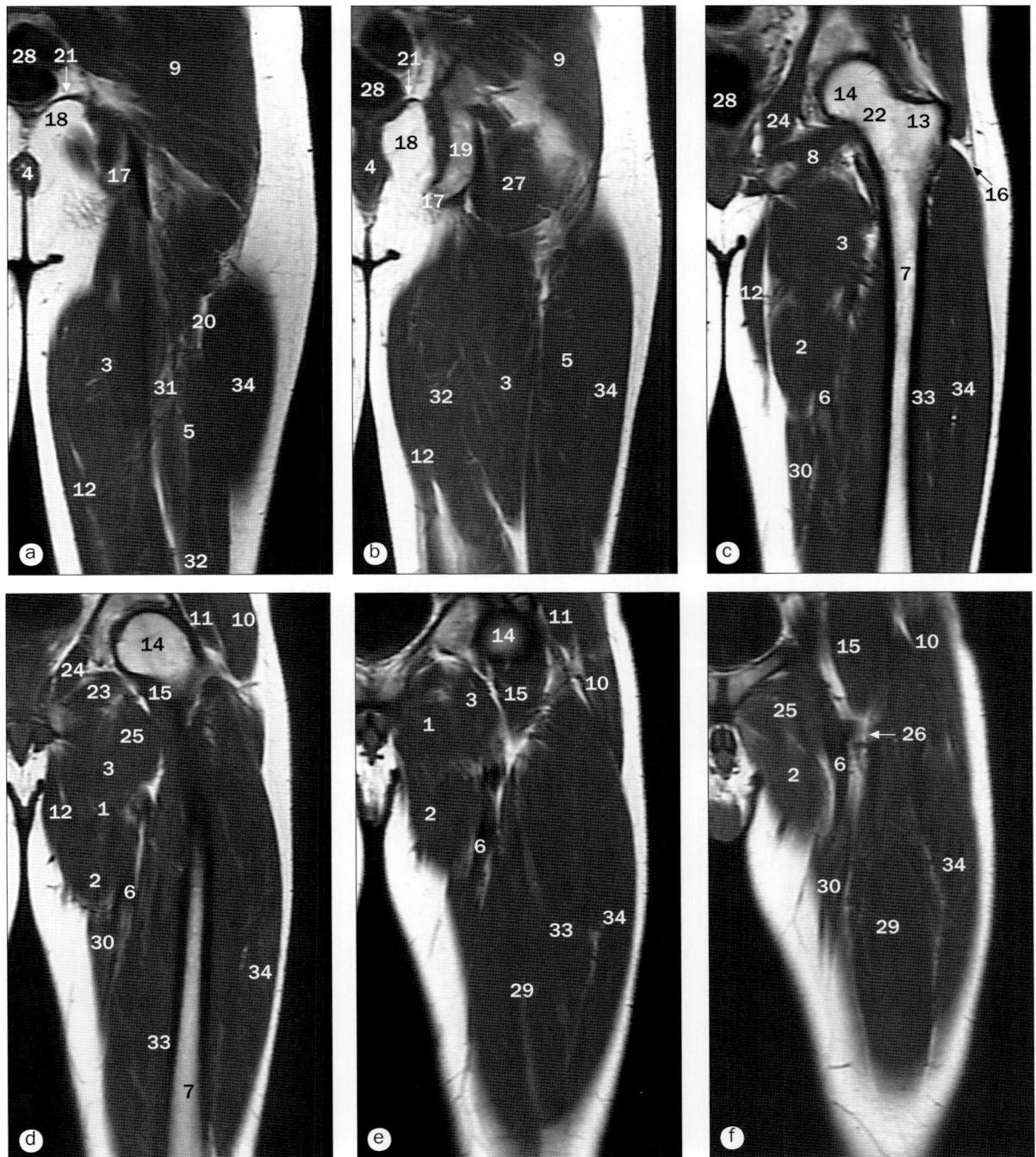

1 Adductor brevis muscle
2 Adductor longus muscle
3 Adductor magnus muscle
4 Anal canal
5 Biceps femoris muscle
6 Femoral artery
7 Femur
8 Gemellus muscle
9 Gluteus maximus muscle
10 Gluteus medius muscle
11 Gluteus minimus muscle
12 Gracilis muscle
13 Greater trochanter of femur
14 Head of femur
15 Iliopsoas muscle
16 Iliotibial tract
17 Ischial tuberosity
18 Ischio-anal fossa
19 Ischium
20 Lateral intermuscular septum
21 Levator ani muscle
22 Neck of femur
23 Obturator externus muscle
24 Obturator internus muscle
25 Pectineus muscle
26 Profunda femoris artery
27 Quadratus femoris muscle
28 Rectum
29 Rectus femoris muscle
30 Sartorius muscle
31 Semimembranosus muscle
32 Semitendinosus muscle
33 Vastus intermedius muscle
34 Vastus lateralis muscle

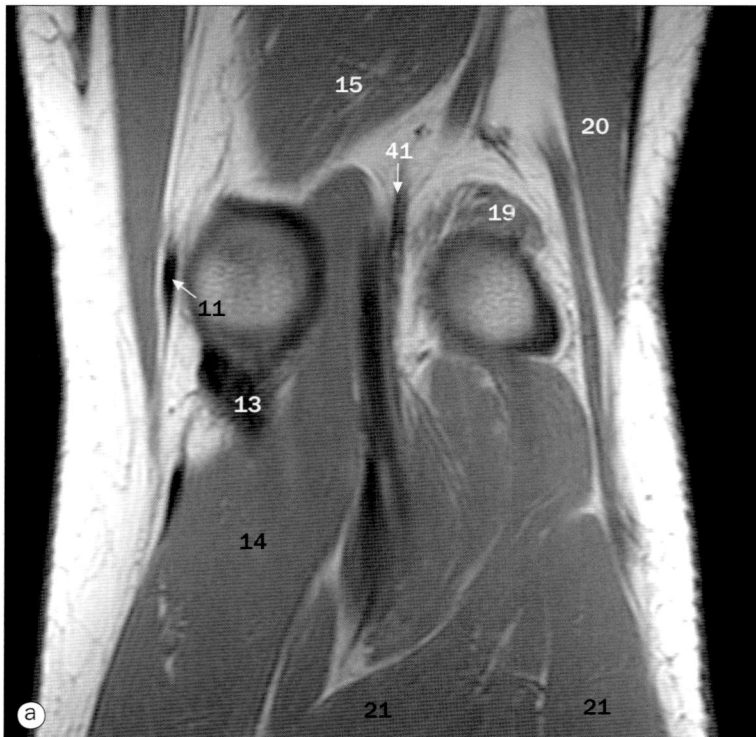

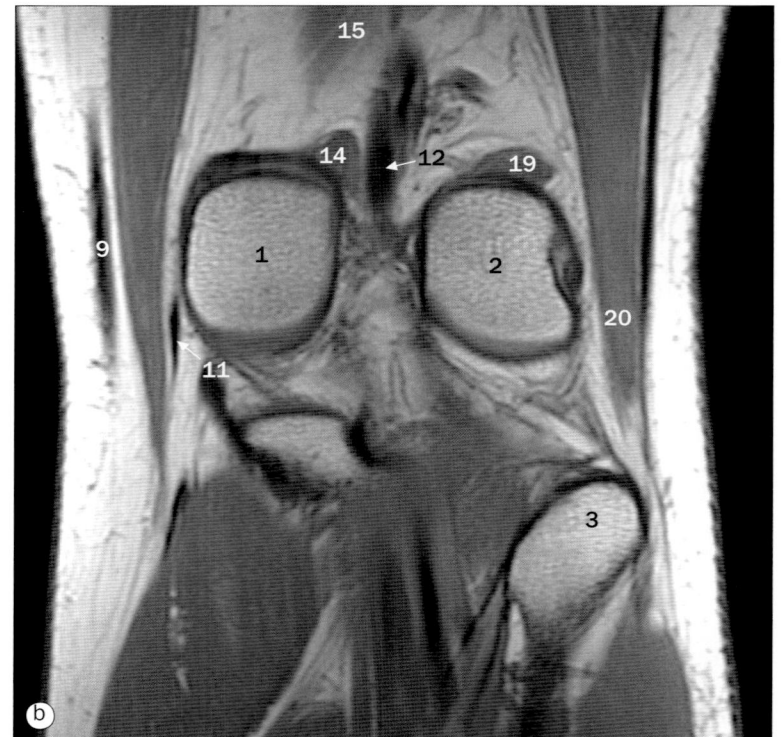

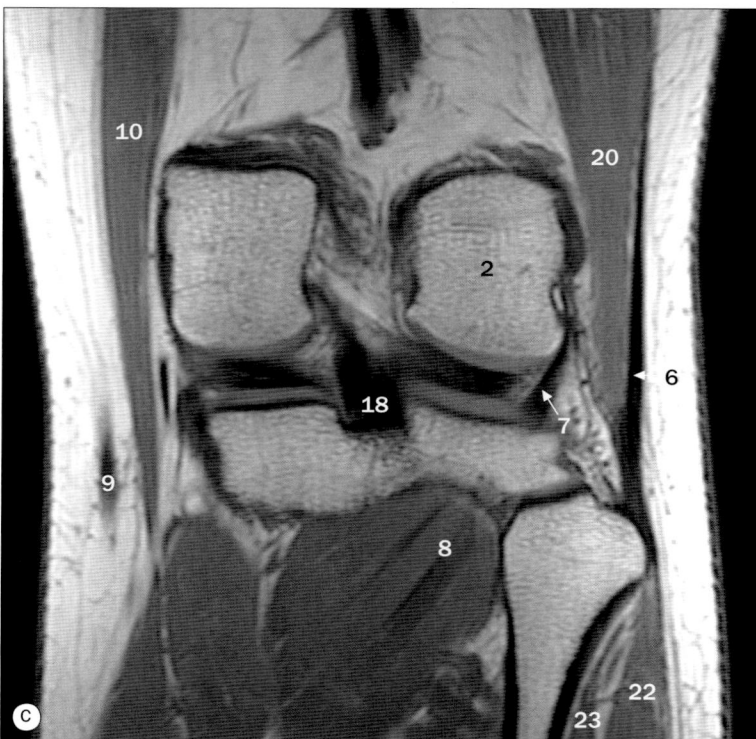

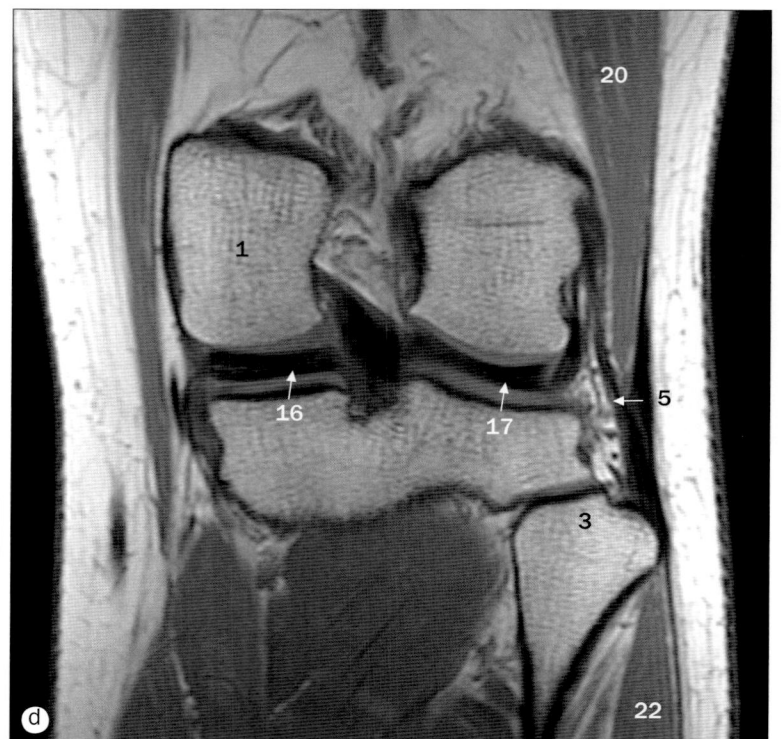

(a)–(h) Knee, coronal MR images, from posterior to anterior.

1 Medial femoral condyle	9 Great (long) saphenous vein	17 Posterior horn lateral meniscus
2 Lateral femoral condyle	10 Sartorius muscle	18 Posterior cruciate ligament
3 Head of fibula	11 Tendon of gracilis muscle	19 Lateral head of gastrocnemius
4 Proximal tibiofibular joint	12 Popliteal artery	20 Biceps femoris muscle
5 Lateral collateral ligament	13 Common peroneal (fibular) nerve	21 Soleus muscle
6 Iliotibial tract	14 Medial head of gastrocnemius muscle	22 Peroneus (fibularis) longus muscle
7 Tendon of popliteus muscle	15 Semimembranosus muscle	23 Extensor digitorum longus muscle
8 Popliteus muscle	16 Posterior horn medial meniscus	24 Anterior cruciate ligament

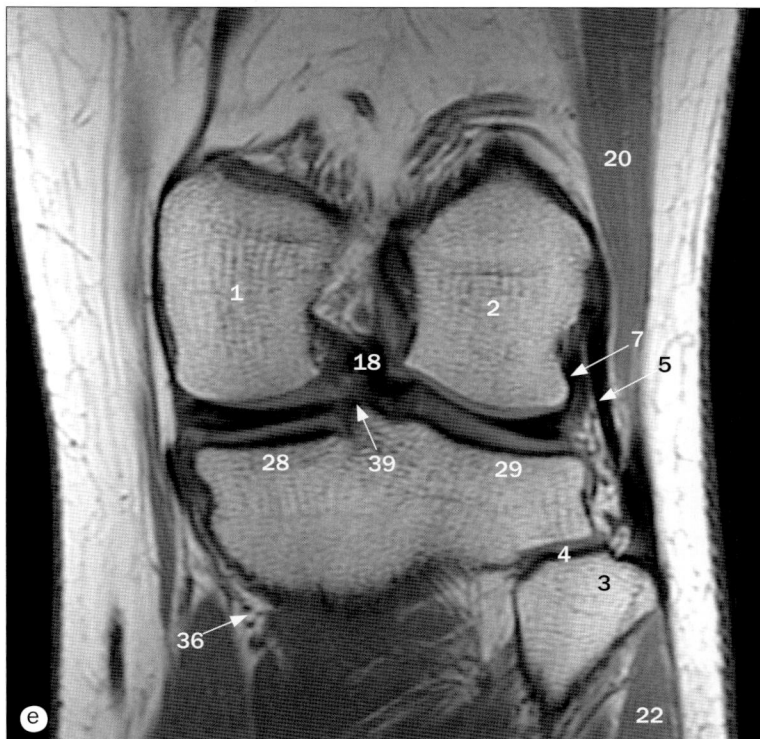

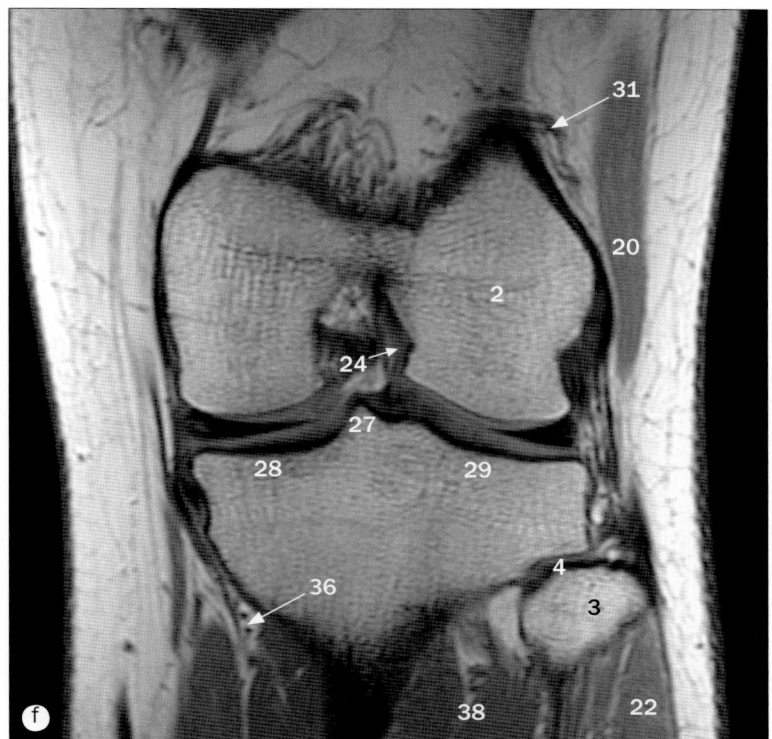

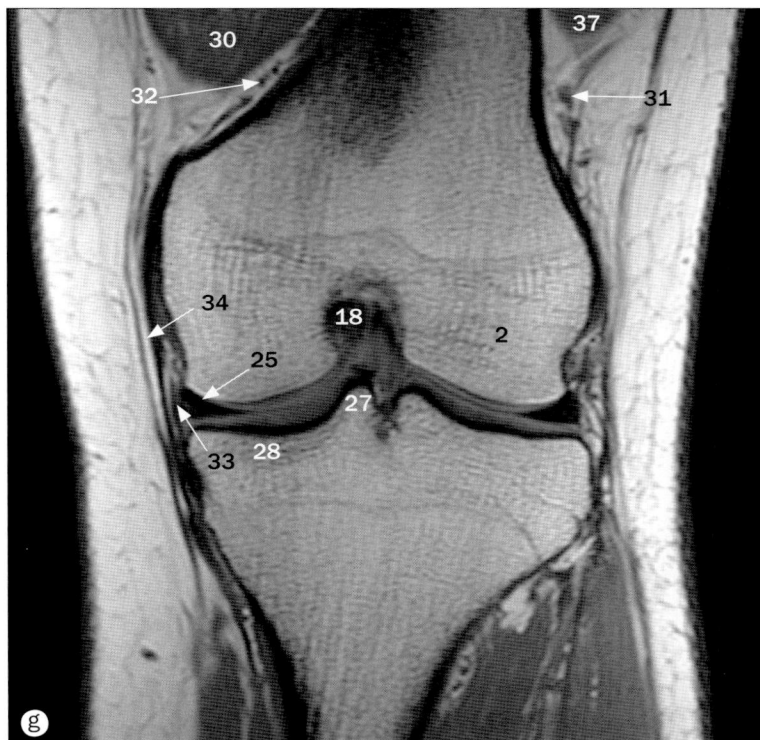

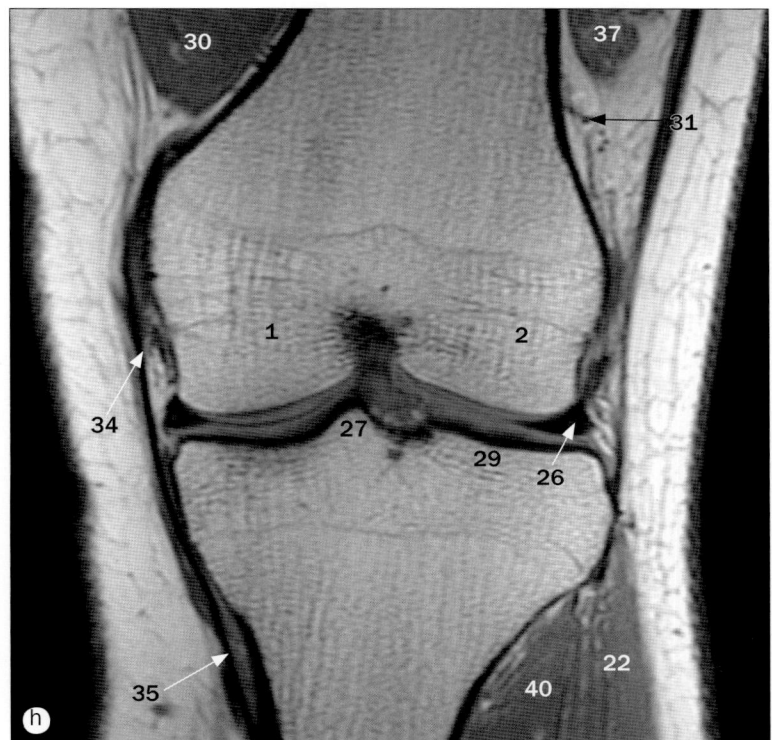

(a)–(h) Knee, coronal MR images, from posterior to anterior.

25 Body of medial meniscus
26 Body of lateral meniscus
27 Tibial spine
28 Medial tibial condyle
29 Lateral tibial condyle
30 Vastus medialis muscle

31 Lateral superior genicular artery
32 Medial superior genicular artery
33 Medial collateral ligament deep portion
34 Medial collateral ligament superficial portion
35 Pes anserinus (muscle attachments)

36 Medial inferior genicular artery
37 Vastus lateralis muscle
38 Tibialis posterior muscle
39 Root of posterior horn, medial meniscus
40 Tibialis anterior muscle
41 Tibial nerve

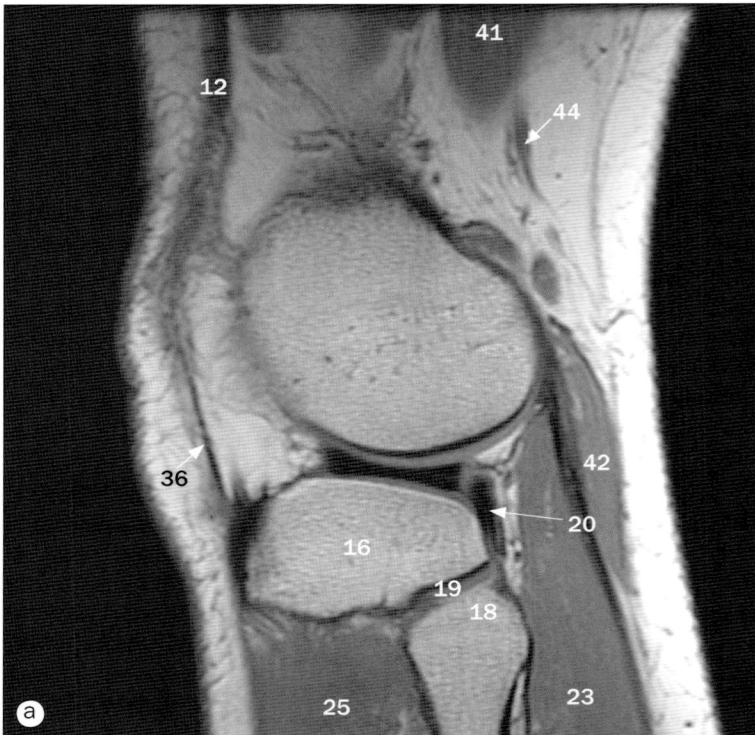

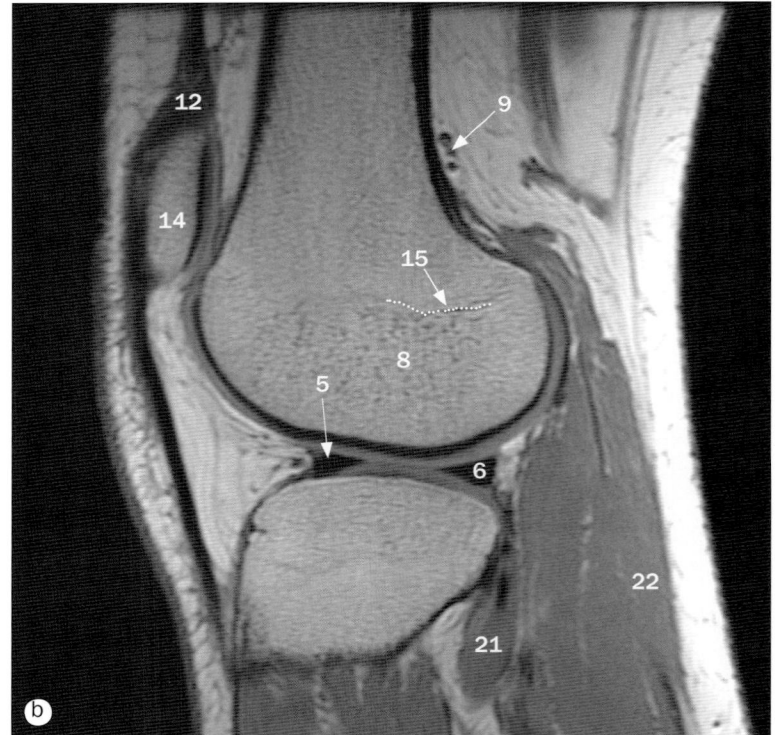

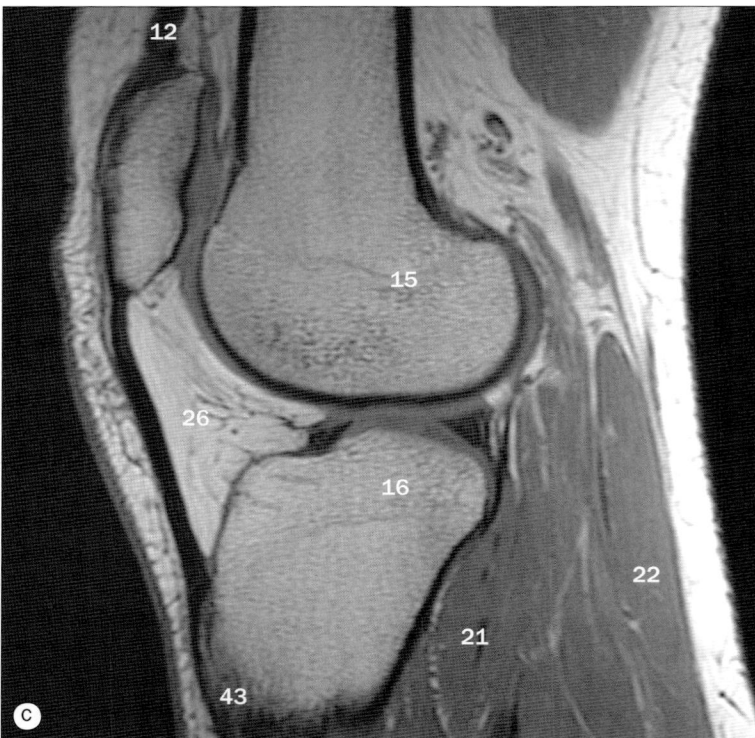

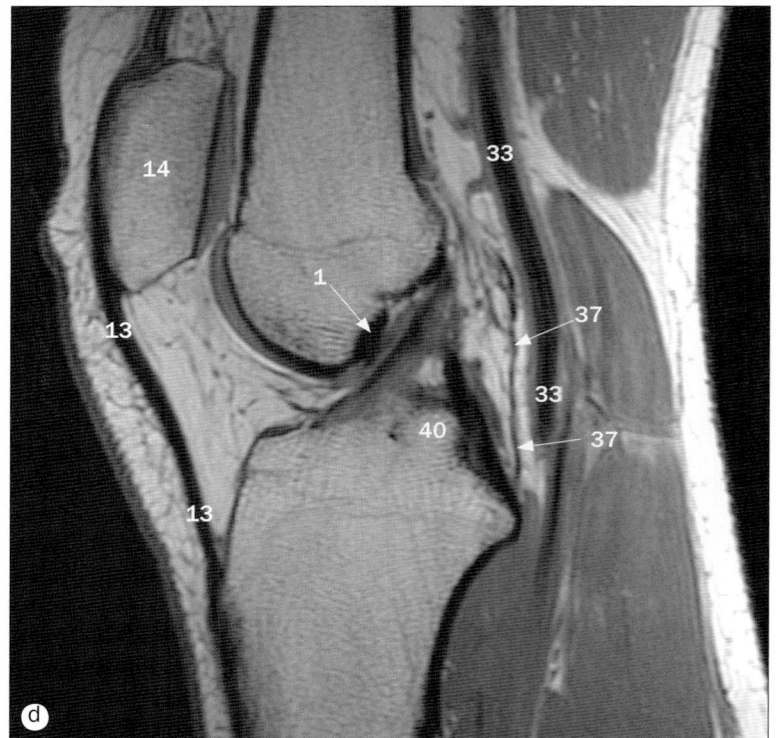

(a)–(h) Knee, sagittal MR images, from lateral to medial.

1 Anterior cruciate ligament	9 Lateral superior genicular artery and veins	17 Medial tibial plateau
2 Posterior cruciate ligament	10 Median intermuscular septum	18 Fibular head
3 Anterior horn medial meniscus	11 Medial superior genicular artery	19 Proximal tibiofibular joint
4 Posterior horn medial meniscus	12 Quadriceps tendon	20 Popliteus tendon
5 Anterior horn lateral meniscus	13 Patellar tendon	21 Popliteus muscle belly
6 Posterior horn lateral meniscus	14 Patella	22 Lateral head of gastrocnemius muscle
7 Medial condyle of femur	15 Epiphyseal line/scar	23 Soleus muscle
8 Lateral condyle of femur	16 Lateral tibial plateau	24 Vastus medialis muscle

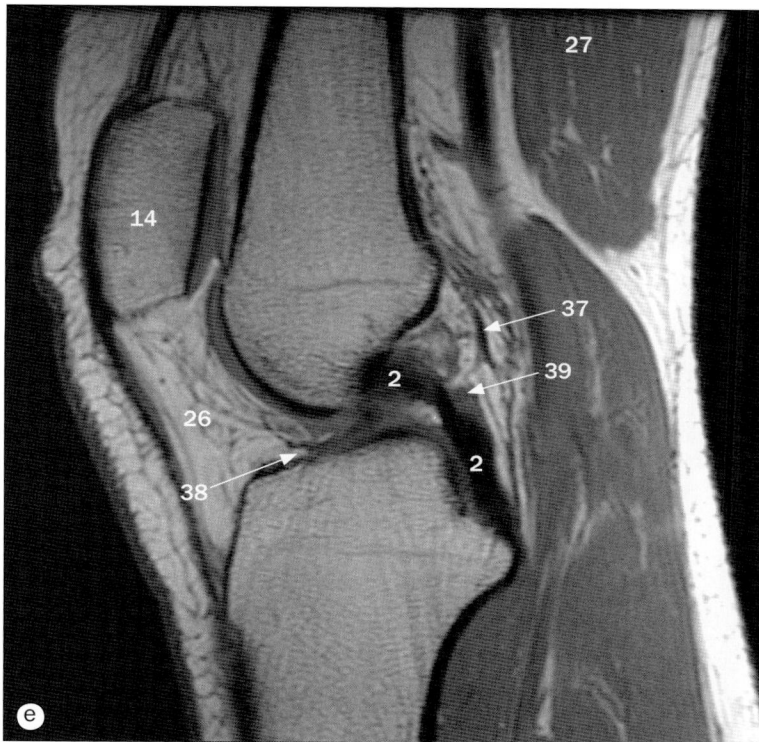

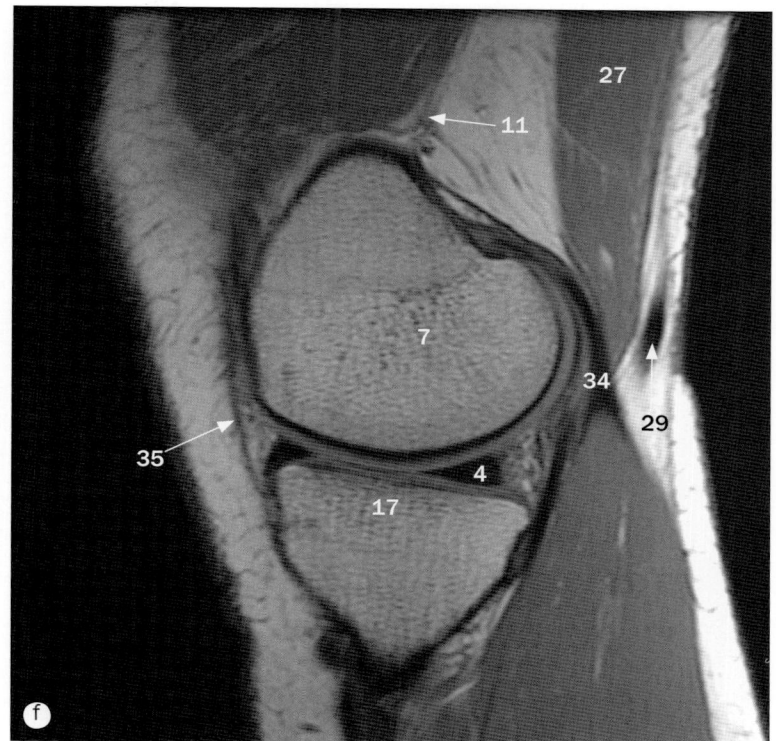

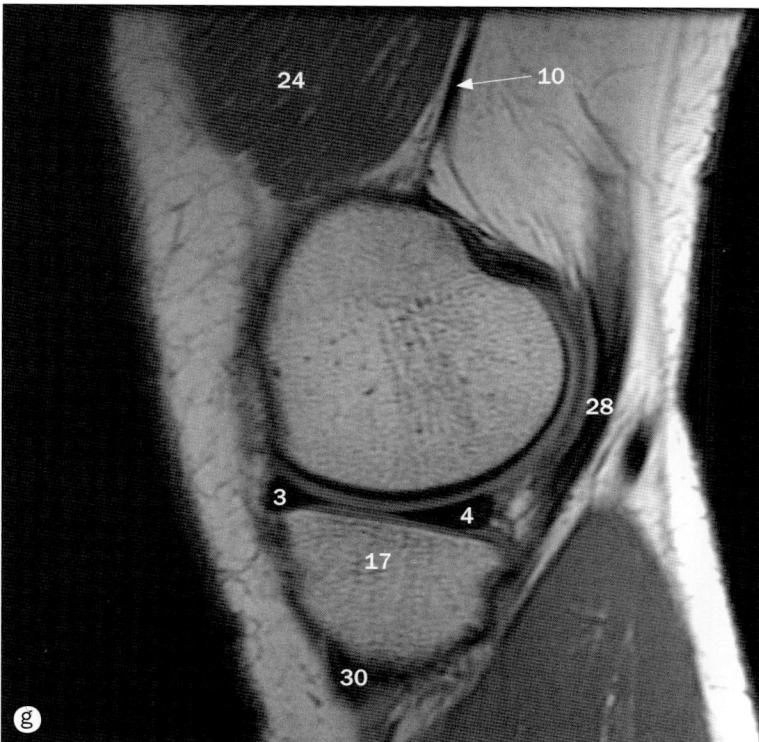

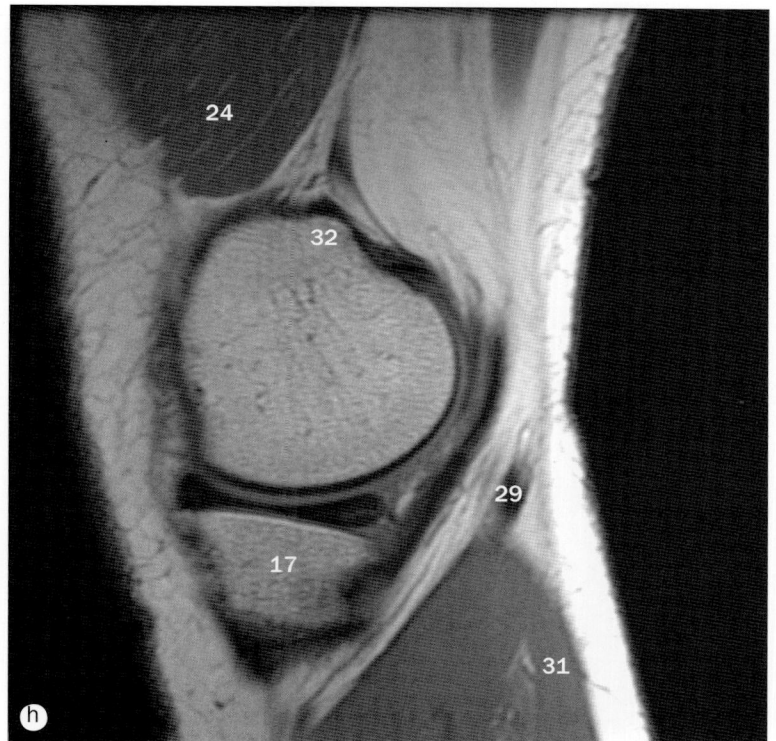

(a)–(h) Knee, sagittal MR images, from lateral to medial.

25 Tibialis anterior muscle	32 Adductor tubercle	39 Meniscofemoral ligament (Wrisberg)
26 Infrapatellar fat pad	33 Popliteal artery	40 Tibial spine
27 Semimembranosus muscle	34 Medial head of gastrocnemius tendon	41 Biceps femoris muscle
28 Semimembranosus tendon	35 Medial patellar retinaculum	42 Plantaris muscle
29 Semitendinosus tendon	36 Lateral patellar retinaculum	43 Tibial tuberosity
30 Sartorius tendon	37 Posterior joint capsule	44 Common peroneal (fibular) nerve
31 Medial head of gastrocnemius muscle	38 Transverse ligament	

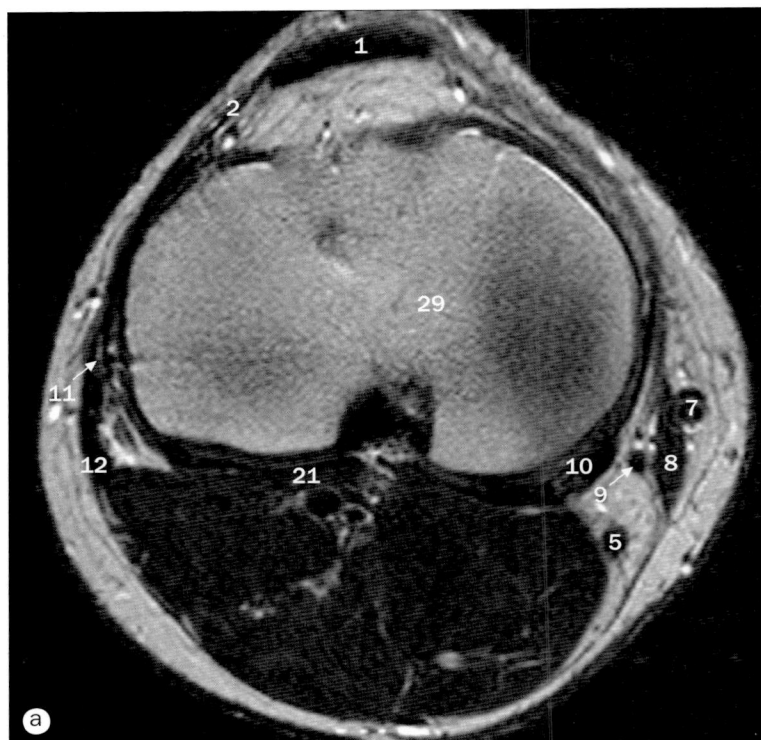

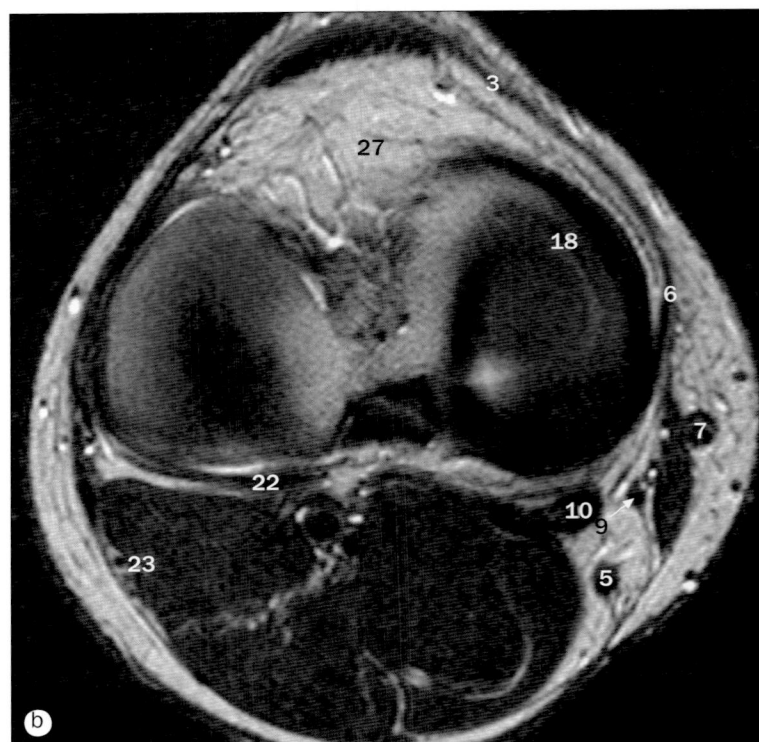

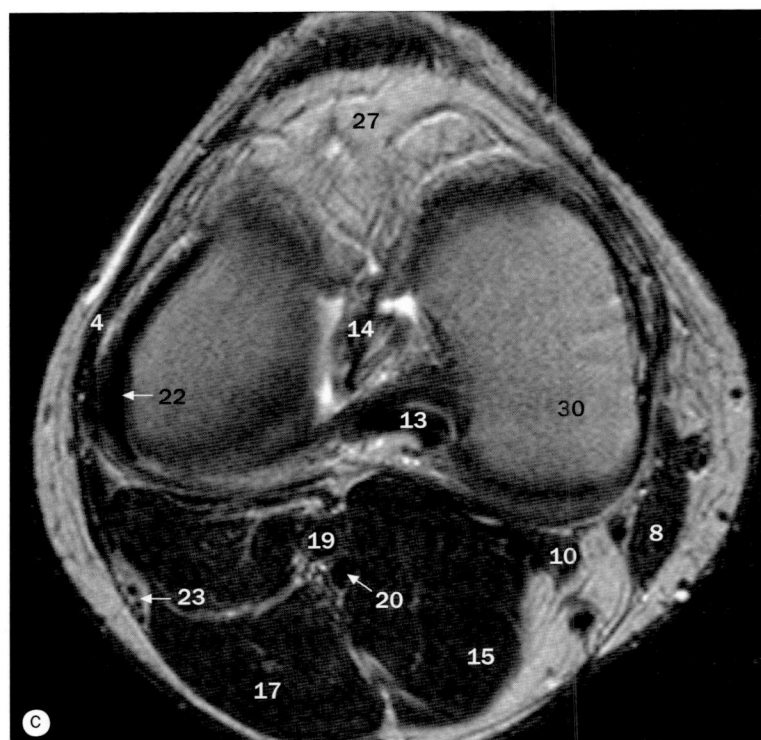

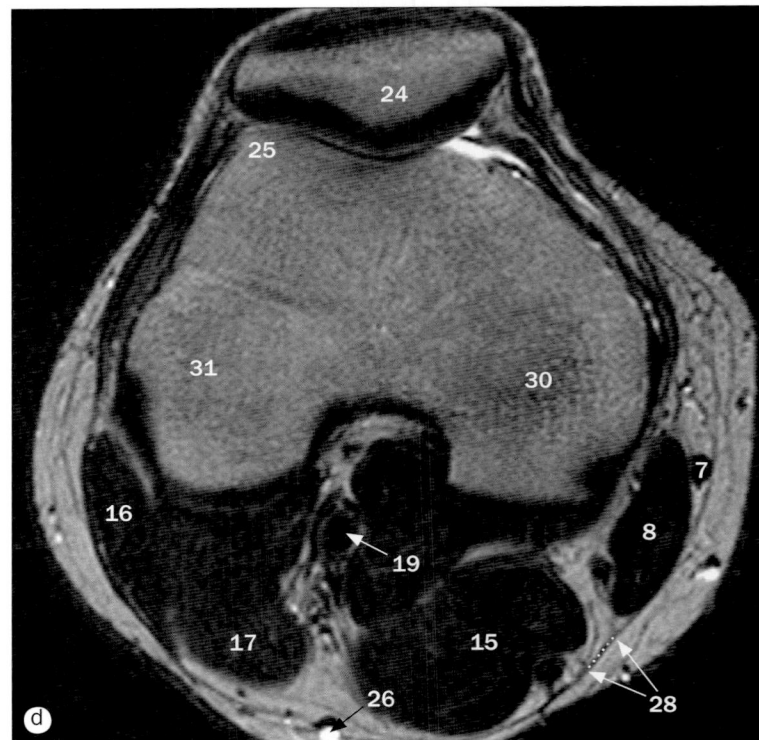

(a)–(d) Knee, axial MR images, from inferior to superior.

1 Patellar tendon	12 Biceps femoris tendon	21 Popliteus muscle
2 Lateral patellar retinaculum	13 Posterior cruciate ligament	22 Popliteus tendon
3 Medial patellar retinaculum	14 Anterior cruciate ligament	23 Common peroneal (fibular) nerve
4 Iliotibial tract	15 Medial head gastrocnemius muscle	24 Patella
5 Semitendinosus tendon		25 Lateral condylar eminence
6 Medial collateral ligament	16 Biceps femoris muscle	26 Short (lesser) saphenous vein
7 Long (great) saphenous vein	17 Lateral head gastrocnemius muscle	27 Infrapatellar fat pad
8 Sartorius muscle		28 Deep fascia (fascia lata)
9 Gracilis tendon	18 Medial meniscus	29 Tibial plateau
10 Semimembranosus tendon	19 Popliteal artery	30 Medial condyle of femur
11 Lateral collateral ligament	20 Popliteal vein	31 Lateral condyle of femur

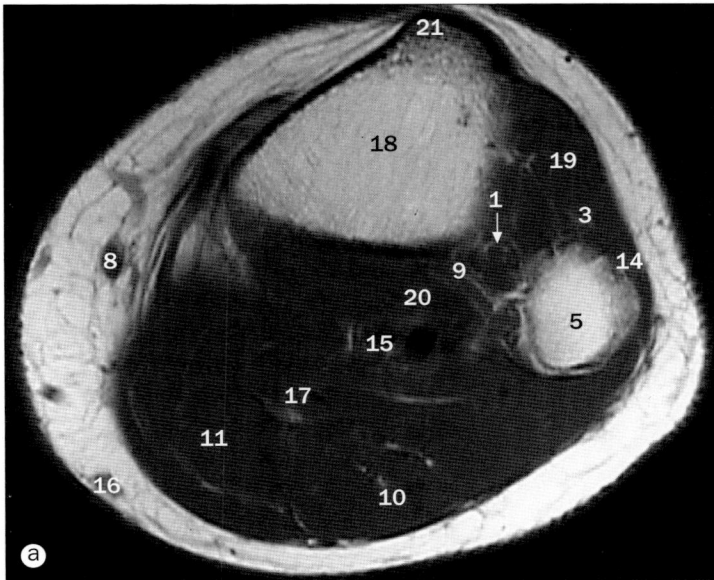

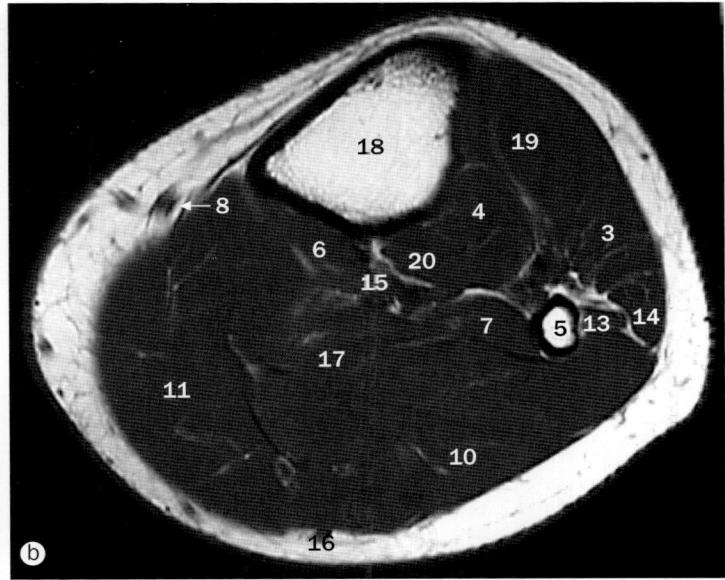

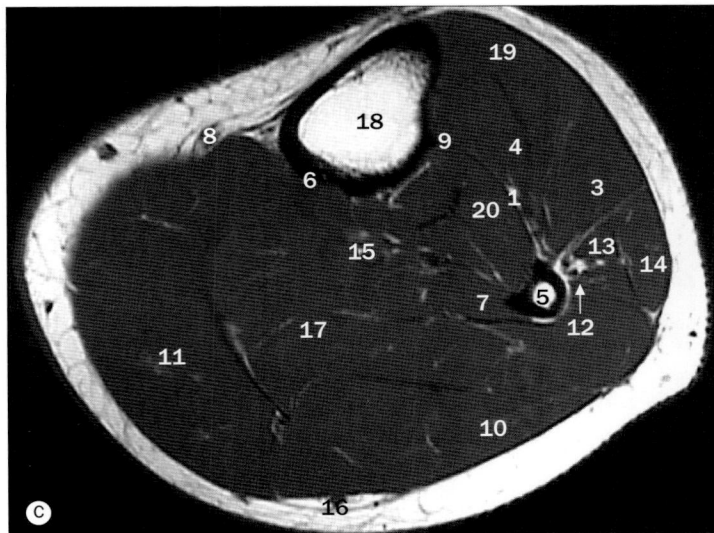

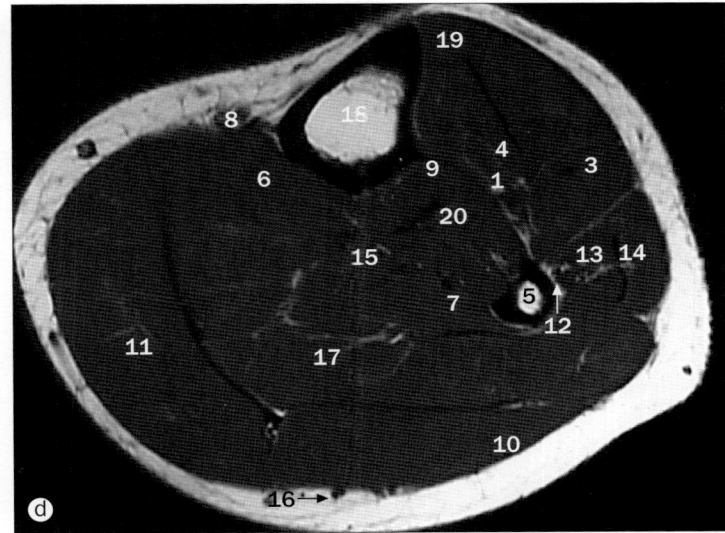

(a)–(e) Calf, axial MR images.

1 Anterior tibial artery
2 Aponeurosis of gastrocnemius muscle
3 Extensor digitorum longus muscle
4 Extensor hallucis longus muscle
5 Fibula
6 Flexor digitorum longus muscle
7 Flexor hallucis longus muscle
8 Great (long) saphenous vein
9 Interosseous membrane
10 Lateral head of gastrocnemius muscle
11 Medial head of gastrocnemius muscle
12 Peroneal artery
13 Peroneus brevis muscle
14 Peroneus longus muscle
15 Posterior tibial artery
16 Small saphenous vein
17 Soleus muscle
18 Tibia
19 Tibialis anterior muscle
20 Tibialis posterior muscle
21 Tuberosity of tibia

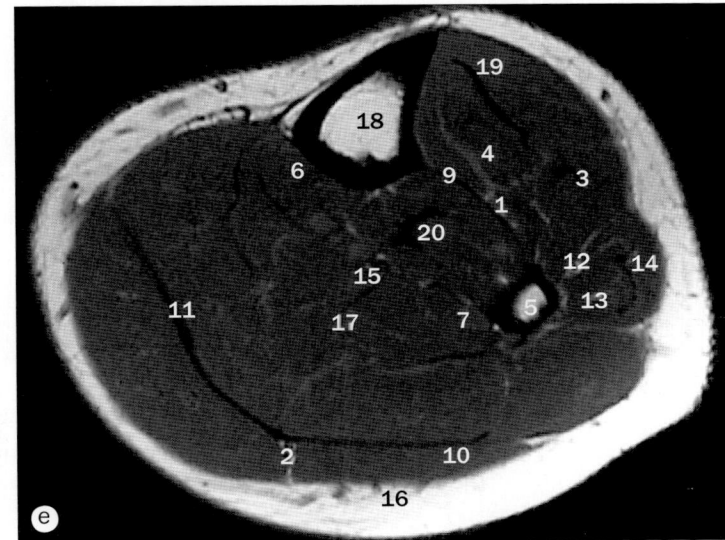

(a)–(h) Axial MR images of the ankle, from superior to inferior.

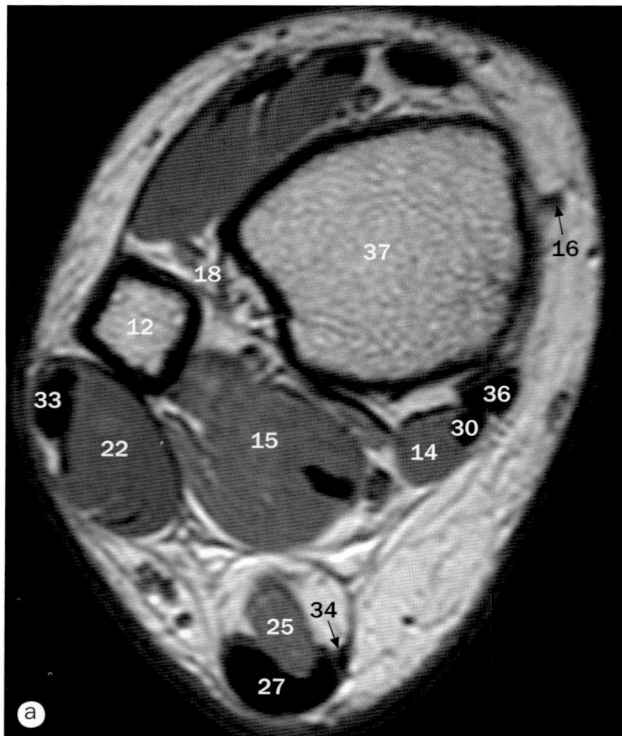

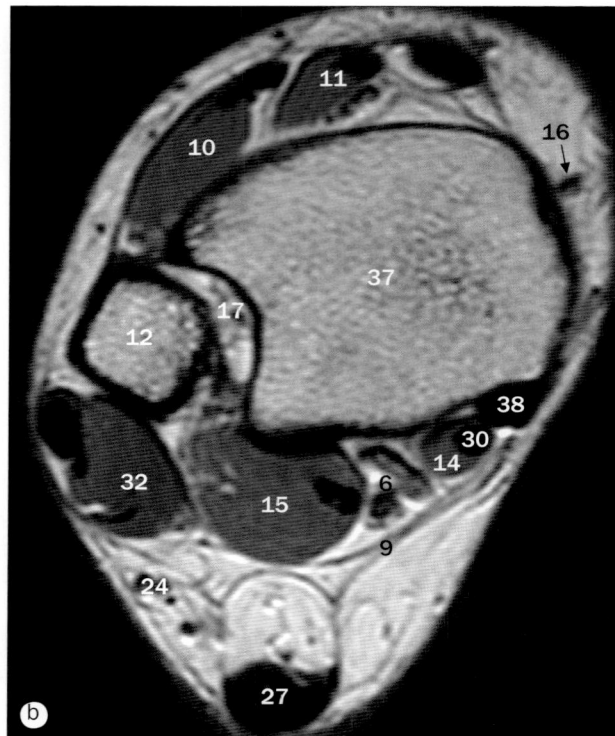

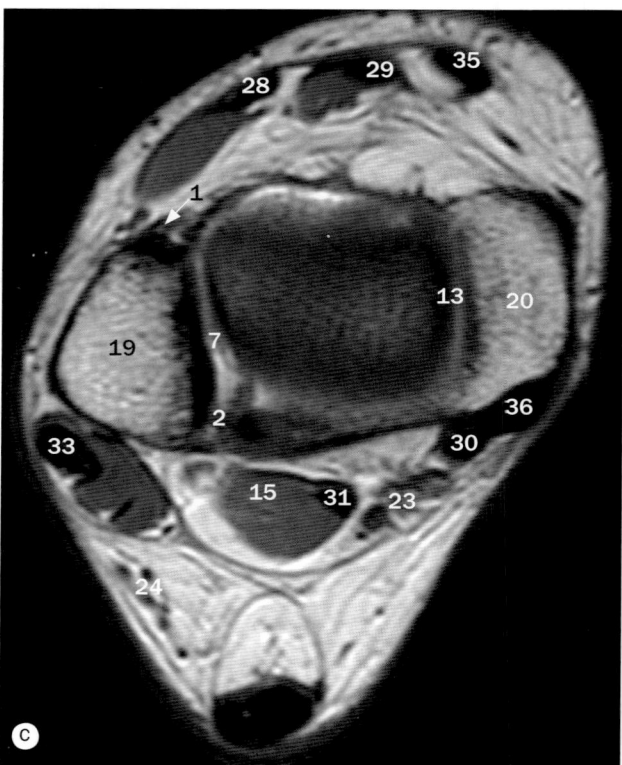

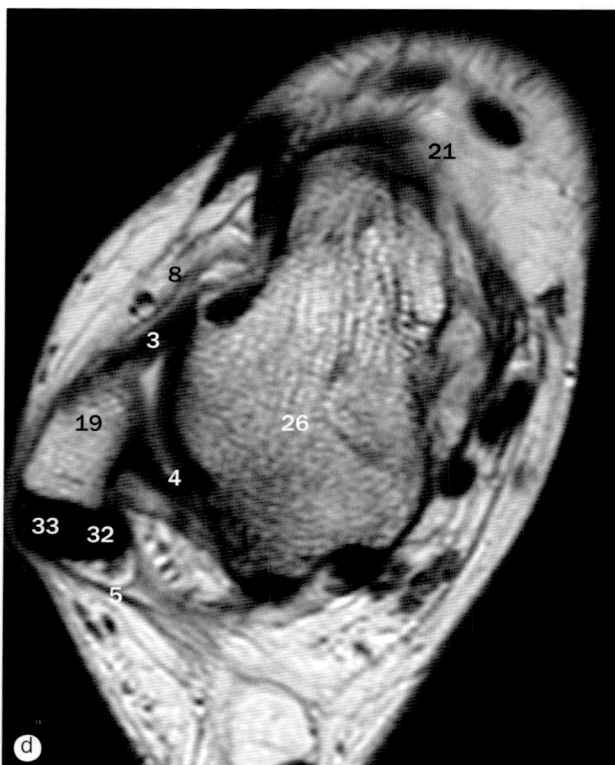

1 Anterior inferior tibiofibular ligament
2 Posterior inferior tibiofibular ligament
3 Anterior talofibular ligament
4 Posterior talofibular ligament
5 Peroneal (fibular) retinaculum
6 Neurovascular bundle
7 Talofibular joint
8 Extensor retinaculum
9 Flexor retinaculum
10 Extensor digitorum muscle
11 Extensor hallucis longus muscle
12 Fibula
13 Talotibial joint
14 Flexor digitorum longus muscle
15 Flexor hallucis longus muscle
16 Great (long) saphenous vein
17 Inferior tibiofibular joint
18 Interosseous membrane
19 Lateral malleolus
20 Medial malleolus
21 Navicular
22 Peroneus (fibularis) brevis muscle
23 Posterior tibial artery and vein
24 Small saphenous vein
25 Soleus muscle
26 Talus
27 Tendo calcaneus (Achilles' tendon)

28 Tendon of extensor digitorum muscle
29 Tendon of extensor hallucis longus muscle
30 Tendon of flexor digitorum longus muscle
31 Tendon of flexor hallucis longus muscle
32 Tendon of peroneus (fibularis) brevis muscle
33 Tendon of peroneus (fibularis) longus muscle
34 Tendon of plantaris muscle
35 Tendon of tibialis anterior muscle
36 Tendon of tibialis posterior muscle
37 Tibia
38 Tibialis posterior muscle

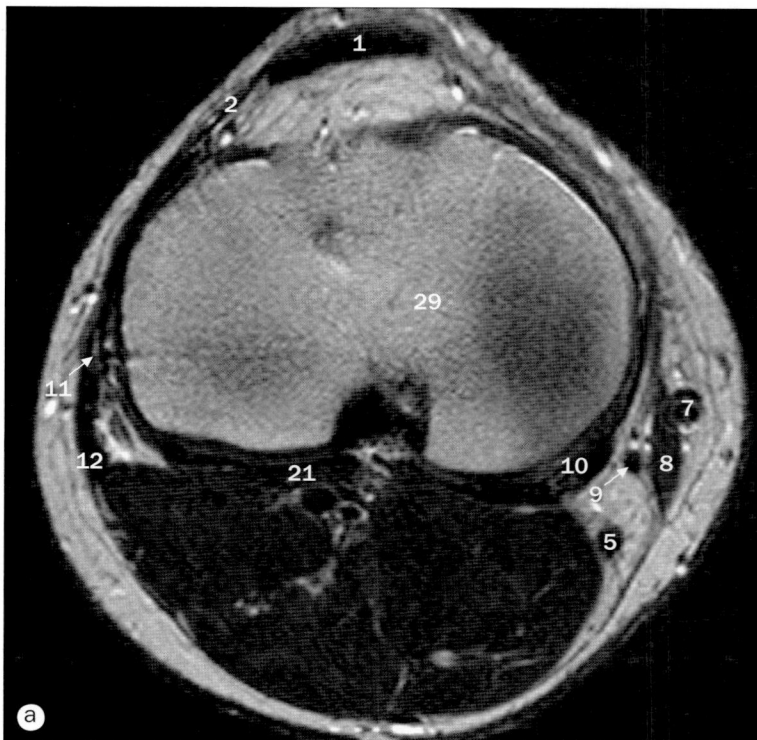

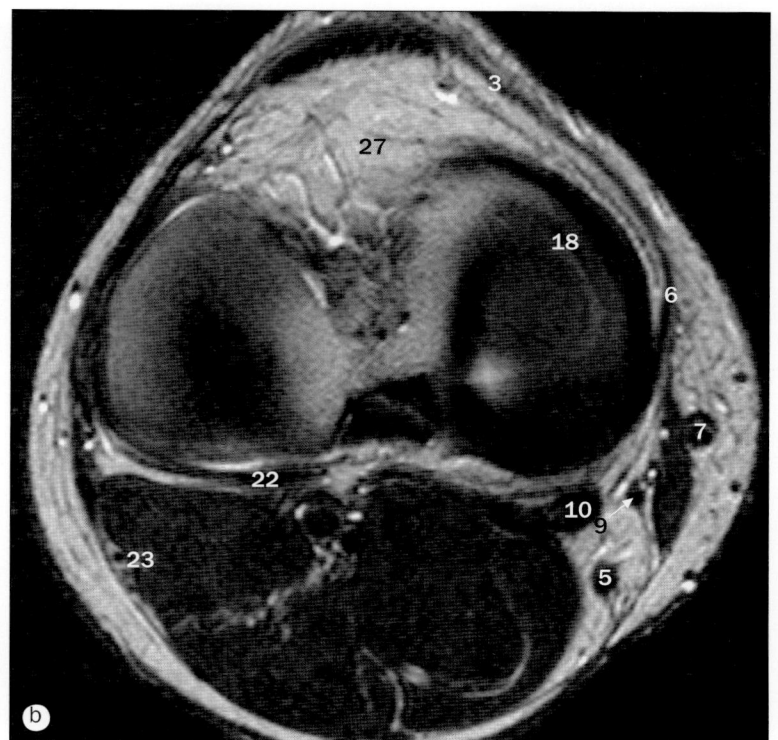

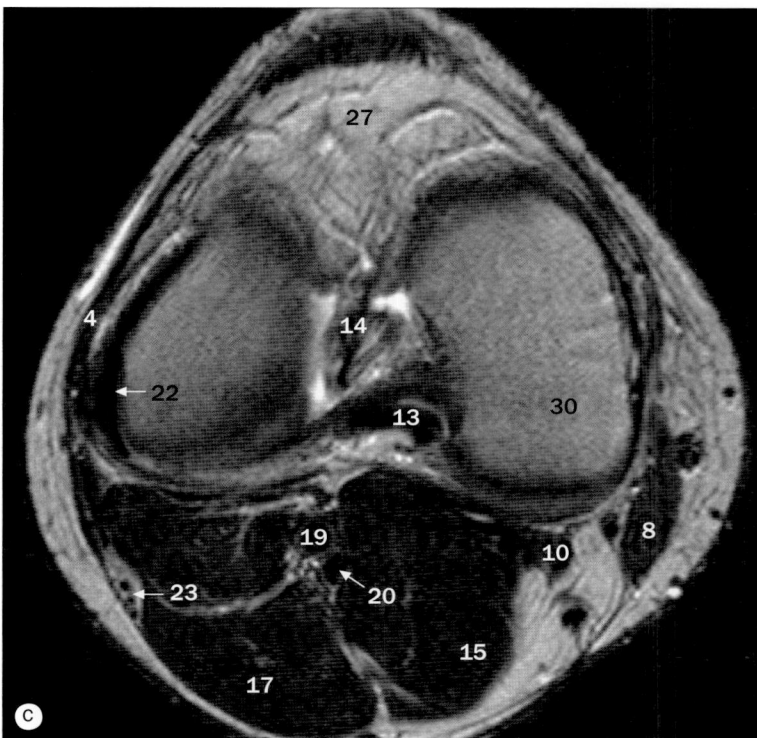

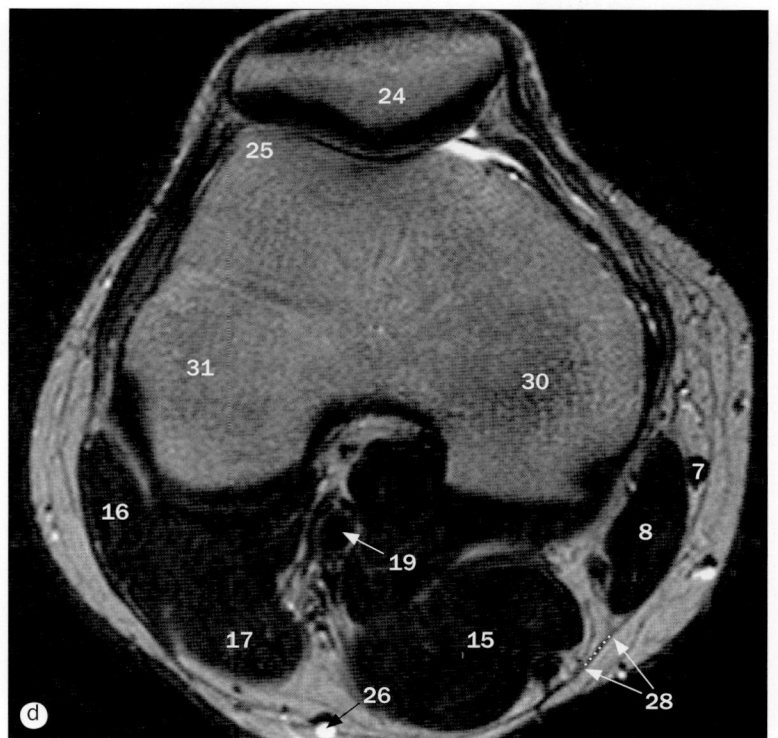

(a)–(d) Knee, axial MR images, from inferior to superior.

1 Patellar tendon
2 Lateral patellar retinaculum
3 Medial patellar retinaculum
4 Iliotibial tract
5 Semitendinosus tendon
6 Medial collateral ligament
7 Long (great) saphenous vein
8 Sartorius muscle
9 Gracilis tendon
10 Semimembranosus tendon
11 Lateral collateral ligament

12 Biceps femoris tendon
13 Posterior cruciate ligament
14 Anterior cruciate ligament
15 Medial head gastrocnemius muscle
16 Biceps femoris muscle
17 Lateral head gastrocnemius muscle
18 Medial meniscus
19 Popliteal artery
20 Popliteal vein

21 Popliteus muscle
22 Popliteus tendon
23 Common peroneal (fibular) nerve
24 Patella
25 Lateral condylar eminence
26 Short (lesser) saphenous vein
27 Infrapatellar fat pad
28 Deep fascia (fascia lata)
29 Tibial plateau
30 Medial condyle of femur
31 Lateral condyle of femur

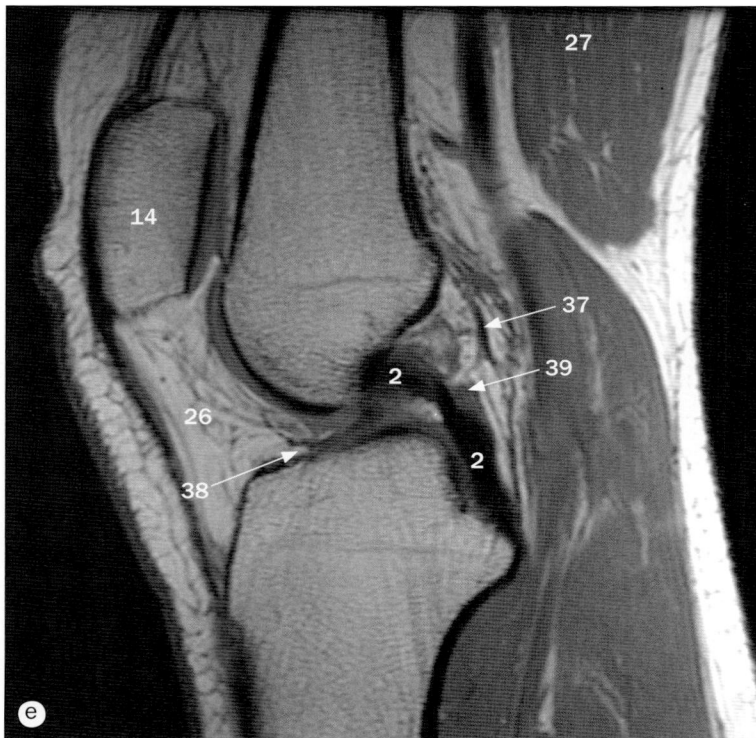

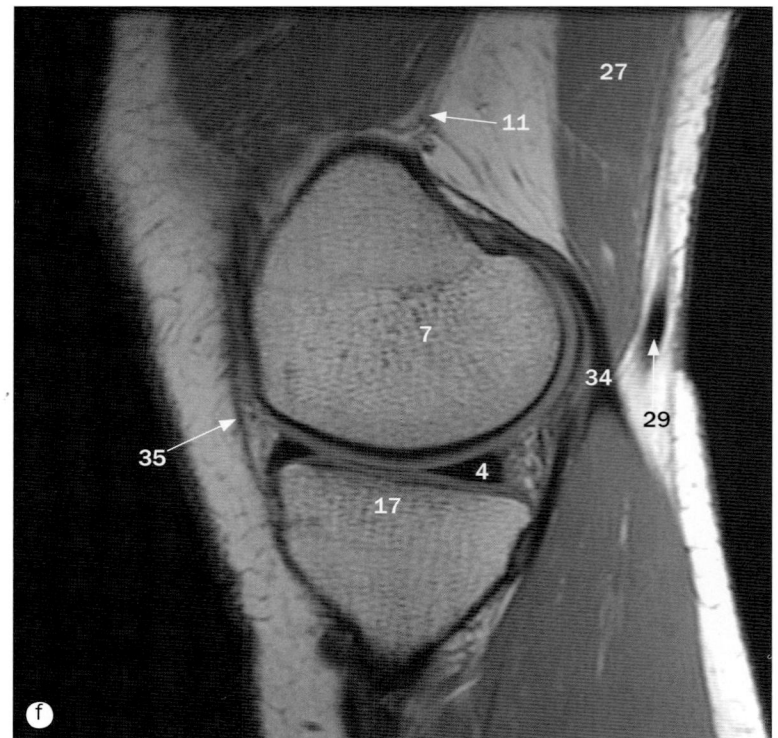

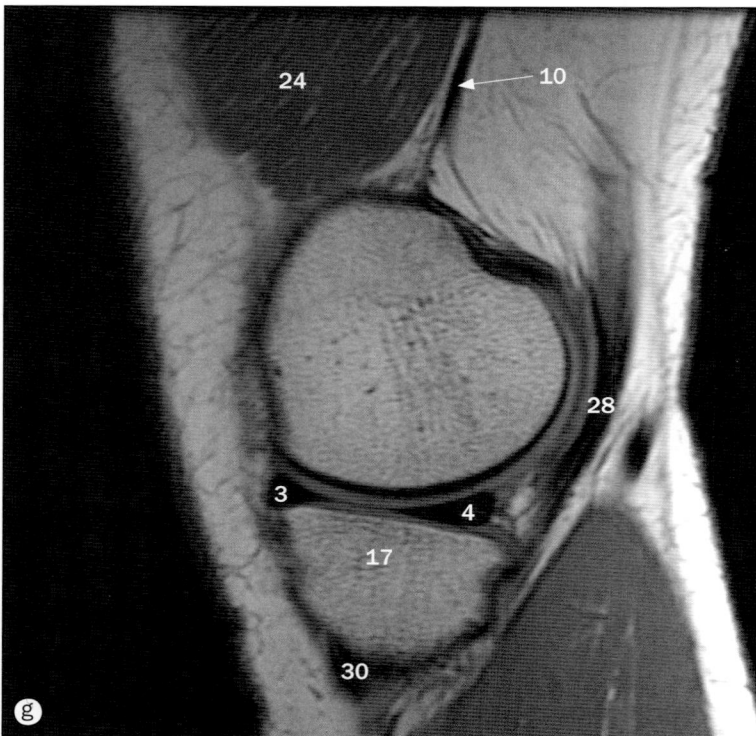

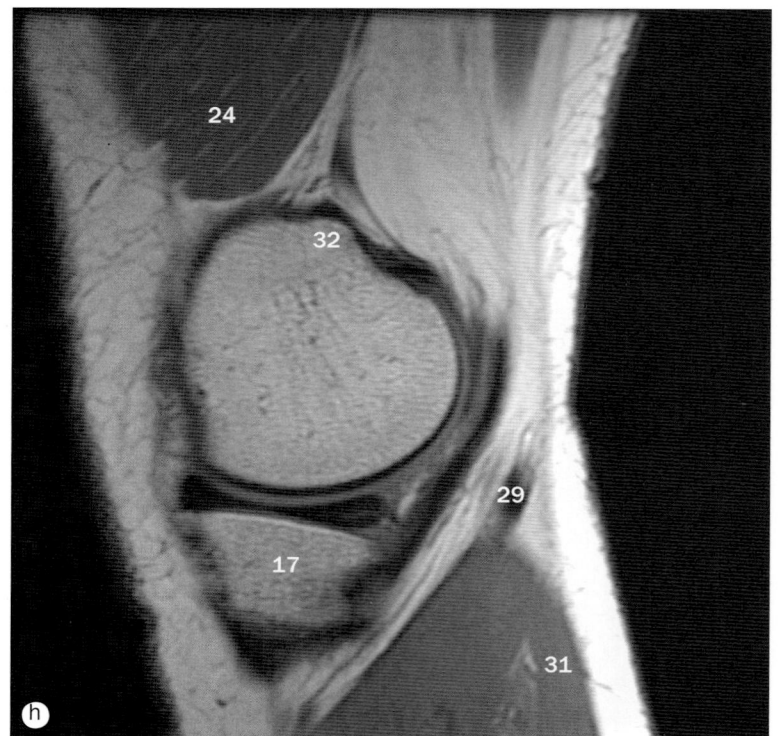

(a)–(h) Knee, sagittal MR images, from lateral to medial.

25 Tibialis anterior muscle	**32** Adductor tubercle	**39** Meniscofemoral ligament (Wrisberg)
26 Infrapatellar fat pad	**33** Popliteal artery	**40** Tibial spine
27 Semimembranosus muscle	**34** Medial head of gastrocnemius tendon	**41** Biceps femoris muscle
28 Semimembranosus tendon	**35** Medial patellar retinaculum	**42** Plantaris muscle
29 Semitendinosus tendon	**36** Lateral patellar retinaculum	**43** Tibial tuberosity
30 Sartorius tendon	**37** Posterior joint capsule	**44** Common peroneal (fibular) nerve
31 Medial head of gastrocnemius muscle	**38** Transverse ligament	

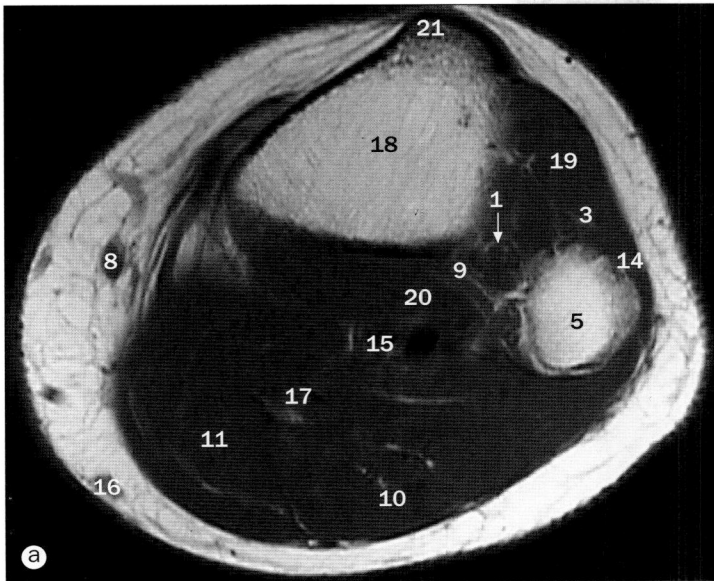

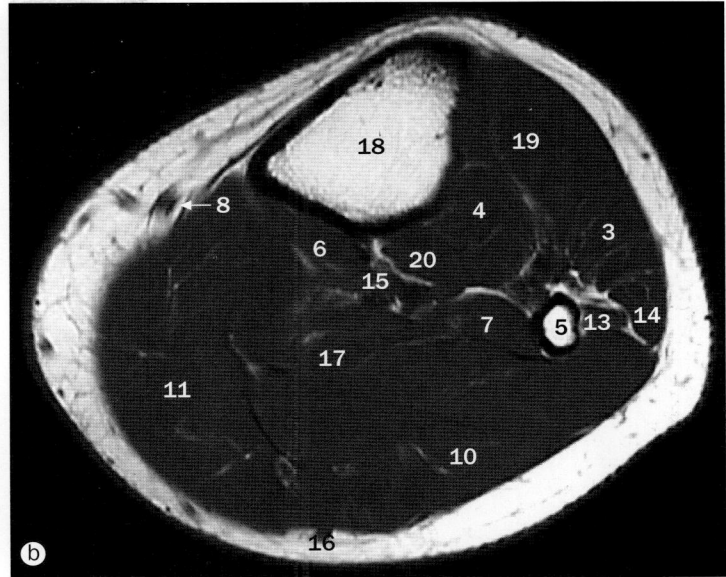

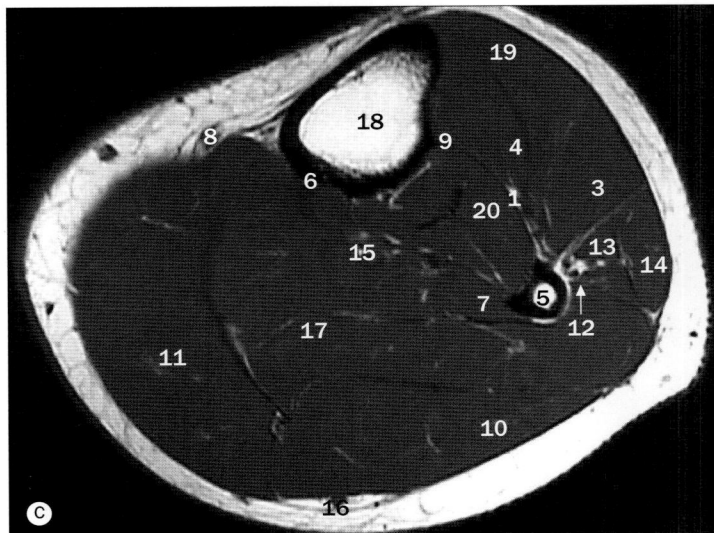

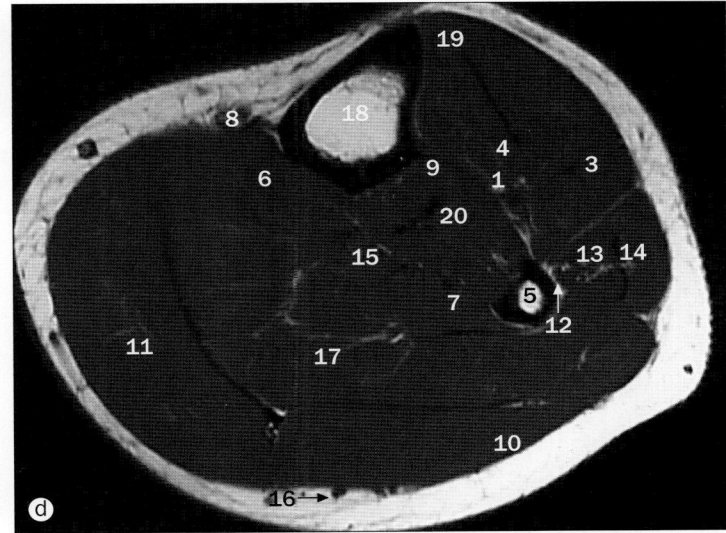

(a)–(e) Calf, axial MR images.

1 Anterior tibial artery
2 Aponeurosis of gastrocnemius muscle
3 Extensor digitorum longus muscle
4 Extensor hallucis longus muscle
5 Fibula
6 Flexor digitorum longus muscle
7 Flexor hallucis longus muscle
8 Great (long) saphenous vein
9 Interosseous membrane
10 Lateral head of gastrocnemius muscle
11 Medial head of gastrocnemius muscle
12 Peroneal artery
13 Peroneus brevis muscle
14 Peroneus longus muscle
15 Posterior tibial artery
16 Small saphenous vein
17 Soleus muscle
18 Tibia
19 Tibialis anterior muscle
20 Tibialis posterior muscle
21 Tuberosity of tibia

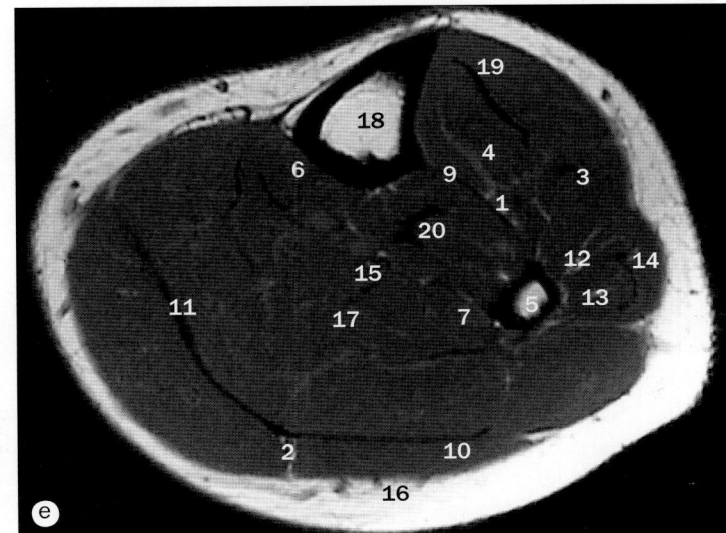

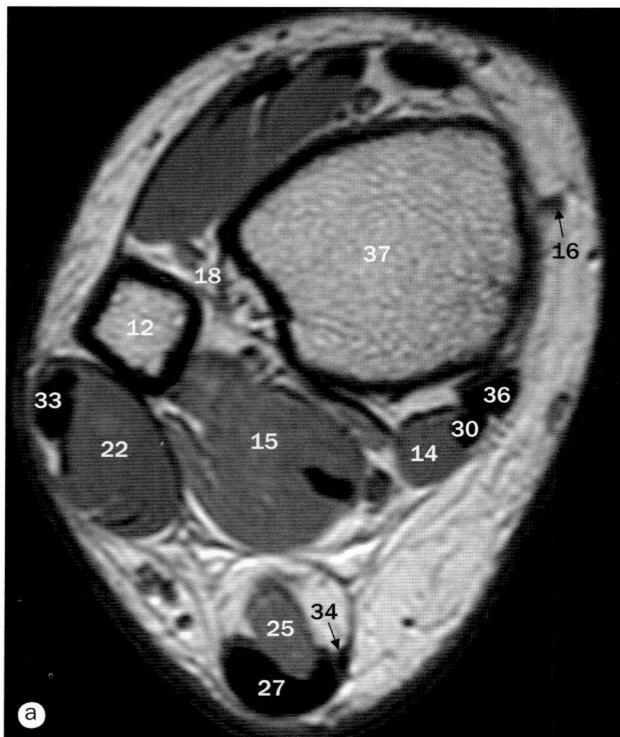

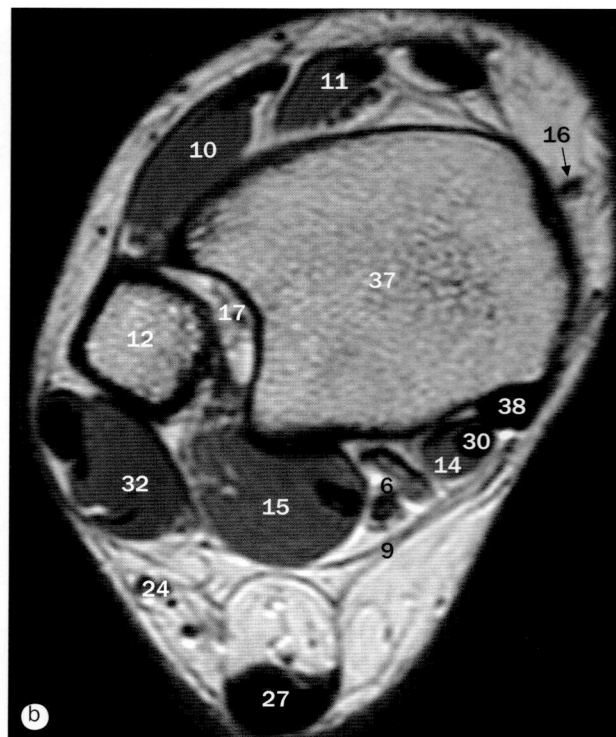

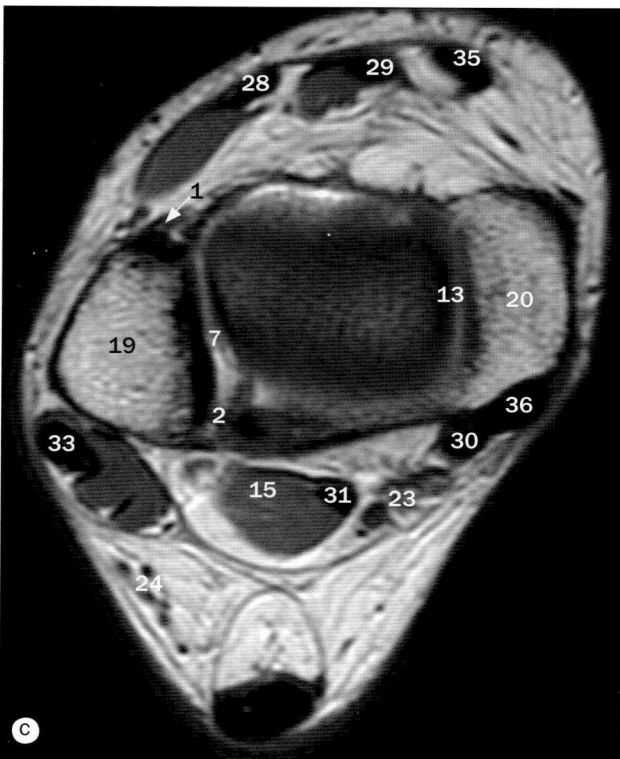

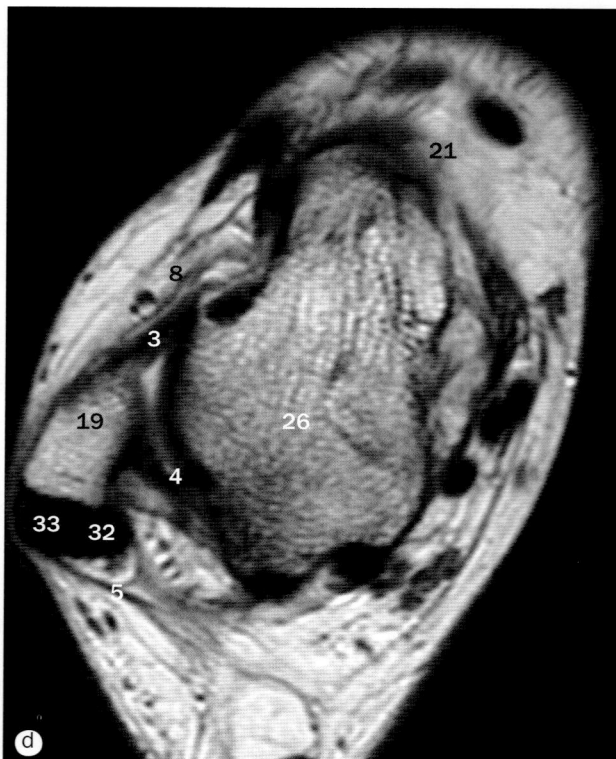

(a)–(h) Axial MR images of the ankle, from superior to inferior.

1 Anterior inferior tibiofibular ligament
2 Posterior inferior tibiofibular ligament
3 Anterior talofibular ligament
4 Posterior talofibular ligament
5 Peroneal (fibular) retinaculum
6 Neurovascular bundle
7 Talofibular joint
8 Extensor retinaculum
9 Flexor retinaculum
10 Extensor digitorum muscle
11 Extensor hallucis longus muscle
12 Fibula
13 Talotibial joint
14 Flexor digitorum longus muscle
15 Flexor hallucis longus muscle
16 Great (long) saphenous vein
17 Inferior tibiofibular joint
18 Interosseous membrane
19 Lateral malleolus
20 Medial malleolus
21 Navicular
22 Peroneus (fibularis) brevis muscle
23 Posterior tibial artery and vein
24 Small saphenous vein
25 Soleus muscle
26 Talus
27 Tendo calcaneus (Achilles' tendon)

28 Tendon of extensor digitorum muscle
29 Tendon of extensor hallucis longus muscle
30 Tendon of flexor digitorum longus muscle
31 Tendon of flexor hallucis longus muscle
32 Tendon of peroneus (fibularis) brevis muscle
33 Tendon of peroneus (fibularis) longus muscle
34 Tendon of plantaris muscle
35 Tendon of tibialis anterior muscle
36 Tendon of tibialis posterior muscle
37 Tibia
38 Tibialis posterior muscle

(a)–(h) Axial MR images of the ankle, from superior to inferior.

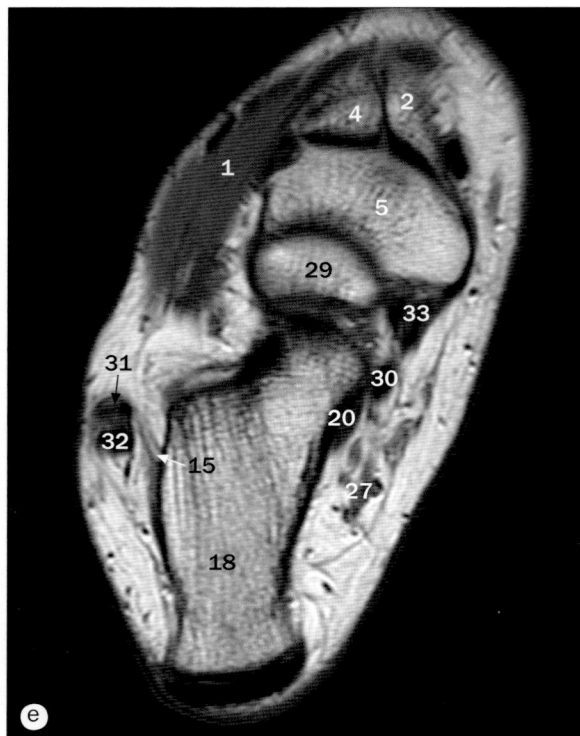

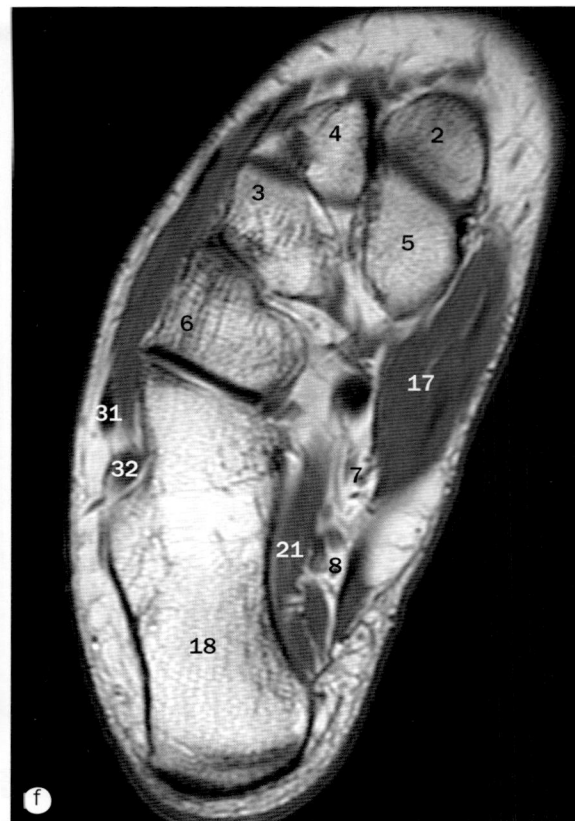

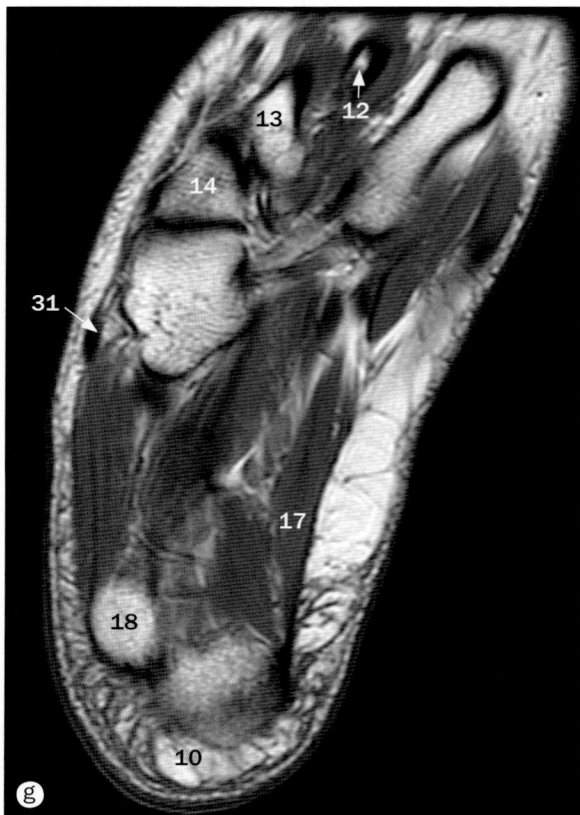

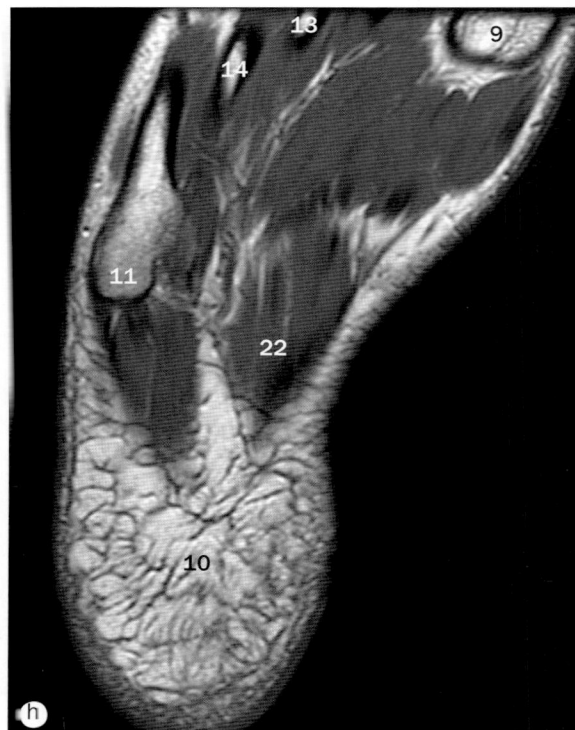

1 Extensor digitorum brevis
2 Medial cuneiform
3 Lateral cuneiform
4 Intermediate cuneiform
5 Navicular
6 Cuboid
7 Medial plantar nerve and vessels
8 Lateral plantar nerve and vessels
9 First metatarsal head
10 Heel fat pad
11 Fifth metatarsal base (tuberosity)
12 Second metatarsal
13 Third metatarsal
14 Fourth metatarsal
15 Calcaneofibular ligament
16 Abductor digiti minimi muscle
17 Abductor hallucis muscle
18 Calcaneus
19 Deltoid ligament
20 Tendon of flexor hallucis longus
21 Flexor accessorius muscle (quadratus plantae)
22 Flexor digitorum brevis muscle
23 Inferior tibiofibular joint
24 Lateral malleolus
25 Medial malleolus
26 Plantar aponeurosis
27 Posterior tibial artery
28 Sustentaculum tali
29 Talus head
30 Tendon of flexor digitorum longus muscle
31 Tendon of peroneus (fibularis) brevis muscle
32 Tendon of peroneus (fibularis) longus muscle
33 Tendon of tibialis posterior muscle

(a)–(d) Ankle and foot, coronal MR images.

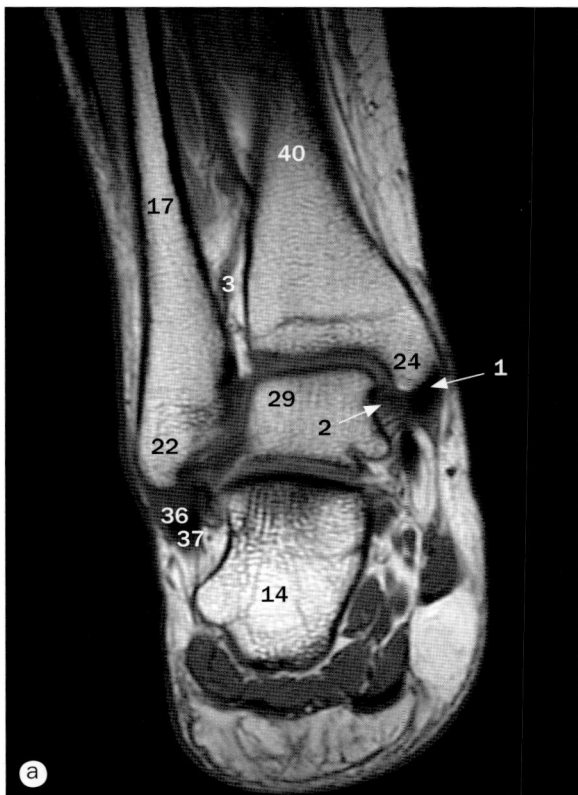

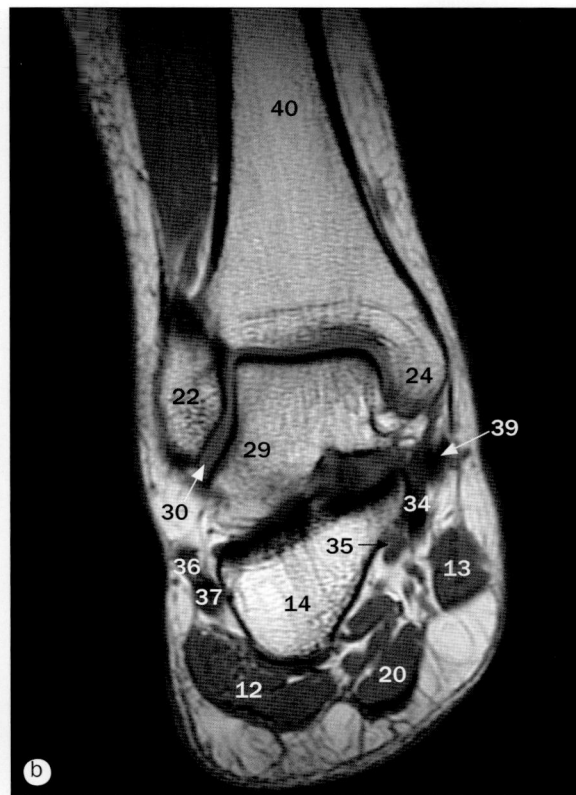

1 Deltoid ligament, superficial portion
2 Deltoid ligament, deep portion
3 Tibiofibular ligament
4 First metatarsal
5 Second metatarsal
6 Third metatarsal
7 Fourth metatarsal
8 Fifth metatarsal
9 Great (long) saphenous vein
10 Plantar calcaneonavicular 'spring' ligament
11 Extensor digitorum brevis
12 Abductor digiti minimi muscle
13 Adductor hallucis muscle
14 Calcaneus
15 Cuboid
16 Extensor digitorum brevis muscle
17 Fibula

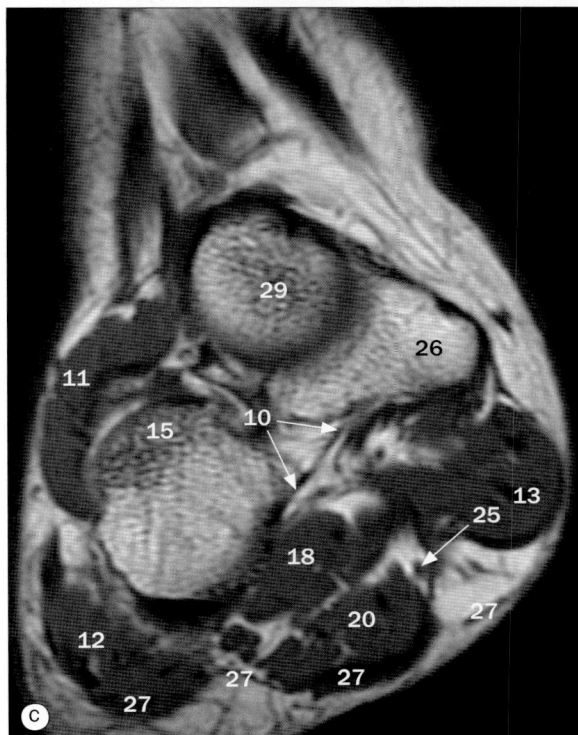

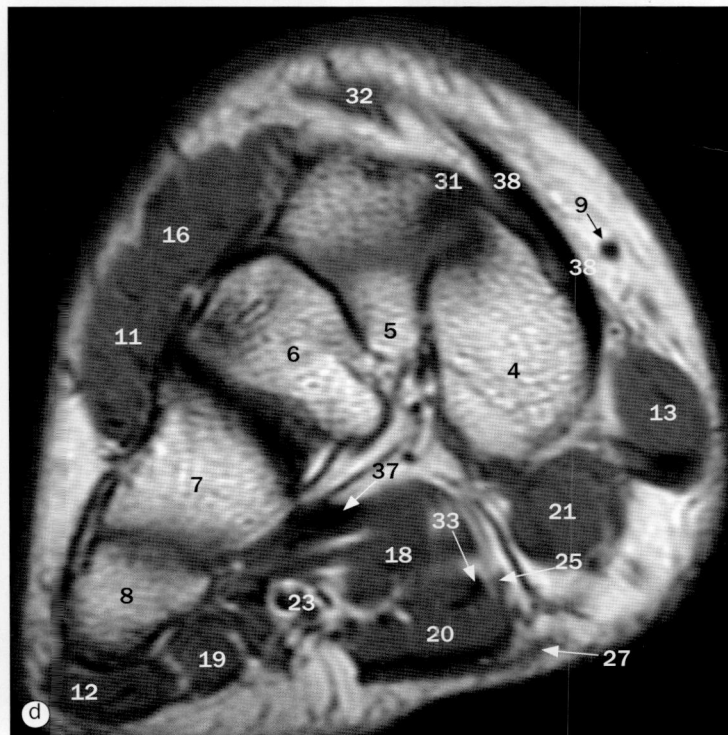

18 Flexor accessorius muscle
19 Flexor digiti minimi muscle
20 Flexor digitorum brevis muscle
21 Flexor hallucis brevis muscle
22 Lateral malleolus
23 Lateral plantar nerve and vessels
24 Medial malleolus
25 Medial plantar nerve and artery
26 Navicular

27 Plantar aponeurosis
28 Sustentaculum tali
29 Talus
30 Talofibular joint
31 Tendon of extensor digitorum longus muscle
32 Tendon of extensor hallucis longus muscle
33 Tendon of flexor digitorum brevis muscle
34 Tendon of flexor digitorum longus muscle

35 Tendon of flexor hallucis longus muscle
36 Tendon of peroneus (fibularis) brevis muscle
37 Tendon of peroneus (fibularis) longus tendon and muscle
38 Tendon of tibialis anterior muscle
39 Tendon of tibialis posterior muscle
40 Tibia

(a)–(d) Ankle, sagittal MR images, from lateral to medial.

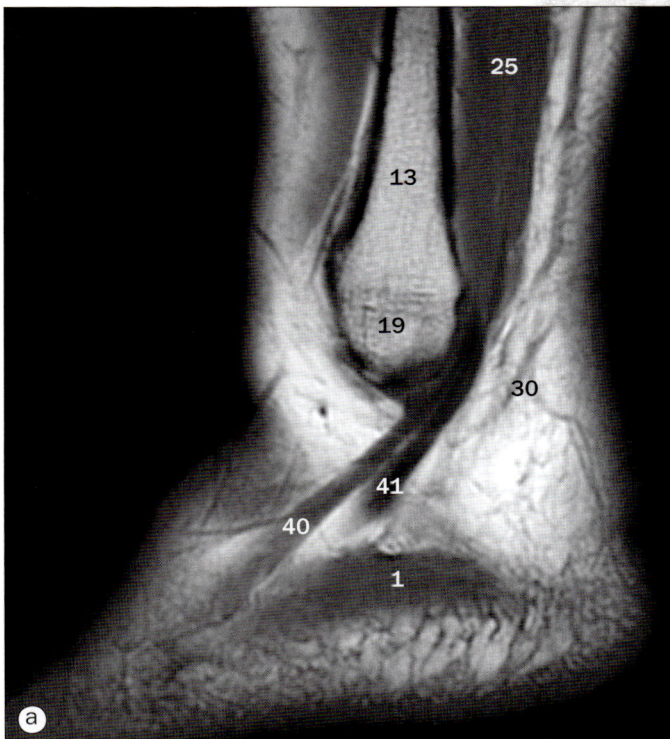

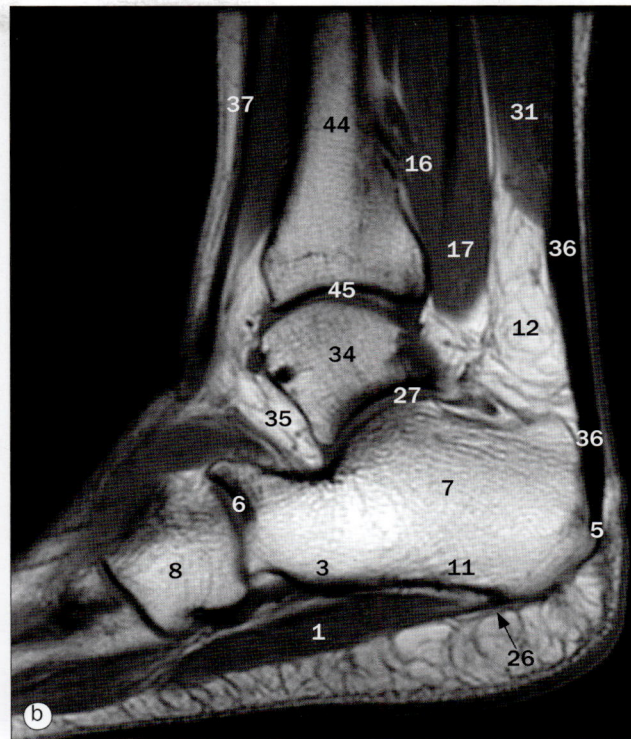

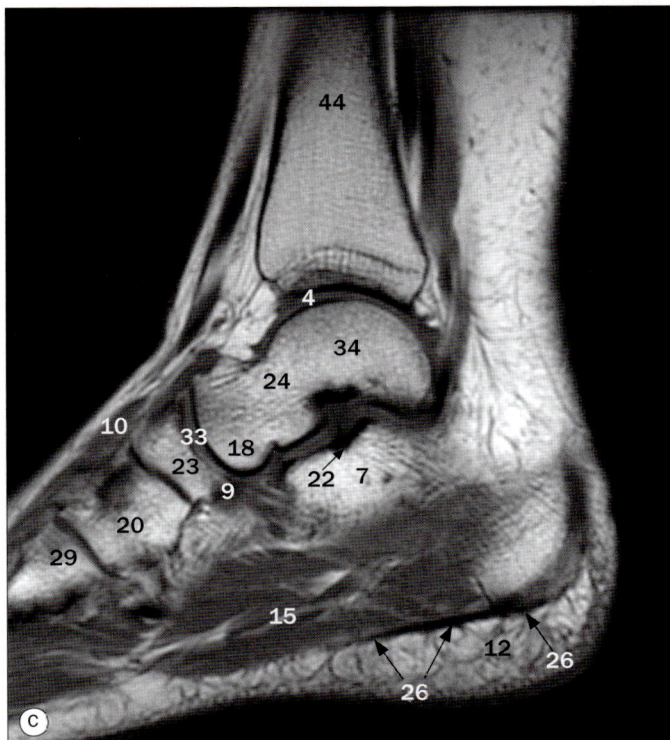

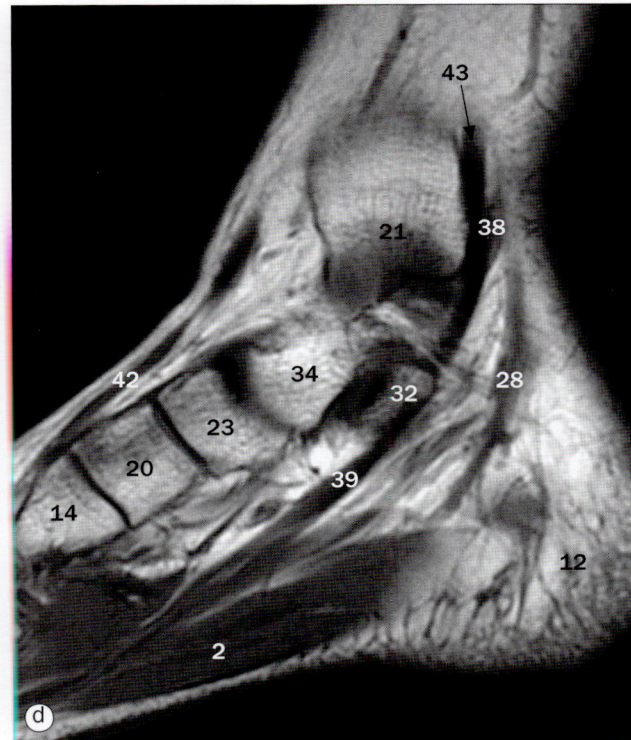

1 Abductor digiti minimi muscle
2 Abductor hallucis muscle
3 Anterior tubercle of calcaneus
4 Articular cartilage
5 Insertion of Achilles tendon
6 Calcaneocuboid joint
7 Calcaneus
8 Cuboid
9 Cuneonavicular joint
10 Extensor digitorum brevis muscle
11 Lateral process calcaneus
12 Fat pad
13 Fibula
14 First metatarsal
15 Flexor digitorum brevis muscle
16 Flexor digitorum longus muscle
17 Flexor hallucis longus muscle
18 Head of talus
19 Lateral malleolus
20 Medial cuneiform
21 Medial malleolus
22 Middle facet, subtalar joint
23 Navicular
24 Neck of talus
25 Peroneus brevis muscle
26 Plantar aponeurosis
27 Posterior subtalar joint
28 Posterior tibial artery and vein
29 Metatarsal base
30 Small (short) saphenous vein
31 Soleus muscle
32 Sustentaculum tali

33 Talonavicular joint
34 Talus
35 Tarsal sinus
36 Tendocalcaneus (Achilles' tendon)
37 Tendon of extensor digitorum muscle
38 Tendon of flexor digitorum longus muscle
39 Tendon of flexor hallucis longus muscle
40 Tendon of peroneus brevis muscle
41 Tendon of peroneus longus muscle
42 Tendon of tibialis anterior muscle
43 Tendon of tibialis posterior muscle
44 Tibia
45 Tibiotalar part of ankle joint

(a)–(b) Foot, coronal MR images.

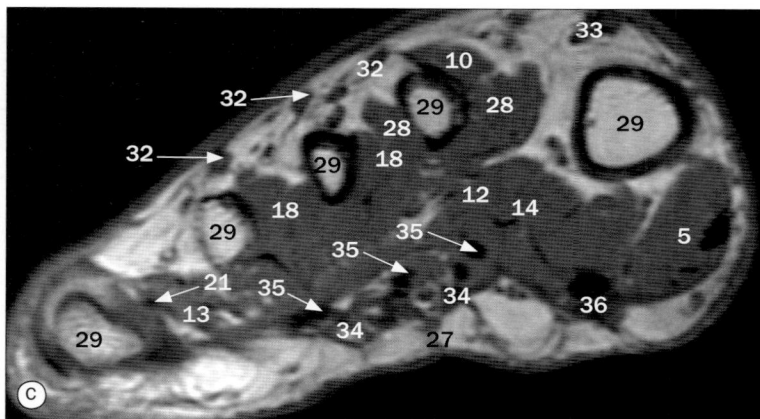

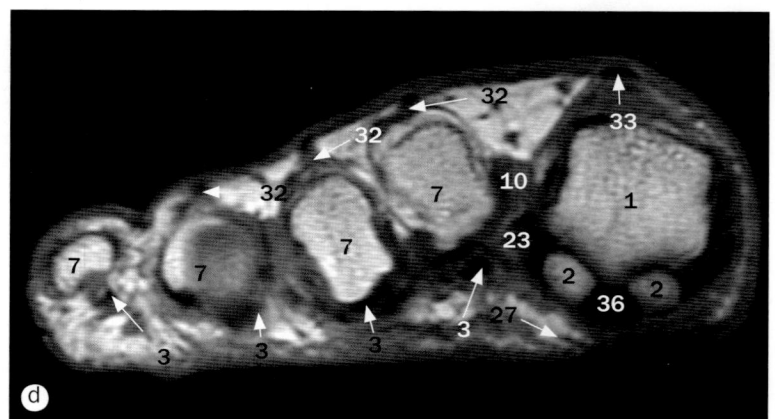

(c)–(d) Foot, axial MR images.

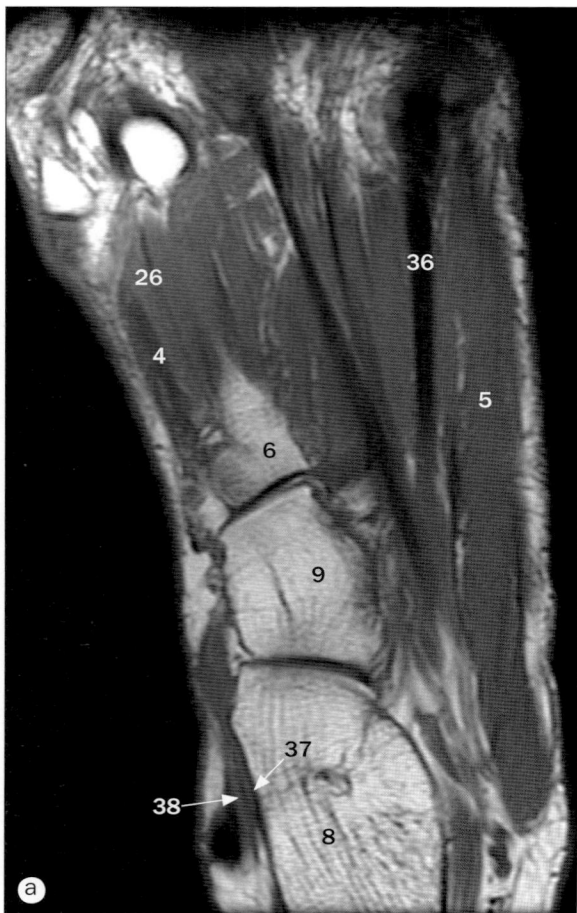

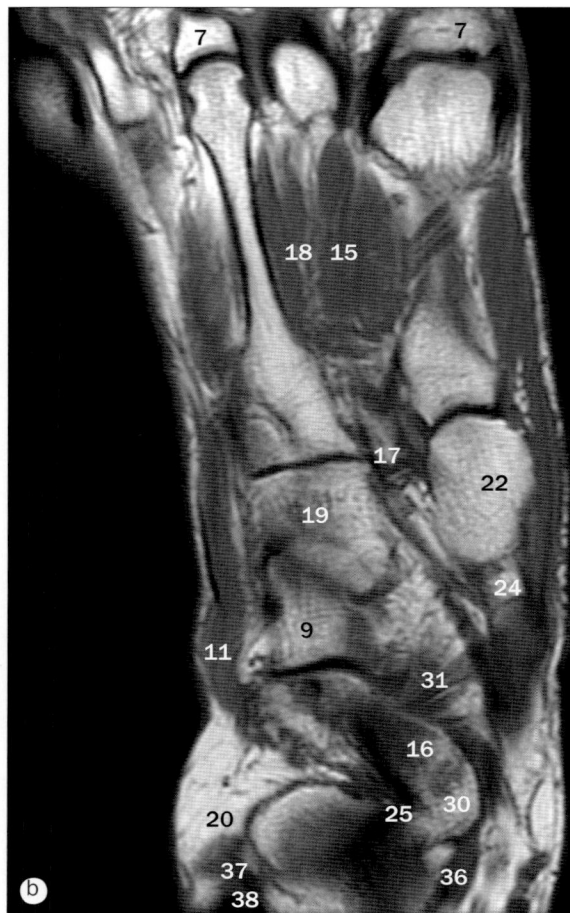

1 Head of first metatarsal
2 Sesamoid bones in flexor hallucis brevis
3 Flexor digitorum longus
4 Abductor digiti minimi muscle
5 Adductor hallucis muscle and tendon
6 Base of metatarsal
7 Base of proximal phalanx
8 Calcaneus
9 Cuboid
10 Dorsal interossei muscle
11 Extensor digitorum brevis muscle
12 Flexor accessorius muscle (quadratus plantae)
13 Flexor digiti minimi muscle
14 Flexor digitorum brevis muscle
15 Flexor hallucis brevis muscle
16 Head of talus
17 Intermediate cuneiform
18 Interossei muscles
19 Lateral cuneiform
20 Lateral malleolus

21 Lateral plantar nerve
22 Medial cuneiform
23 Medial plantar nerve and artery
24 Navicular
25 Neck of talus
26 Opponens digiti minimi muscle

27 Plantar aponeurosis
28 Plantar interossei muscle
29 Shafts of metatarsals 1,2,3,4,5
30 Talus
31 Tarsal sinus
32 Tendon of extensor digitorum longus muscle

33 Tendon of extensor hallucis longus muscle
34 Tendon of flexor digitorum brevis muscle
35 Tendon of flexor digitorum longus muscle
36 Tendon of flexor hallucis longus muscle
37 Tendon of peroneus brevis muscle
38 Tendon of peroneus longus muscle

8 Nuclear medicine

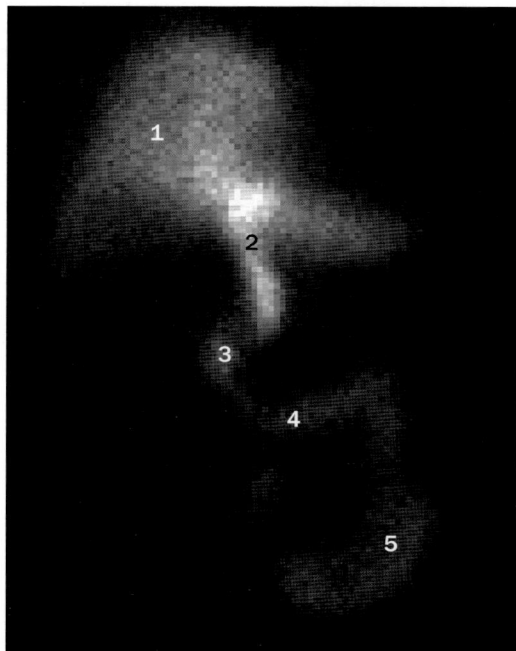

Hepatobiliary scan. The agents injected for this exam are rapidly cleared from the blood. The hepatocytes of the liver extract most of the injected dose and excrete it into the intrahepatic biliary tree. From there, the tracer flows into the hepatic and bile ducts. The agent will often passively fill the gall bladder (not seen in this example for various reasons, e.g. surgically absent, gall bladder is distended or has actively contracted during imaging or patient has had a prolonged fast prior to imaging). The agent then will enter into the duodenum through the ampulla of Vater, and eventually into the small bowel.

1 Liver
2 Bile duct
3 Descending (second) part of duodenum
4 Horizontal (third) part of duodenum
5 Jejunum

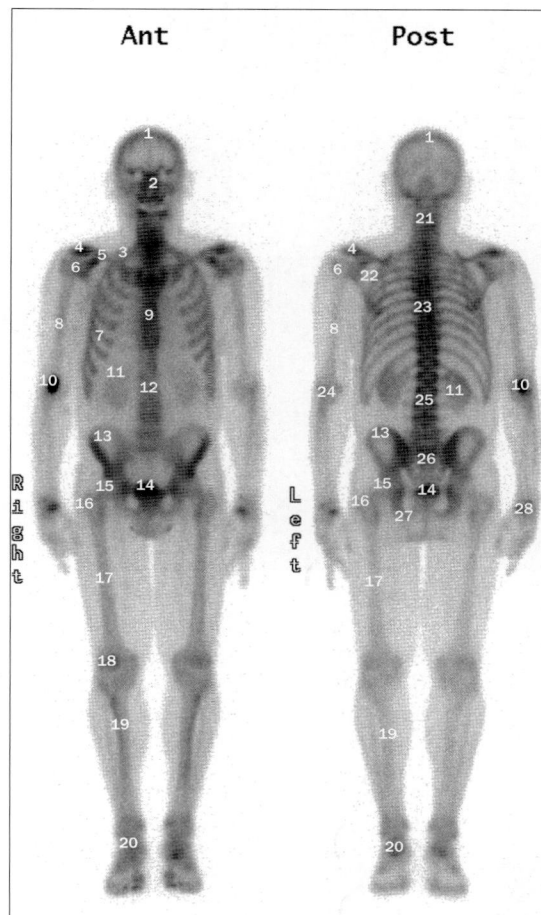

Whole body bone scan. Bone scans use physiologic agents to detect subtle abnormalities in bone metabolism. They are used to define skeletal abnormalities to include infectious, traumatic, congenital, metabolic and malignant conditions. Although the bone takes up the agent, some remains in the blood pool and is eventually excreted by the kidneys.

1 Cranium/skull	14 Urinary bladder
2 Nose and facial bones	15 Femoral head
3 First rib	16 Greater trochanter of femur
4 Acromioclavicular joint	17 Femoral shaft
5 Clavicle	18 Patella
6 Humeral head	19 Tibia
7 Fifth rib	20 Ankle
8 Humeral shaft	21 Cervical spine
9 Sternum	22 Scapula
10 Soft tissue extravasation at injection site in antecubital fossa	23 Thoracic spine
	24 Elbow
	25 Third lumbar vertebral body
11 Right kidney	26 Sacrum
12 Bodies of lumbar spine	27 Ischial tuberosity
13 Iliac	28 Wrist

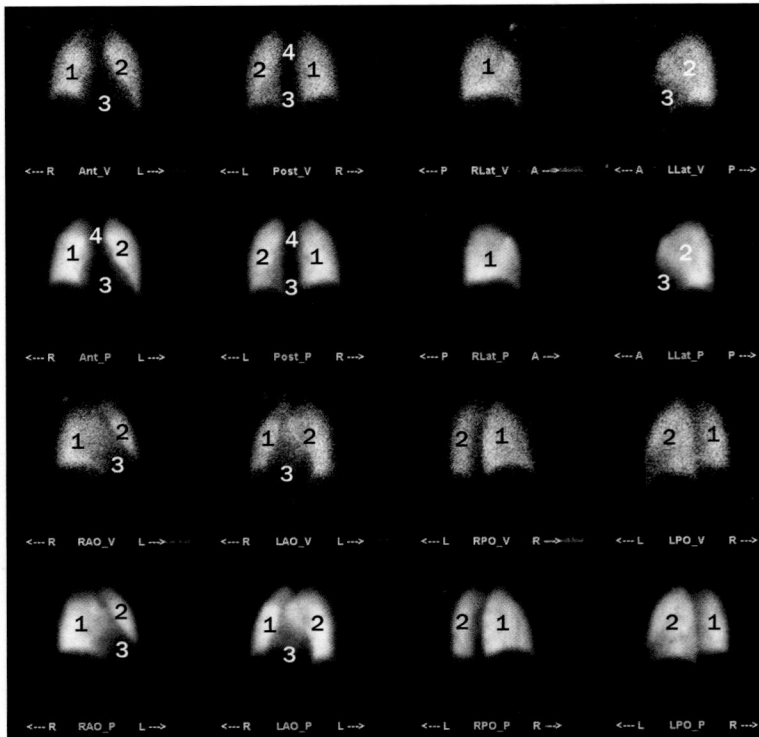

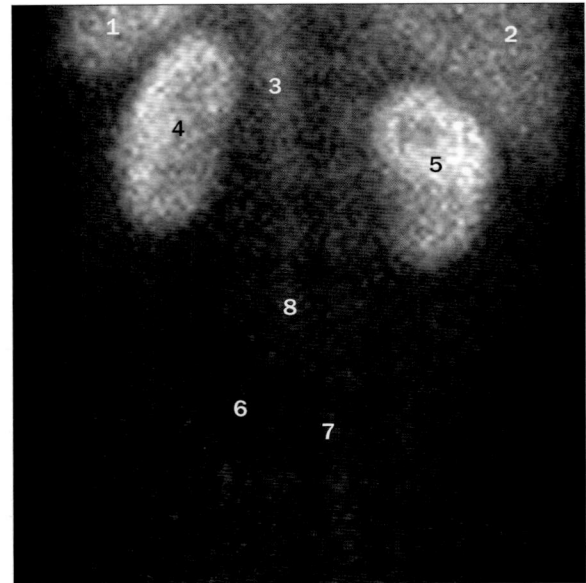

Lung scan. Imaging of the lungs involves both ventilation and perfusion. These two distributions match in the normal state. The order of imaging the ventilation and perfusion depends on the agents being used. Both ventilation and perfusion imaging evaluate the lungs in eight projections (anterior, posterior, right lateral, left lateral, right anterior oblique (RAO), left anterior oblique (LAO), right posterior oblique (RPO) and left posterior oblique (LPO)). The first and third rows are ventilation and the second and fourth rows are the matching perfusion.

| 1 | Right lung | 3 | Cardiac silhouette |
| 2 | Left lung | 4 | Mediastinum |

Renal scan. Renal imaging is performed with the camera placed on the patient's back because the kidneys are closer to the skin surface thus optimising the activity from the kidneys. Depending on the radiopharmaceutical used, relative structure and/or function of the kidneys can be obtained. In general, perfusion and excretion of the agent can be assessed in renal imaging. In the early staging of imaging some of the agent remains in the blood pool allowing visualisation of the surrounding structures.

1	Spleen	5	Right kidney
2	Liver	6	Left common iliac artery
3	Abdominal aorta	7	Right common iliac artery
4	Left kidney	8	Abdominal aortic bifurcation

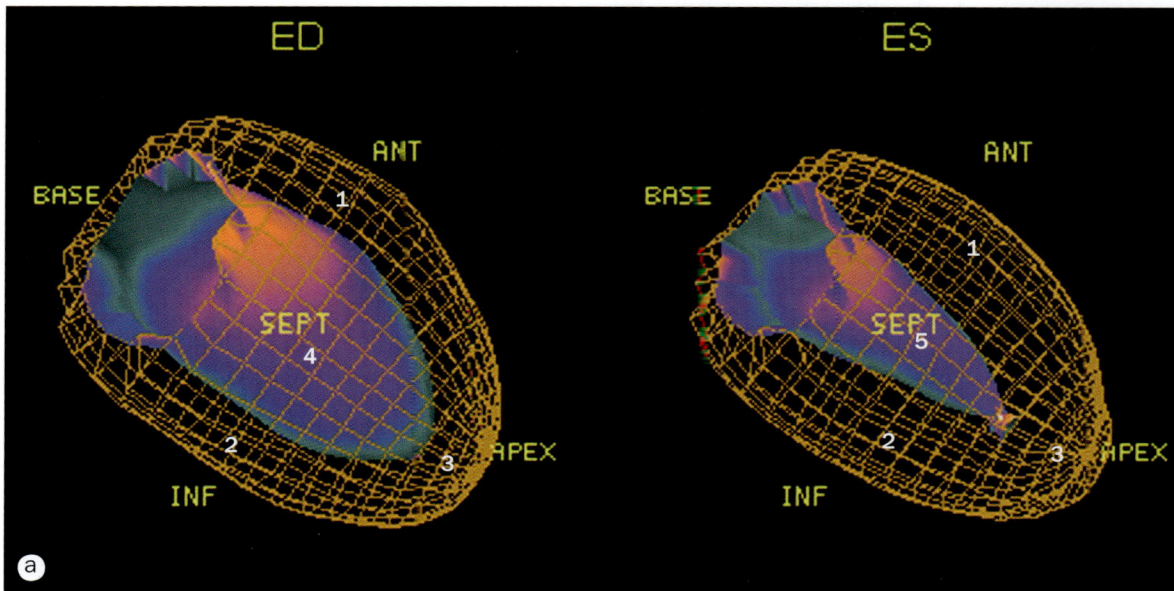

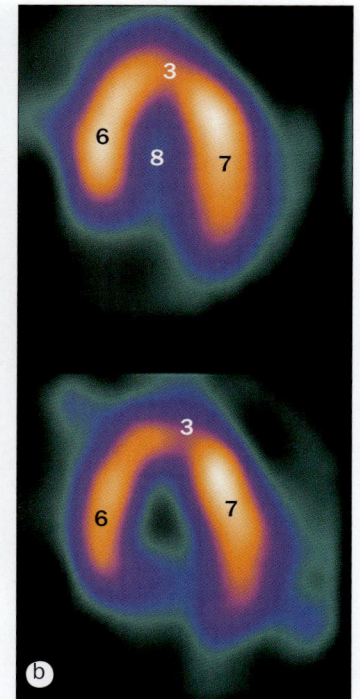

Cardiac scans, (a) 3D reconstructions of the left ventricle at end diastole (ED) and end systole (ES). Subtracting the ventricular volume at end systole from end diastole represents the ejection volume during systole.

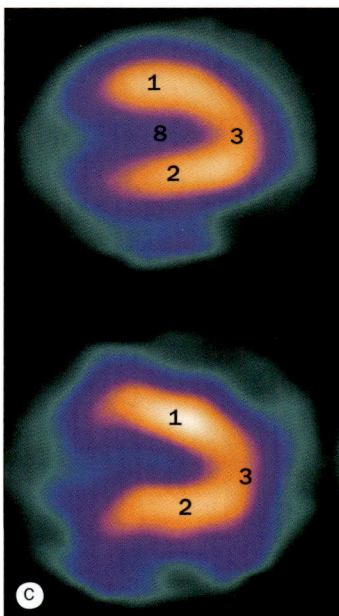

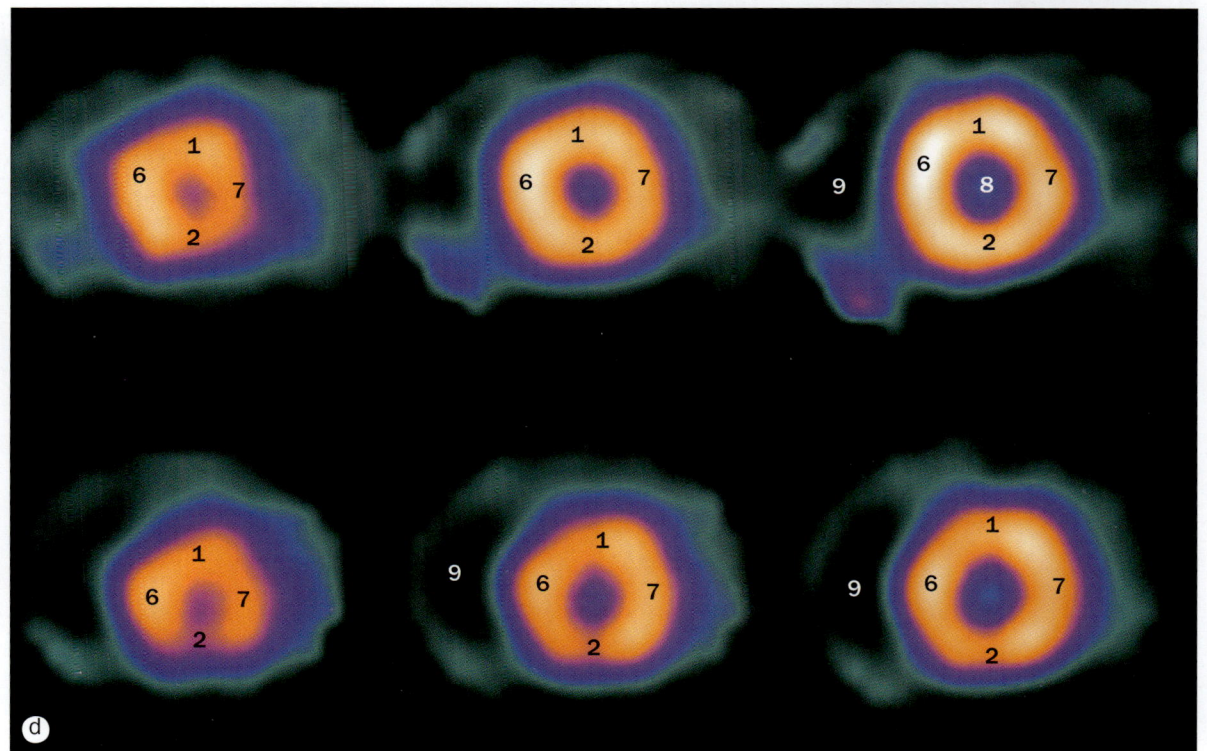

Cardiac scans, (b)–(d), images are obtained during stress (exercise or pharmaceutical) represented by the top row of images and during rest represented by the bottom row of images. Comparison of these can determine alterations in cardiac circulation, from acute ischaemia to an old infarction. After imaging, the heart is sliced in different planes to evaluate the specific walls and the circulation that supplies them. The left ventricle appears as a 'horseshoe' shape on the vertical long axis (b) and horizontal long axis (c), and as a 'donut' on the short axis (d) views. The anterior wall, apex and portion of the septum are supplied by the left anterior descending artery (LAD). The right coronary artery (RCA) supplies the inferior wall and part of the septum, and the circumflex artery supplies the lateral wall.

1 Anterior wall of left ventricle
2 Inferior wall of left ventricle
3 Apical portion of left ventricle
4 Blood pool volume within the left ventricle at end diastole
5 Blood pool volume within the left ventricle at end systole
6 Interventricular septum
7 Lateral wall of left ventricle
8 Left ventricle cavity
9 Right ventricle cavity

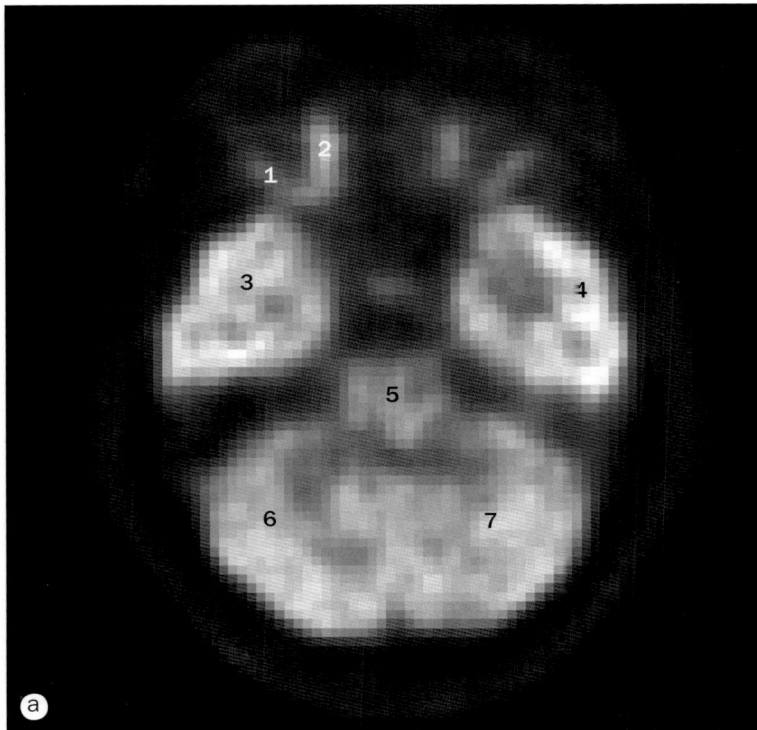

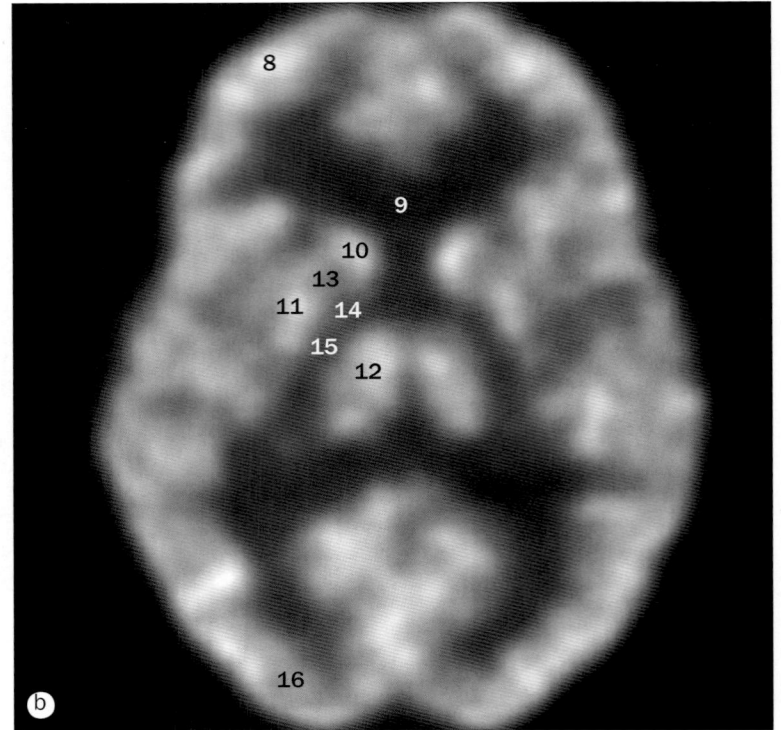

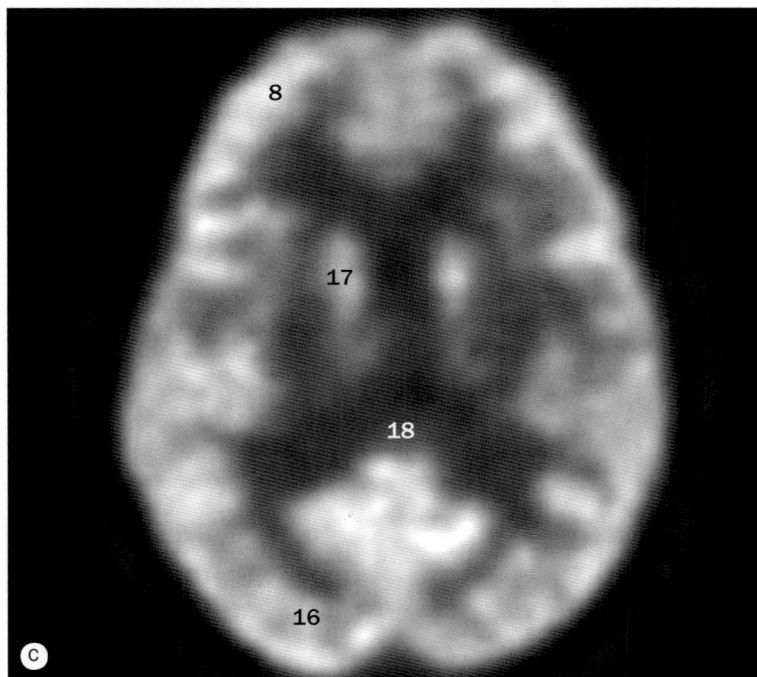

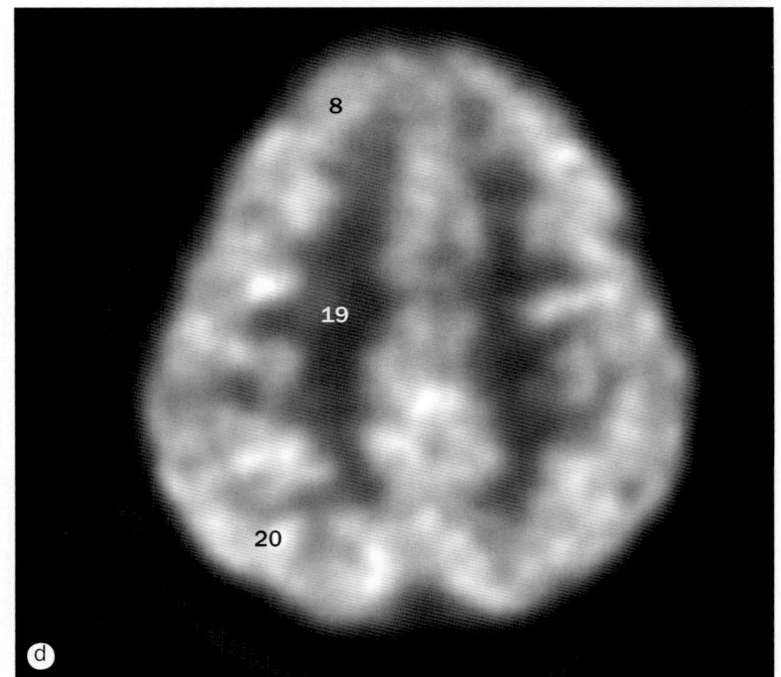

(a)–(d) PET metabolic brain scans. Fluorodeoxyglucose (FDG) is a derivative of glucose. Cells cannot differentiate between glucose and FDG. A major difference is that, once inside the cell, FDG is not metabolised and is trapped. This allows for easy imaging of structures in the body. The brain has high FDG uptake, with grey matter having a higher uptake compared with white matter. The basal ganglia usually have slightly higher uptake than the cortex. It is normal to have areas of increased uptake in the frontal eye fields, visual cortex and Wernicke's region.

1 Lateral rectus muscle	**8** Frontal lobe	**15** Internal capsule, posterior limb
2 Medial rectus muscle	**9** Corpus callosum, genu	**16** Occipital lobe
3 Right temporal lobe	**10** Caudate nucleus, head	**17** Caudate nucleus, body
4 Left temporal lobe	**11** Putamen	**18** Corpus callosum, splenium
5 Brainstem	**12** Thalamus	**19** Corona radiata
6 Right cerebellar hemisphere	**13** Internal capsule, anterior limb	**20** Parietal lobe
7 Left cerebellar hemisphere	**14** Internal capsule, genu	

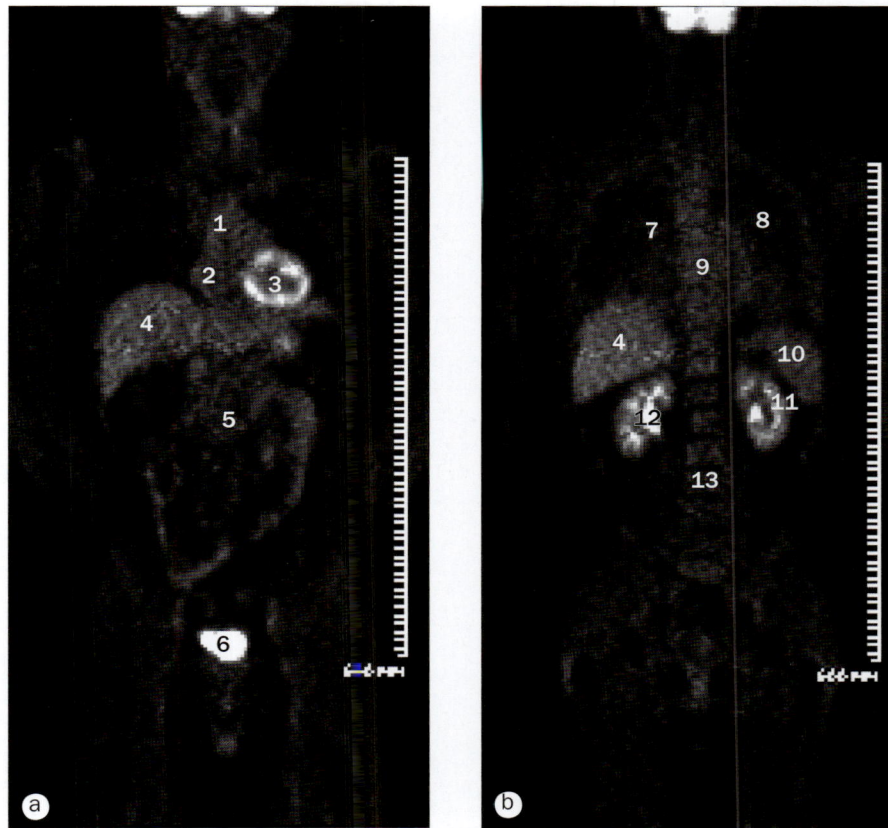

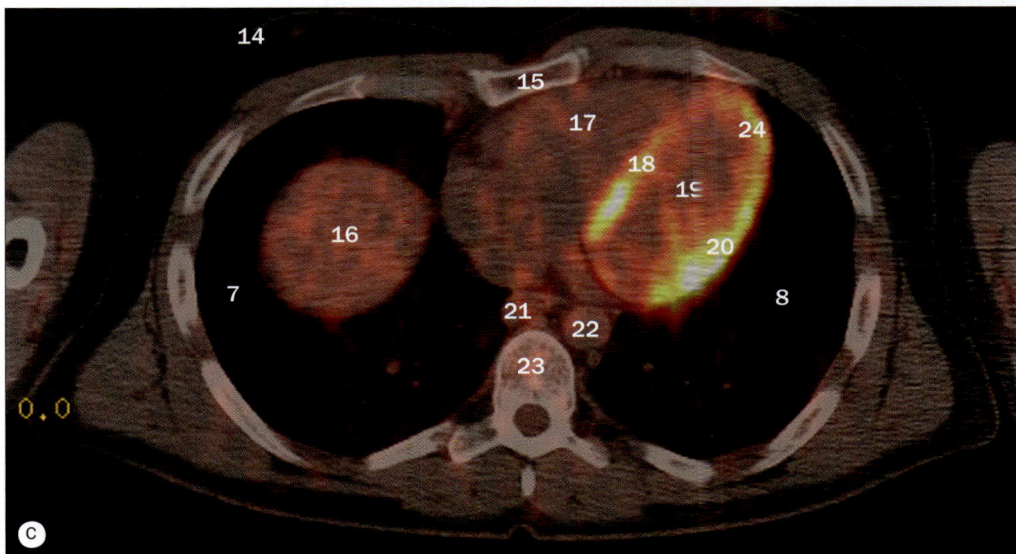

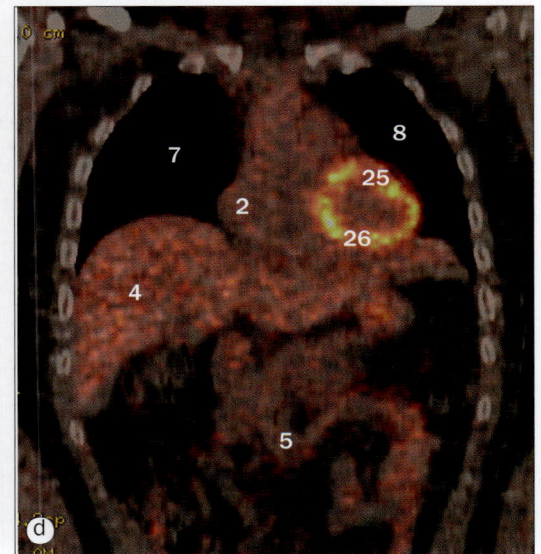

(a)–(d) Whole body PET/CT scans. PET imaging offers physiological function of the tissue and CT offers anatomical information. By fusing these images, precise localisation of areas of interest is made. Figures (a) and (b) are coronal PET images of the body at different depths. Figures (c) and (d) are fused PET/CT images in the axial (c) and coronal (d) projections.

1 Mediastinum	10 Spleen	19 Left ventricle, cavity
2 Right atrium	11 Cortex of kidney	20 Lateral wall of left ventricle
3 Left ventricle	12 Kidney, renal pelvis	21 Oesophagus
4 Liver	13 Lumbar spine	22 Descending thoracic aorta
5 Small bowel	14 Right breast tissue	23 Thoracic vertebral body
6 Bladder	15 Sternum	24 Apex of left ventricle
7 Right lung	16 Liver, dome	25 Anterior wall of left ventricle
8 Left lung	17 Right ventricle	26 Inferior wall of left ventricle
9 Thoracic spine	18 Interventricular septum	

Index

Note: References are to text mentions (mainly in the legends and boxes) rather than the numbers encoding structures in the figures. The most common imaging modalities (radiographs and conventional CT and MRI) have not been indexed.

A

abdominal aorta *see* aorta
abducens nerve (CN6), 16, 18, 49
  in ambient cistern, 50
abductor digiti minimi muscle
  foot, 231, 232, 233, 234
  hand, 86, 87, 88
abductor hallucis muscle, 231, 233
abductor pollicis brevis muscle, 86, 87, 88
abductor pollicis longus muscle, 82, 85
  tendon, 86
acetabular ligament, transverse, 220
acetabulum, 134, 134, 142, 154, 156, 162, 166, 208, 222
  labrum *see* labrum
  notch, 220
  roof, 60, 134, 156
    anterior, 220
    posterior, 220
Achilles tendon, 230, 233
acoustic meatus/canal (auditory canal)
  external, 3, 7, 9, 15, 32, 64
  internal, 2, 4, 9, 13, 15, 18, 43, 50
acromioclavicular joint, 79, 145
  isotope scan, 235
acromion of scapula, 68, 69, 79
Adamkiewicz, artery of, 66
adductor brevis muscle, 134, 153, 155, 157, 158, 161, 164, 165, 167, 219, 221, 222, 223
adductor canal (subsartorial canal), 222
adductor hallucis muscle, 232, 234
  tendon, 234
adductor longus muscle, 134, 153, 155, 157, 158, 161, 164, 165, 167, 219, 220, 221, 222, 223
adductor magnus muscle, 153, 158, 161, 163, 164, 165, 167, 219, 220, 221, 223
adductor pollicis muscle, 87, 88
adductor tubercle, 227
adrenal gland *see* suprarenal gland
Alcock's canal (internal pudendal neurovascular bundle), 152, 154, 159
alveolar bone/process/rim/ridge of maxilla, 8, 11, 30, 34, 46
alveolar foramen, inferior, of mandibular ramus, 61
alveolar nerve, inferior, 49
alveolar recess, 8
alveolar vessels
  inferior, 49
  posterior superior alveolar artery, 33
ambient cistern, 18, 44
  abducens nerve in, 50
  posterior cerebral artery in, 38, 40
amniotic fluid, 202, 203
ampulla
  ductus deferens, 199
  hepatopancreatic/Vater's, 182
  rectal, 154, 159, 160, 165
  terminal, 205, 206
  uterine tube, 195
anal canal, 134, 153, 154, 160, 165, 166, 169, 223
anal sphincter, external, 134, 154, 160
anastomotic artery, great (arteria radicularis magna), 66
anastomotic vein

inferior (vein of Labbé), 37, 41
superior (vein of Trolard), 37
anconeus muscle, 84, 85
angiograms *see* aortogram; arteriogram; magnetic resonance angiogram; venogram; ventricles (heart)
angular artery (angular branches of middle cerebral artery), 36
angular veins, 23
ankle, 212–14, 213, 230–3
  isotope scan, 235
annular epiphysial discs for vertebral body (thoracic spine), 58
annulus fibrosus, 63
anococcygeal raphe, 169
anorectal junction, 153, 163
antecubital fossa, 235
anterior chamber of globe, 20, 23
anus, 164
  see also anal canal; anal sphincter; anorectal junction
aorta, 62, 92, 94, 111, 113
  abdominal, 103, 105, 107, 124, 126, 128, 130, 138, 140, 143, 145, 148, 157, 183, 185
  bifurcation, 139, 236
  catheter introduced via femoral artery into *see* femoral artery
  fetal, 202, 203
  non-cross-sectional views, 174, 176, 183, 202, 203, 236
  pigtail catheter tip in, 183
  arch (aortic knuckle or knob), 33, 90, 91, 96, 100, 104, 105, 106, 108, 111, 117, 140, 142
    fetal, 203
    subtraction angiography, 117
  ascending, 91, 95, 100, 104, 105, 106, 108, 114, 117, 138, 140, 149
    fetal, 203
  descending, 90, 96, 100, 104, 105, 106, 108, 117, 142
    fetal, 203
    PET/CT scan, 239
  root, 115
aortic sinus, 113
  posterior (=non-coronary sinus), 114
aortic valve, 90, 91, 96, 100, 104, 105, 106, 108, 113, 117
aortogram
  abdominal, 183
  subtracted arch, 117
apical artery (superior pulmonary lobe), 110
aponeurosis
  bicipital, 84
  external oblique abdominal muscle, 150
  gastrocnemius muscle, 229
  plantar, 231, 232, 233, 234
appendicular artery, 130, 185
appendix, 131, 179
aqueduct of Sylvius, 21, 45, 47, 51
aqueous humour, 23
arachnoid granulation, 45
arcuate arteries, 194
arcuate eminence of temporal bone, 4, 12, 50
areola of nipple, 120
arteria radicularis magna, 66
arteries *see* blood vessels *and specific arteries*
arteriograms
  chest
    bronchial arteries, 116
    pulmonary arteries, 110–11
  coronary, 113, 114
  gastric artery and vein, 185
  gastroduodenal, selective, 193
  lower limb, 216, 217, 218

mesenteric arteries
  inferior, 186
  superior, 191
  penile, 198
  spinal, 66
  subtraction *see* subtraction angiography
  upper limb, 76
arthrography, MR *see* magnetic resonance arthrography
articular capsule
  knee joint, posterior, 227
  shoulder joint
    anterior, 79
    posterior, 80
articular cartilage, ankle, 233
articular discs of temporomandibular joints, 7
  see also intervertebral discs
articular eminence of temporal bone, 7
articular processes (facets)
  inferior
    C1, 57, 61
    C4, 56
    L2, 59
    thoracic, 58
  superior
    C1, 57
    C2, 57
    C4, 56
    C5, 56
    L3, 59
    sacral vertebrae, 60
    thoracic vertebrae, 58
articular tubercle for temporomandibular joint, 3
aryepiglottic fold, 27
arytenoid cartilage, 28
atlanto-axial joint, 57, 58
atlas (C1), 56
  arch, 4
    anterior, 3, 8, 13, 14, 22, 32, 46, 47, 50, 56, 57, 61, 64
    posterior, 13, 25, 46, 47, 56, 61
  articular processes *see* articular process
  body, 56
  lateral mass, 2, 13, 15, 50, 56, 57, 61, 64
  spinous process, 56
  transverse foramen *see* transverse foramen
  transverse ligament, 61
  transverse process, 12, 13, 15, 57, 61
  tubercles, 13, 64
atrioventricular nodal artery, 113, 114
atrium
  left, 91, 96, 100, 104, 105, 106, 108, 111, 115, 140, 142, 149
    auricle/appendage, 90, 96, 100, 108, 111, 115
    border, 91
    coronary supply, 113
    fetal, 203
  right, 77, 90, 97, 102, 104, 105, 109, 112, 115, 138, 140, 146, 148
    auricle/appendage, 97, 109
    border, 90
    fetal, 203
    PET/CT scan, 239
  septum *see* interatrial septum
auditory canal *see* acoustic meatus
auditory nerve, 18
auditory tube (Eustachian tube), 9, 32
auricle
  atrium *see* atrium
  ear (=pinna), 3, 7, 42
auricular artery, posterior, 33
auriculotemporal nerve, 50
axillary artery, 76, 79, 108

left, 103
axillary fold, anterior, 90
axillary recess, 79
axillary vein, 77, 79, 108
axis (C2), 8, 14
  articular process, superior, 57
  base, 13
  body, 25, 50, 56, 57, 61
  lamina, 61
  lateral, 56
  odontoid process/peg (dens), 2, 4, 6, 8, 13, 14, 22, 25, 46, 47, 50, 56, 57, 61, 64
  pedicle, 61
  spinous process, 56, 57, 61
  transverse foramen, 13
  transverse process, 57
azygos vein, 94, 96, 108, 116, 124, 143
  arch, 92, 116
  superior, catheter tip introduced via femoral vein into, 116
  venogram, 116

B

barium studies
  small intestine, 179
  stomach/duodenum, 178
    barium pooling in stomach, 178
basal vein of Rosenthal, 37, 45, 51
basilar artery, 16, 21, 22, 33, 38, 40, 43, 46, 47, 49
  bifurcation, 45
basilar part
  of occipital bone *see* basi-occiput
  of sphenoid *see* basisphenoid
basilic vein, 76, 78, 83, 84, 85, 86
basi-occiput (basilar part of occipital bone/lower clivus), 2, 3, 14, 50, 56
  basisphenoid and, synchondrosis, 3, 50
basion, 13
basisphenoid, 50
  basi-occiput and, synchondrosis, 3, 50
  marrow of, 41
basivertebral vein, 62, 63, 65
biceps brachii muscle, 82, 83, 84
  tendon, 79, 82, 83, 84
    long head, 79
biceps femoris muscle, 134, 153, 155, 164, 223, 224, 228
  long head, 221
  short head, 221
  tendon, 228
bicipital aponeurosis, 84
bile duct, 235
  common, 126, 174, 176, 182
biliary system, 182
  radionuclide scans, 235
biparietal diameter measurement, 202
bite block, 34
bladder (urinary), 132, 134, 137, 139, 142, 147, 148, 151, 152, 153, 157, 158, 159, 160, 162, 166, 169, 170, 189, 219, 220
  base and neck, 152, 198
  contrast medium in, 188, 198
  fetal, 200, 201, 203
  full, 199
  internal sphincter, 156
  isotope scan, 235
  non-cross-sectional views, 188, 189, 196, 197, 199, 219
  PET/CT scan, 239
  trigone, 153, 156, 159
bone(s), wrist and hand, 74–5
  see also specific bones

brachial artery, 76, 82, 83, 84
  deep (profunda brachii artery), 76, 84
  muscular branches, 76
brachialis muscle, 82, 83, 84
  tendon, 84
brachiocephalic artery, 33
brachiocephalic trunk, 92, 96, 100,
    104, 105, 106, 108, 117, 138
brachiocephalic vein, 77
  left, 92, 96, 100, 108, 138, 149
    site of entry, 77
  right, 33, 93, 97, 102, 109
brachioradialis muscle, 82, 83, 84, 85
brain, 16–17, 36–53
  fetal, 202
  neonatal, new, 52–3
  PET metabolic scan, 238
  vessels, 36–41
brainstem, 52, 53
  PET scan, 238
  superior cerebellar arteries behind,
    38
breast (female), 90, 120–2, 136
  PET/CT scan, 239
broad ligament of uterus, 151, 155,
    156, 159, 161
bronchial arteriogram, 116
bronchial artery, 116
bronchial trunk, common, 116
bronchogram
  left lung, 118
  right lung, 119
bronchus
  anterior basal segmental, 94, 118,
    119
  anterior segmental, 92, 118, 119
  apical (superior) segmental, 118, 119
  apical segment inferior lobe, 94
  apical segmental, 119
  apicoposterior segmental, 118
  carina of trachea bifurcating to, 90,
    96, 100, 108, 142
  inferior lobe, 119
    apical segment, 94
    left, 92, 94, 96, 108
    right, 95, 97, 109
  intermediate, 92, 118, 140
  lateral basal segmental, 94, 118
  lateral segmental, of middle lobe, 94,
    119
  lingular segmental, 92
    inferior, 94, 118
    superior, 95, 118
  main
    left, 58, 90, 92, 96, 100, 101,
      104, 105, 106, 108, 118, 140,
      142
    right, 58, 90, 91, 93, 97, 102,
      104, 105, 106, 109, 118, 119,
      140, 142
  medial basal segmental, 95, 118,
    119
  medial segmental, of middle lobe, 95,
    119
  middle lobe, 95
  posterior basal segmental, 95, 118,
    119
  posterior segmental, 93, 119
  superior lobe
    left, 92, 96, 108
    right, 93, 97, 109, 119
  upper lobe
    left, 140
    right, 140
bulbous urethra, 198

c

C1 see atlas
C1/C2 intervertebral foramen, 61
C2 see axis
C2/C3
  facet joint, 61
  uncovertebral joint, 61

C3
  body, 25
  spinous process, 56
  uncus, 63
C3/C4
  facet joint, 56
  intervertebral disc, 56
  uncovertebral joint, 56
C4
  articular processes see articular
    processes
  body, 25
  lamina, 56
  pars interarticularis, 56
  pedicle, 56
  spinous process, 56
  transverse process, 56
  uncus (posterolateral lip), 56
C5
  articular processes see articular
    processes
  body, 57
  lamina, 57
  spinous process, 57
  transverse process, 56, 57
  uncus, 57
C6
  body, 58
  lamina, 56
  pedicle, 56
C7
  body, 62
  pars interarticularis, 56
  transverse process, 56, 64
C7/T1, intervertebral foramen, 56
C8 nerve roots, 64
  intervertebral foramen, 56
caecum, 131, 132, 137, 139, 141,
    157, 167, 172
  non-cross-sectional views, 172, 179,
    180, 181
calcaneal artery, medial, 217
calcaneal tendon (Achilles tendon), 230,
    233
calcaneocuboid joint, 233
calcaneofibular ligament, 231
calcaneonavicular ligament, plantar, 232
calcaneus, 125, 212, 214, 231, 232,
    233, 234
  anterior tubercle, 233
  girl, 213
  lateral and medial process, 212
  posterior aspect, centre for, 213, 215
  sustentaculum tali, 212, 231, 232,
    233
calcarine artery, 38
calcarine cortex, 21, 44
calf (leg), 229
  arteriogram, 127
  lymphatics, 206
  peripheral lower leg lymphatic
    channels, 206
  venous plexus, 218
calix see calyx
callosomarginal artery, 36, 45, 48
calvarium of skull, 45
  inner table, 45
  outer table, 45
calyx
  major, 196, 197
  minor, 196, 197
  upper pole, 194
canaliculi, lacrimal, 23
canine tooth, 34
capitate, 73, 74, 75, 86
capitulum of humerus, 70, 71, 72, 82,
    83
capsula interna (internal capsule), PET
    scan, 238
capsular veins, 194
  right, 189
capsule
  articular see articular capsule
  of white matter see external capsule;
    internal capsule
cardinal ligament (transverse cervical
    ligament), 151, 159

cardiophrenic angle, left, 90
carina (bifurcation of trachea to left/
    right bronchi), 90, 96, 100, 108,
    142
carotid arteries, 36, 37
  common, 28, 29, 33, 62
    left, 33, 92, 96, 100, 101, 104,
      106, 108, 117, 140
    right, 33, 102, 117
  external, 25, 33
    catheter tip in, 33
  internal, 9, 14, 16, 21, 22, 23, 25,
      32, 33, 40, 42, 43, 48
    bifurcation, 45
    cavernous portion, 9, 36, 44, 46
    cervical portion, 36
    intracranial/supraclinoid, 36, 44
    petrous portion, 33, 36
carotid sulcus, 3
carpus, 75
cauda equina, 62, 63, 65
caudal lumbar thecal sac, 63
caudate nucleus
  body, 45, 50, 52, 53
  head, 45, 46, 48, 52, 53
  PET scan, 238
caudate segment of liver, 125
caudate vein, anterior, 37
caval veins see vena cava
cavernous body of penis see corpus
    cavernosum
cavernous sinus, 23, 37, 48
  dural lateral wall, 48
  internal carotid artery in, 9, 36, 44,
    46
cavum septum pellucidum, 52, 53, 202
  fetal, 202
central sulcus (of Rolando), 45, 46
central sulcus artery, 36
centrum semiovale, 45
cephalic vein, 77, 78, 82, 83, 84, 85,
    86
cerebellar artery
  anterior inferior, 17, 38
  posterior inferior, 38, 64
    hemispheric branch, 38
    inferior vermian segment, 38
    medullary segment, 38
    origin, 38
    retrotonsillar segment, 38
    supratonsillar segment, 38
  superior, 38, 40, 49
    behind brainstem, 38
    hemispheric branch, 38
    thalamoperforating branches, 38
    vermian branch, 38
cerebellar peduncles
  inferior, 46, 51
  middle, 43, 46, 47
  superior, 18, 44, 46, 47, 51
cerebellar vein, precentral, 38
cerebellomedullary cistern see cisterna
    magna
cerebellopontine angle, 43
cerebellum, 46, 47, 52, 53
  dendate nucleus, 51
  fetal, 202
  flocculonodular lobe, 43
  hemispheres, 16, 46, 51
    folia, 42, 46, 47, 51
    PET scan, 238
  nodule, 51
  tent (tentorium cerebelli), 46
  tonsil, 42, 47, 51
  vermis
    inferior, 43
    superior, 44
cerebral aqueduct (of Sylvius), 21, 45,
    47, 51
cerebral artery
  anterior, 36, 40, 45, 46, 47, 48
    internal frontal branch, 36
  middle, 21, 36, 45, 46, 47, 48, 49
    angular branches (=angular artery),
      36
    anterior temporal branches, 36
    genu, 36, 39

  insular branches, 36, 39
  parietal branches see parietal
    artery
  second order branch, 45
  posterior, 19, 21, 36, 38, 44, 49
    in ambient cistern, 38, 40
    in interpeduncular cistern, 38
    posterior choroidal branches, 38
    precommunicating segment, 40
    quadrigeminal portion, 38, 40
    splenial branches, 38
    thalamoperforating branches, 38
cerebral peduncles, 19, 21, 45, 46,
    47, 50
  middle, 51
cerebral sulci
  central (of Rolando), 45, 46
  cingulate sulcus, 46
  lateral (Sylvian fissure), 45, 46, 47,
    48, 52
cerebral veins
  great see Galen
  internal (of Galen), 37, 39, 41, 45,
    46, 47, 51
  superficial, 37, 41
cerebrospinal fluid, spine, 62, 63
cervical artery, ascending, 33, 117
cervical ligament, transverse, 151,
    159
cervical portion of internal carotid
    artery, 36
cervical spinal cord, 25, 46, 47, 61,
    62, 64
cervical spine, 61
  isotope scan, 235
  see also C1; C2 etc.
cervix of uterus, 144, 148, 155, 160,
    195
  in fetal ultrasound, 200, 201
  os, 161
    external, 150, 161
    internal, 150, 161
  wall, 151, 161
chamber of eye see eye
chest see thorax
cholangiopancreatogram
  endoscopic retrograde, 182
  MR, 182
choroid, 23
choroid plexus, 49, 52, 53
  fetal, 202
choroidal artery, anterior, 36
choroidal branches of posterior cerebral
    artery, posterior, 38
choroidal vein, superior, 39
choroidal vessels (unspecified), 45
ciliary body, 21
cingulate gyrus, 45, 46, 47, 48
cingulate sulcus, 46
circumflex artery (circumflex branch of
    left coronary artery), 108, 113,
    114, 115
  obtuse marginal branch see marginal
    branch of circumflex artery
circumflex femoral vessels, 157
  lateral circumflex femoral artery, 187,
    216
  lateral circumflex femoral vein, 218
  medial circumflex femoral artery, 216
circumflex humeral artery see humeral
    artery
circumflex iliac artery, deep, 187
circumflex scapular artery, 76
cistern
  ambient see ambient cistern
  cerebromedullary see cisterna magna
  interpeduncular see interpenduncular
    cistern
  oculomotor, 18
  prepontine, 46, 47, 49
  quadrigeminal, 45
  suprasellar see suprasellar cistern
cisterna chyli, 205, 206
cisterna magna (cerebellomedullary
    cistern), 43, 46, 47, 51, 64
  fetal, 202
claustrum, 45

clavicle, 27, 56, 58, 68, 69, 79, 90,
    96, 100, 108, 136, 138, 145,
    149
    isotope scan, 235
clinoid process, anterior, 3, 11, 13,
    21, 48
clivus, 3, 9, 13, 17, 22, 43, 53, 64
    lower see basi-occiput
coccygeus muscle, 159
coccyx, 60, 159, 197
    female, 148, 151, 160
        segment, 173
    male, 134, 163, 169
cochlea, 9, 15, 43, 50
cochlear nerve, 17
coeliac axis, 105, 107, 140, 148
coeliac trunk, 124, 184
    catheter tip in, 184
    non-cross-sectional views, 174, 176,
        183, 184
    subtracted arteriograms, 184
colic artery
    left, 185, 186
        ascending branch, 186
        descending branch, 186
    middle, 185
    right, 185
colic vein, left, 186
collateral ligaments (of knee)
    lateral, 224, 228
    medial, 228
        deep portion, 225
        superficial portion, 225
collateral vein (in orbit)
    anterior, 23
    medial, 23
colliculus
    inferior, 44, 46, 51
    seminal, 198, 199
    superior, 45, 46, 47, 51
colon, 181
    ascending, 124, 126, 128, 130, 132,
        137, 139, 140, 143, 148
        non-cross-sectional views, 172,
            179, 180, 181
    descending, 62, 126, 130, 137, 139,
        140, 143, 148, 155, 166
        non-cross-sectional views, 172,
            180, 181
    flexures see hepatic flexure; splenic
        flexure
    marginal artery of (Drummond's), 186
    sacculations, 180
    sigmoid see sigmoid colon
    transverse see transverse colon
colonography, CT, 181
commissure
    anterior, 21, 45, 47
    posterior, 45
common tendinous origin
    in elbow
        extensors, 83, 84
        flexors, 83, 84
    hamstrings, 154, 158, 163, 165
communicating artery
    anterior, 36, 40, 45
    posterior, 36, 38, 40
concha, nasal see turbinates
condylar fossa of TMJ, 14
condyles
    femoral, lateral, 210, 224, 225, 226,
        228
        eminence, 228
    femoral, medial, 210, 224, 225, 226,
        228
    mandibular, 3, 4, 12, 32
        head, 7, 8, 14, 34
        neck, 7, 8, 34
    occipital, 8, 13, 42, 61
    tibial, lateral and medial, 210
connecting vein, superficial (in orbit), 23
constrictor muscle of pharynx, superior,
    25
conus arteriosus (pulmonary conus;
    right ventricular outflow tract),
    105, 107, 112, 115, 136, 149
conus artery, 113

right, 114
conus medullaris, 62 63, 65
Cooper's ligament, 121, 122
coracobrachialis muscle, 79
coracoclavicular ligament, 79
coracohumeral ligament, 79
coracoid process of scapula, 68, 69, 79
cornea, 23
corona radiata, 45, 46, 49
    PET scan, 238
coronal suture, 3, 4
    fetal, 202
coronary arteries, 113
    angiogram, 113, 114
    left, 113, 114, 115
        anterior interventricular branch
            (=left anterior descending), 96,
            108, 113, 114, 115
        circumflex branch see circumflex
            artery
        main stem, 113
    right, 105, 107, 109, 113, 114, 115,
        117
        posterior interventricular branch,
            114
coronary sinus, 96
    left, 113
    right, 114
coronoid process
    mandible, 6, 8, 11, 12, 34, 42, 49
    ulna, 70, 82
corpus callosum, 52
    body, 46, 47, 48, 53
    genu, 45, 46, 47, 48, 53
        PET scan, 238
    pericallosal artery extending around,
        36
    splenium, 45, 46, 47, 51, 53
        PET scan, 238
corpus cavernosum, 134, 163, 164,
    167, 168, 169, 170, 198
    cavernosogram, 198
    crus (crus of penis), 134, 164, 167
corpus luteal cyst, 155, 156, 158
corpus spongiosum, 167, 168, 169
cortical veins, 45, 46
    superficial, 37
costal cartilage
    anterior, 103
    female, 136
costocervical trunk, 33, 117
costophrenic angle, left, 90
costotransverse joint, 96
costovertebral joint, 96
cranial fossa
    anterior, floor, 6
    posterior, 16–17
cranial nerves, 18–19
cranium see skull
cribriform plate (of ethmoid bone), 10,
    11, 13
cricoid cartilage, 29, 32
crista galli, 2, 10, 21, 45
crown of tooth, 34
crown–rump length, 200
cruciate ligaments
    anterior, 224, 225, 228
    posterior, 224, 225, 228
crus
    diaphragm see diaphragm
    penis/corpus cavernosum, 134, 164,
        167
cubital vein, median, 77
cuboid, 212, 213, 214, 215, 230, 232,
    234
cuneiform
    intermediate, 213, 214, 215, 230,
        234
    lateral, 212, 213, 214, 215, 230,
        234
    medial, 214, 215, 230, 233, 234
cystic duct, 174, 176, 182

D
deciduous teeth, 34
deep artery of penis, 198

deep artery of thigh (profunda femoris
    artery), 135, 153, 164, 167,
    187, 216, 219, 221, 223
deep brachial artery (profunda brachii
    artery), 76, 84
deep circumflex iliac artery, 187
deep fascia of thigh (fascia lata), 150,
    152, 163, 164, 165, 166, 228
deep femoral vessels see femoral
    artery; femoral vein; femoral
    vessels
deep inguinal nodes, 204, 205
deep palmar (arterial) arch, 76, 78, 88
deep palmar branch of ulnar artery, 78
deep perineal pouch, 156
deltoid branch of thoraco-acromial
    artery, 117
deltoid insertion of levator muscle, 29,
    54
deltoid ligament, 231
    deep portion, 232
    superficial portion, 232
deltoid muscle, 79
    tendon, 79
dendate nucleus of cerebellum, 51
dens (odontoid process/peg) of axis, 2,
    4, 6, 8, 13, 14, 22, 25, 46, 47,
    50, 56, 57, 61, 64
dentition, 34
diagonal arteries (coronary vessels),
    113, 114
diaphragm, abdominothoracic, 124, 194
    left (hemidiaphragm), 96, 137, 141,
        143, 144, 149
        crus, 126, 128, 143, 144
        dome, 90, 91, 105, 107, 174, 176
    right (hemidiaphragm), 97, 137, 141,
        143, 144, 147
        crus, 129, 141, 143, 144, 148
        dome, 90, 91, 105, 107, 175, 177
diaphragm, urogenital, see also
    urogenital diaphragm
diastole
    angiogram of LV in, 113
    end of see end diastole
digastric muscle
    anterior belly, 24, 30
    posterior belly, 24
digitally subtracted arteriograms see
    subtraction angiography
diploë, 3, 45
diploic veins, 47
discs
    articular, of temporomandibular joints,
        7
    intervertebral see intervertebral discs
dorsal artery, foot (dorsalis pedis
    artery), 217
dorsal interosseous muscles
    foot, 234
    hand, 87, 88
dorsal pancreatic artery see pancreatic
    artery
dorsal penile vessels, 163, 170
dorsal root (of spinal nerve)
    cervical, 64
    ganglion, 62
dorsal sacroiliac ligaments, 159
dorsal tubercle of radius, 86
dorsal venous arch
    foot, 217
    hand, 86
dorsum sellae, 3, 4, 13, 14, 21, 22
Douglas' (rectouterine) pouch, 151,
    155, 161
Drummond's (marginal) artery, 186
ductus (vas) deferens, 133, 170, 199
    ampulla, 199
duodenum
    ascending (fourth) part, 129
    descending (second) part, 124, 126,
        128
        non-cross-sectional views, 178,
            179, 182, 235
    double-contrast barium meals, 178
    flexure at junction of jejunum and,
        129

horizontal (third) part, 128, 178
    isotope scan, 235
    superior part (first part; cap), 127,
        139, 178
dural lateral wall of cavernous sinus, 48

E
ear, 14–15
    external
        pinna, 3, 7, 42
        tragus, 50
    inner, 12
    middle, 12
        cavity of see tympanic cavity
        inner, 9
        ossicles (incus and malleus), 67
ejaculatory duct, left, 199
elbow, 71–2, 82–5
end diastole
    3D reconstructions of left ventricle at,
        237
    blood pool volume within LV at, 237
end systole
    3D reconstructions of LV at, 237
    blood pool volume within LV at, 237
endometrium, 161
endoscopic retrograde
    cholangiopancreatography, 182
endotracheal tube, 33
epicondyles
    femoral, lateral and medial, 210
    humeral, 70, 71, 72, 73, 82, 83, 84
epididymis, 134
    body, 169
    head, 168, 169
epidural space, 62, 63
epigastric artery, superficial inferior,
    133
epigastric vessels
    inferior, 163, 168
    superficial, 150
epiglottis, 24, 26, 29, 32, 56, 61
epiphyseal discs, annular see annular
    epiphyseal discs
epiphyseal line/scar
    ankle, 213
    elbow, 72
    femur, 208, 209, 211, 226
    hand, 75
    shoulder, 69
epitympanum, 14
erector spinae muscle, 62, 96, 108,
    124, 126, 128, 131, 132, 140,
    144, 154, 159, 160, 169, 170
ethmoid bone
    cribriform plate, 10, 11, 13
    orbital layer (lamina papyracea), 9, 10
    perpendicular plate, 11
ethmoidal air cells, 2, 3, 21, 43
    anterior, 9, 10
    middle, 9
    posterior, 9
ethmoidal branch of ophthalmic artery,
    36
ethmoidal sinuses, 6, 8, 23
Eustachian (auditory) tubes, 9, 32
extensor carpi radialis brevis muscle,
    83, 84, 85
extensor carpi radialis longus muscle,
    83, 84, 85
    tendon, 85
extensor carpi ulnaris muscle, 85
    tendon, 86
extensor digiti minimi muscle, tendon,
    86, 87
extensor digitorum brevis muscle, 231,
    232, 233, 234
extensor digitorum longus muscle, 224,
    229
    tendon, 232, 234
extensor digitorum muscle
    ankle, 230
        tendon, 230, 233
    wrist/hand, 85
        tendon, 86, 87

extensor hallucis longus muscle, 229, 230
tendon, 230, 232, 234
extensor origin, common, 83, 84
extensor pollicis brevis muscle, tendon, 86, 87
extensor pollicis longus muscle, 84
tendon, 86, 87, 88
extensor retinaculum, ankle, 230
external capsule, 45, 48
extraperitoneal fat (cave of Retzius/ retropubic space), 152, 159, 160, 161, 169
eyeball (globe of eye), 9, 10, 12, 18, 20, 22, 23, 46
anterior chamber, 21, 23
lens, 23, 44
vitreous chamber, and humour, 21, 23
eyelids, 10, 23

F
facet see articular processes
facet (zygapophyseal) joint, 62
C2/C3, 61
C3/C4, 56
L4/L5, 59
L5/S1, 165
facial artery, 33
labial branch, 33
facial bones, 6, 8–13
isotope scan, 235
facial nerve (CN7), 16, 18, 43, 50
in stylomastoid foramen, 17
fallopian tube see uterine tube
falx cerebri, 45, 48, 52
fetal, 202
fascia
pectoralis, anterior, 120, 121
renal, 127, 129
subcutaneous (abdomen), 129
thoracolumbar, 62, 159, 161
Waldeyer's, 151, 159, 161
fascia lata, 150, 152, 163, 164, 165, 166, 228
fat pad
ankle, 233
elbow, anterior, 80
infrapatellar, 227, 228
feet see foot
femoral artery, 134, 139, 219, 220, 221, 222, 223
common, 151, 152, 157, 161, 162, 168, 216
deep (profunda femoris artery), 135, 153, 164, 167, 187, 216, 219, 221, 223
intertrochanteric part, 154
lateral circumflex, 187, 216
left, catheter introduced into distal abdominal aorta via, 216
medial circumflex, 216
right, catheter introduced into distal abdominal aorta via, 187
superficial, 135, 153, 164, 187, 216
femoral canal, 152, 157, 168
femoral nerve, 221
branches, 151, 162
femoral vein, 134, 139, 218, 219, 221
catheter tip introduced via
into left femoral vein, 189
into left internal iliac vein, 188
into superior vena cava and azygos vein, 116
common, 151, 152, 157, 161, 162
deep (profunda femoris vein), 164
lateral circumflex, 218
muscular tributary, 218
superficial, 153, 164
femoral vessels
circumflex see circumflex femoral vessels
common, 147, 167, 168
deep (profunda femoris vessels), 153
left, 149

superficial, 167
femur, 142, 208, 209, 210, 211, 221, 222
condyles see condyles
epicondyles, lateral and medial, 210
epiphysial line, 208, 209, 211
fetal, 202, 203
length measurement, 203
greater trochanter, 134, 145, 151, 152, 158, 163, 166, 208, 219, 220, 223
centre for, 209
sotope scan, 235
head, 134, 139, 141, 149, 152, 162, 163, 165, 167, 193, 208, 209, 219, 222, 223
centre for, 209
fovea of (fovea capitalis), 165, 167, 208
isotope scan, 235
ligament (=ligamentum teres femoris), 135, 163
intercondylar fossa, 209
intertrochanteric, 208
lesser trochanter, 135, 153, 155, 163, 164, 167, 208
centre for, 209
neck, 135, 152, 163, 165, 167, 208, 209, 220, 223
shaft, isotope scan, 235
tubercles of intercondylar eminence, 210
fetal ultrasound, 200–3
fibula, 211, 212, 213, 229, 230, 232, 233
apex/styloid process, 210
distal, centre for, 213, 215
head, 210, 224, 226
centre for, 211
malleolus, lateral and medial, 213
neck, 210
fibular (peroneal) nerve, common, 224, 228
fibular (peroneal) retinaculum, 230
fibularis brevis and longus muscles; see peroneus
filum terminale, 148, 161
flexor accessorius muscle, 230, 231, 232, 234
flexor carpi radialis muscle, 83, 84, 85
tendon, 86
flexor carpi ulnaris muscle, 82, 83, 84, 85
tendon, 86
flexor digiti minimi muscle
foot, 232, 234
hand, 87, 88
flexor digitorum brevis muscle, 231, 232, 233, 234
tendon, 232, 234
flexor dig torum longus muscle, 230, 233, 234
tendon, 230, 231, 232, 233, 234
flexor digitorum profundus muscle, 82, 83, 84, 85
tendon, 86, 87, 88
flexor digitorum superficialis muscle, 82, 83, 84, 85, 86
tendon, 86, 87, 88
flexor hallucis brevis muscle, 232, 234
sesamoids in, 214, 234
flexor hallucis longus muscle, 229, 230, 233
tendon, 230, 231, 232, 233, 234
flexor origin, common, 83, 84
flexor pollicis brevis muscle, 87, 88
flexor pollicis longus muscle, tendon, 86, 87, 88
flexor retinaculum
ankle, 230
wrist, 86
flocculonocular lobe of cerebellum, 43
fluorodeoxyglucose in PET brain scan, 238
foramen
alveolar, inferior (of mandibular ramus), 61

incisive, 13
infraorbital, 6
interventricular (of Monro), 46, 47, 50, 57
intervertebral see intervertebral foramen
jugular, 15, 16, 43
Luschka's, 17, 43, 51
Magendie's, 42, 51
obturator, 173, 208, 209
palatine, greater, 12
sacral, anterior/pelvic, 60, 133, 173
sciatic, 145
sphenopalatine, 11
stylomastoid see stylomastoid foramen
transverse see transverse foramen
foramen lacerum, 9, 14
foramen magnum, 4, 42, 46, 47, 51, 62, 64
foramen rotundum, 2, 9, 11
foramen spinosum, 9
forceps major and minor, 45
forearm, 73, 85
fetal ultrasound, 203
fornix
of brain, 47
of vagina, posterior, 151, 156, 161
four chamber view of fetal heart, 203
fovea capitalis of femur, 165, 167, 208
fovea ethmoidalis, frontal bone, 11
frontal bone, 10
fovea ethmoidalis, 11
orbital plate, 45
orbital roof, 11
zygomatic process, 6, 7
frontal branch of anterior cerebral artery, internal, 36
frontal horn of lateral ventricle, 45, 48
frontal lobe, 45, 48, 53
orbital cortex of, 46, 47
PET scan, 238
frontal process of zygoma, 3, 6
frontal sinus, 2, 3, 10, 44, 46, 47
infundibulum, 44
frontal veins, 21
frontopolar artery, 36, 45
frontozygomatic suture, 6
fundus
gall bladder, 174, 176
stomach see stomach
uterus, 150, 157, 161, 195

G
Galen
great cerebral vein of, 37, 39, 40, 46, 47
cistern of see ambient cistern
internal cerebral vein of, 37, 39, 41, 45, 46, 47, 51
gall bladder, 124, 126, 136, 138, 146
fundus, 174, 176
neck, 182
non-cross-sectional view, 174, 176, 182
gastric artery, 185
left, 140, 183, 184
catheter tip in origin of, 185
oesophageal branch of, 185
right, 185
gastric veins
left, 185
oesophageal branches, 185
short, 185
gastrocnemius muscle
aponeurosis, 229
lateral head, 222, 224, 226, 229
medial head, 224, 227, 228, 229
tendon, 227
gastroduodenal arteriogram, selective, 193
gastroduodenal artery, 184, 192, 193
gastro-omental (gastro-epiploic) artery
left, 184, 191
right, 184, 191

gemellus muscle, 134, 155, 165, 219, 220, 223
genicular artery
lateral inferior, 216, 217
lateral superior, 216, 225, 226
medial inferior, 216, 217, 225
medial superior, 216, 217, 225, 226
genicular vein, lateral superior, 226
geniculate bodies, medial and lateral, 21
genioglossus muscle, 24, 30
geniohyoid muscle, 26, 30
genitalia, external, fetal male, 203
genu
corpus callosum see corpus callosum
internal capsule, PET scan, 238
middle cerebral artery, 36, 39
gestation sac, 200, 201
glans penis, 168, 169, 170
glenohumeral ligament
inferior, 79
middle, 80
superior, 80
glenoid/glenoid fossa, 68, 69, 79
labrum see labrum
globe of eye see eyeball
globus pallidus, 45, 49
glossopharyngeal nerve (CN9), 16, 18
glottis, 28
gluteal artery
inferior, 134, 187
superior, 133, 187
gluteal veins
inferior, 134, 188
superior, 133, 188
gluteal vessels
inferior, 154, 162
superior, 150, 154, 158, 165
gluteus maximus muscle, 133, 134, 141, 144, 147, 148, 150, 152, 154, 158, 161, 162, 164, 165, 167, 170, 219, 220, 221
gluteus medius muscle, 133, 134, 139, 141, 145, 150, 153, 154, 156, 161, 162, 165, 166, 219, 220
gluteus minimus muscle, 133, 134, 150, 155, 156, 161, 162, 165, 166, 219, 220
tendinous insertion, 153
gonadal vessels
female, 155
male, 165
gracilis muscle, 134, 155, 157, 167, 221, 223, 228
tendon, 224
grey matter, brain, 45
spinal cord, 62
Guyon's canal, 86
gyri (cerebral)
cingulate, 45, 46, 47, 48
gyrus rectus, 21
insular, 45, 48
postcentral, 45
precentral, 45

H
hamate, 73, 74, 75, 86
hook, 74, 86
hamstrings, origin, 154, 158, 163, 165
hamulus on medial pterygoid plate, 61
haustrations, colon, 180
heart, 94, 112–15, 120, 121, 237
3D reconstructions, 115, 237
fetal ultrasound, 200, 201, 203
silhouette on lung scan, 236
hemi-azygos vein, 94, 96, 108
accessory, 116
hemidiaphragm see diaphragm
hemisphere, cerebellar see cerebellum
hemispheric branches
posterior inferior cerebellar artery, 38
superior cerebellar artery, 38
hemispheric vein
inferior, 39
superior, 39

hepatic artery, 174, 183, 184
  common, 124, 141, 149
  left, 184
  non-cross-sectional views, 174, 175, 176, 183, 184
  right, 175, 177, 184
hepatic duct
  common, 182
  left, 182
  right, 182
hepatic (right colic) flexure, 127, 129, 136, 139, 140, 146
  non-cross-sectional views, 172, 180, 181
hepatic veins, 140, 142, 147, 148, 190
  branch, 174, 176
    left, 175, 177
    middle, 126, 175, 177
    right, 127, 175, 177
hepatobiliary scan, 235
hepatopancreatic ampulla, 182
hepatorenal recess, 174, 176
Heubner's recurrent artery, 36
hip, 208, 219–20
hip joint, 197
hippocampus, 44, 49
horizontal fissure, 84, 91, 92
  great, vein of the, 39
Houston's fold, 154, 159
humeral artery
  anterior circumflex, 76
  posterior circumflex, 76
humerus, 70, 72, 73, 74, 82, 83, 84
  anatomical neck, 68
  capitulum, 70, 71, 72, 82, 83
  epicondyles see epicondyles
  head, 68, 69, 79
    isotope scan, 235
  intertubercular groove, 68
  olecranon fossa, 70, 82, 83, 84
  shaft, isotope scan, 235
  surgical neck, 68
  trochlea, 70, 72, 82, 83
  tuberosities see tuberosities
Hunter's (subsartorial) canal, 222
hyoid bone, 34, 57
  body, 25, 29
  greater horn, 25, 29
hypoglossal nerve (CN12), 18
hypoglossus muscle, 30
hypopharynx, 24, 26–9
hypothalamus
  mamillary body, 19, 45, 50
hypotympanum, 14
hysterosalpingography, 195

I

ileal branches of superior mesenteric artery, 131, 139, 185
ileocaecal valve, 179
ileocolic artery, 131, 183, 185
ileocolic vein, 191
ileum, 128, 130, 131, 137, 138, 141, 149, 150
  proximal, 179
  terminal, 131, 132, 139, 179, 181
iliac artery, 185
  common, 157, 187
    isotope scan, 236
    left, 131, 132, 138, 236
    right, 131, 132, 138, 147, 236
  deep circumflex, 187
  external, 134, 139, 150, 157, 159, 167, 187, 219, 220
    left, 132
    right, 132, 147
  internal, 159, 187
    anterior trunk of, 187
    branches, 156
    left, 132
    posterior trunk of, 187
    right, 1, 132
iliac bone see ilium
iliac lymph nodes, common and external, 204, 205

iliac lymphatics, efferent, 204
iliac vein
  common, 169, 189, 190
    catheter in, 66
    left, 131, 132, 141, 160
    right, 131, 132, 141, 147
  external, 134, 139, 150, 167, 190
    catheter tip introduced via left femoral vein into, 188
    left, 132, 188
    right, 132, 147
  internal, 159, 190
    anterior division, 188
    left, 132
    right, 132
iliac vessels
  common
    bifurcation, 155
    point of ureteric crossover, 197
  internal
    branches, 155
    left and right, 143, 150
iliacus muscle, 132, 138, 140, 143, 150, 155, 156, 158, 165, 166, 220
iliolumbar artery, 187
iliolumbar ligament, 155
iliolumbar vein, 190
iliopsoas muscle, 134, 137, 138, 146, 151, 153, 157, 158, 161, 162, 164, 219, 220, 222, 223
  tendon, 163, 164
  see also psoas muscle
iliotibial tract, 134, 153, 164, 221, 223, 224, 228
ilium (iliac bone)
  crest, 59, 60, 135, 173, 209, 220
    centre for, 173
    female, 137
  female, 139, 141, 144, 147, 149, 150, 154, 158
    crest, 137, 155, 156
    girl, 206
    isotope scan, 235
  male, 131, 132, 166, 167
  spine
    anterior inferior, 150, 173, 208
    anterior superior, 167, 173
incisive canal, 8
incisive foramen, 13
incisors, 34
incus, 9, 15
infrahyoid strap muscle, 28, 29
infra-orbital artery, 33
infra-orbital foramen, 6
infraspinatus muscle, 79, 96, 145
  tendon, 79
infratemporal fossa, 49
infundibulum
  right ventricle, 91
inguinal canal, 168, 170
inguinal ligament
  female, 152
  male, 168
inguinal lymph nodes, 168, 204, 205
inguinal lymphatics, 204, 205
inion, 3, 43
innominate bone, 209
insular branches/segment of middle cerebral artery in, 36, 40
insular gyrus, 45, 48
interatrial septum, 96, 100, 108
  fetal, 203
intercondylar eminence, tubercles of, 210
intercondylar fossa, 209
intercostal artery, 108, 116, 117
  left 11th, se-ective catheterisation, 66
intercostal muscle, 145
intercostal veins, 116
  right superior, 109
intercostobronchial trunk, catheter tip in, 116
interhemispheric fissure, 45
interlobar arteries, 194
intermuscular septum, femoral

lateral, 221, 223
median, 226
internal capsule
  anterior limb, 45, 48
  PET scan, 238
  posterior limb, 45
internuclear cleft, 63
interosseous artery
  anterior, 76, 85
  common, 76
  posterior, 76
interosseous membrane
  forearm, 85
  leg, 229, 230
interosseous muscles
  foot, 234
    dorsal, 234
    plantar, 234
  hand
    dorsal, 87, 88
    palmar, 87, 88
interpenduncular cistern, 18, 50
  posterior cerebral artery in, 38
interspinous ligament, 63
interthalamic adhesion (massa intermedia) of thalamus, 50
intertrochanteric crest of femur, 208
intertrochanteric line, 208
intertrochanteric part of femur, 154
intertubercular groove of humerus, 68
intertubercular lamella of C4 transverse process, 56
interventricular artery, left anterior, 113
interventricular branch
  anterior, of left coronary artery (=left anterior descending artery), 96, 108, 113, 114, 115
  posterior, of right coronary artery, 114
interventricular foramen of Monro, 34, 46, 47, 50, 57
interventricular septal artery, posterior (=posterior descending artery), 113
interventricular septum, 97, 101, 104, 105, 106, 108, 109
  fetal, 203
  isotope scan, 237
  PET/CT scan, 239
intervertebral discs
  C3/C4, 56
  lumbar
    indentation in anterior thecal margin, 65
    L4/L5, 59, 167, 169
  lumbosacral (L5/S1), 155, 159, 160
  sacral, space for, 60
  thoracic, 58
    T5/T6 nucleus pulposus, 62
intervertebral (neural) foramen
  C7/T1, 56
  cervical, 61
  lumbar, 59, 63
    catheter tip in, 66
intracranial portion
  internal carotid arteries, 36, 44
  optic nerve, 19, 21, 22
intralobular ducts, 182
intravertebral veins, 66
ischio-anal fossa, 223
  female, 151, 152, 154, 158, 161
  male, 134, 163, 164, 165, 166, 169, 170
ischiocavernosus, 164, 167
ischium, 223
  female, 145, 147, 149, 152, 153, 154, 158, 173, 209
    ramus, 173
  male, 134, 135, 163, 164, 165, 167, 173
  spine, 208
    female, 208
    male, 134, 163
  tuberosity, 153, 154, 158, 163, 164, 165, 173, 208, 223
    isotope scan, 235

J

jejunal branches of superior mesenteric artery, 131, 139, 183, 185
jejunal vein, 191
jejunum, 124, 126, 128, 130, 138, 139, 141, 146, 149
  flexure at junction of duodenum and, 129
  isotope scan, 235
  valvulae conniventes (plicae circulares), 179
joints see specific joints and entries under articular
jugular bulb, 33, 37, 39, 41
jugular foramen, 15, 16, 43
jugular vein
  anterior, 26
  external, 24, 26
  internal, 24, 26, 29, 33, 36, 37, 38, 39, 41, 42, 50, 62
    right, 146

K

kidney, 63, 126, 127, 128, 129, 140, 142, 145, 146, 172, 175, 177, 196, 197, 203, 235, 236
  calyx see calyx
  cortex, 127, 128
    PET/CT scan, 239
  fascia, 127, 129
  fetal, 203
  isotope scans, 235
  lower poles, 194
  papilla, 175, 196
  pelvis, 127, 129, 196
  upper poles, 194, 196
  see also entries under renal

L

L1, body, 59, 142
L2
  body, 65
  inferior articular process, 59
  lamina, 59
L3
  body, 63, 235
  spinous process, 59, 65
  superior articular process, 59
  transverse process, 59
L3/L4, lumbar puncture needle in space between, 65
L4, spinal nerve, 65
L4/L5 articular/intervertebral disc, 59, 167, 169
L5, 169, 170
  body, 148, 165, 166, 197
  nerve root, 159, 160, 161, 165
  spinal nerve, 65
  spinous process, 154
  transverse process, 143
L5/S1
  facet joint, 165
  intervertebral disc, 155, 159, 160
Labbé, vein of, 37, 41
labial branch of facial artery, 33
labium majus/majorum, 137, 153, 157
labium minus/minorum, 155, 157
labrum
  acetabular, 219, 220
  glenoid, 28, 79, 80
labyrinthine artery, 43
lacrimal canaliculi, 23
lacrimal gland, 20, 44
lacrimal sac (nasolacrimal sac), 10, 23
lambdoid suture, 2, 3, 4
  fetal, 202
lamina (vertebral), 62, 96
  C2, 61
  C4, 56
  C5, 57
  C6, 56
  L2, 59

lamina papyracea, 9, 10
large bowel see specific regions
laryngeal space, 29
larynx, 26–9, 149
latissimus dorsi muscle, 96, 124, 126, 130, 141, 145
lens, 23, 44
lenticulostriate arteries, 36
lentiform nucleus, 46, 47
levator anguli oris muscle, 25
levator ani muscle, 60, 223
   female, 151, 154, 156, 158, 160
   male, 134, 163, 165, 166
levator labii superioris alaeque nasi, 42
levator muscle (of thyroid gland), 29, 54
levator palpebrae superioris muscle, 20, 22
levator scapulae muscle, 26
levator veli palatini muscle, 32
ligaments
   broad (of uterus), 151, 155, 156, 159, 161
   calcaneofibular, 231
   collateral see collateral ligaments
   coracoclavicular, 79
   coracohumeral, 79
   cruciate see cruciate ligaments
   deltoid see deltoid ligament
   glenohumeral see glenohumeral ligament
   iliolumbar, 155
   inguinal see inguinal ligament
   interspinale, 63
   longitudinal see longitudinal ligament
   meniscofemoral, 227
   nuchal, 25, 62
   petroclinoid, 44
   plantar calcaneonavicular, 232
   round see round ligament
   sacroiliac, dorsal/posterior, 159
   sacrospinal, 135, 151, 163
   supraspinal, 62
   suspensory see suspensory ligament
   talofibular see talofibular ligament
   tibiofibular see tibiofibular ligament
   transverse see transverse ligament
   transverse acetabular, 220
   transverse cervical, 151, 159
   transverse pubic, 163
   uterosacral, 151
ligamentum flavum, 61, 62, 63
   posterior indentation on thecal sac from, 64
ligamentum teres see round ligament
ligamentum venosum, fissure for, 124, 126, 136
limbs see lower limb; upper limb
linea alba, 168
lingual artery, 33
lingual septum see tongue
lingual vein, 33
lingula of mandible, 61
lingular branch (pulmonary artery)
   inferior, 110
   superior, 110
lingular segment (lungs)
   inferior, 94
   superior, 93, 95
lingular segmental bronchus, 92
   inferior, 94
liver, 95, 120, 121, 144, 149, 192, 235
   dome, 239
   fetal, 202, 203
   lobes see lobes
   non-cross-sectional view, 172
      PET/CT scan, 239
      radionuclide scans, 235, 236
   segments 1-8 of, 125
   vessels, 192
lobar arteries, 194
lobes
   brain see frontal lobe; occipital lobe; parietal lobe; temporal lobe
   liver
      left, 124, 126, 136, 138, 175, 177

right, 97, 124, 126, 127, 136, 138, 142, 146, 175, 177
lung
   anterior basal segment inferior, 93
   anterior segment superior, 92, 94
   apical segment inferior, 95
   apical segment right superior, 92
   apicoposterior segment left superior, 92
   lateral basal segment inferior, 94
   lateral segment middle, 92, 94
   lower, right, 140
   medial basal segment inferior, 95
   medial segment middle, 92, 95
   middle, 120
   posterior basal segment inferior, 95
   posterior segment superior, 93
   superior lingular segment, 93
   see also bronchus; pulmonary artery
   thyroid see thyroid gland
longissimus capitis muscle, 25
longitudinal ligament
   anterior, 63
   posterior, 63
longitudinal muscle of tongue, 31
longitudinal vertebral venous plexi, 66
longus capitis muscle, 25, 26, 42
longus colli muscle, 25, 26, 27
lower limb, 207–34
   blood vessels, 216–18
   peripheral lower leg lymphatic channels, 206
lumbar arteries, 130, 183, 185
lumbar chain of lymph nodes
   ascending, 204, 205, 206
   crossover, 204, 205
lumbar plexus, 155
lumbar spinal cord, 62, 63, 65, 66
lumbar spine/vertebrae, 59, 66
   body see vertebral body
   PET/CT scan, 239
   see also L1; L2 etc
lumbar veins, 130, 132
   ascending, 66, 190
lumbosacral trunk, 154, 165
lumbrical muscle, 87, 88
lunate, 73, 74, 75, 86
lungs, 93–6, 118–19, 236
   fissures see horizontal fissure; oblique fissure
   isotope scans, 236
   left, 138, 140, 149, 236, 239
   lobes see lobes
      PET/CT scan, 239
   right, 138, 140, 146, 148, 236, 239
   vasculature, 110–11
Luschka's foramen, 17, 43, 51
Luschka's joints see uncovertebral joints
lymph nodes
   iliac, 204, 205
   inguinal, 168, 204, 205
   lumbar chain see lumbar chain
lymphatics, 204–6

M
Magendie's foramen, 42, 51
magnetic resonance angiogram
   brain, 40
   neck, 33
magnetic resonance arthrography
   hip, 220
   shoulder, 79–81
magnetic resonance cholangiopancreatogram, 182
malar process of maxilla, 3, 6
malleolus
   lateral, 212, 230, 231, 232, 233, 234
   medial, 230, 231, 232, 233
malleus, 7, 9, 15
mamillary body (of hypothalamus), 19, 45, 50
mamillary process (of cervical vertebral transverse process), 59

mammary artery, internal see thoracic artery, internal
mammary branches of lateral thoracic artery, 120
mammary vein, internal, 120
mandible, 4, 6, 30, 35, 46, 47, 54, 57, 149
   alveolar canal within, 34
   angle, 34, 56
   body, 24, 34
   condyle see condyle
   coronoid process, 6, 8, 11, 12, 34, 42, 49
   fossa, 7
   head, 43, 49
   lingula, 61
   ramus, 2, 6, 8, 11, 14, 31, 34, 42, 61
manubrium, 90, 93, 97, 102, 105, 107, 108, 136, 146, 149
marginal (wandering) artery of Drummond, 186
marginal artery of heart, 114
   right, 113
marginal branch of circumflex artery, obtuse, 114
   first, 113
marginal vein
   lateral, 217
   medial, 217
massa intermedia of thalamus, 50
masseter muscle, 8, 11, 12, 24, 31, 42, 48
mastoid air cells, 8, 15, 43, 51
mastoid process/tip of temporal bone, 2, 4, 6, 15, 42, 61
maxilla, 11
   alveolar process/rim/ridge/bone, 8, 11, 30, 34, 46
   anterior nasal spine, 13, 34
   malar process, 3, 6
   orbital floor, 11
   palatine process, 6
maxillary artery, 33, 36
maxillary nerve, 49
maxillary sinus/antrum, 2, 6, 8, 10, 11, 12, 22, 30, 34, 43, 46, 47
Meckel's (trigeminal) cave, 17, 18
   trigeminal ganglion in, 49
median nerve, 84, 85, 86
mediastinum, 96–109
   anterior, 91
   axial CT, 96–9
   axial MR, 108–9
   coronal CT, 100–3
   isotope scan, 236
   PET/CT scan, 239
   sagittal MR, 104–7
medulla oblongata, 16, 42, 46, 47, 51
medullary cone (conus medullaris), 62, 63, 65
membranous interventricular septum, 101, 108
membranous urethra, 135, 198
meningeal artery, middle, 33
meningeal branch of vertebral artery, 38
meningeal vessels, middle, grooves for, 3
meniscofemoral ligament, 227
meniscus
   lateral
      anterior horn, 226
      body, 225
      posterior horn, 224, 225, 226
   medial, 228
      anterior horn, 226
      body, 225
      posterior horn, 224, 226
mental tubercle, 34
mesencephalic vein
   lateral, 39
   posterior, 39
mesencephalon see midbrain
mesenteric artery
   inferior, 130
      arteriogram, 186
      catheter tip in, 186

      non-cross-sectional views, 186, 187
      sigmoid arteries from, 141, 186
   superior, 105, 107, 127, 129, 138, 140, 148, 191
      arteriogram, 191
      catheter tip in, 185, 191
      ileal branches, 131, 139, 185
      jejunal branches, 131, 139, 183, 185
      non-cross-sectional views, 175, 177, 183, 185, 191, 192, 193
mesenteric vein
   inferior, 186
   superior, 127, 138, 148
      non-cross-sectional views, 175, 177
mesentery, small bowel, 137, 138
mesocolon
   sigmoid (=mesosigmoid), 159, 161
   transverse, 137
mesorectum, 151
mesosigmoid, 159, 161
metacarpal artery, palmar, 78
metacarpal bones (metacarpals), 73–88
   fetal, 203
midbrain (mesencephalon), 16–17, 18, 21, 45, 50
   red nucleus of, 19
   tectum of, 51
mitral valve, 90, 91, 97, 103, 104, 105, 106, 109, 111, 113
   fetal, 203
moderator band (septomarginal trabecula), 190
   fetal, 203
molars, 34
Monro's (interventricular) foramen, 46, 47, 50, 57
multifidus muscle, 25
muscles see specific muscles
myelogram, cervical, 64
mylohyoid muscle, 24, 31
myometrium, 150, 156, 157, 161

N
nares, 8
nasal bones, 6, 9, 10, 13
   isotope scan, 235
nasal cavity, 8
   inferior meatus, 8, 10
   middle meatus, 8, 10
   superior meatus, 10
nasal concha/turbinates see turbinates
nasal septum, 2, 4, 6, 8, 10, 30, 34, 42
nasal spine of maxilla, anterior, 13, 34
nasogastric tube tip, 194
nasolacrimal duct, 9, 10, 11, 13, 23, 43
   see also lacrimal sac
nasopharynx, 8, 10, 11, 24, 29, 32, 42, 46, 47, 48
natal cleft, 58, 151, 164
navicular bone, 212, 213, 214, 215, 230, 231, 232, 233
neonatal brain, 52–3
nerve(s) see specific nerves
nerve roots, spinal see spinal nerve roots
neural foramen see intervertebral foramen
neurovascular bundle
   inferior rectal, 155, 164, 165
   obturator, 154, 156, 158, 167
   pudendal, internal, 152, 154, 159
newborn brain, 52–3
nipple, 120
non-coronary sinus, 114
nose, 29, 54
   see also entries under nasal
nuchal ligament, 25, 62
nucleus pulposus, 63
   T5/T6, 62

O

oblique fissure, 93, 95
  left, 91
  right, 91
oblique muscle (abdomen)
  external, 126, 128, 130, 133, 136, 150, 157, 166, 168
    aponeurosis of, 150
  internal, 128, 130, 133, 136, 157, 166
oblique muscle (orbit)
  inferior, 22
  superior, 20
obliquus capitis inferior muscle, 25
obturator externus muscle, 135, 137, 141, 143, 153, 155, 156, 158, 159, 163, 165, 167, 220, 222, 223
obturator foramen, 173, 208, 209
obturator internus, 220
obturator internus muscle, 135, 141, 143, 151, 152, 154, 155, 156, 158, 165, 166, 219, 223
  tendon, 219
obturator nerve, 163, 219
obturator neurovascular bundle, 154, 156, 158, 159, 167
obturator vessels, 135, 150, 152, 163, 187, 188
occipital artery, 33, 36
  medial, calcarine branch (=calcarine artery), 38
occipital bone, 57
  basilar part see basi-occiput
  condyle, 8, 13, 42, 61
  external protruberance, 3
    inion, 3, 43
  squamous, 4
occipital horn of lateral ventricle, 45
occipital lobe, 45, 53
  calcarine cortex, 21, 44
  PET scan, 238
occipital vessels (unspecified), 42
occiput, 64
  see also basi-occiput
oculomotor cistern, 18
oculomotor nerve (CN3), 18, 49
odontoid process/peg of axis, 2, 4, 6, 8, 13, 14, 22, 25, 46, 47, 50, 56, 57, 61, 64
oesophageal branches
  left gastric artery, 185
  left gastric vein, 185
oesophagogastric junction, 141
oesophagus, 27, 93, 96, 109, 140, 142, 148
  entrance, 29
  PET/CT scan, 239
olecranon fossa of humerus, 70, 82, 83, 84
olecranon process (olecranon) of ulna, 70, 71, 72, 82, 83, 84
olfactory cortex, 48
olfactory nerve (CN1), 18, 21, 45
olfactory tract and bulb, 19
operculofrontal artery, 36
ophthalmic artery, 23, 36
  ethmoidal branch, 36
ophthalmic nerve, 49
ophthalmic vein
  inferior, 23
  superior, 20, 23, 44
opponens digiti minimi muscle
  foot, 234
  hand, 87, 88
opponens pollicis muscle, 87, 88
optic canals, 11, 13
optic chiasm, 19, 21, 45, 48
  in suprasellar cistern, 46, 47
optic nerve (CN2), 9, 18, 20, 23, 44, 46, 47, 49
  infraorbital segment, 21
  intracanalicular segment, 19, 21
  intracranial segment, 19, 21, 22
  intraocular segment, 19, 22
optic radiation, 45
optic tract, 21, 45, 49

oral cavity, 29
orbicularis oculi, 22
orbicularis oris muscle, 25, 29, 54
orbit, 20–3
  floor, maxillary bone, 11
  roof, frontal bone, 11
orbital canal, inferior, 10
orbital cortex of frontal lobe, 46, 47
orbital fissure
  inferior, 9, 11, 13
  superior, 2, 6, 9, 11, 13
orbital layer of ethmoid bone (lamina papyracea), 9, 10
orbital plate of frontal bone, 45
orbital wall of zygoma, lateral, 11
orbitofrontal artery, 36
orbitofrontal branch of pericallosal artery, 36
oropharynx, 8, 24, 29, 32, 48
os naviculare (navicular), 212, 213, 214, 215, 230, 231, 232, 233
ossicles of middle ear (incus and malleus), 67
ovarian vessels, 150
ovary
  left, 150, 155
  physiological (corpus luteum) cysts, 155, 156, 158
  right, 150, 155, 158

P

palate
  hard, 8, 10, 23, 30, 42, 48
  soft, 3, 6, 29, 31, 49
palatine bone, horizontal plate, 6
palatine foramen, greater, 12
palatine process of maxilla, 6
palatine tonsils, 24, 32
palatopharyngeus muscle, 31
palmar (arterial) arch, deep, 76, 78, 88
palmar (venous) arch, superficial, 78, 87
palmar branch of ulnar artery, deep, 78
palmar carpal branch of ulnar artery, 78
palmar digital artery
  common, 78, 88
  proper, 88
palmar digital vein, 78
  common, 78
palmar interosseous muscles, 87, 88
palmar metacarpal artery, 78
palmaris longus muscle, 84, 85
  tendon, 86
pampiniform plexus of veins, 186, 189
pancreas, 146
  body, 124, 126, 138, 141, 149, 174, 176
  head, 124, 126, 138, 174, 176
  neck, 126, 138, 177
  non-cross-sectional views, 174, 175, 176, 177
  tail, 127, 141, 149, 175, 177
pancreatic artery
  dorsal, 184
    catheter tip in, 192, 193
  great (pancreatica magna artery), 184
  transverse, 184, 192, 193
pancreatic duct, 126, 174, 182
  accessory, 182
  ampullary part, 182
pancreaticoduodenal artery
  inferior, 185
    anterior branch, 192, 193
    posterior branch, 192, 193
  superior, 184
    anterior branch, 192, 193
    posterior branch, 192, 193
papilla, renal, 175, 196
papillary muscles, 96, 101, 109
papyraceous plate (lamina papyracea), 9, 10
paracentral artery, 36
paraglenoid sulcus, 60
paranasal sinuses, 6, 8–13

plate, 7
  see also specific sinuses
parapharyngeal space, 8
pararenal fat, 126, 128
parietal artery (parietal branches of middle cerebral artery)
  inferior internal, 36
  posterior, 36
parietal lobe, 45, 49, 52, 53
  PET scan, 238
parieto-occipital artery, 38
parotid duct, 42
parotid gland, 24, 31, 35, 49
  deep lobe, 42
  superficial lobe, 42
pars interarticularis
  C4, 56
  C7, 56
  lumbar spine, 59
pars marginalis of orbicularis oris muscle, 29, 54
pars peripheralis of orbicularis oris muscle, 29, 54
patella, 209, 211, 226, 228
  isotope scan, 235
patellar retinaculum, medial and lateral, 227, 228
patellar tendon, 226, 228
pectineus muscle, 135, 137, 152, 153, 158, 164, 165, 167, 168, 170, 219, 220, 222, 223
pectoralis major muscle, 96, 109, 120, 121, 138, 149
  fascia, 120, 121
pectoralis minor muscle, 80, 96, 109, 121, 138
pelvic sacral foramen (anterior sacral foramen), 60, 133, 173
pelvis (pelvic region), 132–49, 154–61, 169–70, 187–9, 209
  axial CT, male, 132–5
  axial MRI
    female, 151–3
    male, 162–4
  coronal CT, female, 136–45
  coronal MRI
    female, 154–8
    male, 165–8
  fetal ultrasound, 203
  girl, 209
  non-cross-sectional views
    anteroposterior projections, 172
    blood vessels, 187–9
    female, 173, 188
    lymphatics, 204
    male, 173, 189, 198–9
  sagittal CT, female, 146–9
  sagittal MRI
    female, 158–61
    male, 169–70
pelvis (renal), 127, 129, 196
pelvi-ureteric junction, 196, 197
penile (spongy) urethra, 167, 168, 198
penile artery, 198
  deep, 198
  dorsal, 198
penile vessels (unspecified)
  arteriogram, 198
  dorsal, 163, 170
penis
  bulb, 134, 164, 167
  corpus cavernosum see corpus cavernosum
  corpus spongiosum, 167, 168, 169
  crus of 134, 164, 167
  glans, 168, 169, 170
  suspensory ligament, 167, 168
perforating artery, 216
perforating branches of internal mammary artery, anterior, 120, 121
perforating vein, 216
pericallosal artery, 36
  extending around corpus callosum, 36
  orbitofrontal branch, 36
pericardium, 97, 101, 104, 105, 106, 109

recesses, 109
  superior, 93, 97
perineal artery, 198
perineal body, 153, 155, 160
perineal pouch
  deep, 156
  superficial, 156
peritoneal cavity, contrast media spillage into, 195
peroneal.../peroneus... see under fibular; fibularis
perpendicular plate, ethmoid bone, 11
pes anserinus, 225
petroclinoid ligament, 44
petrosal sinus, superior, 39
petrosal vein, 39
petrous portion/part
  internal carotid artery, 9, 14, 33, 36
  temporal bone see temporal bone
phalanges
  fingers, 74, 75, 87, 88
  toes, 214, 215, 234
pharyngeal tonsils, 13, 31
pharyngeal vessels, ascending, artery, 33
pharyngobasilar raphe, 50
pharynx, 24–32
  see also hypopharynx; nasopharynx; oropharynx
phrenic artery, 184
  inferior, 194
    catheter tip in origin of, 194
phrenic vein, inferior, 194
pineal gland, 45, 51
pinna of ear, 3, 7, 42
piriformis muscle, 133, 135, 150, 154, 158, 165, 222
  insertion, 154
  slips of origin, 161
pisiform, 73, 74, 86
pituitary fossa see sella turcica
pituitary gland, 18, 44, 46, 47, 48
placenta, 202, 203
plantar aponeurosis, 231, 232, 233, 234
plantar artery
  lateral, 217
  medial, 217, 232, 234
plantar calcaneonavicular ligament, 232
plantar cutaneous venous plexus, 217
plantar interosseous muscles, 234
plantar nerve
  lateral, 231, 234
  medial, 231, 232, 234
plantar venous arch, 217
plantar vessels (unspecified), medial and lateral, 231
plantaris muscle, 227
  tendon, 230
planum sphenoidale, 2
platysma muscle, 24, 26, 30
plicae circulares, jejunum, 179
pons, 16, 21, 22, 43, 46, 47, 50
  tegmentum, 46, 47
pontomesencephalic vein, anterior, 39
popliteal artery, 217, 221, 222, 224, 227, 228
popliteal vein, 222, 228
popliteus muscle, 224, 228
  belly, 226
  tendon, 224, 226, 228
portal vein, 127, 138, 140, 147, 191
  branch, 174, 176
    left, 191
    right, 191
  non-cross-sectional views, 174, 175, 177
postcentral gyrus, 45
pouch of Douglas, 151, 155, 161
preauricular sulcus, 60
precentral cerebellar vein, 38
precentral gyrus, 45
precommunicating posterior cerebral artery segment, 40
preganglionic segment of CN5 (trigeminal), 18
premolars, 34

prepontine cistern, 46, 47, 49
prevertebral muscle, 29
princeps pollicis artery, 78
princeps pollicis vein, 78
profunda brachii artery, 76, 84
profunda femoris artery, 135, 153, 164,
      167, 187, 216, 219, 221, 223
profunda femoris vein, 164
profunda femoris vessels, 153
pronator teres muscle, 82, 83, 84, 85
properitoneal fat line, 172
prostate, 135, 163, 166, 169, 170
      peripheral zone, 199
      rectal ultrasound, 199
      transitional zone, 199
prostatic urethra, 169, 198
psoas muscle, 63, 130, 138, 141, 150
      margin, 172
      psoas major, 62, 127, 128, 132,
            143, 146, 155, 156, 158, 166
      psoas minor, 143
      see also iliopsoas muscle
pterygoid canal (Vidian canal), 10, 11
pterygoid fossa, 8
pterygoid muscle
      lateral, 8, 11, 12, 31, 42, 49
      medial, 8, 11, 24, 31, 42, 49
pterygoid plate
      lateral, 8, 11, 42
      medial, 8, 11, 43, 61
pterygopalatine fossa, 9, 10, 11, 12,
      22
pubic ligament, transverse, 163
pubis (pubic bone), 160
      body, 134, 153, 159, 160, 167, 168,
            169
            non-cross-sectional view, 173
      female, 148, 152, 153, 155, 156,
            157, 158, 159, 160
            girl, 209
      male, 134, 135, 163, 167, 168, 169
            non-cross-sectional view, 173, 208,
                  209
      ramus
            inferior, 134, 155, 156, 167, 173,
                  208
            superior, 60, 135, 139, 152, 157,
                  158, 163, 167, 173, 208
      symphysis see symphysis pubis
      tubercle, 173
      unossified junction between ischium
            and, 209
puborectalis muscle
      female, 151, 152, 155, 160
      male, 169
pubovaginalis muscle, 156
pudendal artery, internal, 198
pudendal neurovascular bundle, 152,
      154, 159
pulmonary artery, 93, 110, 112, 115,
      138
      arteriogram, 110
      catheter in main artery, 110
      fetal, 203
      inferior lobe, 110
      left, 90, 91, 96, 100, 101, 104, 105,
            106, 108, 112, 140, 149
      middle lobe, 110
      right, 90, 91, 97, 102, 105, 107,
            109, 110, 112, 140
            lower lobe, 95
            superior lobe, 97, 102, 109
      superior lobe, 110
            right, 97, 102, 109
pulmonary conus, 136
pulmonary outflow tract (from right
      ventricle; conus arteriosus), 105,
      107, 112, 115, 136, 149
pulmonary trunk, 90, 91, 97, 101, 104,
      106, 109
pulmonary valve, 90, 91, 101, 104,
      105, 106, 109, 112
pulmonary vein
      fetal, 203
      left, 115
            inferior, 96, 103, 108, 111
            superior, 92, 96, 101, 108, 111
      right, 115
            inferior, 95, 97, 103, 105, 107,
                  109
            superior, 97, 102, 105, 107, 109,
                  111
pulp anastomoses (finger), 78
pulp chamber of tooth, 34
putamen, 45, 48
      PET scan, 238
pyloric part of stomach, 127, 128

Q

quadratus femoris muscle, 135, 153,
      155, 164, 165, 220, 222, 223
quadratus lumborum muscle, 123, 130,
      143, 144
quadratus plantae (flexor accessorius
      muscle), 230, 231, 232, 234
quadriceps tendon, 222, 226
quadrigeminal cistern, 45
quadrigeminal plate, 51
quadrigeminal portion of posterior
      cerebral artery, 38, 40

R

radial artery, 76, 78, 84, 85, 86
radial nerve, 84, 85
radial recurrent artery, 76
radialis indicis vein, 78
radicular vessels, 63
      great radicular artery (arteria
            radicularis magna), 66
radius, 70, 71, 72, 73, 74, 75, 77, 82,
      83, 84, 85, 86
      dorsal tubercle, 86
      fetal, 203
      head, 70, 71, 72, 82, 83, 84
      neck, 70
      styloid process, 74
      tuberosity, 70, 83
      ulnar notch, 74
ramus
      of ischium, 173
      of mandible, 2, 6, 8, 11, 14, 31, 34,
            42, 61
      of pubis see pubis
rectal artery, superior, 186
rectal nerve, inferior, 163
rectal vein, superior, 186
rectal vessels
      inferior, 163
      middle, 154
      superior, 154
rectosigmoid junction, 150, 154, 159
      161, 165
rectouterine pouch (of Douglas), 151,
      155, 161
rectum, 60, 133, 135, 143, 144, 147
      148, 152, 154, 162, 166, 169
      170, 223
      ampulla, 154, 159, 160, 165
      folds of Houston, 154, 159
      inferior neurovascular bundle, 155,
            164, 165
      non-cross-sectional views, 172, 180,
            181
      prostatic ultrasonography via, 199
      wall, 199
rectus abdominis muscle, 127, 128,
      130, 132, 133, 135, 136, 149,
      150, 152, 158, 160, 168, 169,
      170
rectus femoris muscle, 135, 157, 161,
      162, 164, 168, 220, 221, 222,
      223
      tendon, 219
rectus muscle
      inferior, 20, 22, 43, 46
      lateral, 20, 21, 23, 44
            PET scan, 238
      medial, 21, 23, 44
            PET scan, 238
      superior, 20, 21, 22, 44
rectus sheath, 161

recurrent artery of Heubner, 36
red nucleus of midbrain, 19
renal artery, 194
      accessory, 183
      catheter tip in, 194
      left, 126, 141
            non-cross-sectional view, 183
      main, 194
      right, 127, 129, 140
            non-cross-sectional views, 175,
                  177, 183
renal organ see kidney
renal pelvis, 127
renal vein
      left, 140
            non-cross-sectional view, 175, 177,
                  194
      right, 127, 129
            non-cross-sectional view, 175
retina, 23
retinaculum
      extensor, ankle, 230
      flexor see flexor retinaculum
      patellar, medial and lateral, 227, 228
      peroneal, 230
retrobulbar fat, 22
retromandibular vein, 24, 32, 42, 49
retropharyngeal soft tissues, 29
retropubic space (cave of Retzius), 152,
      159, 160, 161, 169
retrotonsillar segment of posterior
      inferior cerebellar artery, 38
Retzius' cavity (retropubic space), 152,
      159, 160, 161, 169
ribs, 58, 136, 144, 145, 146
      1st, 56, 57, 58, 64, 90, 146
            isotope scan, 235
      5th, isotope scan, 235
      10th, 145
      12th, 59, 65, 129, 130, 144, 172,
            197
            fetal, 202
            head, 16
Rolando's fissure (central sulcus) 45,
      46
roots
      dental, 34
      spinal nerve see spinal nerve roots
Rosenthal's (basal) vein, 37, 45, 51
rotator cuff, 80
round foramen (foramen rotundum), 2,
      9, 11
round ligament (ligamentum teres)
      of femur (=ligament of head of femur),
            135, 163, 219, 220
      of uterus, 151, 152
rugae of stomach, 178

S

S1
      disc space, 60
      sacral nerve, 154
            root, 159, 160, 161
      see also L5/S1
S1/S2
      sacral foramen, 60
      terminal theca at, 65
S2 nerve root, 159, 160, 161
      sacral foramen for, 60
S3 root, 160
sacculations of colon, 180
sacral artery
      lateral, 187
      median, 187
sacral canal
      central, 150
      upper and lower part, 60
sacral foramen, pelvic/anterior, 60,
      133, 173
sacral nerve
      S1, 154
            root, 159
      S2, root, 159
sacral plexus (of veins), 160, 188

sacral veins, lateral, 66
sacral venous plexus, 66
sacro-coccygeal junction, 160
sacroiliac joint, 59, 60
      female, 142, 144, 154, 158, 173
      male, 133, 165
      non-cross-sectional views, 173, 179,
            197
sacroiliac ligaments, dorsal, 159
sacrospinous ligament, 135, 151, 163
sacrouterine fold (uterosacral ligament),
      151
sacrum, 60, 135, 160, 169, 170
      ala, 60, 133, 154, 158, 165, 197
      body, 159
      crest, 173
            median, spinous tubercle on, 60
      female, 142, 144, 147, 148, 150,
            154, 158, 159, 160, 173
      isotope scan, 235
      male, 133, 135, 162, 165, 169
            non-cross-sectional view, 59, 60, 63,
                  65, 173
      promontory, 59, 60, 63, 65
sagittal sinus
      inferior, 36, 37, 45, 51
      superior, 17, 36, 37, 41, 44, 48
sagittal suture, 2, 4
salivary glands, 35
      see also specific glands
Santorini's duct (accessory duct of
      pancreas), 182
saphenous vein
      long/large/great, 153, 162, 164,
            168, 217, 218, 221, 224, 228,
            229, 230, 232
      short/small/lesser, 217, 228, 230,
            233
sartorius muscle, 133, 135, 137, 152,
      157, 161, 162, 164, 219, 220,
      221, 222, 223, 224, 228
      tendon, 227
scalene muscles, anterior/middle/
      posterior, 28
scaphoid, 73, 74, 75, 86
scapula, 68, 80, 91, 145
      acromion, 68, 69, 79
      coracoid process, 68, 69, 79
      glenoid fossa see glenoid
      isotope scan, 235
      spine, 68, 80, 90
scapular artery, circumflex, 76
sciatic foramen, 145
sciatic nerve, 135, 145, 151, 153,
      154, 158, 162, 164, 165, 221
sclera, 23
scutum, 15
sella turcica (pituitary/hypophyseal
      fossa), 3, 6, 13, 22
      floor, 9
semicircular canal
      horizontal, 50
      posterior, 43, 50
      superior, 44, 50
semicircular canals, 9, 15, 17
      superior, 4
semimembranosus muscle, 135, 153,
      164, 221, 222, 223, 224, 227,
      228
      tendon, 227
seminal colliculus, 198, 199
seminal vesicle, 133, 135, 162, 165,
      166, 169, 170, 199
semi-oval centre (centrum semiovale),
      45
semispinalis capitis muscle, 25, 27
semispinalis cervicis muscle, 27
semitendinosus muscle, 135, 153,
      164, 219, 221, 222, 223
      tendon, 227, 228
septal arteries, 113
      posterior interventricular, 113
septomarginal trabecula see moderator
      band
septum pellucidum, 45, 48
      cavity of see cavum septum
            pellucidum

serratus anterior muscle, 97, 109, 127, 139
sesamoid bones
　ankle, in flexor hallucis brevis muscle, 214
　wrist, 74
sigmoid arteries, 141, 186
sigmoid colon, 133, 135, 139, 140, 143, 144, 147, 148, 150, 155, 156, 158, 161, 166, 168, 169
　non-cross-sectional views, 172, 180, 181
sigmoid mesocolon (=mesosigmoid), 159, 161
sigmoid sinus, 33, 37, 39, 41
sigmoid vein, 186
sinuatrial nodal artery, 113
sinus
　paranasal see paranasal sinuses
　venous, confluence of, 37, 39, 41, 44
　see also specific sinsuses
skull (cranium), 2–5
　calvarium see calvarium
　fetal, ultrasound, 202
　isotope scan, 235
small bowel, 157, 162, 165, 166, 168, 169, 170
　mesentery, 137, 138
　PET/CT scan, 235
　see also specific regions
small (short/lesser) saphenous vein, 217, 228, 230, 233
soft tissues, neck, 29
soleus muscle, 224, 226, 230, 233
spermatic cord, 135, 162, 168, 169, 170
sphenoid bone
　basilar part see basisphenoid
　body, 2, 14, 44, 49
　greater wing, 2, 3, 7, 9, 11, 48, 53
　　temporal surface of, 2
　lesser wing, 2, 6, 11
　planum sphenoidale, 2
sphenoid sinus/antrum, 2, 6, 8, 9, 10, 11, 21, 31, 43, 46, 47, 48
spheno-occipital (basisphenoid–basi-occiput) synchondrosis, 3, 50
sphenopalatine foramen, 11
sphenoparietal sinus, 39
sphincter
　anal, external, 134, 154, 160
　urethral see urethral sphincter
spinal artery, anterior, 38, 64, 65
spinal canal, 97, 143, 144, 148
　fetal, 202, 203
　sacral, 60
spinal column (spine) see vertebral column
spinal cord, 51, 62–6, 144, 148
　anterior median fissure, 65
　cervical, 25, 46, 47, 61, 62, 64
　fetal, 202
　grey and white matter, 62
　thoracic, 62, 64, 65
spinal nerve
　cervical, 63
　lumbar, 65
　S1 (sacral nerve), 154
spinal nerve roots, 62, 63, 65
　C8 see C8
　dorsal see dorsal root
　L5, 159, 160, 161, 165
　sacral see S1; S2; S3
　subarachnoid space lateral extension around, 65
　ventral, 64
spinalis capitis muscle, 25
spinalis cervicis muscle, 27
spine see vertebral column
spinous processes, 56–62, 144
spinous tubercle of median sacral crest, 60
spleen, 95, 139, 140, 142, 149
　non-cross-sectional views, 172, 175, 177, 191
　isotope scan, 236
　PET/CT scan, 239

splenial branches of posterior cerebral artery, 38
splenic artery, 141, 142, 149, 191
　catheter tip in, 191
　non-cross-sectional view, 183, 184, 191
splenic (left colic) flexure, 124, 126, 128, 136, 139, 140
　non-cross-sectional views, 172, 180, 181
splenic vein, 127, 138, 142, 148, 185, 191
　non-cross-sectional views, 175, 177
splenium of corpus callosum see corpus callosum
splenius capitis muscle, 24, 27
spring ligament, 232
squamous occipital bone, 4
sternoclavicular joint, 96, 109
sternocleidomastoid muscle, 23, 27, 29, 32, 42, 50
sternohyoid muscle, 27
sternum, 91, 93, 102, 120, 136, 149
　body of, 96, 104, 105, 106, 108, 136
　fetal, 203
　isotope scan, 235
　manubrium of see manubrium
　PET/CT scan, 239
　xiphoid process see xiphisternum
stomach, 95, 148
　antrum, 137, 178
　body, 124, 126, 137, 172, 178
　double-contrast barium meals, 178
　fetal, 202, 203
　fundus, 90, 91, 124, 137, 140, 142, 149, 172, 178
　　barium pooling, 178
　greater curvature, 124, 178
　lesser curvature, 126, 178
　non-cross-sectional views, 172, 178, 179
　pyloric part, 127, 178
　rugae, 178
straight gyrus (gyrus rectus), 21
straight sinus, 37, 39, 41, 44
striate artery, medial (recurrent artery of Heubner), 36
styloid process
　fibula, 209
　radius, 74
　temporal bone, 8, 12, 14, 24, 61
　ulna, 73, 86
stylomastoid foramen, 15
　facial nerve, 17
subarachnoid space
　cerebrospinal fluid in, 62
　contrast fluid
　　cervical region, 64
　　lumbar region, 65
　lateral extension around spinal nerve roots, 65
　spinal nerves within, 65
subclavian artery, 33
　left, 92, 96, 100, 101, 103, 104, 105, 106, 108, 117
　right, 33, 102, 117
subclavian vein, 77
　left, 103
　right, 33
subcutaneous (abdominal) fascia, 129
submandibular duct, 35
submandibular gland, 24, 26, 31, 35
submental artery, 33
subsartorial canal, 222
subscapular artery, 76
subscapularis muscle, 80, 97, 109, 145
　tendon, 80
substantia nigra, 19
subtalar joint
　middle facet, 233
　posterior, 233
subtraction angiography (incl. digitally subtracted arteriograms and venograms)
　abdomen

coeliac trunk arteriogram, 184
　hepatic arteriogram, 192
　pancreatic arteriogram, 193
　superior mesenteric arteriogram, 185
aortic arch, 117
brain, 36–9
hand, 78
neck, 33
pelvis, 187
sulcus
　carotid, 3
　cerebral see cerebral sulci
　preauricular (paraglenoid), 60
supinator muscle, 82, 84, 85
supraclinoid internal carotid arteries, 36, 44
supracondylar ridge, medial, 83, 84
supraorbital vein, 23
suprarenal arteries, superior, 194
suprarenal gland (adrenal gland), 194
　angiograms, 194
　left, 126, 194
　right, 127, 142
suprarenal vein, left, 194
　catheter tip in, 194
suprascapular artery, 33, 117
suprasellar cistern, 45, 48
　optic chiasm in, 46, 47
supraspinatus muscle, 80, 97, 145
　tendon, 80
supraspinous ligament, 62
supratonsillar segment of posterior inferior cerebellar artery, 38
suspensory ligament
　Cooper's, 121, 122
　lens, 23
　penis, 167, 168
sustentaculum tali of calcaneus, 212, 231, 232, 233
Sylvian (cerebral) aqueduct, 21, 45, 47, 51
Sylvian fissure (lateral cerebral sulcus), 45, 46, 47, 48, 52
Sylvian point, 36
sympathetic chain, pelvis, 155
symphysis pubis (pubic symphysis), 60, 135, 137, 153, 157, 160, 163, 167, 168
　non-cross-sectional view, 173, 209

T
T1, 58
　spinous process, 56
　transverse process, 56
T4, spinous process, 62
T5/T6, nucleus pulposus, 62
T6
　pedicle, 58
　spinous process, 58
T11, vertebral body, 58
T12, vertebral body, 148
talofibular joint, 230
talofibular ligament
　anterior, 230
　posterior, 230
talonavicular joint, 233
talus, 212, 213, 214, 215, 230, 232, 233, 234
　head, 212, 231, 233, 234
　medial tubercle, 212
　neck, 212, 233, 234
tarsal bones, 213
tarsal sinus, 232, 233, 234
tectum of midbrain, 51
teeth, 34
tegmen tympani, 7
tegmentum of pons, 46, 47
temporal artery
　anterior, 36
　inferior, 38
　posterior, 36, 38
　superficial, 33
temporal bone, 14–15

articular eminence, 7, 12
mastoid process/tip, 2, 4, 6, 15, 42, 61
petrous part, 2, 43
　apex, 9
　arcuate eminence, 4, 12, 50
styloid process, 8, 12, 14, 24, 61
zygomatic process, 7
temporal branches of middle cerebral artery, anterior, 36
temporal horn of lateral ventricle, 44, 49
temporal lobe, 7, 9, 43, 46, 47, 48, 52, 53
　left, PET scan, 238
　uncus, 44, 51
temporal process of zygomatic bone, 6
temporal surface of greater wing of sphenoid, 2
temporalis (temporal) muscle, 7, 8, 11, 23, 31, 42, 44, 48
temporomandibular joints, 7, 32
　articular tubercle, 3
　condylar fossa, 7
tendons see common tendinous origin and specific tendons
tensor fasciae lata muscle, 133, 135, 152, 161, 162, 167, 216, 221
tensor tympani muscle, tendon, 15
tentorium cerebelli, 46, 51
teres minor muscle, 80
terminal ampulla, 205, 206
terminal filum, 148, 161
terminal ileum, 131, 132, 139, 179
testicle (testis), 135, 167, 168, 169, 170
　undescended, in inguinal canal, 189
　venogram, 189
testicular artery, left, 129, 131
testicular vein
　left, 129, 131
　　catheter tip introduced via left femoral vein via, 189
　right, 189
thalamoperforating branches
　posterior cerebral artery, 38
　superior cerebellar artery, 38
thalamostriate vein, 37
thalamus, 45, 50, 52, 53
　fetal, 202
　massa intermedia of, 50
　PET scan, 238
theca/thecal sac, 65, 127, 129, 133, 154, 161, 165, 169, 170
　caudal lumbar, 63
　indentation from intervertebral disc, 65
　indentation from ligamentum flavum, 64
thigh, 221–3
　deep artery of (profunda femoris artery), 135, 153, 164, 167, 187, 216, 219, 221, 223
　deep fascia of (=fascia lata), 150, 152, 163, 164, 165, 166, 228
　fetal, 202, 203
thoracic artery
　internal (internal mammary artery), 96, 108, 117, 120, 121
　　anterior perforating branch, 120, 121
　　left, 33, 103
　　right, 33, 103
　lateral, 76
　　intramammary branches of, 120
　superior, 76, 117
thoracic duct, 205, 206
thoracic spinal cord, 62, 64, 65
thoracic spine/vertebrae, 58
　intervertebral discs see intervertebral discs
　isotope scan, 235
　PET/CT scan, 239
　vertebral body see vertebral body
　see also T1; T4 etc.
thoracic vein, internal, 96, 108
thoraco-acromial artery, 76
　deltoid branch, 117

thoracolumbar fascia, 62, 159, 161
thorax (chest), 89–122
  coronal CT, 100–3, 136–45
  fetal, anterior wall, 203
  sagittal CT (sequential), female,
    146–9
  vessels, 116–17
thumb
  artery to radial aspects of, 78
  distal phalanx, 74, 87, 88
  fetal, 203
  proximal phalanx, 74, 88
thyrocervical trunk, 117
  catheter tip in, 33
thyrohyoid muscle, 32
thyroid artery, 33
  inferior, 33, 117
  superior, 33
thyroid cartilage, 29, 61
  lamina, 27
thyroid gland, 27, 29, 32
  isthmus, 29
  lobe, 29
    right, 33
thyroid vein
  inferior, 33
  middle, catheter tip in, 33
  superior, 33
tibia, 210, 211, 212, 213, 215, 230,
    232, 233
  condyles, lateral and medial, 210
  isotope scan, 235
  plateau, 228
    lateral and media, 226
  spine, 227
  tuberosity, 210, 211, 227, 229
tibial artery
  anterior, 216, 217, 229
    muscular branches, 216, 217
  posterior, 216, 217, 229, 230, 231,
    233
    muscular branches, 216, 217
tibial nerve, 221, 225
tibial vein
  anterior, 218
  posterior, 218, 230, 233
tibialis anterior muscle, 225, 227, 229
  tendon, 230, 232, 233
tibialis posterior muscle, 225, 229, 230
  tendon, 230, 231, 232, 233
tibiofibular joint
  inferior (distal), 212, 230, 231
  superior (proximal), 224, 226
tibiofibular ligament, 232
  anterior inferior, 230
  posterior inferior, 230
tibiotalar part of ankle joint, 233
toes, phalanges, 214, 215, 216
tongue, 29, 54, 98
  base, 29
  longitudinal muscle, 31
  septum (=lingual septum), 230
  transverse muscle, 31
tonsil(s)
  cerebellar, 47
  palatine, 24, 32
  pharyngeal, 13, 31
tonsillar vein, 39
torcular Herophilli, 37, 39, 41, 44
torus tubarius, 27
trabeculae of right ventricle, 112
trachea, 28, 29, 32, 57, 58, 62, 90,
    91, 93, 97, 102, 105, 107,
    109, 118, 119, 140, 148
  carina, 90, 96, 100, 108, 142
tragus, 50
transitional zone of prostate, 199
transverse acetabular ligament, 220
transverse cervical ligament (cardinal
    ligament), 151, 159
transverse colon, 127, 129, 130, 136,
    157, 158
  non-cross-sectional views, 179, 180,
    181
transverse fissure (horizontal fissure),
    91, 92, 94
transverse foramen, 64

of C1 (atlas), 61
  vertebral artery exiting, 33
of C2 (axis), 13
transverse ligament
  atlas, 61
  knee, 227
transverse mesocolon, 137
transverse muscle of tongue, 31
transverse pancreatic artery, 184, 192,
    193
transverse perineii see urogenital
    diaphragm
transverse process, 97
  C1/atlas, 12, 13, 15, 57, 61
  C2/axis, 57
  C4, 56
  C5, 56, 57
  C7, 56, 64
  L3, 59
  L5, 143
  thoracic vertebra, 58
    T1, 56
  tubercles of see tubercles
transverse pubic ligament, 163
transverse rectal fold (of Houston), 154,
    159
transverse sinus, 37, 39, 41
  groove for, 4
  left, 39
  right, 37, 39
transversus abdominis muscle, 129,
    130, 133, 136, 157, 166
trapezium, 73, 74, 75, 88
trapezius muscle, 25, 27, 51, 80, 97,
    109
trapezoid, 73, 74, 75, 88
triceps muscle
  lateral head, 82, 83, 84
  long head, 84
  medial head, 82, 83, 84
  tendon, 82
tricuspid valve, 90, 91, 97, 103, 105,
    107, 109
  fetal, 203
trigeminal cave see Meckel's cave
trigeminal ganglion in Meckel's cave, 49
trigeminal nerve (CN5), 18, 50
  maxillary branch, 49
  ophthalmic branch, 49
triquetral, 73, 74, 75
triradiate cartilage, 209
trochanters, femoral see femur
trochlea, humeral, 70, 72, 82, 83
trochlear nerve (CN4), 18–19, 49
trochlear notch of ulna, 70
tubercles
  adductor, 227
  articular, for temporomandibular joint,
    3
  of calcaneus, anterior, 233
  of humerus see tuberosities
  of intercondylar eminence, 210
  mental (of mandible), 34
  of pubis, 173
  of radius, dorsal, 86
  spinous, of median sacral crest, 60
  of talus, medial, 212
  of transverse process
    C1, 13, 64
    C2, 61
    C4, 56
    C5, 57
tuberculum sellae, 3
tuberosities
  humeral (=tubercle)
    greater, 68, 69, 79
    lesser, 68
  ischial see ischium
  metatarsal (5th) base, 212, 214, 231
  radial, 70, 83
  tibial, 210, 211, 227, 229
turbinates (concha), nasal
  inferior, 2, 8, 10, 30, 42
  middle, 8, 10, 13, 30
  superior, 9, 10
tympanic annulus, 15
tympanic cavity (cavity of middle ear), 9

lower part (hypotympanum), 14
roof (tegmen tympani), 6
upper part (epitympanum), 14

U

ulna, 71, 72, 73, 75, 77, 83, 84, 85,
    86
  coronoid process, 70, 82
  distal, 74, 75
  fetal, 203
  head, 74
  olecranon (olecranon process), 70,
    71, 72, 82, 83, 84
  styloid, 73, 86
  trochlear notch, 70
ulnar artery, 76, 78, 85, 86, 87
  deep palmar branch, 78
  palmar carpal branch, 78
ulnar nerve, 84, 85, 86
ulnar notch of radius, 74
ulnar recurrent artery, 76
umbilical cord, 202, 203
umbilical vein, 203
umbilicus, 131, 168, 202
uncovertebral (Luschka's) joints
  C2/C3, 61
  C3/C4, 61
uncus (posterolateral lip)
  C3, 61
  C4, 56
  C5, 57
  temporal lobe, 44, 51
upper limb, 67–84
  vessels, 76–8
ureter, 153, 155, 165, 189
  left and right, 123, 131, 132, 196,
    197
  orifice, 156
urethra
  female, 153, 156, 160
  male, 135, 167, 198, 199
    bulbous urethra, 198
    course of, 199
    distal urethra, 199
    external meatus, 170
    membranous urethra, 135, 198
    penile urethra, 167, 168, 198
    prostatic urethra, 169, 198
urethral sphincter
  external (sphincter urethrae), 156,
    198
  internal (of bladder), 157
urinary bladder see bladder
urogenital diaphragm (transverse
    perineii)
  female, 154, 156, 159
  male, 167
urogram
  3D CT, 197
  intravenous, 196
uterine (fallopian) tubes, 155, 156,
    159, 195
  ampulla, 195
  isthmus, 195
  right, 150
uterine artery, 187
uterine veins, 144
uterosacral ligament, 151
uterus, 143, 144, 148, 187, 195, 196
  body, 156
  broad ligament, 151, 155, 156, 159,
    161
  cavity, 150, 155, 157, 161, 200, 201
  cornu, 195
  endometrium, 161
  in fetal ultrasound, 200, 201, 202
  fundus, 150, 157, 161, 195
  myometrium, 150, 156, 157, 161
  neck see cervix
  round ligament, 151, 152
  transverse cervical ligament of, 151,
    159
uvula, 24, 31

V

vagina, 142, 144, 148, 152, 156, 159,
    160
  posterior fornix, 151, 156, 161
  posterior wall, 155
vagus nerve (CN 10), 16
vallecula (epiglottica), 24, 26, 29, 32,
    61
valvulae conniventes, jejunum, 179
vas deferens see ductus deferens
vasculature see blood vessels;
    lymphatics
vastus intermedius muscle, 135, 153,
    219, 220, 221, 222, 223
vastus lateralis muscle, 135, 153, 157,
    163, 164, 167, 219, 221, 222,
    223
vastus medialis muscle, 157, 221, 222,
    225, 227
Vater's ampulla, 182
veins see blood vessels, specific veins
    and entries under venous
vena cava
  inferior, 62, 90, 91, 94, 96, 100,
    104, 105, 106, 108, 124, 126,
    128, 130, 138, 140, 146, 148,
    189, 190
    non-cross-sectional views, 62, 90,
      91, 174, 176
  superior, 33, 77, 90, 93, 97, 102,
    105, 107, 109, 115, 138, 140,
    146, 148
    catheter tip introduced via femoral
      vein into, 116
venogram
  azygos, 116
  hepatic, subtracted, 192
  lower limb, 218
    foot, 217
  lumbar, 66
  neck, 33
  orbital, 23
  pelvic, female, 188
  suprarenal, 194
  testicular, 189
  upper limb, 77
venous arch
  in foot, dorsal and plantar, 217
  in hand
    dorsal, 86
    superficial palmar, 78
venous circulation of brain, 41
venous ligament, fissure for, 124, 126,
    136
venous plexus
  calf, 218
  plantar cutaneous, 217
  sacral, 66
venous sinuses, confluence of, 37, 39,
    41, 44
  see also specific venous sinuses
venous valves, 218
ventral nerve root, 64
ventricles (brain)
  3rd, 45, 46, 47, 49, 52, 53
  4th, 16, 43, 46, 47, 51, 53
    lateral (Luschka's) foramen of, 17,
      43
    superior recess, 21
  lateral, 46, 47, 52, 53
    body/atrium of, 45, 46, 49
    frontal/anterior horn, 45, 48
    occipital/posterior horn, 45
    temporal/inferior horn, 44, 49
  lateral, trigone of, 45, 51
  medial (Magendie's) foramen of, 42,
    51
ventricles (heart)
  left, 90, 101, 113, 115, 117, 136,
    138, 140, 237
    apex, 113, 237, 239
    border, 90
    cavity, 97, 101, 104, 105, 106,
      108, 113, 237, 239
    coronary supply, 113
    fetal, 203
    outflow tract, 113

ventricles (heart) (continued)
  PET/CT scan, 239
  right, 90, 91, 102, 105, 107, 112,
    115, 136, 138, 149
    cavity, 97, 102, 105, 107, 109,
      237
    fetal, 203
    infundibulum, 91
    outflow tract (=pulmonary outflow
      tract; conus arteriosus), 105,
      107, 112, 115, 136, 149
    PET/CT scan, 239
    trabeculae, 112
  septum see interventricular septum
ventricular branch (of coronary artery)
  lateral, to left ventricle, 113
  right, 114
vermian branch/segment
  posterior inferior cerebellar artery, 38
  superior cerebellar artery, 38
vermian vein
  inferior, 38
  superior, 39
vermis see cerebellum
vertebral artery, 28, 33, 38, 39, 40, 42,
    46, 47, 50, 117, 124
  groove (on atlas), 61
  meningeal branch, 38
  reflux of contrast into, 33

at transverse foramen of atlas, 38
vertebral body, 58, 96, 104, 108, 124,
    126, 130, 175, 177
  annular epiphysial discs for see
    annular epiphysial discs
  C3, 25
  C4, 25
  C5, 57
  C6, 58
  C7, 62
  fetal, 202, 203
  lumbar
    isotope scan, 235
    L1, 59, 142
    L2, 65
    L3, 63, 235
    L5, 148, 165, 166, 197
  sacral, 159
  thoracic, 239
    PET/CT scan, 239
    T6, 58
    T11, 58
    T12, 148
  uncus see uncus
vertebral canal see spinal canal
vertebral column (spine), 55–63
  cervical, 61
  fetal, 202, 203
  isotope scan, 235

PET/CT scan, 239
vertebral notch, inferior
  lumbar, 59
  thoracic, 58
vertebral venous plexi, longitudinal, 66
verumontanum, 198, 199
vesical vessels, superior, 157
  artery, 187
vesicoureteric junction, 153, 196
vessels see blood vessels
vestibular apparatus, vestibule of, 50
vestibular fold, 32
vestibular nerve, 17
vestibulocochlear nerve (CN8), 16, 43,
    50
  see also cochlear nerve; vestibular
    nerve
Vidian canal, 10, 11
visual cortex, primary (=calcarine
    cortex), 21
vitreous chamber of globe and vitreous
    humour, 21, 23, 44
vocalis muscle, 28, 32
vomer, 8, 13, 31

W
Waldeyer's fascia, 151, 159, 161
Wharton's duct, 35

white matter
  brain, 45
  spinal cord, 62
Wrisberg's (posterior meniscofemoral)
    ligament, 227

X
xiphisternum, 97, 103, 105, 106, 136,
    149

Y
yellow ligament see ligamentum flavum

Z
zona orbicularis, 220
zygapophyseal joint see facet joint
zygoma (zygomatic bone), 11, 12, 31
  arch, 3, 4, 5, 6, 8, 9, 11, 12, 14, 31,
    43
  frontal process, 3, 6
  orbital wall, lateral, 11
  temporal process, 6
zygomatic process
  frontal bone, 6, 7
  temporal bone, 7